HEALTH SCIENCE

KENNETH L. JONES

LOUIS W. SHAINBERG

CURTIS O. BYER

MT. SAN ANTONIO COLLEGE

Harper & Row, Publishers

NEW YORK, EVANSTON, AND LONDON

Library of Congress Catalog Card Number: 67-18443

CONTENTS

PREFACE

Health education at the college level is not a technical subject, nor is it merely a requirement of the traditional educational program. It is an academic subject, imparting knowledge that will be useful to an individual preparing to be an informed and conscientious adult. Throughout the elementary and high school years, health education is concerned primarily with personal health. This educational background need not be duplicated in college. Therefore we have omitted information that the student has already reviewed many times. The student in a college health program—with increasing frequency— either is a parent or will be one in the near future. This young person is interested in learning the scientific basis of health practices. *Health Science* is intended as such a scientific guide for the individual and his growing family. It stresses material that is essential for achieving a longer, healthier life. The information presented will help prepare students for the important job of explaining the basic principles of health to their children.

This text is designed to be used in a one-semester lecture course in college health education and also as a reference tool for the student and his family. The text along with the corresponding instructor's manual could easily be adapted to a professional course in college health teacher preparation.

Clean, open drawings are featured. Complete outlines of all chapters are included to be used as study tools, for quick reference, and as refreshers for the busy student. Important words have their pronunciation, derivation, and meaning given in the glossaries following each chapter. Five appendixes of useful information are included as tools for both the student and the instructor.

For a number of years the Health Department of Mt. San Antonio College has experimented with and reworked its health courses, trying to produce a complete, informative, and interesting program. *Health Science* and the companion instructor's materials are the product of this work.

K. L. JONES
L. W. SHAINBERG
C. O. BYER

ACKNOWLEDGMENTS

The authors wish to express their gratitude and appreciation to all of the many people who helped make this book possible. In particular, we are indebted to:

Robert E. Carrel, M.D., Neurologist, Pediatrician, and Mario Valente, M.D., Pediatrician, both of Pacific State Hospital, Spadra, California, for their reviews and comments on Chapters 2 and 3.

Karl Menninger, Director, Menninger Foundation, Topeka, Kansas, for his review of Chapter 2 and permission to use his concepts throughout this chapter.

Norman E. Byer, M.D., Assistant Clinical Professor, Department of Surgery/Ophthalmology, UCLA, for his suggestions and comments on the disorders of the eye.

Bob W., member of Alcoholic Anonymous, for his personal comments and fine insight into the needs and problems pertaining to the abuse of alcohol which were incorporated into Chapter 5.

George T. Roleder, B.D., M.A., Instructor, Mt. San Antonio College, for his interpretation of modern trends in courtship and marriage and his review of Chapter 8.

Garrett Hardin, Ph.D., Professor of Biological Sciences, University of California at Santa Barbara, who provided us with his personal ideas on the critical issue of abortion and the ethics of the modern society.

June H. Vail, M.S., Instructor, Mt. San Antonio College, for her comments and suggestions regarding the nutritional concepts used by the authors.

Paul Dyment, M.D., pediatrician in private practice, whose suggestions were incorporated into the preventive medicine and immunization schedules in this book.

Gary Romig, the artist who prepared the line drawings that illustrate this book.

Lawrence D. Parker, M.A., Instructor, Mt. San Antonio College. We are especially grateful to Mr. Parker for his fine editing of the entire manuscript.

Ralph Grawunder, Professor, San Diego State College, and L. H. Glass, Professor, San Fernando Valley State College for their reviews and comments on the original manuscript.

Morey R. Fields, Dean of Faculty, Nassau Community College, Garden City, Long Island, and Mrs. Joyce B. Friel, Chaffey College, Alto Loma, California, for their excellent reviews of the entire manuscript.

Clay J. Stratton and George A. Middendorf, College Division, Harper & Row, Publishers, for their excellent editorial guidance and constant encouragement.

HEALTH
SCIENCE

CHAPTER 1

A LIFETIME
OF HEALTH

MEANINGS OF HEALTH

FACTORS INFLUENCING
HEALTH

We are now witnessing the most rapid scientific and technological development in the history of man—development that can lead to greater fulfillment than man has ever known. But to achieve this level of fulfillment, man must apply his newly gained skills with care; he must avoid wherever possible the creation of new problems and must find satisfactory solutions for those problems that inevitably do arise.

During the Industrial Revolution machines began to be used for weaving and other tasks that had formerly been done by hand. Some social critics feared that unemployment, with its subsequent social problems, would be the certain result—and for some people for some time this was true. However, in the long run industrialization freed man of many tedious, degrading, menial jobs and, through a raised standard of living, actually decreased the unemployment rate. But this success was possible only through an increase in the average level of education.

1

Today we are facing similar problem-creating situations. Machines (including computers) are doing much of the work not only in factories, but also in the fields, in the homes, in the schools and hospitals. This trend toward automation and increasing application of scientific knowledge is world wide and is, again, being accompanied by increasing urbanization and consequent social dislocation and unrest.

Through our great reduction in the death rate we have increased life expectancy in the United States and many other countries. But this increased longevity has created many actual and potential problems— physical, psychological, and sociological. The chronic degenerative diseases of the elderly have assumed more importance. An increased longevity rate is accompanied by longer periods of retirement; yet our nation is a work-centered one. Therefore, the mental health of the elderly has become a national problem. Questions for which solutions have to be found are: Will the senior citizen be able to maintain his important feeling of independence and personal value? What sociological adjustments will be necessary to compensate for the greater numbers of elderly individuals?

Another result of reduction in death rate is the threat of overpopulation, already a reality in many countries. It is imperative that when parents are provided with the assurance that their offspring will reach maturity, they also be provided with the methods and motivation for limiting the number produced. Only through balanced birth and death rates can the world's standard of living be raised and that of the United States be maintained.

Increase in length of life, migration from village and farm to the city, increasing need for education to meet the standards of today's world—these are only some of the problems we face as we try to improve the quality, as well as the quantity, of man's life.

MEANINGS OF HEALTH

Health is a word with a wide range of meanings and definitions. To the man on the street health means freedom from disease. He and his family consider themselves healthy when they are safe, sound, and whole. His interpretation is the positive meaning of health. He expects health and takes it as an everyday part of life. To the individual who has lost his health his most priceless possession has been lost. He may have every materialistic possession, but without health he has nothing. To the physician health is the normal functioning of the body. He has the knowledge of the ages and the satisfaction of maintaining the health of the individual. To the quack health is a fee, payable in advance. He preys on the public and is maintained by the ignorance and fear generated when health sways toward the negative side. A sick person will often grasp for anything that will give him confidence. The quack relies upon this fear and ignorance. He "guarantees" a cure when the medical profession is unable to make such a guarantee.

To obtain a definition adequate for our purposes, we must define health as it relates to the world and the individual. The World Health Organization's constitution defines health as "a state of complete physical, mental, and social well-being and not merely the absence of disease or infirmity." This is an international definition of health. A "state" may be obtained for someone by someone else. A physician, through medicine, may obtain a state of physical well-being for a patient. Such a definition removes the pressure from the individual and rests it upon health organizations throughout the world. In trying to obtain such a state of health, the American Health Association has visualized four steps or levels of public health. These levels are (1) mortality, (2) serious morbidity, (3) minor morbidity, and (4) positive health.

Level 1. *Mortality* encompasses the first essential of public health— to conserve life, as in the successful fighting of deadly plagues and famines. The United States has obtained this level to a great extent, but many desperately underprivileged nations of the world are struggling below such a level at the present time.

Level 2. *Serious morbidity* is the level at which efforts are made to prevent, control, and treat diseases and conditions that disable, cripple, or produce chronic illness. The introduction of seat belts, the education of automobile drivers, the dissemination of information about harmful drugs, and the early diagnosis and treatment of heart conditions and cancer are examples showing progress toward reaching this level.

Level 3. *Minor morbidity* is the level at which efforts are made to control or alleviate minor illness and disturbances, for example, the efforts made to alleviate or control the effects of smog, the common cold, personal tension, digestive disturbances, and adverse social conditions affecting health.

Level 4. *Positive health* is the level at which complete control of health hazards is reached. At this level the individual could live to his inherited genetic potential. To reach this level, we must overcome levels 1, 2, and 3. If we are successful the world can truly enjoy "a state of complete physical, mental, and social well-being."

Before we can obtain such a national and international level of health, the *individual* must become responsible for a personal level of health that only he may obtain. Doctor E. B. Johns of the Department of Public Health at the University of California at Los Angeles defines health as "a quality to achieve a personally satisfying and socially useful life." An individual develops qualities for himself. Even one who is severely physically handicapped may still have the qualities of a healthy person. And those who enjoy normal good health must make their own efforts to maintain it. This type of health is something one works to maintain or obtain.

Actually what we have stated above are two types of health—*world health* and *personal health*. Both must be obtained before either may work completely. *Health Science* is designed as an individual's guide toward enriched personal health.

FACTORS INFLUENCING HEALTH

MENTAL OUTLOOK ON LIFE

Mental health is recognized today as an essential and inseparable part of one's total health. Poor mental health is at least as handicapping in life as poor physical health. Not only do emotional problems severely limit the pleasure one derives from living, but also they frequently result in physical illness. The abuse of alcohol or drugs is today properly regarded as an emotional health problem.

INTELLIGENT USE OF FOODS

Today's methods of growing, processing, and shipping foods make the achievement of good nutrition by people of even modest income easy. Yet there are people in all income brackets who show signs of poor nutrition. Most commonly observed today are the symptoms of over-nutrition—excessive weight. Nutritional deficiencies are common in the United States, especially among families of low income or poor education, and among those who rely upon nutritional fads.

LIVING WITH OTHERS

Our individual and national welfare depend strongly upon people's understanding each other socially, because social stresses can cloud the lives of millions. A high level of emotional health is essential for pleasant relationships with neighbors, productive relationships with co-workers, and peaceful relationships between different ethnic and social groups. As world population increases, international tensions increase proportionately. The quest for world peace involves finding solutions for many problems relating to physical and emotional health.

Lifelong individual happiness depends upon proper preparation for marriage and careful selection of marriage partners. A stable marriage relationship is still considered basic to a strong civilization. The limitation of family size is important for both individual happiness and national and world welfare.

DISEASE PREVENTION

Among the most traditional of the factors promoting health is the prevention of disease. Methods for the prevention of most communicable diseases are now available. Some of these methods are public health concerns, such as the control of mosquitoes and the assurance of safe foods and drinking water. But much disease prevention remains the responsibility of the individual, for example, the procuring of immunizations and the prevention of venereal diseases. The prevention of the chronic degenerative diseases, now still largely in the research stages, will, when understood, probably rest mainly upon the efforts of the individual.

CHOOSING BEST HEALTH SERVICES

The individual is responsible for selecting the best health services from those available in the community. Individuals must choose their medical practitioner carefully, checking his training, skill, and ethical standards. Quacks still flourish in many cities of the United States. Even among legitimate practitioners, a wide range in skills exists. The choice of hospitals can greatly influence the quality of care received. Many of the nation's hospitals do not meet the minimum standards for accreditation. The choice of a poor practitioner often restricts the patient to a poor hospital, compounding the situation. The quality of care received often depends upon ability to pay, which, for the average family, depends upon the type of health insurance carried. Health insurance policies vary greatly in terms of coverage and value received. Many people unsuspectingly select very poor health insurance plans.

MASTERING THE ENVIRONMENT

Man's continued success as the dominant living organism on earth depends upon his maintaining an environment favorable to his welfare. Fortunately, in recent years there has been an increasing awareness of the relationship between man and his environment. One of the most critical problems is the pollution of that environment. Man can afford no further pollution of his air, soil, and water. Such pollution is not only esthetically unpleasant, but is also a definite health hazard.

Greater attention must be given to the significant problem of world population dynamics. There must be world-wide recognition of the fact that we live on a finite earth with finite resources and that even with the most efficient application of those resources, there is a limit to the number of people the earth can support.

Today's college student has at hand the potential for a lifetime of health and happiness for himself and his family. The remaining chapters of this book will acquaint the reader with the means for attaining such a life.

C H A P T E R 2

COMMON EMOTIONAL PROBLEMS

Emotional health differs from other phases of health science in that we must often deal with opinions rather than with well-established facts. Someday, hopefully, the formula for maintaining emotional health will be as definitely established as the formula for maintaining a balanced diet is today. In the meantime, we must, to some extent, content ourselves with educated guesses. Because of this lack of finality, we must also be prepared to receive different answers from equally competent authorities for a given emotional problem.

THE NORMAL PERSONALITY

It would be very difficult to set up a standard by which an individual's emotional normality could be judged. It is more difficult to describe the normal personality than to define the abnormal personality; certainly,

7

no line can be drawn easily to separate the two. At best, we can only set forth traits or characteristics indicative of the normal person. It should be emphasized that we are portraying the normal mature adult. Clearly, this is a different personality from that found in a normal child, a normal teen-ager, or the emotionally immature adult.

A RELAXED CONSCIENCE

The well-adjusted person has worked out a harmonious relationship between his instinctive desires, his conscience, and his environment, which enables him to make the maximum use of his emotional energies. He is then free to direct these energies toward constructive work, adjustment to the opposite sex, and service to other people. His reactions toward life in general are based upon external reality rather than upon some rigidly constructed internal defense. He has a strong sense of reality and yet continues to grow with experience. He is never rigid and inflexible.

A HEALTHY ATTITUDE TOWARD LIFE

Although each mature person differs from the next person in terms of background and interests, he has a healthy interest in what is going on around him. Such a person expects and accepts happiness and, when a problem does arise, he meets it with a desire to solve it and to learn from it. He attempts to analyze his fears objectively and to master them.

AN ABILITY TO LOVE AND UNDERSTAND OTHERS

The mature person does not have a large number of childish needs that are striving for expression. He has the ability to initiate expressions of affection for other people. Such an ability extends beyond his partners, mate, and children. He can accept people of racial, religious, and cultural backgrounds different from his own. He can afford such feelings because they reflect a sense of inner security.

A REASONABLE DEPENDENCE UPON OTHERS

A mature person will demonstrate reasonable reliance upon the judgment and experience of other people. Although he is capable of making independent decisions and facing the consequences of those decisions, he realizes the value of good counsel from others. He seeks advice from better qualified persons, rather than feeling that he is always right. He can accept fair criticism of his mistakes and faults and does not need to regard these as a threat to his personal security.

MODERATION IN NEGATIVE EMOTIONS

Although it is not unusual for a person to feel reactions of anger and dislike for persons or things, the mature person does not allow such emotions to overpower his rational control over his own actions.

AN ABILITY TO MAKE LONG-RANGE CHOICES

The mature person is willing to sacrifice some immediate pleasures for the sake of long-range goals. He values pleasure, but he plans his life to yield the greatest net satisfaction over the long run. These plans involve choices of career, management of finances, and matters of marriage and children. He looks beyond the immediate situation to the future.

MIND AND BODY

The human being functions as a psycho-physical unit. The mind (*psyche*) is just one aspect of the individual. The physical or organic aspects of the person are expressed as the *soma*. These two terms, combined into the word *psychosomatic*, describe conditions which are caused by the effect of the mind upon the body or of the body upon the mind.

Physical disorders can lead to emotional disturbances. A person who has undergone an amputation or who has been crippled through an accident may experience emotional upsets. A married woman who desires children but cannot become pregnant may become despondent. The individual suffering severe pain can become depressed. Such pain endured over a prolonged period of time may lead to more severe degrees of emotional disturbance. He may become critical of other people, be hard to live with in the home, or find it difficult or impossible to carry out his normal responsibilities. Excessive fatigue may be accompanied by irritability or depression. Keeping the body in good physical health through proper nutrition, rest, and exercise is an essential part of good mental health.

On the other hand, the mind affects the body. Sometimes the effects are harmless and brief, as when a person blushes with embarrassment or when the mouth becomes dry through fear. Other effects may be more severe and may be present for months or years. Where the stress or anxiety continues for long periods of time, physical symptoms may even become a way of life. The symptoms may or may not respond successfully to medical treatment. A person may have vague symptoms such as temporary aches and pains, indigestion, or headaches without apparent organic illness. Others experience distinct organic illnesses such as ulcers, colitis, asthma, high blood pressure, skin rashes, recurrent symptoms of coronary heart disease, obesity, paralysis, deafness, or even blindness.

Although there are many factors in psychosomatic illnesses, all are expressed through some degree of anxiety. The person with psychosomatic disorders seems to have an inability or incapacity to communicate effectively and rid himself of these anxieties. This breakdown of communication may affect any organ of the body. When one set of aches is inadequate as an anxiety-relieving device, there is often a shift in complaints; the conflict of living becomes evident all over again through a new set of symptoms.

EMOTIONS

The newborn child carries within him certain inherited traits. As he grows, these traits develop into elaborate and complicated patterns of reaction to the stimuli he encounters. These patterns are called *emotions.* Examples of emotions are love, anger, and fear.

Emotions are an important part of a person and aid in his survival. They are the spark which can serve to mobilize his psychic and physical resources. Emotions may be used constructively in dealing with oneself and with others. If, however, some emotions are not used constructively, but are given full rein or are unduly suppressed they may become destructive to the personality.

POSITIVE EMOTIONS

The following emotions are constructive in their effect upon a person.

LOVE

An essential emotion in every person is love. It is one of the first needs a child has and is the basis for his physical and emotional security. Without love, the child, who must rely upon others for his needs, has no assurance of life. Children need the love of parents and of other children in the family; parents need the love of each other and of their children. Adults need the love of their associates.

In order for love to flourish there must be a setting of kindness, sympathy, unselfishness, and tolerance. The absence of love in a person's life can lead to unpleasant reactions on his part, such as daydreaming, cruelty, or aggressive actions toward other people.

FAITH

A belief in and reliance upon some power outside oneself is another basic emotional need. Although individuals conceive of this outside power in different ways, it is important for people to believe that the universe and the life in it exist for some useful purpose. The acceptance of this idea becomes an important element in maintaining emotional stability.

ACHIEVEMENT

A sense of personal worth and ability to perform as a useful person in society is another emotional need. Depending upon the situation, one attempts to satisfy this need by performing well scholastically, by doing a job well, by establishing a good home for one's family, or by taking part in activities that are of service to other people. Failure to satisfy this need can lead the person to feel depressed and rejected by his family, friends, or colleagues.

A person will commonly find more satisfaction in one type of work than in another. Thus the area of endeavor to which he gives himself is of great importance. Various occupations have high social prestige (and financial compensations) at any given time. Others less prestigious may offer great satisfaction through their contribution to social welfare or to art. Each individual should try to choose an occupation in which *he* has special interests and abilities.

NEGATIVE EMOTIONS

If the person has emotional needs which go unsatisfied, he has to try to make adjustments for them. All of us at times fail to make sufficient adjustment, and frustrations and unhappiness result. We react to these unsatisfied emotional needs with various negative emotions.

ANGER

Although a normal response to frustration, anger represents a primitive response. It is a "fight" instinct and represents the desire, and perhaps the attempt, to aggressively settle an issue by destroying it, attacking it, killing it, or in some other way trying to neutralize it. Although all human beings feel angry at times, it is necessary that angry reactions be controlled. If repressed, the anger may afflict us in some other manner. Thus it is important that we learn ways to direct those energies aroused by feelings of anger into constructive activities. A minor irritation may be "worked off" by playing a hard game of tennis, cleaning house, or vigorously mowing the lawn. Deep-seated anger should be analyzed for its cause, so that the individual can set about to alter the conditions that make him angry. He may be able to change the external circumstances or his attitude toward them or both. In any case, he accepts anger as the symptom of a problem that needs to be solved.

FEAR

Another reaction to emotional frustration is the "flight" instinct, or fear. Fear may be resorted to as a way of survival or it may represent the decision to try to evade an issue. Fears, if allowed to develop uncontrolled, can lead to over- or under-response to a situation—to panicking or to freezing up. It is important, therefore, that we approach our fears as symptomatic of a problem. Like anger, fear is a warning that some problem needs to be met. And, as with anger, the individual must try to understand *why* he fears, whether fear is the best way of reacting to the situation, and what he can do to overcome this negative emotion.

MENTAL PROCESSES

As we have said, the human being functions as a unit. The separation of mind and body, once thought to be so important, is now considered to be a convenient scheme for describing various activities of the single organism. Modern psychologists describe mind as "the organization of behavior" and they define behavior as "the functioning of the *entire* organism."

Some psychologists, following the pioneer work of the psychoanalyst Sigmund Freud, have (again, for schematic purposes) postulated two levels of mind, the conscious and the unconscious. According to this scheme, the conscious mind is the surface, or "skin," which is observable and which covers the great bulk of the mind, the unconscious.

This theory, although it is arbitrary, is of value for describing the processes in people that we call mind. The processes of *id, ego,* and *super-ego* are the psychoanalytical ways of describing the varieties of human behavior.

THE ID PROCESSES

At the time of birth the child brings with him a bundle of inborn tendencies necessary for survival. These inborn tendencies represent the *unconscious* strivings of the human organism to live and enjoy life. Since the id processes work for the individual's biological survival, they are aggressive and selfish. They operate for his pleasure and gratification. The id does not distinguish between good and evil, between what is realistic and what is not. Since these processes operate under the pleasure principle ("whatever brings pleasure is good"), the child must be educated in control of these processes. The maturing of the individual and pressure from society are necessary to taming of the aggressive id.

THE EGO PROCESSES

The ego processes represent the *conscious* self. It is through the ego that we are aware of reality. The ego processes act as regulators, controlling and balancing the needs of the id with the demands of society and of the superego, or conscience. The ego maintains contact with the outside world by means of the individual's perceptual and motor apparatuses; the conscious self responds on the basis of what it hears, sees, feels, tastes, and smells. Since the individual at birth is untrained emotionally, the processes of the ego develop gradually and gain strength as the individual grows older and responds to the pressures of society.

Instinctive, aggressive impulses which arise in the id must be accepted or rejected for expression by the ego. The ego processes can be thought of as the rational thinking resulting from experiences of trial and error. Therefore there is constant communication between the id and the ego. If an impulse is unwelcome in terms of the ego's experience with reality, the ego processes place barriers against the impulse's entering into consciousness; they strive to restrict us to what is possible. The ego can be described as a controlling agency which recognizes, receives, stores, discriminates, integrates, and acts by restraining, releasing, modifying, and directing impulses. Thus the ego processes can be considered the guardian of the vital balance of the person.

THE SUPEREGO PROCESSES

The superego sits as the advisor, admonisher, encourager, or threatener to the ego. These processes hold the judiciary role in the *unconscious* mind. They are a sort of reference book which the ego uses in regulating impulses stemming from the id. The superego can be considered the conscience, the still small voice which helps us to decide between the rightness and wrongness of actions. It also represents the ideal the ego would like the self either to become or to appear as to others. While the ego processes decide which impulses are possible, as far as society is concerned, the superego processes decide what is permissible.

The superego processes are formed during infancy and childhood. During these early years the child, of necessity, strongly identifies himself with his parents and family. Their attitudes, restrictions, and admonitions, because of his dependence upon and identification with them, become his basis of judging the morality of situations. Since social values change over a period of time, years after an individual has become an adult he may still be carrying these childhood values as a part of his superego in spite of the fact that they may be outdated. For instance, individuals whose parents were overly strict during childhood may be controlled by values which are no longer reasonable. Or, they may be compelled to try to strive for an unattainable ideal if their parents have developed too high and unrealistic an ideal in them during childhood.

METHODS FOR COPING WITH EMOTIONAL CONFLICTS

Within the mind conflicts rage between the various processes— between the id and the ego, the superego and the ego, the id and the superego. Since the primary character in this drama is the ego, it becomes the center for most conflicts. It must be receptive to the impulses from the id and yet control them; it must integrate the person and maintain the vital balance. Conflicts may place considerable pressure on the processes of the ego.

If the ego is under too much pressure from the id, or is being punished by the superego, the individual will experience anxiety. Although it is not always possible for us to pinpoint the exact source of our anxiety, we plainly experience it. Anxieties are both painful and unpleasant. They may express themselves in ways such as guilt, feelings of inferiority, isolation, "bullishness," or even as physical symptoms. Since the ego is thus in jeopardy, it will often seek to find some "crutch" or device with which it can bolster or defend itself. Such a crutch is called by psychologists a *defense mechanism.*

Psychological defense mechanisms are ego processes that are largely unconscious. All of us use them to a greater or lesser extent to cope with difficult situations. They may be acceptable so long as we do not overuse them. The overuse or abuse of defense mechanisms may indicate serious unresolved conflicts in the unconscious mind which could lead to further stress if they go unresolved. Although there are many ways in which the unconscious mind defends a weak ego, we will list only several of the more important ones in the following discussion.

RATIONALIZATION

In an attempt to find reasons to justify one's own failures and short-comings a person may resort to rationalization, a kind of mental deception. Rationalizing his behavior seems to leave him blameless. The student rationalizes his poor performance on an examination on grounds that it was an unfair test or that he was unprepared for it (although he may have studied thoroughly). The use of this mechanism helps to ease the letdown he may feel from failure.

Although the use of rationalization at times helps one to feel more comfortable with himself and may even be justified, the overuse of this kind of thinking may encourage him to put off solutions to problems. It is better to admit one's shortcomings and then either accept them or work out a plan to correct them.

SUBSTITUTION

Everyone has his strengths and weaknesses. In order to satisfy emotional needs, a person can substitute the satisfactions he gains from some activities for the disappointments he experiences in others. An individual who is particularly apt in some athletic activity, for example, may substitute the pleasure he gets from it for the disappointment he feels in his chosen profession. Everyone practices some substitution, but it is important not to choose substitutes for disappointments one has the ability to overcome. It is equally important not to choose substitutes that can harm the individual or others, such as using harmful drugs or resorting to alcoholism.

REGRESSION

Regression is a reversion to childlike and immature behavior when one is faced with difficult situations. It represents a retreat from the present frustrations to the fancied security of some time in the past. A person displays regression when reacting to a situation in the way he would have done as a child—going into a tantrum when he cannot have his way, not playing unless he is the captain, or throwing his bat away if an unfavorable call is made against him in a baseball game. Although such regression rarely gains a person the kind of treatment he wants, the ego temporarily feels more comfortable.

PROJECTION

Projection is the denying of one's own weakness by placing the blame for a situation on another person or persons. For example, an executive may fire a subordinate for a mistake the executive himself has made and for which he is responsible. Some people who have certain weaknesses are very apt at seeing these weaknesses in other people and are quick to condemn others for their own omissions. Children show projection by running to their parents and tattling on a brother or sister who has done something they themselves have done. We tend to project those feelings that bother us most. If we despise someone, we may not find it difficult to think that he despises us, so that we can easily "justify" becoming mean, sarcastic, and distorted.

REPRESSION

Repression is a process of selectively forgetting. A person unconsciously tries to forget those events in his past or present that may cause him pain or discomfort—a kind of emotional block. The individual tries to repress these feelings from being expressed; in other words he feels one way while trying to act another. His feelings are not to be denied, however, and will seek expression in one way or another. They may express themselves as dreams, amnesia, slips of the tongue, or purposeful forgetting. Since such repressed feelings can create anxiety and guilt, many psychologists feel it is better for a person's emotional health that he find reasonable ways of expressing his feelings.

IDENTIFICATION

Identification is a kind of hero worship by which a person identifies himself with persons or institutions that represent ideal qualities. This process can be very helpful to developing children who identify themselves with persons or groups representing high goals and ideals. College students frequently seek to be identified with individuals or groups who can bring them attention and prestige. Identification is desirable if the ideal represents high standards and, on the whole, can be one of the most satisfying mental mechanisms. However, overidentification or overreliance upon one's family, school, or other group may hinder one's own personal development and may detract from good mental health.

FANTASY AND DAYDREAMING

Daydreaming can be helpful if it is not overdone. The fantasy a child creates is an important part of his development. Adults use it in constructive imagination, as shown by the artist. We can escape from the pressures of reality through the pleasures of fantasy. It is possible to relax by entering the world of illusion found in fiction, drama, and poetry. This mechanism can become harmful, however, when it is overused as a means of escaping from the problems and disappointments of the real world. It may be used to the point where an individual cannot distinguish between reality and fantasy, and thus become a serious disturbance to his emotional health.

EMOTIONAL DYSORGANIZATION

It has been indicated how the ego processes go about the task of trying to regulate events that tend to disturb a person's adjustment inside himself and with society. The ego tries to level off the disturbances as best it can. Sometimes, however, an individual experiences situations which disturb him deeply. He experiences frustrations or alarm; the primitive, aggressive impulses of the id, over which the ego has maintained control, are aroused and threaten that control. From the other side, the superego's ideal may be so high as to be impossible, and the ego, which tries to regulate the self with regard to the *possible,* may give way. The inability of the ego processes to maintain normal control constitutes what is commonly called emotional, or mental, illness (the two are synonymous).

Instead of using the older, traditional concept of mental illness complete with definite labels and diagnoses, the authors of this text follow the lead of Dr. Karl Menninger, co-founder of the Menninger Clinic, a psychiatric hospital in Topeka, Kansas. His is a simple, yet broad approach which sees emotional illness as a continuum which ranges from relative emotional normalcy to emotional collapse or death. Dr. Menninger has coined the word *dysorganization* to describe the increasingly painful or disturbing experiences the ego goes through in trying to maintain successful control over the id processes. The prefix *dys-* means "painful"; thus this word refers to the pain or disturbance the person experiences in trying to maintain an organized emotional balance. (Do not mistake this word for *disorganization,* which means the state of being disarranged.) In dysorganization the organization is only impaired; it is neither lost nor destroyed.

Starting with a relatively normal adjustment, Menninger describes increasing degrees of emotional dysorganization to represent increasing degrees of mental illness. As the pressure from anxiety becomes greater, one's whole self becomes more and more threatened. At the extreme, the person may even die, since the whole system, both emotional and physical, may collapse under the unbearable strain of dysorganization.

According to Menninger's concept, the entire range of mental illness, extending from the so-called "emotionally normal person" to the most severe cases (terminal collapse or death) can be conveniently divided into five levels or groupings. The text will describe each of these five levels or steps of increasingly severe mental illness (see Fig. 2.1).

FIRST LEVEL OF DYSORGANIZATION

The person with the beginnings of emotional dysorganization experiences a somewhat more than normal amount of tension and shows it through "nervousness." The ego is aware of an increase in aggressive impulses coming from the id—fear, anger, frustration. Although the person may not recognize these as a threat to the ego, he knows that he is using more than an average amount of will power to master his internal reactions. He may respond by determining not to notice these rising tensions or may even try to convince himself that everything is all right. Normally the person is able to manage these problems by using one or more of the defense mechanisms previously described. But, just as a person who is physically ill may be conscious of his breathing or the beating of his heart (activities we normally take for granted), the emotionally disturbed person becomes aware of emotional disturbances and is made uneasy by them. He may be forced to exert conscious effort to control these problems, minor as they are.

At the same time the ego processes become increasingly alert, or *hyperalert*, to events around the person. A hyperalert person may hear

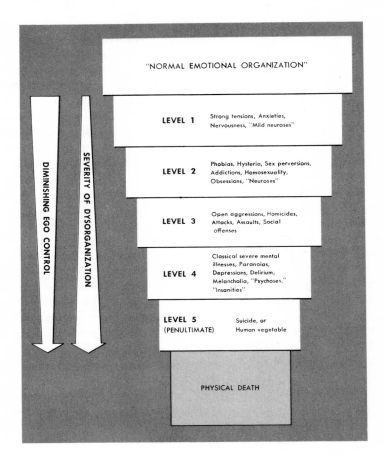

Fig. 2.1 Levels of emotional dysorganization.

mysterious noises in the night or detect the slightest irregularity in the appearance of something. Although some alertness is a normal reaction, in the first level of dysorganization alertness becomes exaggerated. The individual looks for possible dangers—sounds are exaggerated, lights are more intense, and his entire perception is keener. The person unconsciously refuses to relax at night during sleep. There may be increased touchiness, tearfulness, irritability, nervous laughter, moodiness,

or depression. Sometimes this person may appear overactive by display-
ing restlessness—walking the floor, biting his fingernails, or driving
aimlessly about in his car. He may worry, or think obsessively about
something, anxiously reflecting on it time and again. He may daydream
excessively and thus impair realistic thinking and effective action, or
be overzealous in identifying with some cause. This person may experience certain psychosomatic ailments—itching skin, twitching eyes, diarrhea, upset stomach, or pain for which aspirin or sleeping pills produce
remarkable results.

All of these actions are tools the ego processes use to deal with
emergencies. Because these actions represent a type of illness, they can
also be considered as symptoms, although the person does not consider
himself ill (yet he does not feel quite well). Such symptoms are both
uncomfortable and expensive in terms of medical treatment. Yet they
may serve to protect a person's ego and thus save him.

Although designated here as the first level of dysorganization, the
degree of disturbance we have just described is sometimes labeled *mild
neurosis* or, with some, *mild hypochondriasis*. The presence of one or
several of these symptoms surely would not indicate positive proof of
illness, yet the presence of several such symptoms over a period of days
or weeks could well indicate some inability to cope satisfactorily with
life situations.

Usually the emergency device will disappear the moment the stress
which originally caused it disappears. Many persons showing such simple
dysorganization over a period of time eventually recover, although some
remain as chronic cases and some become worse. If these symptoms continue for too long a period of time, they are physically wearing. A headache can be endured for a few hours, but one lasting for days or weeks
could lead the individual into more severe dysorganization. If a person
who is already undergoing some stresses runs into new ones, deeper
dysorganization could result. If the ego is unable to control behavior
with the mild devices suggested here, the ego processes are led to increased activity. Something else must be done; other ego-saving devices
must be called upon, which lead the person to the more severe second
level of dysorganization.

SECOND LEVEL OF DYSORGANIZATION

The increased emotional changes that occur at this level are still
slight, yet they may cause definite detachment of the person from his
environment. He becomes a little more unrealistic. Although his actions
may or may not appear changed in the eyes of others, he further shuts
off the real world. This isolation means a lessened contact with the
normal flow of stimulation and information. The ego processes become
more impaired. At this stage the person is aware that his emotional

state is neither comfortable nor pleasant. He may feel a sense of failure, uselessness, or disappointment with himself or others; he has less joy in productive work. Other people begin to appear deliberately provocative or indifferent. The person keeps doing things he does not want to do and saying things he does not want to say. Saint Paul made a related comment when he wrote, "The good which I would, I do not; but the evil which I would not, that I practice."

SYNDROMES CHARACTERIZING THE SECOND LEVEL

This management of aggressive impulses is handled with one of several emergency devices. Some emergencies are acute and last only for a short time. Some are chronic and become a permanent part of the personality. A group of symptoms that occur together and characterize a disease is called a *syndrome*.

1. *Blocking the aggressive impulse through withdrawal.* A person may unconsciously sever contact with the outside world temporarily. He can do it by fainting, having total lapse of memory, sleepwalking, selective blindness, selective deafness, selective amnesia, or through phobias. Phobias are the attaching of strong negative feelings to objects or situations, such as thunderstorms, cars, high places, snakes, cats, or public speaking. Sometimes individuals with phobias express their anger and fear by embracing, rather than withdrawing from, that which they fear. They may become pathologically daring, for example, playing "chicken" (a game in which cars approach each other head on at high speed; the first driver to swerve is defeated). This extreme boldness is typical of the second level of dysorganization.

2. *Controlling the aggressive impulse through affliction.* Some people have such intense hostility toward a person, group, or situation that they can not get it out of their systems merely by swatting flies or playing a hard game of tennis. Instead, they take out their hostility on themselves. Usually the self-punisher operates quietly. He expresses aggressions unconsciously in accidental injury, peptic ulcers, hypertension, or obesity. Although physically painful, these expressions probably provide him with salvation because he actually feels jeopardized.

Some go through vivid fantasies accompanied by real pain or psychosomatic illnesses (a kind of hypochondriasis). Some women demonstrate *pseudocyesis,* a false pregnancy characterized by interruption of menstruation, enlargement of the abdomen, and increased pigmenting of the nipples. Menninger cites the following psychosomatic case history.

A psychiatrist in Columbus, Georgia, last week detailed the amazing case history of a woman who spent seventeen of her twenty-eight years in a *psychosomatic marathon.* Her ailments included hives, headaches, hacking cough, constant sore throat, nausea, earaches, muscular soreness, and numbness in her right leg. The patient was never without some of these symptoms. She had paid 602 visits to 22 physicians and one chiropractor and was hospitalized five times. She received 33 different kinds of medication, 600 tests, and 1,500 injections. Nothing helped. Finally, the last physician advised her that she was "emotionally ill" and needed psychiatric help. After 32 consultations spread over eight months, her symptoms had all but disappeared, and she was dismissed. The patient's total bill: some $2,700 for medical care, $500 for psychiatry.[1]

Physiological reactions are in all instances considered to be accompanied by psychological reactions and vice versa.

3. *Controlling the aggressive impulse by compensating acts*

Rituals. All of us use some rituals or ceremonies every day. They may be acts which bring us pleasure although, in some cases, they may be accompanied by discomfort and inconvenience. They may include such things as calisthenics, dietary fads, daily enemas, abdominal massage, or even certain religious practices. These are symptoms of a problem when they become ends in themselves, when a ritual is no longer essential to another purpose, but the mere doing of it becomes a kind of release.

Compulsions. These are acts which seem to be quite unreasonable and unnecessary to a rational person, but which are irresistible to the person doing them. Examples could be craving for more food than one needs or hoarding items above and beyond the amount required for a secure and comfortable future. Although everyone does some of these things, when carried to excess compulsions can indicate advancing emotional dysorganization.

Obsessional thinking. In spite of having the appearance of thoughtful consideration in preparation for action, obsessional thinking actually takes the place of action. As such thinking becomes more intense, effective actions and productivity diminish. Obsessional thinking may be another device for handling increasing emotional problems.

Sexual perversion. Sexual perversion and promiscuity, like other psychiatric symptoms, represent an emotional compromise. Among the various forms of perversion are *homosexuality,* obtaining gratification by practicing intimacies with a member of the same sex; *fetishism,* deriving erotic satisfaction from objects instead of people, such as an article of a person's clothing or a lock of hair; *pedophilia,* obtaining satisfaction by the seduction of children; *exhibitionism,* obtaining gratification by exposing one's sexual organs to the gaze of others; *sadism* and *masochism,* obtaining gratification by inflicting pain and cruelty upon another person or by having such pain inflicted; and *voyeurism,* obtaining gratification by looking at other people's sexual activities. Psychiatrists believe that behind these acts there is hate, so that the perversions represent a type of cover-up for deeper aggres-

[1] K. Menninger *et al., The Vital Balance: The Life Process in Mental Health and Illness,* New York, Viking, 1964, pp. 187–188.

sions. The person has to get his sexual experience at any cost, so he engages in actions which are condemned by our society and which may be very destructive to him.

A further word should be said regarding homosexuality. This type of compromise for neutralizing aggressive impulses is accepted as a legitimate device by some therapists but not by others. A few authorities feel it ought to be legally allowed among those afflicted, even though it is not the behavior of an emotionally normal person. If homosexual practice is accompanied by violence, or if innocent people are plainly made to suffer, this ego compromise obviously cannot be condoned by society. If it does not involve harm to others and is a relationship between adults, our traditional attitude toward it ought to be more lenient according to some therapists. The authors do not, of course, recommend homosexuality; yet it has worked for some people as an emotional compromise and has allowed some of them to make significant contributions to society.

4. *Personality deformities.* In some cases, defensive devices become a permanent part of one's personality. Society's tolerance of him will likely depend on his social standing, power, and wealth. Whether the person is considered sick or not depends on society's opinion of him. If he is wealthy, he may be considered eccentric; if he is poor, he may be rejected or even judged criminal. Not knowing causes, other people may find it easy to assign motives.

Of the various kinds of such personality deformities, such as the infantile (beautiful but useless) and the narcissistic (excessively vain and selfish), only the addictive personality will be discussed here.

In light of the 5,200,000 Americans who are addicted to alcohol, narcotics, and other drugs, this category represents the largest single psychiatric affliction in the United States. In spite of the fact that addiction is painful and can disable a person, there is a common misunderstanding among people in general about this kind of illness or disease. It is too often considered simply a vice that the victim has voluntarily chosen. In reality it often represents a "chemically induced escape from reality" which may be innocent in its beginnings, but may later become a successful substitute for the things from which the victim wishes to escape. Thus it represents a degree of ego failure.

Traditionally, the second level of dysorganization has been described by such familiar terms as neurosis, psychoneurosis, or hysteria. Dr. Menninger strongly suggests that these old names are wrong and obsolete in that ailments of this second level are not the result of inflammation of the nerves, excess sexual activity, or exhaustion of the mind. The devices used on this second level represent an attempt to control and reduce an increased state of tension. Their use may avert more serious consequences. If they tide one over the emergency, they may disappear with *reduced* anxiety. If these devices are not sufficient, however, stress and tension may continue to *increase* and the threat to the person continue. Such a person may move on to the third level of dysorganization.

THIRD LEVEL OF DYSORGANIZATION (OPEN AGGRESSION)

In the third level of dysorganization the uncontrolled aggressive impulse is expressed directly on the things around the individual. The ego will likely rationalize itself into believing this expression is actually a way of self-defense. Are not all wars fought, in the eyes of either side, for self-preservation? Individuals use the same reasoning. The aggressive individual will not usually go to the point of trying to give logical reasons for his behavior, either to himself or to others. He may not even know why he carried out the act of vengeance or perpetrated the assault.

Society today no longer considers open aggression an acceptable evidence of manliness or as necessary for survival. Capital punishment, for instance, is interpreted by many as being a kind of corporate aggressive expression which is socially undesirable and, furthermore, ineffective as a deterrent to crime. Other critics believe that if it is to be a deterrent to potential criminals, capital punishment should be conducted openly for all to see, rather than in its usual setting of almost complete secrecy.

The muggings, clubbings, and shootings displayed each day on television represent a kind of reverting to the past when such aggression was more acceptable. This type of expression is highly satisfying to the weak individual. Thus, as present-day society becomes more and more civilized, not only should the reasons for personal violence become fewer, but also such physically aggressive people should become less tolerated. Cases of open aggression today often give strong evidence of ego failure. The sick individual who commits an aggressive act is showing that all or nearly all restricting control has been lost.

In general such an individual may be described in the following manner:

1. The aggressive impulse is no longer concealed.
2. He shows disregard for laws and social customs and little heed for conscience.
3. His judgment, consciousness, and perception may be impaired during the aggressive act.
4. After the aggressive act is over, the emotional tension is relieved.

SYNDROMES CHARACTERIZING THE THIRD LEVEL

The following grouping lists some types of aggressive behavior typical of the third level.

1. *Chronic, repeated aggressions.* Some people are rebels in search of never-found causes; they do not know what they are against, but whatever it is, they are against it. Their behavior is self-damaging, and they do not seem to learn from experience. A typical example would be the boy who seems to make all the wrong turns throughout school life, however long that may last. Although seemingly a promising student, he seems to go from bad to worse. Once out of school he cannot hold down a job because he is always breaking some trust or responsibility.

The characteristics of such "antisocial" behavior are similar for all ages, differing only in the nature of one's work and play activities. These persons are more lacking in common sense, more unrealistic, more detached from a sense of the past, more lacking in a reasonable vision of the future, and slower in seeking help than are individuals on the second level.

2. *Occasional violence.* There are also the spectacular, once-in-a-lifetime, or very infrequent outbursts of violence. These may, nevertheless, be severe enough to lead to corrective measures of some type, perhaps even capital punishment. Example of these would include such things as senseless beatings, suicide, and murder.

Regarding murder, although the episode may be bizarre and senseless, the murderer is usually just as puzzled as anyone as to why it all happened. Even though such acts are often violent, the murderer has been successful in putting off something he fears more—his own destruction. The murder is a substitution used by him to preserve his own life, which he prizes more highly than that of his victim. At the moment the murder was the only solution which the crippled ego of the murderer could find.

Some patients in this category have the syndrome called *hypomania,* a type of runaway acceleration of the processes of the mind. Such persons may talk too much, go too fast, and sleep too little. As one such patient said, "My wife thought I was on Cloud Seven all the time. First I was worried half sick, then everything was just rosy. My wife thought maybe I wasn't crazy, but I was driving all the rest of them crazy."

3. *Convulsive reactions.* It was early observed that victims of epileptic convulsions gained a sudden release from the convulsion. It was this observation that led to the development of convulsive shock therapy, by both insulin and electricity, among nonconvulsive psychiatric patients. Although the causes of convulsions are wide ranging, all of them result in the release of unbearable tension.

It is felt by some psychiatrists that rising, unresolved psychological tensions are one of the factors leading up to the onset of a given seizure. Loss of consciousness may be an unconscious reaction of the victim when faced with some demand for action which endangers his acceptable pattern of behavior.

Thus, in summary, the expression of open, direct aggression, except in certain socially acceptable forms, is evidence of acute or chronic ego failure. These acts are often explosive and destructive and in some cases are accompanied by a loss of consciousness. Open aggression represents a weaker ego situation than that of the second level of dysorganization. There is more detachment from reality and more injury to the victim, to the environment, and to the perpetrator. Yet these aggressions are thought to represent an attempt by the individual to avoid even greater ego failure.

FOURTH LEVEL OF DYSORGANIZATION

The preceding three levels represent lesser examples of emotional illness. Formerly, people dismissed these three lesser degrees of dysorganization as eccentricity, perversion, or viciousness. Thus, in the past such people were not often under the care of a physician. Such illness does not generally happen suddenly, but may develop over a span of years. If the condition worsens, it may lead to the fourth level of dysorganization, sometimes called *psychosis* (also known in the past as lunacy or insanity). These illnesses may have various causes. Certain forms may develop gradually, resulting from increasing stress. However there is evidence that other forms have a biochemical or hereditary basis. Regardless of the causes, the effects may appear similar.

In the fourth level pretense of control is no longer effectively maintained. Aggressive impulses break into consciousness and into action so easily that the ego processes appear to have lost their control. The person loses contact with the world of reality and the sense of loyalty he has felt toward it. To him the outside world appears distorted, and he responds with emotional reactions which are out of place, exaggerated, and unpredictable. Effective productivity, either in the home or on the job, is lost. Sometimes the patient appears scarcely human. Although he may appear odd, senseless, or fantastic, a therapist can see some pattern in the patient's talk which matches his past experience.

SYNDROMES CHARACTERISTIC OF THE FOURTH LEVEL

Various recognizable groups of symptoms are typical of the fourth level. Although the names assigned to these may be helpful in treatment, in legal decisions, and for general communication, it should never be concluded that specific "diseases" are being described. These are not diseases, but rather various forms of dysorganization within patients. Although we refer to various syndromes, we should think of all of them as one general "illness" which may take upon itself one of the following forms:

1. The individual may have feelings of sadness, guilt, despondency, and hopelessness, with convictions of inadequacy, incompetence, unworthiness, or wickedness. Physical reactions may be retarded. Delusions, with feelings of guilt, defection, unworthiness, and self-abasement, along with fantasies of imaginary offenses and punishments, are common. (This has been called melancholia and depression.)

2. He may demonstrate erratic and disorganized excitement, or excessive talking, acting, elation, and excitement. His actions may be self-injuring, bizarre, exhibitionistic, or annoying. A characteristic feature is the great and continuing overflow of poorly controlled energy. (This has been called mania, delirium, furor, or frenzy.)

3. He may be overly absorbed with himself, silly, or he may have bizarre delusions with irrelevant and incoherent speech and apparent indifference to social mores or standards. The patient may be inert or mute, have hallucinations, or have occasional sudden impulsive outbursts of speech or actions. (This condition has been called chronic delirium, chronic deterioration, or autism.)

4. He may have a preoccupation with persecution, accompanied by defensiveness, resentment, and suspiciousness. Still, the person may appear dignified and sensible at times. (This condition is called paranoia.)

5. He may appear confused, delirious, bewildered; he may be suffering from amnesia or hallucinations. These are commonly connected with severe injury, intoxication, or brain inflammation. Inflammation may be brought on by conditions such as encephalitis, arteriosclerosis, Huntington's disease, and poisonings. (This condition has been called dementia or delirium.)

Once again, according to the concept used in this text, these are not separate diseases, but varieties of one disease. In other words, this is one illness with various expressions. These symptoms are reversible (except in cases of brain injury). People with such advanced cases may recover when favorable situations once again surround them. Then the evidence of extreme crisis and dysorganization may well be left behind. When circumstances are not favorable, patients rarely die, but instead continue to live in a world of chronic, long-term maladjustment. Some modern psychiatrists believe this condition is the result of the neglect or ignorance of the society.

FIFTH LEVEL OF DYSORGANIZATION

Some patients are beyond help, and some remain disabled in spite of the best efforts. A few deteriorate until they eventually die, but the percentage of such patients is small. Emotional illness is not an invasion, but a defensive reaction. Consequently, there can be no predetermined course of development. Although most patients improve, a few proceed on to complete emotional collapse. As desperate as some of the above syndromes appear, there is an even lower point to which the emotions may be carried. At that level the patient seems to have little real consciousness, although he maintains certain basic life functions such as breathing, digesting, and excreting. In some cases even these will fail.

The fifth level clearly represents the greatest extremity to which the ego processes can be pushed. It is also described as being the penultimate level of emotional dysorganization—in other words, the step before the last. In this "way out" situation, the ego disintegrates and repudiates life itself. All that is left is a self-destructive determination to end it all. The spark of life goes out; hope and effort end in futility.

Suicide, for instance, is a biological paradox in which the ego processes appear to die. We are not speaking here of the half-hearted suicide attempts which are arranged to test the love of someone with hopes for a last-minute rescue. It is undoubtedly highly rewarding to some apparent suicides to be rescued, with much pleading, from rooftops or open windows. Earnest suicides come about for various reasons. Some represent a kind of self-offering for sins committed; some, a sort of loyalty (such as family suicides, or suicide pacts between lovers). Suicide may be revenge on those who will remain. With some cases, it appears the victim is carrying out an actual aggression, even to the point of murdering *with* suicide—as in airplane bombings in which others are also killed. Suicide may represent a flight from pain, incurable disease, or condemnation to death. In some countries suicide is not even known; in others, it is rather common; in most, it is considered an irrational act. Its impact is felt by everyone associated with the victim.

Suicide, although often vividly reported by news media, actually represents one of the lesser causes of death. For example, in the age group 15–24, suicide is the third major cause of death and yet represents only about 5 percent of the total deaths within this age group.[2]

Thus where the ego processes cannot easily cope with daily emotional situations, their failure leads first to mild dysorganization, then to open aggressive actions which may give some relief from pressure, but which, if unresolved, finally lead to total self-destruction.

All of these described conditions are merely varying expressions of the process of dysorganization, which may be an outgrowth of the demands placed upon human beings in a tension-filled and constantly changing world.

2 *The Facts of Life and Death, Selected Statistics on the Nation's Health and People,* Washington, D.C., U.S. Department of Health, Education, and Welfare, Public Health Service, 1965, p. 14.

SCOPE OF THE PROBLEM OF MENTAL ILLNESS

The problem of mental illness can be considered from several vantage points. In addition to the incidence of mental illness and the number of patients in hospitals, we must also consider the personnel providing mental care, facilities available for providing this care, and the methods of therapy being used.

PREVALENCE OF MENTAL ILLNESS

The incidence of mental illness will depend somewhat upon how "mental illness" is defined. According to the concept of mental illness used in this text, even the early stages of emotional dysorganization, beginning with symptoms of anxiety and nervousness (which may not impair a person), can constitute mental illness. Thus everyone could be considered as being mentally ill at some time in his life. In the opinion of Dr. Menninger, everyone *is* mentally ill at some time. Anxiety and stress are widespread. A study conducted in New York City compared life stress and mental health. Of those tallied, 70.8 percent evidenced mixed anxiety and 51.7 percent reported some psychosomatic symptoms. The majority of these, however, were not impaired by their stresses.[3] It is estimated that perhaps as many as 10 percent of the United States population are now suffering from some form of *serious* mental illness or will be at some time in their lives.

There are other ways of measuring the prevalence of mental illness. More than half of the hospital beds in the country are occupied by mental patients.[4] Each year over 1 million persons receive treatment in our mental hospitals and in the psychiatric wards of general hospitals.

Since 1900 the rate of hospitalization for mental illness has more than doubled. This is not evidence of an increased prevalence in mental illness. It is considered to be the result of a growing awareness of the problems of mental health, a higher percentage of people living in urban areas, the gradual aging of the population, and a significant increase in mental health facilities. Although the rate of hospitalization for mental illness in this country is one of the highest in the world, this does not indicate that there is a higher percentage of mental illness in the United States than in other countries. This country has more facilities for the care of such illness and has, in comparison with many other countries, made greater attempts to understand it. In some countries relatively little is done to care for mental illness.

Fortunately, the number of resident patients in mental hospitals has

[3] Louis A. Dublin, *Factbook on Man, From Birth to Death,* New York, Macmillan, 1965, p. 317.
[4] *Ibid.,* p. 316.

been decreasing since 1955. This decrease has occurred in spite of an increase in the general population. Although the number of new admissions to mental hospitals has been increasing, the net number of releases from these hospitals has been increasing faster, according to the Mental Health Statistics of the U.S. Department of Health, Education, and Welfare. These developments are the results of the new drugs being used in therapy (see the discussion on methods of treatment, p. 31). Over all, it does not appear that the rate of mental illness is increasing in this country.

PROFESSIONAL WORKERS WITH THE MENTALLY ILL

Most patients today are treated by a specially trained group of people, rather than by one individual. This group is known as the psychiatric team. In addition to physicians and nurses, it may include social workers, psychologists, occupational therapists, physical therapists, and others who are concerned with specialized aspects of the patient's rehabilitation.

1. *Psychiatrist.* The psychiatrist is a physician who has been qualified by the American Board of Psychiatry and Neurology. As the leader of the psychiatric team he is responsible for diagnosing the case, prescribing treatment, administering psychotherapy, and supervising and directing the work of other members of the team. He delegates much of the total program to various members of the team.

2. *Clinical psychologist.* Although not a medical doctor, the psychologist commonly holds either a doctor of philosophy or masters degree in psychology. His most effective contribution to the psychiatric team is his work in association with the psychiatrist. He helps to develop and refine diagnostic devices for the detection of maladjustments, studiesthe personality structure, helps in recognition of the symptoms of disease, and develops new therapeutic techniques. He may share the actual psychotherapy in some institutions.

3. *Psychiatric social worker.* This person will usually hold a masters degree in social work with emphasis on psychiatry. He will maintain contact with relatives, friends, employers, and others connected with the patient. He assists them in making such changes in the environment as are indicated as desirable or necessary for the mutual benefit of the patient and his surroundings.

4. *Psychiatric technician.* The technician is charged with the actual physical custody of the patient. This person is important because of the personal influence he has over the patient. Strong personal contacts between the technician and the patient can greatly enhance the psychiatric treatment process. He must be a high school graduate and will usually be given on-the-job training.

Even with the recent improvements in the care of the mentally ill, the psychiatric team is still hard-pressed. Of the more than 15,000 psychiatrists in the United States, approximately half of them work in mental hospitals and clinics, with a case load of about 111 patients per doctor. Such a case load forbids adequate treatment for all hospitalized patients. Although more than half of all hospitalized patients in the United States are mental patients, less than one-fortieth of all registered nurses are involved in psychiatric care. There is a corresponding deficiency in the available numbers of clinical psychologists and psychiatric social workers.

CLINICAL FACILITIES

1. *State hospitals.* The traditional pattern for medical care for the mentally ill in this country has been the providing of humane custodial care for patients through prolonged hospitalization. In most states during the past century this has been made a responsibility of the state government. Commonly, states have provided "insane asylums." Patients have commonly been admitted either voluntarily or involuntarily through court order.

It has been increasingly apparent that there have been omissions in this type of care. Many times the patient has not been treated until the illness is severe, so that he is no longer responsible for himself and requires a court order to be committed to receive help. After treatment, during the acute period, the patient has been discharged without further thought or responsibility. In other cases, patients have become chronically acute cases and have stayed in institutions for the remainder of their lives. Such hospitalization has been expensive, even when figured on a cost per day of $5 to $10 per patient.

Various state hospitals for the mentally ill have been successfully experimenting with new approaches, such as instituting programs to get chronic patients out of the "asylum," following them up, and making it easier for patients to commit themselves.

2. *Psychiatric sections of general hospitals.* There is an increasing trend to treat disturbed patients in sections of general hospitals reserved for such care. Here the patients evade the stigma attached to the conventional state hospital. In this setting their illness is treated very much like any other ailment. Patients can either confine themselves to their rooms or socialize with other patients who have physical illnesses.

An increasing number of private hospitals are establishing psychiatric facilities on the same basis. Although the cost is somewhat greater, the patient has the advantage of being in the hospital of his choice, possibly under the continuing care of his own physician, and in a setting of general illness rather than of mental illness only.

3. *Community care.* There is growing support for care of psychiatric

patients within a community. Such a program for community care is based upon the following principles:

> Whenever possible, patients should be kept in their home communities and treated there.
>
> Hospitalization, if required, should be short-term and only for the acute phase of the illness, following which the patient should be returned home with continuing care on an outpatient basis.
>
> Local facilities should be provided for earlier diagnosis and treatment of patients, thus preventing a worsening of the condition and possibly avoiding hospitalization.

Around the country programs built upon such principles are being set up and are proving successful. Some have been organized by local communities; others are outgrowths of state hospital programs in the area. They may provide the following kinds of services:

a. *Emergency treatment.* A number of facilities have been organized to offer prompt emergency treatment for psychiatric patients. They offer a kind of community care. At one such clinic, the Albert Einstein School of Medicine in New York City, the patients are seen the day they apply to the clinic for help. Under the circumstances, it has been found that many patients require no more than a half-dozen psychiatric interviews. Along somewhat narrower lines, suicide-prevention centers have been set up in Los Angeles, Boston, New York City, Miami, and other cities. All these centers offer prompt professional help for individuals who are seriously contemplating suicide.

b. *Part-time service.* Many patients need not be hospitalized around the clock. Day hospitals, night hospitals, and clinics that offer treatment for several hours during the day serve patients who fall into this category. Often such homes, operated for patients discharged from state hospitals, are under the supervision of a social worker or nurse. Halfway houses for narcotic addicts are kinds of part-time hospitals.

c. *After-care service.* A cornerstone in the development of community care for psychiatric patients is the establishment of adequate after-care services to complement the preadmission services already mentioned. The obvious purpose of the follow-up or after-care clinic is to offer to patients who have been successfully treated and discharged from an institution additional treatment in the traditional medical sense. Even small, rudimentary after-care programs have succeeded in cutting the readmission rate to some institutions by as much as 50 percent.

METHODS OF TREATMENT

Many different forms of treatment have been used in psychiatry to help the mentally ill patient. Some of these are administered in an institution; others are carried out by the physician in his office. These forms of treatment may be divided into several main categories.

PSYCHOTHERAPY

In psychotherapy the patient, to achieve better adjustment, talks with a specially qualified person—usually a psychiatrist or clinical psychologist. Psychotherapy may be administered in the therapist's office, an outpatient clinic, a hospital, or a school. The therapist intentionally establishes a professional relationship with the patient with the hope of removing, modifying, or retarding existing symptoms and of promoting positive personality growth and development. Therapy should result in the patient's having a better understanding of himself, enabling him to handle his affairs more effectively.

GROUP THERAPY

Group therapy involves verbal sharing among a group of patients and the therapist. The group functions somewhat like a family and provides the same kinds of opportunities and frustrations. It teaches the individual both to share and to participate. He learns to get back from the group what he puts into it. He has to give love, for example, in order to receive help. Some individuals are able to work out problems in a group that they could not work out in individual psychotherapy.

DRUG THERAPY

The discovery of the ataractic drugs (those that free one from confusion), also known as the major tranquilizers, has been an outstanding therapeutic development in recent years. These drugs have become primary means of treatment in mental hospitals. In fact, their use has stopped the increase in the number of hospitalized patients. Tranquilizing drugs suppress emotional disturbance, make the patient more docile, cooperative, and accessible for psychotherapy. The so-called major tranquilizers have been most effective with the more severely disturbed patients. Milder drugs, known as minor tranquilizers, have been widely used to reduce mild forms of anxiety. Although the milder drugs have fewer undesirable side effects than do the major ones, they have a stronger tendency to become habituating. One of these, meprobamate, has been marketed under the trade names Equanil and Miltown. Their distinct advantage is that they neither interfere with the clarity of consciousness nor cause drowsiness as do the sedatives, such as phenobarbital. Other drugs stimulate depressed patients. Combinations of these are used with some patients.

In some cases, sedative drugs such as phenobarbital are used to combat anxiety, overactivity, and insomnia. Although tranquilizers have cut down on the widespread use of sedative drugs, they have not eliminated the use of sedatives.

ELECTROCONVULSIVE THERAPY

Owing to the discovery of the ataractic and antidepressive drugs, electroconvulsive therapy (ECT) has greatly declined. It is of value for certain types of severe depression, as well as for patients who do not respond well to drugs.

Other forms of physical therapy used in the past, in addition to ECT, include hydrotherapy, massage, and insulin shock therapy. These are rarely, if ever, used today. Insulin shock therapy may be helpful for certain types of disorders that do not respond well to other forms of treatment.

PSYCHOSURGERY

Psychosurgery is used today only when all else fails, and even then reluctantly. A number of techniques have been tried, but the most frequently used is the *lobotomy,* in which nerve tracts between the frontal lobes and the thalamus of the brain are severed. At best it is used for patients whose condition is very poor and in whom any improvement is better than their present condition. Once severed, nerve tracts will never replace themselves in the brain.

PREVENTING MENTAL ILLNESS

COMMUNITY ASSISTANCE

Much more can be done by both individuals and the community as a whole to foster mental health.

Each individual should make a conscious effort to lead a well-balanced life, attempting to understand both himself and others. As a parent, he can provide his children with a balance of loving care and consistent discipline. As a citizen in the community he can give matters of mental health his active support.

Members of the community who come into close contact with people— for example, teachers, social workers, lawyers, public health workers, and housewives—should learn to detect emotional stress in themselves and others. Upon such early detection the individual should be referred to a community clinic or local physician. Mass tests of students in schools can be used to detect certain cases of mental illness before they become acute. Such prevention requires cooperation between voluntary and public agencies on all levels.

NATIONAL ASSISTANCE

Under the Mental Health Act of 1946, a mental health program was set up within the Public Health Service. The act created the National Institute of Mental Health to handle research. It also provided funds for grants to states to create and expand clinics and for schools to expand psychiatric and mental hygiene training. This program accounts for many of the new developments in community mental health services.

In 1963 Congress approved a new National Mental Health Program. It has provided grants-in-aid to states to improve their state programs in mental health. Money has been made available to construct nearly 150 community mental health centers for improved local services. Funds have been appropriated to improve existing hospital programs and to provide in-service training programs for staffs in mental hospitals.

Voluntary organizations continue to play an important role in mental health. These include the American Psychiatric Association and the National Association for Mental Health. Voluntary organizations serve to promote adequate care and treatment for the mentally ill and to improve the training programs for the psychiatric professions.

SUMMARY

I. The normal personality may be described as being well-adjusted, free from idiosyncrasies, and having the following traits:
   A. A relaxed conscience.
   B. A healthy attitude toward life.
   C. An ability to love and understand others.
   D. A reasonable dependence upon others.
   E. Moderation in negative emotions.
   F. An ability to make long-range choices.

II. Mind and Body
   A. Humans function as psycho-physical units consisting of:
      1. Psyche—the mind or psychological aspects.
      2. Soma—the body or physiological aspects.
   B. The mind and body are interrelated so that disorders within one can lead to disorders in the other.
      1. Physical disorders can lead to depression, irritability, or despondency.
      2. Psychological disorders may:
         a. Lead to disorders of any organ of the body.
         b. Arise from some degree of anxiety a person is unable to rid himself of.

III. Emotions begin as the newborn child brings into life innate traits which will develop into complex emotions.
   A. Positive emotions effect a person constructively.
      1. Love.

     2. Faith.
     3. Achievement.
  B. Negative emotions are used as adjustments for unsatisfied emotional needs.
     1. Anger.
     2. Fear.
  C. Mental processes determine the behavior of the organism; for descriptive purposes they may be considered as three subdivisions.
     1. Id processes.
     2. Ego processes.
     3. Superego processes.
  D. Methods for coping with emotional conflict:
     1. Conflicts arise when the *ego* (regulator for possible acts) is under pressure from the *id* (impulses toward pleasurable acts) or is being punished by the *superego* (arbiter of permissible acts).
     2. Conflicts, not easily resolved, may result in anxiety, frustration, and fear.
     3. Defense mechanisms may be unconsciously used when the ego is having difficulty coping with emotional conflicts.
       a. Rationalization.
       b. Substitution.
       c. Regression.
       d. Projection.
       e. Repression.
       f. Identification.
       g. Fantasy and daydreaming.

IV. Emotional Dysorganization
  A. Results from the inability of the ego processes to maintain normal control of emotional matters.
  B. Is commonly called mental (emotional) illness.
  C. Has levels representing varying degrees of relative emotional adjustment or of mental illness.
     1. First level of dysorganization—mild neurosis.
     2. Second level of dysorganization—sometimes described as neurosis, psychoneurosis, or hysteria.
     3. Third level of dysorganization—open aggression.
     4. Fourth level of dysorganization—loss of contact with and loyalty toward the real world.
     5. Fifth level of dysorganization—the *penultimate,* the last step before destruction.

V. Scope of the Problem of Mental Illness
  A. Prevalence of mental illness. When mild states of emotional dysorganization, such as anxiety, are included, everyone is mentally ill at some time in his life.
  B. Professional workers with the mentally ill are:
     1. Psychiatrist.
     2. Clinical psychologist.
     3. Psychiatric social worker.
     4. Psychiatric technician.
  C. Clinical facilities include:
     1. State hospitals.
     2. Psychiatric sections of general hospitals.
     3. Community care—provides psychiatric care in the local community.

    a. Emergency treatment—providing community care for emergencies such as attempted suicide or other acute conditions.

    b. Part-time service—clinics offering facilities during the day or night for recently discharged patients (from hospitals) or those not hospitalized full time.

    c. After-care service—a kind of service for the care of patients after their release from an institution (acute care).

D. Methods of treatment

  1. Psychotherapy—effective conversation between the patient and a specially qualified person, in order to achieve a better adjustment with the patient.

  2. Group therapy—verbal sharing between a group of patients and one or more therapists.

  3. Drug therapy—drugs used to combat anxiety, overactivity, and insomnia.

  4. Electroconvulsive therapy—used for patients with severe depression or those not affected by drugs.

  5. Psychosurgery—rarely used, but if used, a last resort in which certain nerve tracts are severed.

E. Preventing mental illness can be accomplished through:

  1. Community assistance

    a. Individuals and families can help by striving for good balance in personal attitudes and family life.

    b. People of the community can learn to detect emotional stress in themselves and others and refer such individuals to physicians or local clinics.

  2. National assistance

    a. National Institute of Mental Health provides funds for research, clinics, and psychiatric training.

    b. National voluntary organizations.

Glossary

If you cannot find the word you wish in this glossary, check the index for text and glossary references.

addiction (ə dik'shən) (L. *addictio,* to give over or surrender). The state of being given over to some habit, creating a physical dependency and often a psychological dependency as well.

aggression (ə gresh'ən) (L. *ad-,* to; *gradi,* to step). A forceful, attacking action, either physical, verbal, or symbolic. It may be realistic and self-protective or unrealistic and unprovoked. It may be directed outward to other things or directed inward to oneself.

amnesia (am nē'zhə) (G. *amnesia,* forgetfulness). A loss of memory due to brain injury, disease, shock, or repression.

ataractic drugs (at ə rak'tik) (G. *a,* not; *taraktos,* disturbed). A group of drugs used to decrease anxiety. Essentially the same as tranquilizers.

autism (aw'tizm) (G. *autos,* self; *ismos,* state of). A form of thinking which gratifies unfulfilled desires without regard to reality; a form of fantasy thinking.

compulsion (kəm pul'shən) (L. *compellere, compulsum,* to drive, to compel).

An insistent, irresistible urge to perform an act which is contrary to a person's ordinary conscious wishes or standards.

continuum (kən tin'yoo əm) (L. *continuus,* continuous). A series in which the discrete parts are united by a common character.

convulsion (kən vul'shən) (L. *convellere,* to tear up, to shake). A violent involuntary contraction or series of contractions of the voluntary muscles.

delirium (di lēr' ē əm) (L. *de-,* from; *lira,* furrow or track, thus, "off the track"). A temporary mental state characterized by confusion, disorientation, and illusions.

dementia (di men'shə, di men'shē ə) (L. *de-,* from; *mens,* mind). An old term denoting madness or insanity; now used to denote organic loss of intellectual functioning.

depression (di presh'ən) (L. *de-,* down; *premere,* to press). In psychology a morbid sadness, dejection, or melancholy.

dysorganization (dis or gə ni zā'shən) (G. *dys,* difficult or painful; G. *organon,* instrument for work). A state of impaired and inefficient emotional organization resulting from a person's inability to cope with internal conflicts and external reality.

ego processes (ē'gō pros'es əz) (L. *ego,* I; *pro-,* forward; *cedere,* to go). According to Freudian theory, one of the three major divisions of the psychic apparatus, which consciously acts as mediator for the impulses of the id, the prohibitions of the superego, and the demands of reality.

fetish (fet'ish) (L. *facticius,* artificial). A material object—natural (such as a foot or other part of the body) or artificial (such as an article of clothing)— which is symbolically endowed with special meaning; sometimes necessary for the completion of the sexual act.

hallucination (hə loo si nā'shən) (L. *hallucinatio,* to wander mentally). A false perception of sounds, sights, etc., that are not actually present; may occur in any of the senses.

homosexual (hō'mō sek'shoo əl) (G. *homos,* same; L. *sexualis,* sexual). Sexual attraction or relationship between members of the same sex.

hyperalert (hī'pər ə lurt') (G. *hyper,* above; It. *all' er ta,* on the lookout). Abnormally and excessively watchful of activities around oneself.

hypochondriasis (hī'pō kən drī'ə sis) (G. *hypo,* under; *chondros,* cartilage). Persistent overconcern with the state of one's health, accompanied by various body pains without evidence of disease. It is so called because the area of the abdomen called the hypochondrium was once thought to be the seat of the disorder.

hypomania (hī'pō mā'nē ə) (G. *hypo,* under; *mania,* madness). A mild form of manic activity. (Manic behavior is characterized by unusual motor activity, elation, and general overreaction to stimuli.)

id processes (id pros'es əz) (L. *id,* it; *pro-,* forward; *cedere,* to go). According to Freudian theory, one of the three main divisions of the psychic apparatus; the id harbors the unconscious instinctive desires and strivings of the person.

impulse (im'puls) (L. *in,* on; *pellere,* to drive). A psychic striving to act; usually referring to an instinctive urge.

instinct (in'stingkt) (L. *in,* on; *stinguere,* to prick). An inborn drive which includes self-preservation, sexuality, aggression, and certain social patterns.

lobotomy (lə bot'ə mē) (G. *lobos,* lobe; *temnein,* to cut). Incision, or cutting, into a lobe of the brain, severing all the fibers connecting that lobe to the rest of the brain.

mania (mā'nē ə) (G. *mania*, madness).   A mental disorder characterized by a preoccupation with some desire, idea, or activity; a morbid compulsion.

masochism (mas'ə kizm) (named after Sacher-Masoch, 1835–1895).   Sexual perversion in which one finds pleasure in receiving physical or psychological pain.

melancholia (mel ən kō'lē ə) (G. *melas*, black; *chole*, bile; *-ia*, condition). Severe depression with inhibition of mental and bodily activity.

narcissism (nahr'si sizm) (from Narcissus, a character in Greek mythology who fell in love with his own image reflected in the water).   Self-love rather than love of another person.

neurosis (no͞o rō'sis) (G. *neuron*, nerve; *-osis*, a process).   A psychic disorder due to unresolved unconscious conflicts; sometimes considered a major category of emotional illness. Also called *psychoneurosis*.

obsession (əb sesh'ən) (L. *obsessio*, obsession).   A persistent, unwanted idea or impulse that cannot be eliminated by logic or reasoning.

pedophilia (pē'də fil'ē ə, ped'ə fil'ē ə) (G. *pais, paidios*, child; *philein*, to love). A morbid interest in children, often expressed in sexual behavior.

phobia (fō'bē ə) (G. *phobos*, fear).   A persistent, unrealistic fear of an external object or situation.

pseudocyesis (so͞o'dō sī ē'sis) (G. *pseudes*, false; *kyesis*, pregnancy).   A false pregnancy.

psyche (sī'kē) (G. *psyche*, soul).   The mind; the mental life, including both conscious and unconscious processes.

psychiatry (sī kī'ə trē) (*psych-; iatreia*, healing).   That branch of medicine which deals with disorders of the mind.

psychiatrist (sī kī'ə trist). A physician trained in psychiatry.

psychoanalysis (sī'kō ə nal'i sis) (G. *psyche*, soul; *ana-*, backward; *lysis*, dissolution).   A psychological theory of human development and behavior that dreams, emotions, and behavior can be traced to the repressed instinctual drives of the id and the defenses of the ego against them.

psychologist, clinical (sī kol'ə jist, klin'i kal) (G. *psycho-; logos*, reason; *klinikos*, pertaining to a bed).   A psychologist with a graduate degree (usually a Ph.D.) who specializes in research, diagnosis, and psychotherapy in the field of emotional disorders.

psychosis (sī kō'sis) (G. *psych-; -osis*, a process).   A major mental disorder of organic or emotional (functional) origin in which there is a departure from normal thinking, feeling, and acting; commonly characterized by loss of contact with reality, lessened control over impulses, and distortion of perception.

psychosomatic (sīkō sə mat'ik) (G. *psycho-; soma*, body).   Pertaining to the interaction of the mind and the body.

psychosurgery (sī'kō sur'jə rē) (G. *psycho-*; L. *chirurgia*, from G. *cheir*, hand; *ergon*, work).   Brain surgery for the treatment of psychiatric disorders by removal or interruption of certain nerve pathways.

psychotherapy (sī'kō ther'ə pē) (G. *psycho-; therapeia*, to nurse).   Any type of treatment based primarily upon verbal or nonverbal communication with the patient, in contrast to other forms of treatment, such as the use of drugs.

sadism (sā'dizm) (named after Marquis de Sade, 1740–1814).   Sexual perversion in which pleasure is derived from inflicting physical or psychological pain on others.

schizoid (skit′soid, skiz′oid) (G. *schizein*, to divide; *oeides*, like, in the form of). Describing traits of shyness, introspection, and introversion.

schizophrenia (skit′sə frē′nē ə, skiz′ə frē′nē ə) (G. *schizein*, to split; *phren*, mind). A severe emotional disorder often characterized by a retreat from reality accompanied by delusions, hallucinations, regression, and emotional disharmony. Once called *dementia praecox*.

soma (sō′mə) (G. *soma*, body).   The body as distinguished from the mind.

superego processes (soo′pər ē′gō pros′es əz) (L. *super*, above; *ego*, I; *pro-*, forward; *cedere*, to go).   According to the Freudian theory, one of the three main divisions of the psychic apparatus, associated with ethics, standards, and self-criticism; these standards help form the conscience.

syndrome (sin′drōm) (G. *syndrome*, concurrence).   A group of symptoms which occur together and whose occurrence indicates a recognizable illness.

unconscious (un kon′shəs) (AS. *un-*, not; L. *conscius*, aware).   In psychological theory, that part of the mind which is only rarely subject to awareness; it includes data which was never conscious or was once conscious but has been repressed.

voyeurism (vwah yur′iz əm, voi yur′iz əm) (Fr. *voir*, to see; G. *ismos*, the act). A compulsive, often sexually motivated, interest in watching or looking at the genitals and/or sexual behavior of others; roughly the same as a "peeping Tom."

CHAPTER 3

STRUCTURE AND DISORDERS OF THE NERVOUS SYSTEM

STRUCTURE OF THE
NERVOUS SYSTEM

THE EYE

THE EAR

SIGNS AND SYMPTOMS
OF NEUROLOGICAL
IMPAIRMENT

KINDS OF NEUROLOGICAL
DISORDERS

SUMMARY

In Chapter 2 we examined the problems that can arise from emotional conflict. The various levels of emotional dysfunction described there seem to have no definite organic basis, although prolonged or severe emotional conflict can certainly affect the body. Such emotional disorders are spoken of as *functional* by psychologists.

In this chapter we will examine the nervous system, including the sensory apparatus which *receives* stimuli, the nerves and central nervous system which *transmit* nervous impulses, and the *effectors* which convert impulses into action. Impairment or disorders of this system are *organic;* not only the functions but the structures of the organism are damaged. However, organic damage to the nervous system can produce symptoms of mental illness very much like those discussed earlier so that, once again, we see that mind and body act as a unit and that mental health is dependent on both.

STRUCTURE OF THE NERVOUS SYSTEM

As dynamic living organisms, humans are continuously carrying on physical activities—transforming food into energy, metabolizing stored food into available energy, maintaining respiration, balancing themselves against gravity, or recoiling from pain. All these activities are under the continuous control and coordination of the nervous system. The over 12 billion nerve cells, or *neurons,* which make up the human nervous system are organized into brain, spinal cord, nerve tracts, and sense organs. The work of this system has been appropriately compared to that done by an electronic computer—but far more efficient and concise than any man-made computer yet developed.

The nervous system in general is divided into *central* and *peripheral* portions. The central nervous system consists of the *brain* and the *spinal cord.* The peripheral nervous system consists of *cranial nerves* that carry messages to and from the brain and *spinal nerves* that carry impulses to and from the spinal cord. Certain peripheral nerves that control specific internal functions are further grouped as the *autonomic nervous system.*

There are also the highly developed and important structures called the *sense organs.* These organs receive messages or sensations from outside or from within the person. Some of these organs, such as the eye, ear, nose, and tongue, are able to receive special kinds of stimuli which are then transmitted to the brain. Others (e.g., the skin) are more generalized. In this chapter two special sense organs, the *eye* and the *ear,* will be described.

THE NEURON

The most important part of the entire nervous system is the neuron. Neurons are the most specialized cells of the body. Like other cells the neuron has a *nucleus* located within the *cell body* (Fig. 3.1). If this nucleus is destroyed, the nerve cell dies and is never restored. The neuron also has fibers that extend out from the cell body. Those nerve fibers which carry impulses from sense organs and other neurons to the cell body are called *dendrites;* those which transmit impulses from the cell body to other neurons or effectors are called *axons.* The axon of one neuron leads to the dendrite of the next. The junction between nerve cells is called a *synapse.*

Nerve fibers often run parallel to each other. Some individual fibers are several feet long. A bundle of them is called a *nerve.* It has been estimated that a nerve an inch in diameter contains approximately 25,000 fibers. When a nerve is severed, therefore, a great many nerve fibers may be broken. Damage to the nerve fibers of the nervous system can be serious and, temporarily or permanently, will probably disrupt communication to and control of some portion of the body. However, if the cell body is not destroyed, a neuron can gradually regenerate some new fibers.

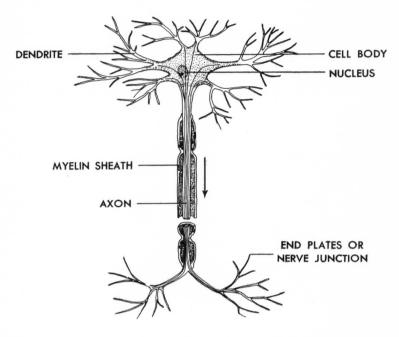

Fig. 3.1 Typical neuron. Arrow indicates the direction of nerve impulses in the cell.

THE CENTRAL NERVOUS SYSTEM

The brain consists of three divisions—the *cerebrum,* the *cerebellum,* and the *brain stem* (Figs. 3.2 and 3.3).

The largest part of the brain is the cerebrum, which is divided into two *cerebral hemispheres,* a right and a left. These two halves are connected by tracts of nerve fibers. The surface, or *cortex* (Fig. 3.4), of the cerebrum is composed of *gray matter,* which in turn is made up of millions of neurons. The cortex of each of these hemispheres is divided into four lobes—*frontal, parietal, temporal,* and *occipital* (Fig. 3.2). In studying these cerebral lobes, *neurologists* have been able to locate areas of the cortex which are responsible for certain body functions— such as vision control, speech, hearing, motor activity, and other sense perceptions. Internally the cerebral hemispheres are made up largely of *white matter*. This white matter surrounds a few islands of gray matter called *basal ganglia*, nerve cell groups located at the base of each cerebral hemisphere which regulate motor impulses that arise in the cerebral cortex and are transmitted to various parts of the body.

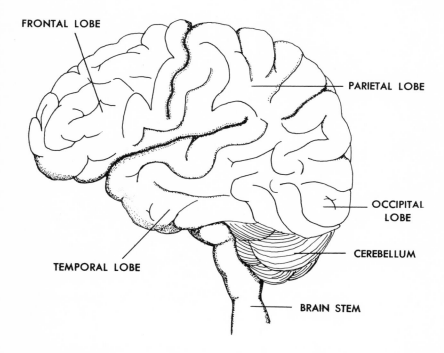

Fig. 3.2 Diagram of the divisions of the brain and the lobes of the cerebral hemisphere (lateral view).

Inside the hemispheres are several cavities filled with *cerebrospinal fluid* (Fig. 3.3). The functions of the cerebrum include control of the voluntary muscles, the interpreting of impulses from the sensory organs, and the control of learned behavior. The cerebrum serves as the center for all intellectual and rational activities.

The *cerebellum* is located below the back or hind portion of the cerebrum; it has the function of coordinating motor impulses between the cerebrum and other parts of the body and helping to maintain body balance and muscle tone. The surfaces of the cerebrum and cerebellum are extensively wrinkled and folded into ridges. These wrinkles and folds allow for a maximum amount of surface area without increasing the brain's total size.

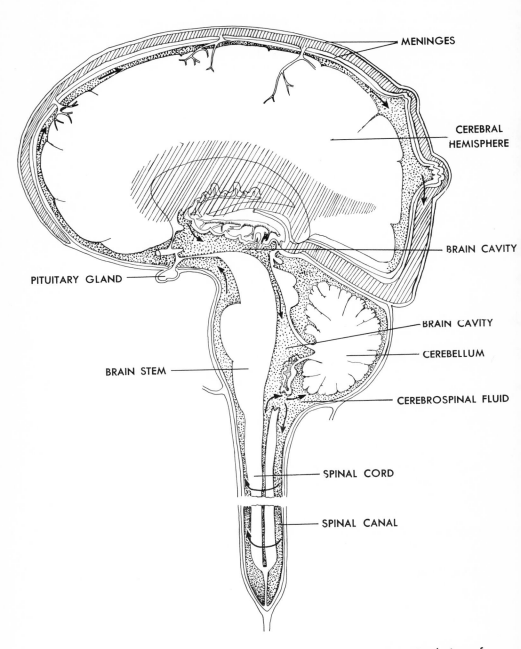

Fig. 3.3 Midsection of the brain and the spinal cord showing circulation of the cerebrospinal fluid. Arrows indicate the direction of the circulation.

The *brain stem* may be thought of as the core of the brain, surrounded by the cerebrum and cerebellum. It contains many nerve tracts for the transmission of impulses and nerve centers for controlling respiration, heartbeat, blood pressure, digestion, and body temperature.

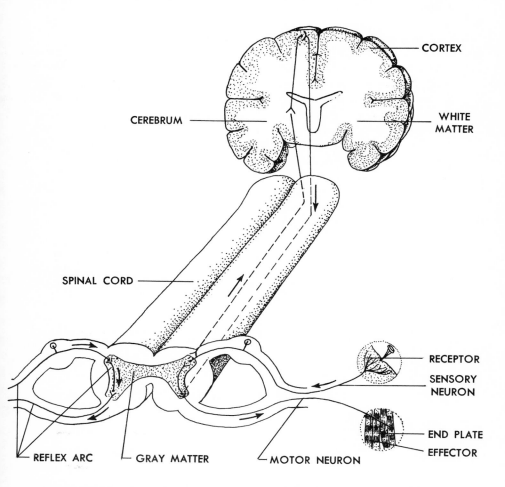

Fig. 3.4 Diagram showing nerve pathways. Shown are impulses passing through a reflex arc. Note impulses passing from a receptor along a sensory neuron to the brain and returning along a motor neuron to a muscle.

Although human brains vary to some extent, they are more highly developed than the brains of lower animals. In particular, the human cerebrum shows the highest level of development of any living thing; it is responsible for man's ability to learn and to reason.

The spinal cord occupies the *spinal canal* inside the *vertebral column* (Fig. 3.3). This cord serves as a main line connecting the brain and the spinal nerves. In cross section the spinal cord can be seen as made up of a large center section of gray matter and an outer sheath of white matter (Fig. 3.4).

THE PERIPHERAL NERVOUS SYSTEM

The peripheral nervous system (Fig. 3.5) is made up of nerves which relate the central nervous system to all other parts of the body. The various cranial and spinal nerves occur in pairs. The cranial nerves transmit impulses which control functions such as speech, smell, vision, eye motion, hearing, and equilibrium. The cranial nerves relay impulses between the brain stem and the organs of the head and neck. The spinal nerves transmit impulses between the spinal cord and the skin and muscle areas that are below the level of the brain.

An impulse from a special sense organ travels over a neural pathway, or circuit. A simple example of a neural pathway is the *reflex arc* (Fig. 3.4). A reflex arc involves two or more neurons and some other organs. It includes (1) a *receptor,* a specialized ending of a sensory nerve fiber associated with a special sense organ; (2) a *sensory neuron* which carries the impulse to the spinal cord; (3) a *motor neuron* which carries the impulse from the spinal cord to an effector organ; (4) *end plates* at the endings of the motor nerve; and (5) an *effector,* such as a muscle or a gland, that carries out the response. All of this action happens while an impulse goes to the brain. The physician often uses this reaction to test the condition of certain nerve tracts. For instance, by tapping the knee area, he can test the nerves between the knee and the spinal cord.

THE AUTONOMIC NERVOUS SYSTEM

The autonomic nervous system (Fig. 3.5) is responsible for those body functions which are generally self-regulating. Activities such as heartbeat, respiration, digestion, endocrine secretion, and bowel elimination are maintained by this system. The autonomic nerves come from nerve centers which extend down the brain stem, inside the body, and along the spinal cord. Although the cranial and spinal nerves generally account for conscious activities, and the autonomic nerves for unconscious activities, this specialization is not true in all cases; there is some mixing of functions.

There are two parts to the autonomic system which act in contrast to each other, the *sympathetic* and the *parasympathetic* divisions. An example of their functions can be observed in the actions of the eye and the salivary glands. The sympathetic nerves dilate the eye, and the

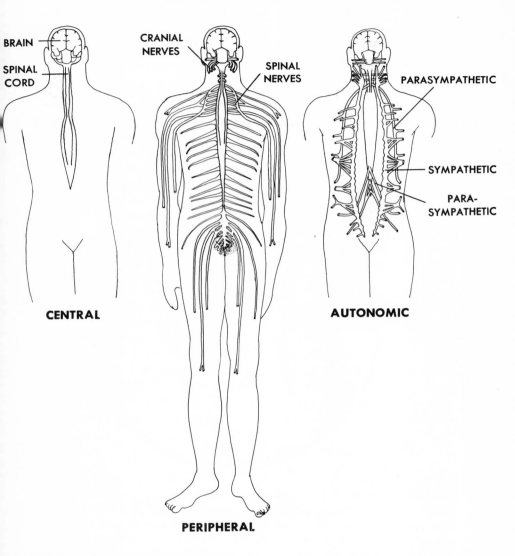

Fig. 3.5 Nervous systems of the body.

parasympathetic nerves constrict it. The salivary glands are relaxed by the sympathetic nerves but contracted by the parasympathetic. Generally, the sympathetic nerves stimulate and increase activities, and the parasympathetic nerves restore and conserve energy.

THE EYE

STRUCTURE OF THE EYE

The eye (Fig. 3.6) is a complex organ about an inch in diameter and
nearly spherical in shape. Its essential features are a lens mechanism
formed by the curved transparent front of the eye, the *cornea,* and a

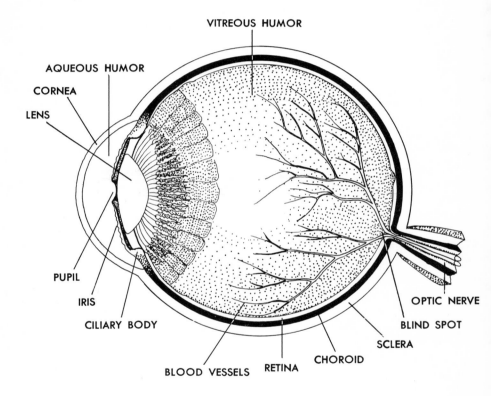

Fig. 3.6 Structure of the eye.

crystalline lens inside. The lens, together with the cornea, focuses an
image on the light-sensitive back wall of the eye, the *retina.* The cavity
between the cornea and the lens contains a watery fluid, *aqueous humor;*
and the cavity between the lens and the retina contains a jelly-like
material called *vitreous humor.*

The wall of the eyeball is made up of three layers of tissue. The outermost layer, called the *sclera,* is a strong, fibrous connective tissue; it is commonly spoken of as the white of the eye. The anterior, or front portion of the sclera, is the transparent cornea.

The middle layer, the *choroid,* lines the inner surface of the sclera and is composed almost entirely of blood vessels which supply the outer layers of the retina. As the choroid extends forward and nears the lens, it merges into a structure known as the *ciliary body.* This body is composed of some muscle, which surrounds and contracts the lens, and some epithelium, which produces the aqueous humor. The ciliary body also extends forward over the front edges of the lens to become the *iris.* The iris is pigmented with *melanin,* thus giving color to the eye. The iris consists of blood vessels, and smooth muscles which are responsible for dilating and constricting the *pupil,* the round opening in the center of the iris. The pupil, which appears black, acts as an adjustable light diaphragm.

The innermost layer of the eye, the *retina,* is light-sensitive and contains photoreceptors. It is composed of a layer of pigmented cells and three layers of neurons. The pigmented cells are those farthest from the lens, next to the choroid layer. In front of the pigmented cells is a layer of receptor cells. Light entering the eye travels to the back of the retina and then reflects out to the receptor neurons. There are two types of receptor neurons, *rods* and *cones,* so named because of their shape. The rods perceive achromatic colors (white, black, and gray) and the cones perceive both achromatic and chromatic color (red, green, etc.). The area of the retina directly back of the lens, the *fovea,* contains only cones. This area is the most active during daylight vision. Outside the fovea are both rods and cones. The rods are most active in adaptation of the eye to darkness. Impulses from the photoreceptors are transmitted to one side of the back of the eye and out the *optic nerve,* which leads away from the eye to the brain. Since there are no photoreceptors at the point where the optic nerve joins the eye, there is a so-called *blind spot* there.

Nature has provided the eye with various structures to protect it from injury or infection. The eye is set in a bony socket, which surrounds and protects it. At the anterior end of the socket the eye is protected by eyelids, which are fringed with protective hairs, the eyelashes. Lining the eyelid and covering the exposed surface of the eyeball is a delicate membrane, the *conjunctiva.* The conjunctiva is kept moist by secretions of the *tear glands (lacrimal glands).* The tear fluid given off by these glands not only washes away foreign particles, but also kills bacteria. Normally just enough tear fluid is secreted to keep a thin film of moisture over the exposed portion of the eye, but when excess fluid is given off, it ordinarily drains into lacrimal ducts, which discharge into the nasal cavity.

DISORDERS OF THE EYE

The good health of the eyes is of incalculable importance. Accordingly, any structural defects, injuries, or diseases which limit or affect the usefulness of the eyes should be given proper medical care. Following are some of the conditions which may affect the eye and reduce its usefulness.

REFRACTIVE DEFECTS

In refractive defects images are focused improperly on the retina (see Fig. 3.7). The most common are myopia (nearsightedness), hyperopia (farsightedness), presbyopia (decreased accommodation as a result of aging), and astigmatism (defective curvature of the cornea).

1. *Myopia.* This is a defect of development that results in an eyeball which is too long, so that usually images are being incorrectly focused in front of the retina. Objects that are far away appear blurred; those nearby are clear. This condition is corrected by the use of concave lenses ground thick at the edges and thin at the center, which throws the point of focus back so that it strikes the retina correctly.

2. *Hyperopia.* This condition occurs when the eyeball is too short or the lens of the cornea is flattened. It causes light rays to come to focus behind the retina. As a result the eye cannot focus properly on nearby objects. The ciliary muscles may be able to compensate by thickening the lens; however, this compensation can be a source of eyestrain. To correct this condition, a convex lens which is thin at the edges and thick in the center is used. The eyes of a person wearing convex lenses may appear larger than their actual size.

3. *Presbyopia.* This disorder is caused by a loss of elasticity of the lens. As a result distant objects are clearly seen, but close objects are blurred. This condition develops as a person grows older. It too can be corrected with prescribed lenses.

4. *Astigmatism.* Because of an irregularity in the curvature of the cornea or the lens, these surfaces do not refract the light uniformly. As a result vision is blurred or distorted to some degree, and the eyes are strained. Astigmatism can be corrected with lenses which are ground to compensate for the distortion.

COLOR BLINDNESS

Color blindness is a hereditary, sex-linked condition, appearing almost entirely in the male. Several recognized types are red blindness, green blindness, violet blindness, red-green blindness, red-violet blindness green-violet blindness, and red-green-violet blindness. The last type is

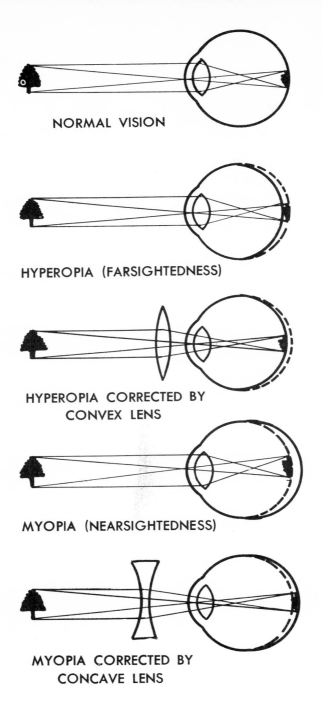

NORMAL VISION

HYPEROPIA (FARSIGHTEDNESS)

HYPEROPIA CORRECTED BY
CONVEX LENS

MYOPIA (NEARSIGHTEDNESS)

MYOPIA CORRECTED BY
CONCAVE LENS

Fig. 3.7 Normal and defective focusing. In the normal eye light is focused exactly on the retina. In the farsighted (hyperopic) eye light focuses behind the retina until corrected by a convex glass lens. In the near-sighted (myopic) eye light focuses in front of the retina until corrected by a concave glass lens.

achromatic, or total, color blindness, and a person having this type sees objects as black, gray, or white. The most common type is red-green blindness, and the least common is total color blindness.

Since there is no way to prevent or correct color blindness, the individuals who inherit this kind of abnormality must learn to contend with it. Yet this condition need not limit their usefulness. Most color-blind people are able to detect some subtle differences between the shades they perceive normally and those they perceive abnormally. Some color-blind people have been successful in fields where color detection is important, such as in medicine. There is usually no other physical abnormality connected with this condition.

DISEASES AND INFLAMMATIONS

Despite all the protection given to the eyes, they are usually open to irritation and infection. The following infections are some of the most common:

1. *Conjunctivitis.* Conjunctivitis is an inflammation of the conjunctiva. The blood vessels become engorged and usually visible, giving the eye a bloodshot appearance. Newborn babies may develop it because of infections they have picked up in their passage through the birth canal. This condition can be controlled by treatment with antibiotics or other solutions.

2. *Cataracts.* Cataract is one of the common causes of blindness. Occurring principally in older people, it is the development of a cloudiness or opacity of the lens which reduces its normal transparency. When a cataract obscures light transmission so greatly that it seriously impairs vision, the condition may have to be corrected by the surgical removal of the entire lens, causing the eye to lose some of its refractive power. This power can be replaced, however, through the use of powerful convex lenses.

3. *Glaucoma.* Glaucoma is the most common cause of blindness. This condition is characterized by an excessive *intraocular* pressure. Aqueous humor is constantly produced from the blood, circulated through the eye, and reabsorbed into the blood stream. If the outflow of aqueous humor is reduced, it cannot escape from the eye rapidly enough, and thus the fluid pressure inside the eye begins to rise. As the pressure rises, the contents of the eye compress backwards against the retina and, in particular, against the optic nerve. As a result the cells of the optic nerve atrophy and are destroyed, causing permanent blindness.

Symptoms of glaucoma include headaches, loss of peripheral vision, need for frequent changes of glasses (particularly in older people), and the seeing of halos around lights. Some forms of the disease progress very rapidly; others develop slowly. Early diagnosis is essential. The malady can often be effectively treated through surgery or the administration of drugs.

Public clinics are sometimes conducted in some areas to test for excessive inner eye pressure. Testing is done painlessly with an instrument called a *tonometer,* which is placed over the surface of the eye. Everyone over the age of 30 should have this test performed by an ophthalmologist. After the age of 40, he should have this test every two years at least; it is a part of every complete eye examination given by an ophthalmologist to people of this age.

CARE OF THE EYES

We have seen how complicated the eye is and the kinds of disorders to which it is subjected. Because the eye is so essential to a person, it should be given the best of professional care. Various professional services are available for the care of the eyes. A physician who specializes in treating diseases, and defects of the eye, as well as injuries to it, is an *ophthalmologist.* He is a physician who is trained to examine the eyes and prescribe lenses, to prescribe medication, to give treatment, and to perform eye surgery. An *optometrist* is trained to examine the eyes for refractive errors and to prescribe appropriate lenses. He is not a physician, and thus is neither trained nor permitted to perform eye surgery or prescribe drugs for the eye. An *optician* is trained to grind lenses and mount them in frames to conform to the face of the patient.

CONTACT LENSES

Lenses that are placed directly on the front of the eyeball under the eyelid have been used for a long time by those in the performing arts and in contact sports. Recent improvements in their construction have increased their popularity. Today they are made of lightweight plastic and are unbreakable. They are small and virtually invisible to other people.

Certain types of visual defects can be corrected satisfactorily with contact lenses; others cannot. They are more suited to the eyes of some people than others. Although they may be desirable for the sake of appearance, they do have drawbacks. They must be placed in the eye and taken out. They can be easily lost. The length of time a person may wear them varies with the sensitivity of his eye to them. Some people find them too irritating to wear at all. Sometimes their cost is excessive.

Contact lenses should be purchased only upon the recommendation of a qualified eye specialist. He will be able to do an exact fitting and to carefully observe the eye afterwards to check its sensitivity to them.

Since he writes a prescription for an oculist to fill, he does not profit from their sale.

SUNGLASSES

Light glare striking the eye can produce eyestrain. Sunglasses can help in producing eye comfort. Although they come in many styles and shapes, most sunglasses can be considered safe for wear. Sunglasses purchased without prescription should be checked first for optical flaws that may create eyestrain. The prices of sunglasses will vary from very cheap to very expensive. It is wise to pay a little more for a good pair of sunglasses that can give the eye the greatest comfort. A person who normally wears prescription lenses should either have sunglasses ground to his prescription or have the type that clip on to his normal glasses. Many sunglasses interfere with color perception. It is not advisable to wear them indoors or on a cloudy day. Sunglasses should never be worn for nighttime driving or for looking directly at the sun.

EYE EXERCISES

Although much has been said by some people in the past concerning the value of eye exercises, they may be of no value unless the patient has muscular imbalance. They are of no value in restoring diseased eyes or in changing the proportions of the eyeball. If such exercises are needed, they should be prescribed by an eye specialist.

EYE IRRITANTS AND INJURIES

The eye is vulnerable to foreign objects and injury. Stray objects that get into the eye, such as dirt, should always be carefully removed. Debris that becomes embedded in the eye should be removed only by a physician.

Many women today use various cosmetic products to enhance the appearance of the eye. Some of these may cause irritation to the edge of the conjunctiva at the edge of the eyelid, as well as irritating the skin. Hairsprays that get into the eye can cause irritation of the eyeball. Anything that causes irritation to the eye should be discontinued.

Eyedrops or eyewashes meant to clear the appearance of the white of the eye, reduce soreness, or clean the eye of dust should be used only upon the recommendation of a physician. The eye is sensitive and such washes may damage the eye.

Eye injury is frequently caused by flying objects or sharp instruments and toys. Anyone working near a grinding wheel or other type of high-speed machine or with caustic or explosive chemicals should wear protective goggles made of safety glass. Children should be advised concerning the correct handling of scissors and sharp-edged toys.

PROPER LIGHTING

Improper lighting while a person is reading or watching television, although not a cause of blindness, may create eye fatigue. Good reading light should be bright enough, evenly distributed, and without glare. Television viewing should properly be done in a partially lighted room to avoid undue eye fatigue.

THE EAR

STRUCTURE OF THE EAR

The ear is a combination sense organ related to both hearing and equilibrium. Structurally it may be divided into three parts: *external ear,* which includes the outer projection and a canal; *middle ear,* which is an air space containing three small bones; and *internal ear,* the most important part, which contains the sensory receptors for hearing and equilibrium (see Fig. 3.8).

The external ear is composed of the *auricle* (ear) and the *external auditory canal.* Together these two structures assist in picking up sound and directing it toward an opening in the skull. At the end of this auditory canal is the *tympanic membrane* (eardrum), which serves as a physical barrier between the external auditory canal and the middle ear cavity. The tympanic membrane is a taut, thin membrane which vibrates in response to intercepted sounds.

The middle ear contains three small bones (*ossicles*) for the transmission of sound to the internal ear. The three small bones within this cavity—the *malleus,* the *incus,* and the *stapes* (Latin for "hammer," "anvil," and "stirrup," and commonly called by the English names)— are united by joints to form a lever system that amplifies vibrations picked up from the tympanic membrane many times over and transfers them to a membrane, the *oval window,* of the internal ear. Air is brought into the middle ear cavity through the *eustachian tube.* This tube connects the lower part of the middle ear cavity with the *pharynx,* and has the function of keeping the air pressure on the inside of the eardrum equal to that on the outside. When air pressure changes rapidly, as in going through a tunnel or up in an airplane, the person may yawn or swallow. This allows the pressure in the middle ear to be equalized by way of the eustachian tube. The mucous membrane which is continuous from the pharynx through the eustachian tube and into the middle ear cavity is susceptible to infections, particularly in children. At the back of this cavity is an opening into the *mastoid air cells,* spaces inside a portion of the temporal bone of the skull.

The internal ear is the area of sensory reception for hearing and equilibrium. It contains the *cochlea* for hearing, and the *semicircular canals* and several other structures for the sense of balance and position.

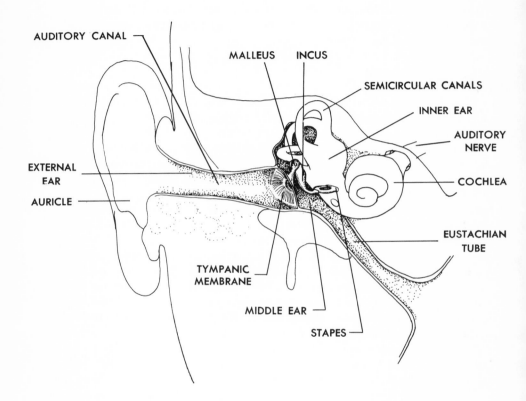

Fig. 3.8 Structure of the ear.

The cochlea is a coiled duct filled with fluid; one portion of the cochlea, the *organ of Corti,* has over 15,000 hair cells that receive sound. As the fluid within the cochlea is set in motion, it stimulates the hair cells, which transmit impulses to the *auditory nerve* which, in turn, sends them on to the cerebrum. Generally a young person can detect sounds with frequencies as low as 30 cycles per second and as high as 20,000 cycles per second.

DISORDERS OF THE EAR

Hearing is one of the special senses necessary for maintaining accurate contact with the outside world. The ear is very sensitive and can be easily injured. Although embedded within the skull, it is exposed to the outside through both the external ear canal and the eustachian tube. If its ability to conduct and perceive sound is impaired, partial or complete loss of hearing may result. One of the major causes of impaired hearing is infection.

INFECTIONS

Infections can occur rather easily in the middle ear. These may result from boils or pimples in the outer ear that have been improperly treated. They may arise from infections of the throat or nose that have traveled through the eustachian tube, or they may be caused by bacteria and viruses which have come from some general body infection, such as influenza, measles, or scarlet fever.

Inflammation in the middle ear may affect the structures used for the transmission of sound, and thus reduce hearing. The inflammation may also move to the mastoid cells, causing *mastoiditis,* with the possibility of spreading through the skull and infecting the brain.

Damage from infections can often be prevented by obtaining prompt treatment from a physician. Antibiotics are effective against most of them. Infections can sometimes be prevented by not tampering with boils or pimples in the outer ear, by keeping the ear free from wax, by keeping objects out of the ear canal, and by being careful not to blow the nose so hard that infectious material might be forced up the eustachian tube into the middle ear.

DEAFNESS

Anything that interferes with the transmission of sound waves or their interpretation may be responsible for loss of hearing. There are two basic types of hearing loss—the conductive and the perceptive types. *Conductive deafness* occurs because there is some kind of interference with the passage of sound through the outer and middle ear. This loss of hearing is greatest in the lower and middle range of the hearing scale. It can be caused by obstruction of the external ear canal, destruction or damage to the ear drum, inflammation of the middle ear resulting in swelling and abscesses, or *otosclerosis,* an immobilizing of the stapes of the middle ear or impairment of the auditory nerve. If a person is aware of persistent "fullness" in the ears, buzzing or ringing sounds, or dullness in hearing, it would be wise to see an otologist, a physician who specializes in ear disorders. He will be able to determine whether there is an actual hearing loss; diagnose the condition; and, if possible, perform the necessary treatment.

Perceptive deafness is caused by damage to the sensory cells of the cochlea or of the auditory nerve. Loss of hearing with this type of deafness is greatest at the higher range of the hearing scale. This form of deafness has numerous causes and is very common among older people. It may be the result of prolonged exposure to loud noises, as in industrial plants, or to viral or bacterial infections of mumps, scarlet fever, or measles. Injuries, such as blows to the head, or the effects of certain drugs, such as excessive dosages of aspirin, quinine, or some of the antibiotics, may also lead to perceptive deafness.

AIDS TO HEARING

Many people have profited from the development of new medical and surgical techniques for the restoration of hearing. For others, restoration is not possible. For some of these the greatest help in hearing has come from hearing aids. At one time hearing aids were clumsy, obvious, and unpredictable in their operation. The new ones available today are compact, efficient in operation, and inconspicuous. Some are built into the earpieces of eyeglasses. Although hearing aids are of little help to those who are totally deaf, they are often useful to people who are partially deaf.

SIGNS AND SYMPTOMS OF NEUROLOGICAL DISORDER

DISTINCTIONS

Impairments of the nervous system, like other bodily ailments, are generally evident first to the individual, his parents, or his friends. An individual may feel different or be aware of increasing difficulty in speaking, walking, or moving his arms. Such *functional* evidence of a disorder is a *symptom;* it may or may not identify the specific disorder. A person with such symptoms should see a physician.

During a medical consultation, the physician will note any general symptoms the patient can relate. Going further, the physician will conduct a clinical examination and attempt to find *objective* evidence of the disorder. Usually a specific disorder can be recognized by the presence of certain *signs*. Sometimes a symptom may be the same as a sign, or it may be unrelated. For instance, a patient may be aware of pain or other symptom somewhere in his body. Such pains may be caused by one of several conditions. For the physician to accurately diagnose the disorder he will need to conduct certain tests. The results of such tests may constitute signs.

GENERAL SIGNS

Some general signs of neurological impairment may be relatively easy to recognize. The following kinds of physical changes may give warnings of neurological disorder.

1. *Mental and emotional state*—lapses of consciousness, shifts in mood and emotional reaction, lapses of memory, disruptions in speech and stream of thought, stupor or coma.
2. *Posture and gait*—changes in posture or inability to stand with the feet together, abnormality in a person's gait, such as waddling, clumsiness, or jerkiness, as seen when he walks.
3. *Limbs*—disrupted reflex actions, lack of coordination, loss of power, wasting away of muscles, failure of a limb to develop, tremors or shaking.
4. *Head and neck*—deformities in size, shape, or symmetry, and painful or stiff neck movements.
5. *Cranial nerves and special senses*—difficulty in smelling, vision, reactions of the eye to light, eye movements, sensations of the face, motor movements of the face, hearing, movements of mouth parts, taste, rotation of the head, or use of the tongue.
6. *Trunk and spinal column*—muscular weakness in the trunk, breathing limitations, lack of sensation, muscle spasms, or limitation of movements.

KINDS OF NEUROLOGICAL DISORDERS

There are many different kinds of neurological disorders. Some of these are the result of a single known cause. Others may be the result of various causes or the cause may be unknown. These disorders may occur during embryonic development, as the result of accident, faulty metabolism, disease, or other causes. A few of the more commonly known neurological disorders are discussed below; they are arranged by cause.

DEVELOPMENTAL

During the time of embryonic development, prior to birth, malformations occasionally occur. These may be due to faulty inheritance or to some sort of developmental accident.

DOWN'S SYNDROME (MONGOLISM)

An unfortunate inherited brain malformation occurring in approximately 0.2 percent of Caucasian live births results in mongolism.
Victims are characterized by physical abnormalities of the face, eyelids,
tongue, and hands, along with general physical and mental retardation.
Because of the similarity in a fold of the eyelid between these victims
and members of the Mongoloid race, the term mongolism has been
misapplied to this condition.

The appearance of the disease in a child is related to the age of the
mother. As the age of the mother increases, the chances of her bearing
an affected child are increased considerably; the age of the father seems to
have no bearing on the disease. The number of pregnancies the mother
may have had preceding birth of the affected child again is not considered a cause for the condition.[1] It is possible for a mongoloid parent
to give birth to a normal child; but if such a mother were to be mated
to a normal partner, the chances would be 50 percent that their children would be mongoloid.

Mongolism occurs in two forms. In the first there is an extra chromosome, giving a total chromosome count of 47 instead of the customary
46. In the second form a part of a chromosome breaks off and reattaches
to another chromosome. In either case an imbalance of genetic material
can lead to maldevelopment of the child.

HYDROCEPHALUS

Hydrocephalus, meaning "water in the head," results in an enlargement of the head. Normally, cerebrospinal fluid is derived from blood
circulating through the cavities inside the brain. This clear fluid passes
from these cavities, down past and around the spinal cord, then back
up around the outside of the brain, where it is finally absorbed by the
veins lining the meninges surrounding the brain (Fig. 3.3). If this fluid
is obstructed from leaving the brain, it accumulates inside the brain
cavities and causes enlargement of the head.

Although due to malformation, it has also been known to result
from infection or tumors. This condition can now be treated by removing the obstructions or by creating artificial openings that allow circulation to resume.

TRAUMATIC

Traumatic disorders arise from wounds or injury. These can be the
result of injury to an infant during the process of being born, to auto-

[1] Curt Stern, *Principles of Human Genetics*, 2nd ed., San Francisco, Freeman,
1960, p. 470.

mobile accidents, falls, assaults, bullet wounds, or other accidental causes. Accidents of all kinds are the leading cause of death up through the age of 24. Accidental injury to the brain and spinal cord are important factors leading to death and disability.

HEAD INJURIES

In a minor head injury the patient may suffer only momentary loss of consciousness without any brain damage (*concussions*). In moderate injury there may be longer periods of unconsciousness, some actual brain damage, and small hemorrhages of blood vessels around the brain, resulting in clotting and pressure on the brain. Severe injury may lead to prolonged unconsciousness and even laceration of the brain.

Complications may be many and varied; they may include shock, convulsions, motor disabilities, respiratory difficulties, bleeding around the meninges, and infection. Severe cases may culminate in death.

SPINAL INJURIES

Spinal injuries are usually the result of accident. Spinal injuries commonly also involve injury to the vertebral column. Such injury may result in paralysis of body parts below the area of damage. Additional complications can occur in the form of shock, respiratory failure, pneumonia, and secondary infections.

METABOLIC

In some instances, disrupted chemical and physical processes in the body can lead to mental defects or nervous disorders.

PHENYLKETONURIA (PKU)

PKU is a hereditary disease which, if untreated, usually brings on mental retardation during the first several years of life. Found in either sex, PKU is transmitted by a recessive gene. About one in every 10,000 babies is a victim.

Although children with this disease appear normal at birth, they lack a liver enzyme which is needed to convert *phenylalanine* (an essential amino acid found in many foods) into *tyrosine* (Fig. 3.9). Because of the absence of this enzyme, phenylalanine accumulates in the body in 20 to 40 times the normal amount. This excessive amount interferes with the movement of other important amino acids into the brain, causing incomplete brain development that is permanent and irreversible.

Owing to the fact that brain development goes on for several years after birth, early detection of PKU is vital. Between the ages of 4 and

24 months, affected children show a progressive decline in mentality. In untreated cases most patients show an IQ of less than 50.

Melanin, the pigment responsible for hair and skin color, is usually less evident in PKU children than in normal children, victims often having blue eyes, blond hair, and fair skin. Victims may not be toilet trained or learn to feed themselves until they are 8 to 10 years of age, if then. About 1 percent of the patients in institutions for the mentally retarded are PKU victims.

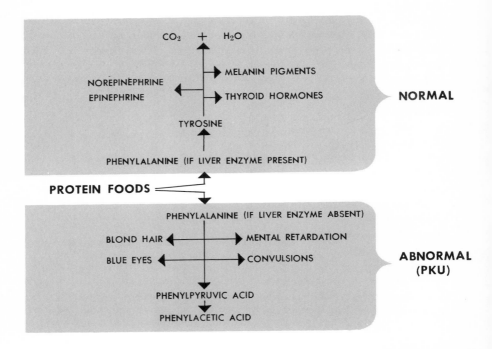

Fig. 3.9 Chart showing the chemical events in the disease phenylketonuria (PKU).

Various detection tests have been developed. One recently developed can be carried out four to five days after birth, before the baby comes home from the hospital.

PKU treatment must begin early. The older the age of the victim before treatment is begun, the greater the amount of damage. Treatment begun after the age of 2 is usually futile. Treatment consists of restricting the patient's dietary intake of phenylalanine. This diet needs to be adjusted as the child matures, but it is not yet known how long such a diet needs to be continued.

With recent developments for early detection and therapy, an increasing number of states are now requiring that all newborn infants be screened for PKU.

DEGENERATIVE

Some disorders arise as the result of tissue deterioration. Tissues and organs that were once active lose their ability to function. Examples of neurological degeneration include the following conditions.

MULTIPLE SCLEROSIS

Multiple sclerosis is a progressive disease resulting in the loss and destruction of the fatty myelin sheaths (see Fig. 3.1) that surround and insulate nerve cells. Scar tissue forms in the damaged areas, causing the nerve tracts to be "short-circuited," distorted, and eventually blocked. This demyelinization occurs in scattered areas of the brain and spinal cord. Once scar tissue is laid down, the nerve cells can never be restored to normal function and sometimes they die. Thus the communication system of the body is permanently damaged. Messages from the brain to the muscles are either distorted or blocked, and bodily movements the individual wants to make are hampered or prevented. The location and extent of the nerve damage is unpredictable.

This disease is characterized by such symptoms as paralysis and numbness of different parts of the body, loss of coordination, tremor of the hands, double vision, dragging of the feet, impairment of the speech, and loss of bladder and bowel control; any of these symptoms can be significant. The disease usually strikes those between the ages of 20 and 40 years, and it may appear at irregular intervals. It may progress gradually or rapidly. It is of equal incidence among both sexes. Although in some cases the disease is fatal, the life expectancy of most patients is approximately that of the rest of the population. Possible causes of the disease are suspected but still unproved.[2] At the present time there is no known cure for this disease. However, many victims of multiple sclerosis are able to adjust to the impairment and live useful lives.

The Multiple Sclerosis Society and the United States Public Health Service's National Institute of Neurological Diseases and Blindness are pursuing research on this disease. It is estimated that approximately 500,000 Americans are afflicted with multiple sclerosis today.

[2] *Understanding the Brain and Nervous System: Research Advances in Neurological and Sensory Disorders*, Washington, D.C., U.S. Dept. of Health, Education, and Welfare, Public Health Service, 1963.

PARKINSON'S DISEASE

Also known as "shaking palsy," this is a disease in which the normal functioning of the basal ganglia of the cerebrum is disrupted. When the functions of the basal ganglia are interfered with, the motor areas of the brain release nerve impulses more easily than they normally would, causing rapid involuntary contractions of the muscles. The muscles usually affected are those controlling the head, the hands, and the fingers. As a result the head and hands shake gently when the body is at rest. Along with this shaking, other muscles of the body become abnormally immobile, causing the facial expression to become unchanging and masklike, the walking to become stiff, and the arms to remain motionless when the person is walking. Because of the rigidity of his body muscles, the victim hates to move. He slumps and his speech becomes inarticulate. As the disease progresses, muscles all over the body become affected and movements of any kind become labored.

Some cases of Parkinson's disease are relatively mild, but others become progressively worse, eventually resulting in death. Although the disease is occasionally found among young people, most of the 1,500,000 victims in this country are older people. Treatment includes drugs, physical therapy, and surgery. Through the use of alcohol or pinpoint freezing (using liquid nitrogen at $-50°C.$), neurosurgeons locate and deaden certain ganglia. In some cases such surgery is successful in reducing or stopping tremor and lessening muscular rigidity. However, since such surgery is destructive, the nerve cells destroyed are never restored.

HUNTINGTON'S CHOREA

Also called *hereditary chorea,* Huntington's chorea is characterized by involuntary jerking movements of body and limbs. The word "chorea" comes from a Greek word meaning "dancing," and the victims of the disease display a dance-like movement. Named after an American physician, this malady consists of a progressive degeneration of the nervous system and leads to gradual physical and mental impairment and the eventual death of the individual. The disease generally appears in adults; on an average it begins in adults between the ages of 30 and 45. It has, however, appeared in victims as early as 1 year and as late as 60 years of age.

Although the disease consists of damage to the basal ganglia of the brain in somewhat the same manner as that found in Parkinson's disease, the damage results in a more spasmodic and extensive involuntary muscular movement than that found in Parkinson's disease.

The disease is inherited and is transmitted from parent to child through a single dominant gene; consequently children of affected parents have a 50 percent chance of inheriting the disease. Since the age of onset is variable, the ailment has been known to develop in children before it has shown up in their parents. However, in such cases one of the parents will be expected to show the disease if he or she lives long enough.

It is essential that parents who know of hereditary defects in their lineage tell their children about them. Failure to pass on such information can result in situations similar to the following account: A man developed Huntington's chorea after he had raised his own family of children; only then was it pointed out to him that his mother had died from the same condition. This information given to him earlier could have helped him decide to refrain from having children, thus averting possible suffering in the next generation.[3]

TUMORS

Tumors may arise in any of the tissues of the nervous system, such as the cells of the structures within the cranium—the meninges, blood vessels, nerve cells, or cranial glands (pituitary or pineal). Tumors may be either benign or malignant (see Chapter 13), but because of their vital location, even benign tumors may have drastic effects.

Tumors also occur within the vertebral column and affect the spinal cord. Although similar in nature to cranial tumors, they occur much less frequently. When malignancies do occur here, they metastasize to the bones of the vertebrae more commonly than do the cranial tumors metastasize to the skull. (*Metastasis* is the transfer of disease from one organ or part to another.) The treatment for intravertebral tumors is surgical, since they tend to compress the spinal cord against the inside of the vertebral canal.

The effects and symptoms of intracranial tumors vary, depending upon the exact location and condition of the tumor. Also, the development of the signs may be gradual or rapid. The parts of the body normally controlled by the affected part of the brain will also be affected and impaired. If treatment is not successful, these tumors are fatal.

With certain kinds of brain tumors some forms of radiation may be used. Other tumors should be removed surgically. A combination of treatment is effective in others.

Any tumor originating in any structure adjacent to the central nervous system which could metastasize is of importance to the nervous system.

[3] Stern, *op. cit.,* p. 677.

INFECTIONS

Several nervous disorders occur as the result of infections. These include poliomyelitis, neuritis, abscess, meningitis, and encephalitis. The last two will be discussed here as examples of infectious causes of neurological disorders.

MENINGITIS

Meningitis is an infection of the meninges due to the presence of specific organisms. These linings (Fig. 3.3), become inflamed; the cerebrospinal fluid becomes cloudy, owing to the presence of increased white blood cells; brain tissues become congested; and some nerve cells degenerate. The patient may suffer from fever, headache, pain and stiffness of the neck, and sometimes convulsions. Treatment depends on the organism responsible. Drugs are used, along with blood transfusions and drainage of cerebrospinal fluid.

Since meningitis usually occurs following a primary infection, effective treatment of other body infections and good nutrition are important in its prevention.

ENCEPHALITIS

Encephalitis is an inflammation of the brain, usually caused by a virus. It may be either the result of a primary infection or a complication of viral diseases such as measles, chickenpox, or mumps. The victim may show headache, fever, and lethargy, progressing into stupor and coma. Although recovery is usual there is permanent damage in some cases. Because of this danger, it is most important that immunizations against diseases such as measles be given to all people, particularly to children.

MULTIPLE OR UNKNOWN CAUSES

Most of the neurological disorders discussed so far are the result of a single known cause. Some disorders, however, are known to arise from a number of causes. Others have causes yet unknown. Following are several examples.

CEREBRAL PALSY

Cerebral palsy denotes the symptoms arising from damage to the central nervous system, usually before or during birth, but sometimes as long as three years after birth. The damage may come about as the result of one of a number of things—trauma or head injury during or following birth, premature birth, prenatal anoxia (oxygen deficiency), congenital malformations, malnutrition, encephalitis, meningitis, German measles in the mother during the first trimester of pregnancy, or Rh incompatibility between mother and fetus.

The symptoms of cerebral palsy range from mild muscular incoordination to severe spasm or violent convulsions. No two patients have identical symptoms. The most common symptom is an awkward, irregular walk. The patient may lack muscular control and/or balance. From 25 to 50 percent of cerebral palsy victims have seizures, more than 60 percent are mentally retarded, and 10 percent to 30 percent have hearing difficulties. The United Cerebral Palsy Association estimates that there are over 550,000 victims of cerebral palsy in the United States and that 1 baby in every 170 newborn has cerebral palsy.

This damage need not necessarily have a bearing upon a patient's intelligence, but he is in need of understanding and special education to fit him for tasks in which he can be useful.

EPILEPSY

Epilepsy is a symptom of certain forms of neurological impairment. Although it has been known to occur in all animals with brains, it is most common among humans. Ancient physicians thought that a person suffering from an epileptic attack had been seized by the devil or by an evil spirit, hence the name epilepsy (which means "seizure" in Greek). These attacks—also called "fits" and "blackouts"—involve a disturbance or impairment of consciousness. Often seizures result in *convulsions,* which are uncontrolled muscular spasms.

Knowledge of the causes of epilepsy is far from conclusive. It is now believed that epileptic seizures may be inherited, represent a chemical imbalance, be acquired from a brain injury, or result from tumors. Most commonly, seizures start during childhood or adolescence.

Convulsion occurs as the result of a disorderly discharge of brain cell impulses. During the period of seizure the muscles of the patient undergo involuntary contractions or spasms. These convulsions may be mild and may not result in loss of consciousness, or they may be severe and leave the patient unconscious.

Convulsions, however, are not unique to epileptics. They can be induced in any individual. It was early observed that patients with emotional conflicts who had experienced convulsions obtained some relief from their emotional conflicts thereby. It was thought, therefore, that if convulsions could be artificially induced, some patients with emotional illnesses could be benefited. Thus *electroshock* (*electroconvulsive therapy*), insulin, and Metrazol have been used to induce convulsions in some types of emotionally disturbed individuals. **Shock** therapy, rarely used today, has been replaced by various psychiatric drugs.

Although more than 30 types of epilepsy have been described, the disorder is usually defined in one of the following categories.

1. *Grand mal.* With this type the victim shows the most severe effects. He usually screams because of the constriction of his chest as the air is forced out through his throat. He falls, all of the voluntary muscles of the body stiffen, and jerking actions follow. Finally the spasm subsides. If a person is having a grand mal attack, it is important to keep him from hurting himself. A firm object may be placed between his teeth to keep him from biting his tongue. Clothing should be loosened around his neck. Persons who are subject to grand mal attacks should be encouraged to lie down when they feel an attack coming on. Drugs useful in reducing the frequency of these attacks include Dilantin, Mesantoin, phenobarbital, and the bromides.

2. *Petit mal.* This minor seizure differs from the major seizures in that its victim has only small (petit) blackouts. The victim, though not falling, becomes suddenly unaware of his surroundings. The attack may last only a few seconds. The victim may go for years without knowing he is an epileptic, unaware he is having petit mal seizures.

3. *Psychomotor epilepsy.* In this type an attack will result in illusions and disorganized movements, short periods of amnesia, abnormal rage, sudden anxiety, discomfort, fear, incoherent speech, or hallucinations.

Unfortunately, there is still considerable misunderstanding and stigma surrounding epilepsy. In spite of the fact that known epileptics have contributed significantly to science, government, and art (Julius Caesar and Feodor Dostoyevsky, for example), some states still prohibit a known epileptic from marriage, from attending public school, or from certain community programs for youngsters. Some states prohibit an epileptic from obtaining a driver's license, even though it can be established medically that his seizures are under control.

Far from being rare, epilepsy has been estimated to occur in about 1 percent of the United States' population. There appears to be little relationship between the incidence of epilepsy and intelligence, occupation, economic and social level, age, or sex.

Electroencephalography (EEG) has been of great help in diagnosing epilepsy. All living tissue of the body has some electrical activity. Variations in electrical activity of brain cells can be picked up from the scalp with electrodes. When amplified and recorded on paper, these fluctuations appear as a wavy line. Neurologists now can recognize a normal wave and certain abnormal ones (see Fig. 3.10). Thus the waves are classified according to their frequency and amplitude and can be used to detect epileptic conditions as well as other brain disorders.

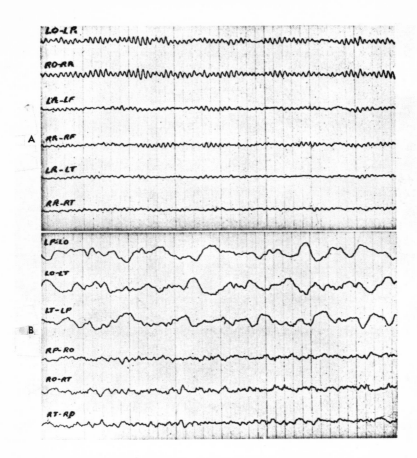

Fig. 3.10 Electroencephalographic tracings. (A) Normal tracings. (B) abnormal tracings.

Electroencephalography is not a perfect diagnostic tool, however. Normal individuals produce an abnormal EEG in 5 to 10 percent of cases tested. On the other hand, abnormal persons may produce normal EEG's.

HEADACHE

Headaches constitute one of the most common, yet most baffling of physical problems. The precise causes of only a few types are known. Where a headache is felt will not necessarily indicate the actual location of the disorder or inflammation. The disorder may be located inside the cranium (*intracranial*) or outside the cranium (*extracranial*).

1. *Intracranial causes.* Since the brain itself is almost totally insensitive to pain, headaches generally arise outside the brain. Disorders of the blood vessels around the brain or of the membranes (meninges) lining the surface of the brain can lead to headache. The pain may be localized or general. For example, inflammation of all the meninges can cause a severe headache over the entire head. This may be due to meningitis, brain surgery, a brain tumor, or a drop in the pressure of the cerebrospinal fluid around the brain. Other causes include high blood pressure, alcoholic binges, or injections of histamine.

Migraine headache is a special type of headache brought on by temporary disturbances in the arteries supplying the inside of the head. It is believed to be caused by prolonged emotion or tension. It often begins with preliminary sensations such as nausea or partial loss of vision. The vascular disturbance results in a reduced blood supply to the head, followed by dilation of the vessels and intense pulsations for 24 to 48 hours. Certain drugs administered during beginning symptoms tend to restore normal blood flow and prevent the intense pains of migraine.

2. *Extracranial causes.* Headaches can arise as a result of various conditions outside the cranium. Spasms in the muscles of the head, scalp, or neck brought on by emotional tension can cause a headache in those areas. Infection or irritation in parts of the nasal structures can cause a headache behind the eyes, above the nose, or in the face. Headaches can originate with the eyes, being brought on by excessive strain on the muscles which focus the eyes, imbalance in eye muscles, or exposure of the eyes to excessive irradiation from the sun or an arc light.

Headache constitutes a vast economic problem. Chronic recurring headaches are responsible for approximately as much economic loss as that from the common cold—costing millions of dollars annually in lost work time. They lead to the spending of over $300 million annually in the United States for popular nonprescription "headache remedies."[4]

SUMMARY

    I. Structure of the Nervous System
       A. Neuron
          1. Most specialized kind of body cell.
          2. Consists of:
             a. Cell body containing nucleus.
             b. Fibers leading to and from the cell body, called:
                (1) Dendrites.
                (2) Axons.
          3. Serves various functions:
             a. Sensory neurons.
             b. Motor neurons.

[4] *Understanding the Brain and Nervous System,* p. 31

B. Central nervous system consists of:
   1. Brain
      a. Cerebrum.
      b. Cerebellum.
      c. Brain stem.
   2. Spinal cord
C. Peripheral nervous system consists of:
   1. Cranial nerves.
   2. Spinal nerves.
D. Autonomic nervous system—responsible for control of body functions which are generally self-regulating.
   1. Extends from nerve centers down the brain stem and spinal cord.
   2. Consists of two divisions which act in contrast to each other:
      a. Sympathetic nerves.
      b. Parasympathetic nerves.

II. The Eye
   A. Structure of the eye
      1. Essentially includes:
         a. Lens mechanism formed by the curved transparent cornea and an internal crystalline lens which focuses an image on the back wall (retina) of the eye.
         b. Two internal cavities.
            (1) One between the cornea and the lens (anterior chamber) filled with a watery fluid (aqueous humor).
            (2) One between the lens and the retina (posterior chamber) filled with a jelly-like material (vitreous humor).
         c. Wall consists of three layers of tissue:
            (1) Sclera—outermost layer.
            (2) Choroid—middle layer.
            (3) Retina—innermost layer; consists of light-sensitive receptor cells called:
               (a) rods.
               (b) cones.
         d. Optic nerve—bundle of neurons which leads from the retina to the brain.
         e. Eye protected from injury and infection by the conjunctiva, a delicate membrane lining the eyelid and covering the exposed eyeball surface, which is kept moist by secretions from the tear (lacrimal) glands.
   B. Disorders of the eye include
      1. Refractive defects—improper focusing of images on the retina, such as:
         a. Myopia—nearsightedness.
         b. Hyperopia—farsightedness.
         c. Presbyopia.
         d. Astigmatism.
      2. Color blindness—hereditary, sex-linked condition.
      3. Diseases and inflammation, which include the following most common types:
         a. Conjunctivitis.
         b. Cataract.
         c. Glaucoma.

C. Care of the eye
   1. May include the professional services of an:
      a. **Ophthalmologist.**
      b. **Optometrist.**
      c. **Optician.**
   2. Contact lenses—placed directly on the front of the eyeball.
   3. Sunglasses—reduce eyestrain caused by excessive light glare.
   4. Eye exercises are of value only in cases of eye muscle imbalance.
   5. Eye irritants and injuries may be prevented by protecting the eye from flying objects or sharp instruments.
   6. Proper lighting is necessary to prevent eye fatigue.

III. The Ear
  A. Structure of the ear
    1. Sensory organs both for *hearing* and *equilibrium.*
    2. May be divided into three structural parts:
      a. External ear consists of:
        (1) auricle.
        (2) external auditory canal.
        (3) tympanic membrane (eardrum).
      b. Middle ear
        (1) Consists of three small bones (ossicles).
          (a) malleus (hammer).
          (b) incus (anvil).
          (c) stapes (stirrup).
        (2) Is adjacent to:
          (a) eustachian tube.
          (b) mastoid air cells (spaces back of the middle ear cavity).
      c. Internal ear consists of:
        (1) cochlea.
        (2) semicircular canals.
  B. Disorders of the ear most often involve the middle ear cavity and sometimes the inner ear as well.
    1. Infections—occur most easily in the middle ear.
    2. Deafness—caused by anything interfering with the transmission of sound waves or their interpretation in the ear.
    3. Aids in hearing—include surgical restoration and the use of some type of hearing aid.

IV. Signs and Symptoms of Neurological Disorder
  A. Distinctions exist between the following terms:
    1. Symptoms—functional evidence of a disorder which is most apparent in the way the patient feels.
    2. Signs—objective evidence of a disorder most apparent to the physician as the result of clinical tests.
  B. General signs often give warnings of neural impairment; they include:
    1. Mental and emotional changes.
    2. Posture and gait.
    3. Limbs.
    4. Head and neck.
    5. Cranial nerves and special senses.
    6. Trunk and spinal column.

V. Kinds of Neurological Disorders
  A. Developmental—malformations occurring prior to birth, due to faulty inheritance or a developmental accident.

B. Traumatic—arise as the result of injury during birth or by accidental means.

C. Metabolic—result of disrupted chemical and physical processes.

D. Degenerative—result in deterioration of the tissues and organs of the nervous system.

E. Tumorous
   1. May arise in any of the tissues of the nervous system, but often in the spinal cord.
   2. May be either benign or malignant, but in either case may cause drastic effects, depending upon the location.

F. Infectious—result in a number of disorders.

G. Multiple and unknown causes—responsible for some of the more baffling neurological disorders.

Glossary

If you cannot find the word you wish in this glossary, check the index for text and glossary references.

achromatic (ak rə mat′ik) (G. *achromatos*, without color).   Colorless.

aqueous humor (ā′kwē əs hyoo′mər) (L. *aqua,* water; *humor,* fluid).   The fluid filling the anterior chamber in front of the lens.

astigmatism (ə stig′mə tizm) (G. *a-,* without; *stigma,* point).   A structural defect of the cornea or lens that prevents light rays from meeting at a single point, thus forming indistinct images.

auricle (aw′ri kəl) (L. *auricula,* a little ear).   The part of the external ear not contained within the head.

autonomic nervous system (aw tə nom′ik) (G. *autos,* self; *nomos,* law).   The division of the nervous system that controls the glands, and smooth and cardiac muscles.

axon (ak′son) (G. *axon,* axis).   The portion of a neuron fiber which carries the impulse away from the cell body.

basal ganglia (bā′səl gang′glē ə) (G. *basis,* base; *ganglion,* knot).   A group of nerve centers located within the cerebrum, below the cortex, which serve as a center for the transmission of nerve impulses.

blind spot.   The small area, insensitive to light, in the retina of the eye where the optic nerve enters.

brain (brān) (AS. *braegen,* brain).   The mass of gray and white nerve tissue in the cranium which includes the cerebrum, cerebellum, and brain stem.

brain stem (brān stem).   All of the brain except the cerebrum and cerebellum; it includes the cranial nerve nuclei and sensory and motor tracts.

cataract (kat′ə rakt) (G. *kata-,* down; *rhegnynai,* to break).   A disease in which the crystalline lens becomes opaque, causing partial or total blindness.

central nervous system.   That division of the nervous system that includes the brain and spinal cord.

cerebellum (ser′ə bel′əm) (L. dim of *cerebrum,* the brain).   The division of the brain behind and below the cerebrum; it is the coordinating center for muscular movements.

cerebral hemisphere (ser′ə brəl hem′i sfēr) (L. *cerebrum,* the brain; G. *hemi,* half; *sphaira,* sphere).   One lateral half, or side, of the cerebrum.

cerebral palsy (ser'ə brəl pawl'zē). Paralysis due to a lesion of the brain, usually suffered at birth.

cerebrospinal fluid (ser'ə brō spīn' əl, sə rē'brō spīn'əl) (L. *cerebrum,* the brain; *spina,* a thorn; *fluidus,* fluid). Fluid that occupies spaces in the brain and circulates through the brain and down the spinal canal.

cerebrum (ser'ə brəm, sə rē'brəm) (L. *cerebrum,* the brain). The main portion of the brain occupying the upper part of the cranium.

choroid (kor'oid) (G. *chorion,* leather; *eidos,* form). The dark, vascular layer of the eye between the sclera and retina.

chromatic (krō mat'ik) (G. *chroma,* color). Pertaining to color.

ciliary body (sil'ē er ē) (L. *cilium,* eyelid). A structure of the eye which regulates the convexity of crystalline lens.

cochlea (kok'lē ə) (G. *kochlias,* snail). A spiral-shaped part of the internal ear which receives sound waves and produces nerve impulses for the auditory nerve.

concussion (kən kush'ən) (L. *concussio,* from *con-,* together; *quatere,* to shake). A brain impairment resulting from a violent blow or jar.

cone (kōn) (G. *konos,* cone). The sensitive cell end of the retina that perceives chromatic color.

conjunctiva (kon jungk tī'və) (L. *con,* with; *jungere,* to join). The mucous membrane lining the inner surface of the eyelid and the front part of the eyeball.

conjunctivitis (kən jungk'tə vī'tis). An inflammation of the conjunctiva.

cornea (kor'nē ə) (L. *corneus,* horny). The transparent part of the outer layer of the eyeball, covering the iris and pupil.

cortex (kor'teks) (L. *cortex,* bark of a tree). The outer layer of the brain, consisting of gray matter.

cranial nerves (krā'nē əl) (G. *kranion,* skull). Any peripheral nerve connected with the brain; arranged in twelve pairs.

cranium (krā'nē əm). The skull, especially that part containing the brain.

crystalline lens (kris'tə lin) (G. *krystallos,* ice; L. *lens,* "lentil"). The transparent lens of the eye, located behind the pupil; serves to focus light on the retina.

dendrite (den'drīt) (G. *dendron,* tree). The branched portion of a nerve cell which carries impulses toward the cell body.

effectors (i fek'tər(z)) (L. *ex-,* out; *facere,* to do). A nerve end organ which serves to distribute impulses which activate a muscle or gland.

electroconvulsive (or **electroshock**) **therapy** (i lek'trō kən vul'siv, i lek'trə shok) (G. *elektron,* amber; L. *con-,* together; *vellere,* to pull). The treatment of emotionally disturbed patients by inducing convulsions; this is done by passing an electric current through the brain.

electroencephalography (i lek'trō en sef'ə log'rafē) (G. *elektron,* amber; *encephalos,* the brain; *graphein,* to write). The recording of electric currents developed in the brain.

encephalitis (en sefə līt'is) (G. *encephalos,* the brain; *-itis,* inflammation). Inflammation of the brain.

end plate. A disc-like expansion at the ending of a motor nerve in a muscle.

epilepsy (ep'i lep"sē) (G. *epolepsia,* seizure). A disease characterized by convulsions, and sometimes spells of unconsciousness.

eustachian tube (yoo stā′shən) (after Bartolommeo Eustachio, an Italian anatomist 1520–1574). A tube connecting the middle ear with the pharynx.

external auditory canal (ek stur′nəl aw′di tor′ē kə nal′) (L. *externus,* outside; *audire,* to hear; *canalis,* a channel). The narrow passage of the external ear leading from the auricle to the tympanum. Also called the external auditory meatus.

external ear (ek stur′nəl ēr). The part of the ear that includes the auricle, the auditory canal, and the tympanic membrane (eardrum).

extracranial (ek′strə krā′nē əl) (L. *extr-,* outward; G. *kranion,* skull). Pertaining to something outside the cranium or the skull.

fovea (fō′vē ə) (L. *fovea,* a pit). The area of the retina directly back of the lens; it contains only cones.

frontal lobe (frun′təl lōb) (L. *frontalis,* forehead; G. *lobos,* lobe). One of the four main divisions of the brain, lying directly behind the forehead.

gene, dominant (jēn, dom′i nənt) (G. *gennan,* to produce). The gene, of a pair of genes, that produces an effect in a person, regardless of the nature of the other gene.

gene, recessive (ri ses′iv) (L. *re-,* back; *cedere,* to yield). One of a pair of genes that produce an effect in the person only when they are inherited from both parents.

glaucoma (glaw kō′mə, glou kō′mə) (G. *glaukos,* gleaming). A disease marked by intense pressure inside the eye, resulting in a hardening of the eyeball and eventual blindness.

grand mal (grahn mahl) (Fr. *grand,* strong, great; L. *malum,* ill). The most severe form of epilepsy in which there are convulsions preceded by periods of unconsciousness.

gray matter (grā mat′ər). Grayish nerve tissue of the brain and spinal cord, made up of nerve cells and nerve fibers.

Huntington's chorea (hunt′ing tənz kə rē′ə) (G. *choreia,* dance). A convulsive nervous disease characterized by involuntary and jerking movements and progressive dementia. Also called *hereditary chorea.*

hydrocephalus (hī′drō sef′ə ləs) (G. *hydor,* water; *kephale,* head). A condition characterized by an abnormal amount of fluid in the cranium, causing an enlargement of the head, atrophy of the brain, and convulsions.

hyperopia (hī′pə rō′pē ə) (G. *hyper,* above; *ops,* eye). A vision defect in which distant objects are seen more clearly than near ones; *farsightedness.*

incus (ing′kəs) (L. *incus,* anvil). The middle of the three ossicles of the middle ear. Also called *anvil.*

internal ear. The part of the ear that includes the cochlea and semicircular canals. Also called *inner ear.*

intracranial (in trə krā′nē əl) (L. *intra-,* within; G. *kranion,* skull). Situated within the cranium.

intraocular (in trə ok′yə lər) (L. *intra-,* within; *oculus,* eye). Situated within the eye.

intravertebral (in trə vur′tə brəl) (L. *intra-,* within; *vertebra,* vertebra). Within the vertebrae, or spine.

iris (ī′ris) (G. *iris,* rainbow). The round, pigmented diaphragm surrounding the pupil of the eye.

lacrimal gland (lak'ri məl) (L. *lacrima,* tears; *glans,* acorn).   A gland, located above the eye, that produces tears.

malleus (mal'ē əs) (L. *malleus,* a hammer).   The outermost of the three ossicles of the middle ear. Also called *hammer.*

mastoid air cells (mas'toid) (G. *mastos,* breast; *eidos,* form).   Spaces inside a part of the temporal bone behind the ear.

mastoiditis (mas toi dī'tis).   Inflammation of the mastoid.

melanin (mel'ə nin) (G. *melas,* black).   A dark pigment found in the skin, hair, iris, and other parts.

meninges (me nin'jēz) (G. *meninx,* a membrane).   The three membranes covering the brain and spinal cord.

meningitis (men in jī'tis).   An inflammation of the membranes covering the spinal cord or brain.

metabolic (met ə bol'ik) (G. *meta,* beyond; *ballein,* to throw).   Pertaining to the sum total of physical and chemical changes occurring in the body and the transformations by which energy is made available to the body.

metastasis (mə tas'tə sis) (G. *meta,* beyond, over; *stasis,* stand).   The transfer of disease from one part of the body to another not directly connected with it.

middle ear.   The cavity interior to the tympanic membrane, including the ossicles, and connecting to the mastoid air cells and eustachian tube.

migraine headache (mī'grān) (G. *hemi,* half; *kranion,* skull).   A type of periodically recurring headache, often confined to one side of the head.

mongolism (mon'gə lizm).   A kind of congenital mental deficiency, accompanied by facial characteristics resembling those of Mongols. Also called *Down's syndrome.*

motor neuron (mō'tər nyoor'on) (L. *movere,* to move; G. *neuron,* nerve).   A neuron carrying impulses from the brain or spinal cord to a muscle or gland.

multiple sclerosis (skla rō'sis) (L. *multiplex,* many folded; G. *sklerosis,* a hardening).   A disease in which there is hardening in various portions of the nervous system.

myelin sheath (mī'ə lin) (G. *myelos,* marrow).   The sheath of fatlike material around certain nerve fibers.

myopia (mī ō'pē ə) (G. *myein,* to shut; *ops,* eye).   A visual defect in which near objects are seen more clearly than distant ones; *nearsightedness.*

nerve (nurv) (G. *neuron,* nerve).   A cordlike bundle of nerve fibers surrounded by a protective sheath; carries impulses from one part of the body to another.

nerve fiber.   An extension of the cell body of a neuron covered with one or more sheaths.

neurologist (nyoo rol'ə jist) (G. *neuron,* nerve; *logos,* word; *-istes,* one skilled in).   An expert in the branch of medicine dealing with the nervous system, both normal and in disease.

neuron (nyoor'on) (G. *neuron,* nerve).   A nerve cell, including its cell body and processes or fibers.

nucleus (nyoo'klē əs) (L. *nux,* a nut).   A spherical body in most plant and animal cells necessary to growth and reproduction.

occipital lobe (ok sip'i təl lōb) (L. *occiput,* back of head; G. *lobos,* lobe).   The hindmost lobe of the cerebral cortex.

oculist (ok'yə list) (L. *oculus,* eye; G. *istes,* one skilled in).   A physician specializing in the treatment of diseases of the eye. An *ophthalmologist.*

ophthalmologist (of thal mol'ə jist) (G. *ophthalmos,* the eye; *logos,* word; *-istes,* one skilled in). A specialist in the branch of medicine dealing with the structure, functions, and diseases of the eye. The old term was *oculist.*

optic nerve (op'tik nurv) (G. *optikos,* pertaining to the eye; *neuron,* nerve). The nerve that arises from the retina of the eye and connects it to the cerebrum.

optician (op tish'ən). A person who makes or sells eyeglasses.

optometrist (op tom'ə trist) (G. *opto-,* vision; *metron,* measure). An expert in the profession of testing the vision and fitting glasses to correct eye defects.

organ of Corti. The terminal portion of the cochlea, containing many auditory cells.

ossicles (os'i kəl[z]) (L. *ossiculum,* little bone). Any small bones. The *auditory ossicles* are the three tiny bones in the middle ear cavity, the *malleus, incus,* and *stapes.*

otologist (ō tol'ə jist) (G. *otos,* ear). A physician specializing in the branch of medicine dealing with the ear and its diseases.

otosclerosis (ō'tə sklə rō'sis) (G. *otos,* ear; *sklerosis,* hardening). A condition characterized by chronic progressive deafness. Caused by the formation of spongy bone around the oval window and stapes.

parasympathetic (par'ə sim pəthet'ik) (G. *para,* beyond; *syn,* with; *pathos,* suffering). A division of the autonomic nervous system in which fibers arise from the midbrain, medulla, or the sacral region of the spinal cord.

parietal lobe (pə rī'ə təl lōb) (L. *paries,* a wall; G. *lobos,* lobe). A lobe of the cerebral cortex located centrally between the frontal and occipital lobes and above the temporal lobe.

Parkinson's disease (pahr'kin sənz) (James Parkinson, English physician, 1755–1824). A chronic disease of the nervous system characterized by a fine, slowly spreading tremor, muscular weakness, and rigidity. Also called *shaking palsy.*

peripheral nervous system (pə rif'ə rəl) (G. *peri,* around; *pherein,* to bear). That division of the nervous system which includes the cranial and spinal nerves and their branches.

petit mal (pə tē' mahl) (Fr. *petit,* little; L. *malum,* ill). A minor form of epilepsy in which there may be a brief blackout of consciousness, and which may even go unnoticed by the victim or others.

pharynx (far'ingks) (G. *pharynx*). The pouchlike structure between the mouth and nasal passages and the esophagus.

phenylalanine (fen'il al'ə nēn, fēn'il al'ə nēn). An essential amino acid found in protein foods.

phenylketonuria (fen'il kēt'ə nyoor"ē ə, fēn'il kēt'ə nyoor"ē ə). A congenital faulty metabolism of phenylalanine, resulting in the appearance of phenylpyruvic acid in the urine. If untreated, phenylketonuria usually brings on mental retardation. Sometimes called *PKU.*

presbyopia (prez"bē ō'pē ə) (G. *presbys,* old; *ops,* eye; *-ia,* a disease). A visual defect caused by loss of the ability to adjust the eye to varying distances due to the hardening of the crystalline lens.

psychomotor epilepsy (sī"kō mō'tər) (G. *psyche,* soul; L. *motor,* mover; G. *epilepsia,* seizure). A form of epilepsy characterized by purposeful motor

and/or psychic activity which is irrelevant to the time and place. The patient
is amnesic afterwards.

pupil (pyoo′pəl) (L. *pupilla,* girl).   The opening at the center of the iris of the
eye for the transmission of light.

receptor (ri sep′tər) (L. *recipere,* a receiver).   A sense organ; a nerve ending
specialized for the reception of stimuli.

reflex action (rē′fleks) (L. *reflexus,* bend back).   A reflected action or movement; an action induced by the stimulation of a receptor and carried on
without the intervention of the will.

refractive defect (ri frak′tiv) (L. *refringere;* to break apart; *agere,* to do).   A
defect in the ability of the eye to refract, or bend, light rays entering it, so
that a distinct image on the retina is not formed.

retina (ret′ə nə) (L. *rete,* a net).   The innermost layer of the eye which is stimulated by light.

rod (rod) (AS. *rodd,* club).   The sensitive element of the retina that perceives
dark and light and generates visual impulses.

sclera (sklē′rə) (G. *skleros,* hard).   The outer, tough, white layer of the eyeball,
except the area of the cornea.

seizure (sē′zhər) (ME. *seizen,* to take possession of).   An attack of epilepsy.

semicircular canal (sem′i sur′kyə lər kə nal′) (L. *semis,* half: *circularis,* a ring;
canalis, a channel).   Any of the three looped tubular structures of the inner
ear that serve to maintain balance in the person.

sense organ (sens or′gən) (L. *sensus;* G. *organon,* an instrument).   An organ
that receives a stimulus and transforms it into a sensation.

sensory neuron (sen′sə rē nyoor′on) (L. *sensus,* sense; G. *neuron,* nerve).   A
neuron carrying impulses from the sense organs to the spinal cord and
cerebral cortex.

sign (sīn) (L. *signum,* sign).   Any objective evidence of a disease.

spinal canal (spīn′əl kə nal′) (L. *spina,* a thorn; *canalis,* a channel).   The passage surrounded by the vertebrae, which contains the spinal cord.

spinal cord (spīn′əl kord).   That part of the central nervous system which is
lodged in the spinal canal.

spinal nerve (spīn′əl nurv).   Any peripheral nerve arising from the spinal cord
and passing out through the vertebrae; arranged in thirty-one pairs.

stapes (stā′pēz) (L. *stapes,* "stirrup").   The innermost of the three ossicles of
the middle ear, shaped like a *stirrup* and sometimes so called.

sympathetic nerve (sim pə thet′ik) (G. *syn,* with; *pathos,* suffering).   A division of the autonomic nervous system in which fibers arise from the thoracic
and lumbar regions of the spinal cord.

symptom (simp′təm) (G. *syn-,* together; *piptein,* to fall).   Any functional evidence of a disease or of a patient's condition; a change in a person's condition which indicates a physical or mental change.

synapse (sin′aps) (G. *synapsis,* a connection).   The region of contact between
adjacent neurons, the junction where an impulse is transmitted from one
neuron to another.

tear gland (tēr gland).   See lacrimal gland.

temporal lobe (tem′pər əl lōb) (L. *tempora,* the temples; G. *lobos,* lobe).   A
lobe of the cerebral cortex located laterally and below the frontal and occipital lobes.

tonometer (tō nom′i tər) (G. *tonos,* tension; *metron,* measure). An instrument used for measuring intraocular pressure.

trauma (trou′mə, traw′mə) (G. *trauma,* wound). A wound or injury.

tympanic membrane (tim pan′ik mem′brān) (L. *tympanum,* drum; *membrana,* membrane). The eardrum.

tyrosine (tī′rə sēn, tir′ə sin). An amino acid essential to the diet.

vertebral column (vur′tə brəl) (L. *vertebra*). The spinal column; bony column of vertebrae.

vitreous humor (vit′rē əs hyoo′mər) (L. *vitreus,* glassy; *humor,* fluid). The semifluid, transparent substance which lies between the lens and the retina of the eye.

white matter (hwīt mat′ər). White nervous tissue, composed mostly of myelinated nerve fibers; the conducting portion of the brain and spinal cord.

C H A P T E R 4

DRUG ABUSE

Treatment of disease is any effort to cure disease, arrest its course, lessen its severity, or alleviate the pain and inconvenience it causes. Treatment includes the administration of drugs and medicines such as vaccines and serums, antibiotics, sulfa drugs, narcotics, and others. These drugs constitute the most important segment of disease treatment.

When used under medical direction, drugs serve mankind, often performing what seem to be miracles in combating disease, relieving pain, and saving life. But when misused or abused, these same drugs can become man's worst enemies. For example, the dangers resulting from the overuse of antibiotics, as shown in Chapter 15, cannot be overstressed. But here we are concerned with the drugs which are purposely abused, the stimulant and depressant drugs.

THE HISTORY OF DRUG ABUSE

In America, narcotics started coming to our shores even before the founding of the Republic. In the late 1800s the volume increased, and just before the Civil War, with the invention of the hypodermic needle, patients were encouraged to buy this new device and apply narcotics on a do-it-yourself basis. Medicines, "elixers," and "tonics" which contained easily obtainable narcotics and which claimed to cure anything started to spread over the nation.

By the end of the Civil War, many thousands of soldiers had received large and numerous injections of narcotics to relieve their suffering from wounds and sickness. Many were addicted and relied on drugs. With the growth of advertising and the promotion of patent medicines containing narcotics, great segments of the population took such medicines and became dependent upon them. Later, individuals found out about the specific narcotic ingredient contained in these medicines and started using the narcotic directly.[1]

This situation is shown in Fig. 4.1, a history of narcotics addiction in the United States. Statistics shown in this table are not considered accurate, because when taken they were not carefully compiled. But the indications are that there were at least 200,000 addicts in 1900—probably many more. Today's estimated total is 60,000, of whom about 46,000 have been officially reported. The geographical distribution of the reported addicts varies from New York, reporting over 10,000 addicts, to such states as Alaska and Vermont, reporting no addiction problems at all.[2]

DRUG HABITUATION

Generally, the public's understanding of the use of drugs is limited to "drug abuse," that is, the use of drugs for purposes other than those intended in medicine. Such abuse is usually associated with dosages many times in excess of those used in legitimate medical care. In all cases of drug abuse there develops in the user a psychological de-

[1] T. T. Brown, *The Enigma of Drug Addiction,* Springfield, Ill., C. C Thomas, 1961.
[2] *Prevention and Control of Narcotic Addiction,* Washington, D.C., U.S. Treasury Department, Bureau of Narcotics, 1964.

Thousand Addicts

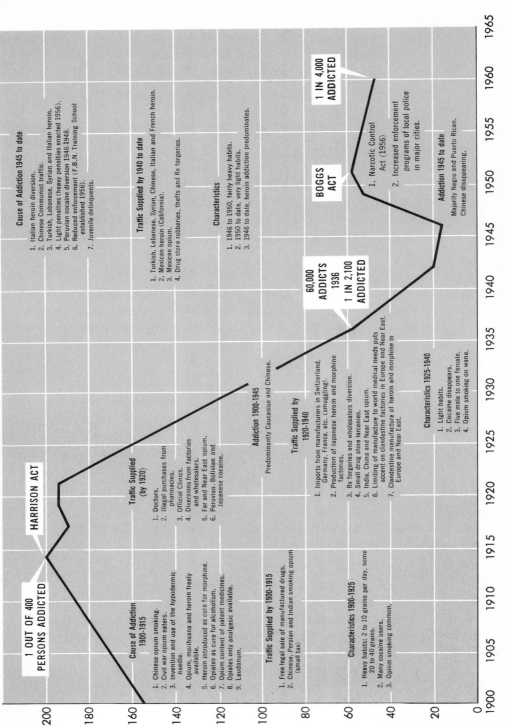

Fig. 4.1 History of narcotics addiction in the United States. (U.S. Department of Narcotics.)

1 OUT OF 400 PERSONS ADDICTED

HARRISON ACT

Cause of Addiction 1900-1915
1. Chinese opium smoking.
2. Civil war opium eaters.
3. Invention and use of the hypodermic needle.
4. Opium, marihuana and heroin freely available.
5. Heroin introduced as cure for morphine.
6. Opiates as cure for alcoholism.
7. Opium content of patent medicines.
8. Opiates only analgesic available.
9. Laudanum.

Traffic Supplied (by 1920)
1. Doctors.
2. Illegal purchases from pharmacies.
3. Official Clinics.
4. Diversions from factories and wholesalers.
5. Far and Near East opium.
6. Peruvian, Bolivian and Japanese cocaine.

Traffic Supplied by 1900-1915
1. Free legal sale of manufactured drugs.
2. Chinese, Persian and Indian smoking opium (small tax).

Characteristics 1900-1925
1. Heavy habits: 2 to 10 grains per day, some 20 to 40 grains.
2. Many cocaine users.
3. Opium smoking common.

Addiction 1900-1945
Predominantly Caucasian and Chinese.

Traffic Supplied by 1920-1940
1. Imports from manufacturers in Switzerland, Germany, France, etc. (smuggling).
2. Production of Japanese heroin and morphine factories.
3. Rx forgeries and wholesalers diversion.
4. Small drug store larcenies.
5. India, China and Near East opium.
6. Limiting of manufacture to world medical needs puts accent on clandestine factories in Europe and Near East.
7. Clandestine manufacture of heroin and morphine in Europe and Near East.

60,000 ADDICTS 1936 1 IN 2,100 ADDICTED

Characteristics 1925-1940
1. Light habits.
2. Cocaine disappears.
3. Five male to one female.
4. Opium smoking on wane.

Cause of Addiction 1945 to date
1. Italian heroin diversion.
2. Chinese Communist traffic.
3. Turkish, Lebanese, Syrian and Italian heroin.
4. Light penalties (heavy penalties enacted 1956).
5. Peruvian cocaine diversion 1946-1948.
6. Reduced enforcement (F.B.N. Training School established 1956).
7. Juvenile delinquents.

Traffic Supplied by 1940 to date
1. Turkish, Lebanese, Syrian, Chinese, Italian and French heroin.
2. Mexican heroin (California).
3. Mexican opium.
4. Drug store robberies, thefts and Rx forgeries.

Characteristics
1. 1946 to 1950, fairly heavy habits.
2. 1950 to date, very light habits.
3. 1946 to date, heroin addiction predominates.

BOGGS ACT

1 IN 4,000 ADDICTED

Addiction 1945 to date
1. Narcotic Control Act (1956)
2. Increased enforcement programs of local police in major cities.

Majority Negro and Puerto Rican, Chinese disappearing.

1900 1905 1910 1915 1920 1925 1930 1935 1940 1945 1950 1955 1960 1965

0 20 40 60 80 100 120 140 160 180 200

pendence upon the drug or the conditions associated with its use. The intensity of such dependency varies with individuals and with the motivation behind the abuse of a drug. In its most intense form dependency represents an uncontrollable craving or compulsion to experience the drug's euphoric effects at almost any cost. Medically, these "users" are considered to have an habituation to drugs. Table 4.1 examines the similarities and differences between drug habituation and drug addiction.

TABLE 4.1 DEFINITIONS OF THE EXPERT COMMITTEE ON ADDICTION-PRODUCING DRUGS OF THE WORLD HEALTH ORGANIZATION

Drug Addiction	Drug Habituation
Drug addiction is a state of periodic or chronic intoxication produced by the repeated consumption of a drug (natural or synthetic). Its characteristics include:	Drug habituation (habit) is a condition resulting from the repeated consumption of a drug. Its characteristics include:
1. An overpowering desire or need (compulsion) to continue taking the drug and to obtain it by any means	1. A desire (but not a compulsion) to continue taking the drug for the sense of improved well-being it engenders
2. A tendency to increase the dose	2. Little or no tendency to increase the dose
3. A psychic (psychological) and generally a physical dependence on the effects of the drug	3. Some degree of psychic dependence on the effect of the drug, but absence of physical dependence and hence of an abstinence syndrome
4. Detrimental effect on the individual and on society	4. Detrimental effects, if any, primarily on the individual

SOURCE: Modified from Maurice H. Seevers, "Medical Perspectives on Habituation and Addiction," *Journal of the American Medical Association,* Vol. 181, No. 2, July 14, 1962, pp. 92–98 (Table 93).

MEDICAL DEFINITION OF DRUG ADDICTION

In addition to causing psychological dependence, some drugs evoke biochemical and physiological adaptations in the user known as tolerance and physical dependence. Tolerance is a fundamental survival mechanism which permits body cells to be exposed continuously to toxic substances without evoking dangerous responses. Drug addictive tolerance occurs in the phenomenon that successive doses of the same amount of drug produce decreasing effects and that larger and larger doses are necessary to achieve the effects of the first dose; thus there is a tendency to increase the dose.

Tolerance is relative, but with repeated administration of increasing doses, the brain is exposed to concentrations of the drug which bring about a physical dependence within the body. This physical dependence in an individual is shown or proved when the drug is suddenly withdrawn from him. Sudden withdrawal brings about a *withdrawal illness* or *abstinence syndrome*.

The symptoms of withdrawal from opiates and their derivatives include irritability, depression, extreme nervousness, pain in the abdomen, and nausea—all to an agonizing degree. Sudden withdrawal from alcohol for a man physically dependent may cause delirium tremens. A sudden withdrawal of barbiturates from a person with physical dependence may cause convulsions, delirium tremens, and frequently death.

Based on the preceding information, the World Health Organization has medically defined addiction as

> . . . a state of periodic or chronic intoxication produced by the repeated consumption of a drug (natural or synthetic), which produces the following characteristics: (1) an overpowering desire or *compulsion* to continue taking the drug and to obtain it by any means; (2) a tendency to *increase the dosage,* showing body *tolerance;* (3) a *psychic* and generally a *physical dependence* on the effects of the drug; and (4) the creation of an individual and social problem.

The terms "addict" and "user" can be ambiguous. We use the term addict to describe those misusing opium and its derivatives, synthetic narcotics, barbiturates, alcohol, and solvents. The user is one who has an habituation for cocaine, amphetamines, marijuana, or LSD.

LEGAL DEFINITION OF ADDICTION

The legal definition of drug addiction rests upon the illicit or illegal *possession* of a narcotic or dangerous drug, not upon the evidence of use of such substances. The United States Supreme Court (*Robinson vs. California,* No. 554, October term, 1961) ruled that the California law making addiction a misdemeanor is unconstitutional. This precedent-setting legal decision affected similar state laws throughout the United States. The Supreme Court based its decision on the contention that addiction is a disease and that an addict is a person who needs medical and psychological treatment, not imprisonment for a specific length of time.

Federal laws include opium and coca leaves or their derivatives marijuana and peyote (mescaline) as "habit-forming narcotic drugs." There is no attempt by the government to legally define narcotics in a general sense, but by Presidential proclamation, specific synthetic substances listed by chemical and common names are declared to be narcotics when, after testing, they have been found to produce sleep or stupor and at the same time relieve pain (The Narcotic Manufacturing Act of 1960).

Dangerous drugs are declared and listed by the Federal Pure Food and Drug Administration after they have been tested and found to be unsafe for self-medication. All medical preparations of this nature bear the following legend on the label: "Federal law prohibits dispensing except upon the written order of a physician."

Most states, having no clinics or laboratories to evaluate possible dangerous drugs or narcotic substances, rely upon the recommendations made by the federal government. State legislatures enact laws against the abuse of those substances that federal laws have declared to be dangerous drugs and narcotics.

LEGAL CONTROL OF NARCOTICS AND DANGEROUS DRUGS

FEDERAL CONTROL OF NARCOTICS

The first federal measure seeking control over narcotics was enacted by Congress on February 9, 1909. It prohibited the importation of opium, its preparations, and its derivatives, except for medicinal purposes. Initially, this act had very little effect on the sale of drugs within the United States, because of public apathy and lack of an agency to enforce the measure.

For all practical purposes there were no limitations on the sale of narcotic drugs within the United States until the enactment and enforcement of the federal statute known as the Harrison Narcotic Act. This statute was approved December 17, 1914, and an amendment in 1930 provided for the establishment of the Bureau of Narcotics to enforce the provisions of the Harrison Act and to apprehend violators.

The Harrison Narcotic Act restricted the importation, manufacture, sale, and dispensing of opiates. It required the keeping of accurate records and inventories of narcotics and made the possession of narcotics a criminal offense. It required physicians to dispense opiates "in the course of their professional practice only" for bona fide medical

TABLE 4.2   **COMPARISON OF MEDICAL CHARACTERISTICS PRODUCING DRUGS, WITH THEIR**

Drugs	Psycho-genic Dependence	Uncontrolled Compulsion to Continued Abuse	Physical Dependence	Tolerance
Opiates and morphine-like analgesics	X	X	X	X
Barbiturates and other hypnotics	X	X	X	X
Alcohol	X	X	X	X
Bromides	X	X		
Cocaine	X	X		
Amphetamines and related stimulants	X	X		X
Marijuana	X	X		?
Solvents	X	X	X	X
Nicotine	X			X
Caffeine	X			X

SOURCE: Modified from Maurice H. Seevers, "Medical Perspectives on
Vol. 181, No. 2, July 14, 1962,

purposes. It limited the selling of narcotics only to licensed druggists after they receive a lawful written prescription issued by a qualified medical practitioner.

The next federal statute, approved in 1922, was an extensive revision of the Harrison Act. It is known as the Narcotic Drugs Import and Export Act. This revision and subsequent revisions are now considered the official position of the federal government with regard to the legal and illegal possession, importation, manufacture, and exportation of narcotics. These acts now authorize the importation of only such quantities of crude opium and coca leaves as the Commissioner of Narcotics shall find necessary to provide for medical and legitimate needs. It prohibits the importation of any form of narcotic drugs, except the prescribed limited quantities of crude opium and coca leaves. Also, the importation of opium for smoking or for the manufacture of heroin is specifically prohibited. And the exportation of manufactured drugs is permitted only under a rigid system of controls.

The third federal law, known as the Marijuana Tax Act, was enacted in 1937. This act has since become part of the Internal Revenue Code. This statute requires the registration and payment of a tax by all

OF COMMON HABIT-FORMING AND ADDICTION-
LEGAL AND REGULATORY STATUS

Psychotoxic Effects During Administration	Psychotoxic Effects During Withdrawal	Regulatory Control: Specific Laws	Regulatory Control: Prescription Only	Available "Over the Counter"
	X	X	X	
X	X		X	
X	X			X
X				X
X		X	X	
X			X	
X		X		
X	X			X
				X
				X

Habituation and Addiction," *Journal of the American Medical Association,* pp. 92–98 (Table 94).

persons who import, manufacture, produce, compound, sell, deal in, dispense, prescribe, administer, or give away marijuana.

The fourth principal federal statute controlling drugs is known as the Opium Poppy Control Act; it was approved in 1942. This act prohibits the cultivation, in the United States, of the opium poppy, except under license. The issuance of this license is conditioned by a determination of the necessity of supplying the medical and scientific needs of the United States for opium and opium products. No such necessity has arisen nor is likely to arise.

These four laws (see Table 4.2) form the basis for federal control over the narcotics traffic in the United States. Anyone illegally dealing in narcotics is subject to federal penalties. Most actions involve investigations and prosecutions under the Harrison Narcotic Act. Other actions are usually left to the individual states.

FEDERAL STATUTORY PENALTIES

In 1956 Congress passed the Narcotics Control Act (Bogg's Act), which set forth a range of stringent mandatory minimum sentences and fines for violation of federal narcotics laws. For the first offense of unlawful sale of narcotics (between adults), the sentence is not less than 5 years or more than 20 years, with an optional fine of up to $20,000 and with no possibility of probation, suspension of sentence, or parole. The minimum for the second or for subsequent offenses is 10 years. The penalty for the first offense of possession of narcotics is not less than 2 years nor more than 10 years, with an optional fine of up to $20,000. In this instance, however, there is the possibility of probation, suspension of sentence, or parole. A minimum of 5 years is imposed for a second offense, and a minimum of 10 years for any subsequent offenses, without the possibility of probation, suspension, or parole.

This law also provides that any person having attained the age of 18 years, who knowingly sells, gives away, furnishes, dispenses, or conspires to sell, give away, furnish, or dispense any heroin unlawfully imported or otherwise brought into the United States, to any person who has not attained the age of 18 years, may be fined not more than $20,000 and shall be imprisoned for life, or for not less than 10 years, except that the offender shall suffer death if the jury in its discretion shall so direct. In other words, this law provides an extremely heavy penalty for the sale of heroin to a minor.

The Bureau of Narcotics maintains that these severe penalties act as a powerful deterrent. Medical groups do not agree. They do not believe that a narcotics addict who is physically and psychologically dependent on a drug will forego satisfaction of this craving for fear of a long prison sentence, or that a marijuana user will be deterred by fear of the penalty that awaits him if he is caught possessing it. Both positions are valid, but the deterrent position would be much stronger if the potential victim understood the penalties prior to his first introduction to marijuana or narcotics.

FEDERAL AND STATE CONTROL OF DANGEROUS DRUGS

The control of dangerous drugs has not been consistent with the corresponding controls of narcotics. In 1938 the Federal Food, Drug and Cosmetic Act was enacted. In essence, all drugs which were unsafe for self-medication were to be dispensed only upon the written order of a physician. Enforcement of these laws is under the jurisdiction of the Federal Food and Drug Administration, and statutory penalties consist of fines and misdemeanor charges against offenders.

In 1951 the prescription requirements of the 1938 law, along with controls on distribution, were strengthened and clarified by the Durham–Humphrey Amendment. The controls of this amendment were directed mainly against the barbiturates and amphetamines. Federal law still restricts these drugs, making it illegal to dispense them without a prescription, but under the federal law mere possession is not a violation. The state laws supplement this federal law with corresponding misdemeanor charges for the illegal possession of barbiturates and amphetamines.

CONTROL OF NARCOTICS BY STATES

In 1932 a model uniform state narcotics law patterned after the Harrison Narcotic Act was submitted to several states. Since that time this law, with minor changes in some states, has been enacted by 47 state legislatures, by Puerto Rico, and by Congress for the District of Columbia. California and Pennsylvania have enacted laws that appear to be comparable in scope and effectiveness. New Hampshire is the only state that has a narcotics law which is not considered to be equal in scope to the uniform State Narcotic Law.

In drug control there has always been cooperation between federal, state, and local law-enforcement officers. Until a few years ago, the problem of enforcement was left largely to the Federal Bureau of Narcotics. Now there are separate narcotics units in local police departments of all large cities and a large proportion of narcotics cases are prosecuted in local and state courts. State authorities are recognizing the importance of heavier penalties as a necessary means of reducing violations of their narcotics laws. In 1955, Ohio, for instance, enacted legislation providing for more drastic penalties, including a 20-year minimum penalty for the unlawful sale of narcotics. Since the enactment and enforcement of such penalties in the Ohio courts, illicit drug peddling in the state has become exceedingly rare. During 1957, heavier penalties were enacted in Alabama, Colorado, Illinois, Minnesota, Missouri, Pennsylvania, and Texas. These penalties ranged from 2 to 10 years of imprisonment for a first offense of unlawful possession to 5 to 20 years for the unlawful sale of narcotics.

ECONOMIC ASPECTS OF DRUG ABUSE

For many years the principal sources of illicit narcotics have been Burma, China, Malaya, India, Turkey, Thailand, Iran, Lebanon, Syria, Italy, and Mexico. China, a large producer of opium and manufacturer of morphine and heroin, is not a member of the United Nations and therefore not subject to any control.[3] Communist China manufactures heroin on such a gigantic scale that it is flooding the world market; it has been estimated by the California State Bureau of Narcotic Enforcement that more than 20 percent of the heroin used on the West Coast of the United States is from Communist China; the rest comes from Mexico. The bulk of the heroin on the illicit market is shipped

3 United Nations, *Bulletin on Narcotics,* Vol. XVII, No. 1, January–March, 1955.

from Italy, France, Iran, and Hong Kong; Peru and Bolivia, through Cuba, supply the greater part of the cocaine used. The majority of the marijuana used in the United States is grown in Mexico and smuggled over the border.

Legally manufactured narcotic drug preparations such as barbiturates, amphetamines, and tranquilizers enter the illicit market in many ways. The variety of medicinal drugs (as shown in the section on barbiturates) is extremely large and rising daily. These legally manufactured pills are diverted in many ways, such as by the burglarizing and robbing of doctors' offices, drugstores, and pharmaceutical houses; the pilfering of doctors' bags left in automobiles; and the smuggling of very large quantities of such drugs from foreign ports, where controls on manufacture and distribution are less rigidly enforced.

The main reason why opium is diverted from legal cultivation into illicit channels is that illicit traffickers offer substantially higher prices than those paid by the national opium monopolies. If estimates are reasonably correct, there can be little doubt that the quantity of opium entering the illicit traffic from opium-producing regions of the world exceeds the total legal production for legitimate purposes.[4]

Heroin is bought in foreign lands for approximately $2500 a kilo (35½ ounces) or about $70.00 per ounce.[5] When smuggled into the United States, it will net the seller in the initial transaction $9000 or $10,000. In Eastern cities, after it has been diluted many times by adding quantities of milk sugar, this cut heroin is then sold to the street trade for about $1.00 per grain (437.5 grains to the ounce). So, the retail value of a kilo of pure heroin may amount to more than $300,000 for the diluted heroin and milk sugar on the New York streets. On the West coast, "bindles" (small folded papers containing 1 to 1½ grains of heroin) and capsules (#5, 1½-grain gelatin capsules), heavily diluted, sell for $5.00 to $10.00 each, depending on the quality and the quantity of the product. A single ounce of "pure" heroin cut to injection strength and sold in papers or capsules will bring in as much as $32,000.[6]

The price of heroin varies in different parts of the country but stays as high as the traffic will bear. Regardless of the prevailing price, it is always far beyond the legitimate income of addicts. An addict must take an injection of heroin three or four times daily. He will use up to three or four capsules for each injection, depending on the tolerance that has been produced by the drug. His injections of heroin will cost from $20.00 to $40.00 a day.

The prices of other illicit drugs vary downward from heroin. Marijuana is usually smuggled into the United States in bricks (marijuana is compressed into a brick by an adobe brick-making machine), paper

4 *Ibid.*
5 T. T. Brown, *op. cit.*
6 *Ibid.*

bags, and gunny sacks. These usually contain about a kilo (2.2 pounds) of marijuana. In California, marijuana sells for about $100 a pound. Approximately 800 cigarettes can be made from a pound of bulk marijuana. A kilo selling at $.50 a cigarette would clear, for the pusher, about $660.[7]

Prices of barbiturates and amphetamines vary with the age of the addict and the availability of the supply. Younger potential users buy pills at a much lower price than addicted older people buy them. At a junior high school these pills may sell for as low as $.05 a pill. This price will then increase to $.65 or more when the individual becomes addicted.[8]

Crimes of violence are often committed by people who are under the influence of stimulant drugs. Sex crimes and violent assaults are rarely committed by those under the influence of opiates or barbiturates, because these depressants quiet the users and lessen their sex drive. However, the use of depressant drugs can lead to violent assaults, hold-ups, and even murder when approaching withdrawal symptoms lead the addict to desperation; he will then take any risk to obtain drugs or the money to buy them.

PUBLIC HEALTH ASPECTS OF DRUG ABUSE

There are at least two distinct philosophies concerning individuals who use drugs. One philosophy sees the drug offender as a person whose criminality manifests itself in drug offenses after he has had an initial exposure to some other form of criminality. His involvement in the use, possession, sale, or theft of drugs is regarded as part of a predicted criminal behavior. The California Board of Corrections reports that the typical heroin addict-prisoner is 27 and was first arrested for violation of the narcotics laws when he was 21. He first began using opiates when he was 20, he received his first commitment for a criminal or delinquent offense when he was 18½ and his first arrest was when he was 16.3 years old.

The other philosophy views the drug user as an unfortunate or sick person who must be protected from himself and prevented from spreading his disease to others. According to this philosophy, active addicts in the community represent a reservoir of infection; narcotic drugs, the infecting agents; and pushers, the vectors. From this idea it follows that the smaller the reservoir (fewer number of addicts), and the scarcer the infecting agent (illicit supplies of narcotics) and vectors (pushers), the less the danger of spread of the disease. This philosophy suggests three ways of controlling or eradicating addiction: (1) complete control of narcotics supplies; (2) elimination of pushers; (3) the isolation and

[7] Ibid.
[8] J. D. Williams, Narcotics, Dubuque, Iowa, Wm. C. Brown, 1963.

elimination of the narcotics users. Doctor D. P. Ausubel, in his book *Drug Addiction*, lists a fourth approach, which is research into the nature, causes, treatment, outcome, and epidemiology of drug addiction.

The first philosophy does not attack the problem but interns the offenders. It is obvious that drug addiction is a public health problem with legal consequences. The abuse of drugs should be attacked as such a problem by our research into the minds of people who become addicts; by finding the environment and conditions that spawn addiction; and by finding workable methods of treatment, rehabilitation, and control.

Law enforcement is the means of control we can use until research gives us the knowledge we need for preventing the illness. Civil government is justified in applying preventive measures here for social ends, but the services now available are far from meeting the present needs. The present reduction in the number of addicts seems to be due to many factors, some being the new federal laws and their enforcement. These laws have proved to be highly desirable, especially since their reinforcement by similar state legislation.

SOCIAL ASPECTS OF DRUG ABUSE

Drug abuse and all the destruction that goes with it—physical, mental, moral, occupational, and social—is plainly a problem that cannot be solved by its victims alone. It is a social problem that concerns all of us. The use of narcotics among adolescents is nothing new. Many teen-agers were addicted in 1900 and an increase in the number was noted immediately after World War I. It gradually decreased and then rose again through 1948.

The assistance of relatives and friends of youngsters and others suspected of sampling drugs can be invaluable in stamping out the traffic. Like the parents of delinquents, the parents of a teen-age drug victim sometimes pay little attention to their child's associates, habits, and the places he frequents.

In 1963 the Los Angeles County Board of Supervisors published the booklet *Darkness on Your Doorstep*. This booklet says that although it is difficult for parents to recognize the effects of narcotics addiction in children, there are eight questions that parents can ask about their children's actions.

1. *Has your youngster become secretive about his friends and his activities?* Does he seem to be involved in some private business? in making appointments? in meeting people? Does he suddenly disappear? Does he make unlikely excuses for all these actions? Has he picked up drug users' terms such as *stash, pot, connection, fix, grass, hay, yellow jackets, red devils, reefers, sticks,* and others?

2. *Is he developing bad attitudes?* Does he make fun of parents, teachers, or police officers? Does he label most people as "squares"? Does he make fun of the good standards of people he used to like?

3. *Is he slipping in school?* Has he dropped the athletics he used to enjoy? Has he given up clubs and social life? Has his interest in the opposite sex grown less instead of greater?

4. *Has he begun to have drowsy spells during the day?* Have there been times when it was difficult to awaken him? Has he seemed "knocked out" rather than sleepy?

5. *Does he go through periods of undue excitement?* Is he sometimes "walking on air"? Does he seem drunk? Can you smell solvent on his clothing? Does he have burns about the nose and mouth which could come from "sniffing"?

6. *Does he have an excessive need of money?* Is he always hunting jobs, losing jobs, or changing jobs? Does he talk about leaving school to make better wages? Are household things disappearing? Is money missing from your purse or wallet? Yet does he seem to be spending so little that you can't imagine where his money goes?

7. *Has he gone in for long-sleeved shirts,* which may hide needle marks or the scars of injections? Does he have skin sores or severe constipation which some drugs produce?

8. *Does he have a stash*—a collection of pills or powders, an outfit or injection equipment, or a packet of weedy-smelling leaves and stems?

These eight danger signals are for the recognition of drug misuse, but whether or not an individual chooses to try and then continue to use drugs depends upon his personality, the availability of drugs, and the attitudes toward drugs prevailing in his immediate and overall social group. Before he ever comes into contact with drugs, he often has an attitude either for or against them. This attitude in general corresponds to that of his neighborhood or community. In areas where the incidence of drug addiction is low, the availability is low and the attitude for the use of drugs is low.

Equally crucial to the person's continued use of drugs is the reaction of his social group to his initial experience—approval or disapproval, reward or punishment, praise or ridicule. If he decides upon the further use of drugs, two consequences are inevitable: (1) he will progressively become disillusioned with values and standards of non-drug users and begin to feel abused and misunderstood by their standards, and (2) his identification and ties with the standards of the drug world will increase.

Advance knowledge of both the properties of drugs and the social reactions to their use can influence the course of an individual's addiction. Although an individual may be addicted, if he does not know about dependence and withdrawal symptoms and if no one points these out to him as evidences of addiction, he may never actually admit to himself that he is an addict. Mature personality needs, strong social pressures, or the availability of adult guidance may reverse the course of his addiction even after a user establishes a physiological dependence upon them.

MEDICAL ASPECTS OF DRUG ABUSE

PHYSICAL ASPECTS OF NARCOTICS ADDICTION

Recognition of opiate drug addicts, especially when they are regularly obtaining a daily dosage, is extremely difficult. Addicts will not reveal their condition, and experience makes them very adept at disguising it.

Very early in the addiction to heroin, morphine, or other opiate, before much tolerance has developed, the pupils of the eyes will present a contracted pinpoint condition, as in Fig. 4.2. These pupils will not react to light, that is, the pinpoint will not change in strong light even if it is flashed directly into the eyes. This condition of the eyes is termed "frozen." After tolerance to the drug has developed to some degree, pupillary constriction may not be as pronounced, but reaction to light will be the same. When addicts have been without a dose for a short period of time, from four to six hours or overnight, they begin to enter withdrawal, in which the pupils of their eyes will be found to be dilated and will have a sluggish reaction to light. Because of the reaction of the addicts' eyes to light, many of them wear dark glasses most of the time.

Long-term addicts tend to be pale and emaciated and to suffer from severe constipation. Their appetites are poor and they show little or no sex interest. While under the influence of a narcotic, addicts are lethargic, semistuporous, dreamy, and not particularly dangerous—this state is ordinarily referred to as "doped." However, if deprived of a regular and necessary supply, addicts will become extremely dangerous, ready to commit any crime necessary to procure the price of a "fix." They suffer excruciating pain if their injections are not taken three to four times daily.

Because of fear, haste, and general disregard, addicts are not careful about sterilizing their equipment, and, as a result, infections and diseases such as syphilis, hepatitis, and malaria are passed on to people using the same "outfit" (Fig. 4.3).

TREATMENT FOR NARCOTICS ADDICTION

The current medical-psychiatric methods of treatment employed at various institutions in America are almost complete failures. Although occasionally a successfully rehabilitated addict can be found, the overall

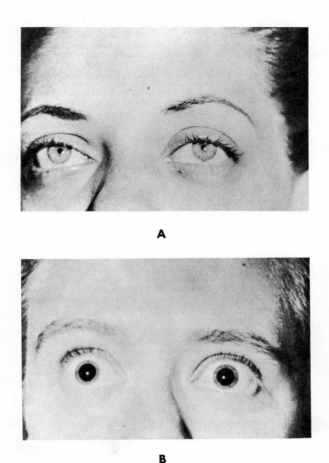

A

B

Fig. 4.2 (A) Contracted pupil reaction to a depressant drug. (B) Dilated pupil reaction to a stimulant drug. (California State Bureau of Narcotic Enforcement.)

results are extremely poor. There are no proven techniques for the effective treatment of drug addicts applicable to the total addict population.

The only known cure for drug addiction is abstinence. Law enforcement temporarily takes the addict out of his usual environment; and, for the period of his incarceration, he is "cured," simply by being forced to abstain from drugs. The same treatment is given in private or public hospitals; the addict is withdrawn from drugs, given a period of recuperation and psychiatric therapy, and then released. The post-institutional follow-up, which should be the most important part of the treatment, is almost nonexistent.

Accepted medical procedures for treating addicts include withdrawal from the drug by a gradual reduction in dosage. Abrupt withdrawal, the

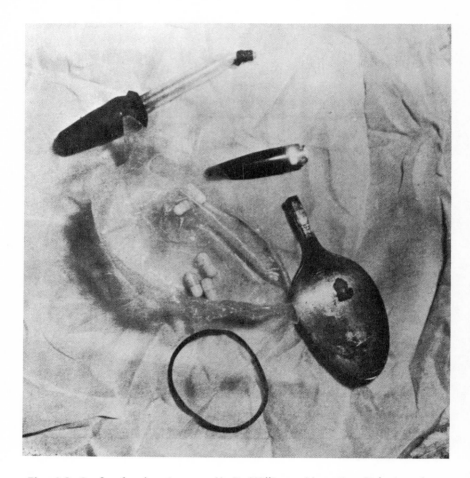

Fig. 4.3 Outfit of a heroin user. (J. D. Williams, *Narcotics,* Dubuque, Iowa, Wm. C. Brown Company, 1963.)

so-called "cold turkey" treatment, is very painful and can be dangerous. During withdrawal the addict experiences a range of symptoms— nausea, watering of the eyes, muscle spasms in the stomach and legs, and hot and cold flashes. In barbiturate withdrawal, convulsions and delirium tremens may occur. In both barbiturate and opiate addiction, abrupt withdrawal has sometimes been fatal.

In opiate cases, the synthetic drug methadone is usually substituted for the addicting drug, and complete withdrawal takes a week or two in most cases. In barbiturate withdrawal, pentobarbital is generally used, and withdrawal takes several days or weeks.

After withdrawal, a slow rehabilitation can begin. A special treatment center, such as a hospital or institutional facility, may be used for the first steps. The addict should be retained in such a treatment center for several months before he is returned to the community. The treatment program must provide many rehabilitative services—medical, physical, vocational, and educational. The return should be made in stages. Short visits home should be made first; then a halfway house, a work camp, or a day-night hospital may be useful if it can provide the addict with social, therapeutic, and vocational services to give him controlled contacts with his community.

LEGAL COMMITMENT FOR DRUG ADDICTION

The federal government treatment centers are maintained by the Public Health Service. The two narcotics treatment centers are at Lexington, Kentucky, and Fort Worth, Texas. These hospitals accept patients addicted only to opiates, cocaine, or marijuana. Three classes of patients are admitted: (1) voluntary patients, (2) prisoners—addicts convicted of violating federal narcotic laws, and (3) probationers—addicts convicted of the same offenses but given suspended sentences on condition that they accept hospital treatment. The Lexington hospital accepts female patients from any section of the country and male patients from east of the Mississippi River. The Fort Worth Hospital accepts only male patients from west of the Mississippi and the New Orleans area. A minimum of four and one-half months of treatment is required. Indigent patients are treated free of charge; others pay a nominal charge. An application for treatment is made directly to the Medical Officer in charge at either hospital.

Individual states almost without exception lack proper facilities and adequate programs for treatment of narcotics addiction. A majority of states attempt treatment in state-operated mental or general hospitals. The few that have posthospital programs recognize the inadequacies and indicate a pessimistic attitude toward the programs.

A promising step in the right direction was taken by New York with the opening of Riverside Hospital in the Bronx in 1952. This hospital received juvenile addicts only; its research on preadult addiction increased the knowledge so desperately needed in this field. It has since been closed. In New York there are also a variety of narcotics programs, both state and municipal.

California has also instituted a program for the control and treatment of narcotics abusers who have been convicted of a felony (the felony need not be a narcotics offense) or are committed through civil action. And Detroit and Chicago have experimented with rehabilitation services for addicts who voluntarily seek help.

States with a small drug-abuse problem face a special problem. It may be prohibitively expensive for such states to establish special rehabilitation facilities and programs. These states might explore with neighboring states the feasibility of establishing regional facilities.

CIVIL COMMITMENT FOR DRUG ADDICTION

Civil commitment is a legal mechanism utilized in lieu of a criminal commitment to ensure control over addicts and potential addicts during rehabilitation, first in an institution, later in a halfway house, and still later in the community under the close supervision of a probation or parole officer. The significant step in this program is that the victim does not establish a criminal record when seeking treatment and help. The Civil Commitment program was pioneered by California and New York.

The California program. The California law provides for the civil commitment of people who are addicted to narcotics or who are in imminent danger of becoming addicted. The law distinguishes three categories of people who may be civilly committed: (1) those convicted of a misdemeanor; (2) those convicted of felonies other than crimes of violence; and (3) those who report to the district attorney their belief that they are, or are about to become, addicted, or who are reported to the district attorney by relatives, friends, or others.

In the case of those convicted of a misdemeanor or felony, further criminal proceedings are suspended after a conviction or plea of guilty; then a petition for civil commitment may be filed and a hearing held. If it is found that the defendant is addicted or in imminent danger of becoming addicted, the court may commit him to the Director of the State Department of Corrections for a maximum period of seven years. On a finding that the defendant is not an addict nor in danger of becoming an addict, the commitment court will return him to the criminal court for sentencing. If at any time after 60 days the Director of Corrections concludes that a committed defendant is not a fit subject for treatment, he is returned to the criminal court for sentencing.

In the case of those who are not charged with the commission of a crime, the commitment court may, after a medical examination and a hearing, deny the petition and discharge the person, or order him committed to the Director of Corrections. When the person has voluntarily sought commitment, the maximum period of commitment is two and one-half years. The Director of Corrections may discharge the patient if the Director concludes at any time after 60 days that the patient is not a fit subject for the program.

The New York program. Under the New York civil commitment law, popularly known as the Metcalf-Volker Act, there are three categories of addicts eligible for admission to the rehabilitation program. The process of commitment, the length of time for which an addict can be held, and the procedures of the program differ with respect to each category.

The largest category covers narcotics addicts who have been arrested for narcotics law violations or other criminal offenses, with the exception of certain serious crimes, but have not yet been convicted. There must be no extensive history of prior felonies or of failures under prior commitments, and there must be no objection from the district attorney.

The addict-offender must request commitment within 10 days of his arrest. If he does, he may be committed for treatment only if the above conditions are met, if the Commissioner of Mental Hygiene is willing to accept him, and if there are adequate facilities available. The total period of commitment may not exceed 3 years, whether spent in a treatment facility or in the community under supervision. If in the course of treatment it is found that the addict offender is unresponsive or uncooperative, he is returned to the court. If he completes the treatment program successfully, he is discharged and the criminal charge dismissed.

The second category includes narcotics addicts who voluntarily commit themselves to a treatment facility or, if under the age of 21, are committed on application by their next of kin. They may be held without a hearing and given treatment for a period of at least 45 days, and longer *if they consent*. Where there has been a hearing, they may be held and given treatment for a period of not more than one year. The addict may be discharged before the expiration of a year if he has recovered or if he is not responsive to treatment.

The third category covers addicts convicted of a crime who are placed on probation by the court on condition that they submit to treatment. Again, the Commissioner of Mental Hygiene must be willing to accept the addict for treatment and adequate facilities must be available. The entire course of treatment cannot exceed the period of probation imposed by the court. If he has recovered or if he is unresponsive or uncooperative, the addict may be returned to the court before the expiration of the probationary period.

EFFECTS OF NARCOTICS AND OTHER DRUGS

Psychological dependence is the one effect which exists in all commonly used or abused drugs that affect the central nervous system. Some substances, such as nicotine and caffeine, can also produce psychological dependence in the user, but these do not produce abnormal psychic behavior in him. The drugs which create problems within society are the drugs which induce psychic manifestations and cause abnormal social behavior. In an attempt to point out the *effects* of drugs rather than to just classify them, Dr. M. H. Seevers suggests that the term "psychotoxic" be used to express such a condition. Table 4.2 is an attempt to present the scientific facts concerning drugs having psychotoxic effects and their relationships with legal and regulatory controls.

The most commonly abused drugs are classified as to their effects on the central and autonomic nervous systems. The following is such a classification.

DEPRESSANTS

The most widely publicized drugs which are abused to a great extent throughout the world are the *opiates* and the *synthetic narcotics*. Their depressant actions include analgesia (relief of pain), sedation (freeing the mind from anxiety, relaxing the muscles, and calming the body), hypnosis (drowsiness or sleep), and euphoria (an exaggerated sense of well-being and contentment).

The main use of narcotics in medicine is for their ability (unlike anesthetics) to produce marked analgesia without excessive drowsiness, muscular weakness, confusion, or loss of consciousness. The narcotics, however, cannot be used effectively as anesthetics, owing to the fact that they depress the respiratory center.

OPIUM

Opium is the juice obtained by cutting the unripe capsule of the Oriental poppy (*Papaver somniferum,* Fig. 4.4). Since each plant yields little juice, large areas of poppies must be planted to produce any large amount of opium. They can be grown profitably only where climate conditions are favorable (hot and dry) and land and labor are cheap—as in India, Turkey, and in certain parts of Russia, China, Egypt, and Mexico.

In opium-producing areas, after the heat of the day has passed the workers go through the fields and make incisions into the capsules or pods of the poppy flower (Fig. 4.5). During the cool night the milky white juice of the pods oozes to the surface. As it comes in contact with the air, it oxidizes, thickens, and takes on a reddish-brown color. The following morning the workers again go among the plants, scrape off the now heavy molasses-like fluid, and collect it on poppy leaves. This material gradually hardens, forming gum-like balls, almost black in color; this is opium in its raw state.

This sticky mass has a bitter taste and a heavy, sweet odor. When opium is being smoked, the odor greatly resembles that of wet, smouldering eucalyptus wood. Opium is generally smoked in an opium pipe or eaten. American drug addicts seldom use opium but do use its derivatives.

Morphine and codeine are the only important narcotic substances obtainable directly from opium, which contains 10 percent morphine

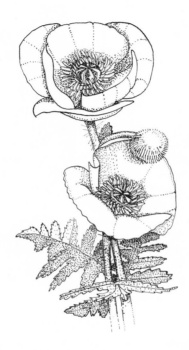

Fig. 4.4 Oriental poppy (*Papaver somniferum*). (J. D. Williams, *Narcotics*, Dubuque, Iowa, Wm. C. Brown Company, 1963.)

and 0.5 percent codeine.[9] The other opium derivatives—such as heroin, Dilaudid, Metopon, and Nalline—are obtainable by chemical modifications of morphine and codeine.

MORPHINE

Morphine is the chief derivative of opium. It is produced by chemically refining opium. It can be pure white, light brown, or off-white; and it may be in the form of a cube, capsule, tablet, powder, or solution. On the illegal market morphine that comes in a gelatin capsule is known

[9] P. G. Stecher, ed., *The Merck Index,* 7th ed., Rahway, N.J., Merck & Co., Inc., 1960, p. 756.

as a "cap." The powder folded into a paper is known as a "deck" or "package." Morphine is about 10 times stronger than opium; therefore, its attack upon the mentality and physical condition of the user may be swift and strong. Unlike heroin, very little morphine is sold by peddlers. When morphine is unlawfully possessed, it usually has been stolen from a physician or pharmacist or obtained by means of forgery on a prescription form stolen from a physician.

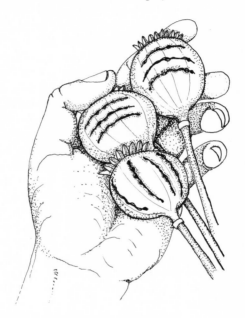

Fig. 4.5 Capsules, or pods, of the poppy flower.

Although morphine is taken into the body mostly by hypodermic injection, some addicts use it orally. This latter method, called a "stomach habit," is not common, since oral ingestion necessitates a larger quantity of narcotic to obtain the desired euphoric effect and the action is slower.[10]

A physician administering drugs will give a subcutaneous injection (injection under the skin). This method which may be used by some addicts at first is known as a "skin pop." It gives too slow an action for the confirmed addict, so he resorts to taking intravenous injections, that is, injections directly into the blood stream through the vein, which immediately gives the desired effect. This type of injection is known as a "mainline."

[10] J. D. Williams, *op. cit.*

HEROIN

Heroin is produced from morphine. It is from 20 to 25 times stronger than morphine, with twice morphine's addictive powers; thus it is a very dangerous drug. In the pure state it is a grayish-brown powder. But, because of its great strength, the peddler is able to dilute it many times with milk sugar (lactose) and still deliver a potent drug to the addict. Consequently the heroin is "cut" in this manner and loses its grayish-brown color, becoming white or off-white, greatly resembling morphine. Seizures of heroin often test 4, 3, or even 1 percent or less in purity. Heroin is odorless and has a distinctly bitter flavor.

The wholesale peddler sells heroin by the kilogram or in 1 ounce or smaller glassine paper bags. The retailers or "pushers" handle it in paper "decks" or "bindles" and in clear or red "caps."

Beginners may introduce the drug to their bodies through the nostrils by "sniffing," but they are soon forced to inject it, due to the inflammation of the nose that "sniffing" produces and the greater "kick" obtained by injection. They begin by injecting it into the fleshy parts of the arm or body, but their rapidly mounting tolerance necessitates injection directly into the veins for the desired euphoric effects. At this point the addict is referred to as a "mainliner." A standard hypodermic needle attached to a syringe or common medicine dropper, as shown in Fig. 4.3, may be used. When a needle is not available, the drug may be forced into the body by opening a blood vessel with a pin or razor blade and the heroin "shot" in directly with the medicine dropper. Generally a tourniquet is attached to the upper arm to bring the main vein into prominence. With constant injection, the blood vessels break down and scars form over the veins, causing the addict to seek new areas for injection until the entire length of the arms are marked by needle punctures. Prolonged addiction results in the necessity to inject between the fingers, in the legs and the neck, above the hairline, and even inside the mouth.

Heroin is about four times more toxic than morphine, and its action has a more demoralizing effect. The danger of addiction to heroin is greater than that to any other drug because the body's tolerance to the drug builds very rapidly. The addict requires increasingly larger doses in a short time in order to secure the original effects. Addicts prefer heroin to morphine and take morphine only when they cannot get heroin.

Heroin is considered the most dangerous of the narcotic drugs, and because of its effects, the manufacture and sale of heroin in the United States and its importation from abroad are prohibited by federal law (Opium and Narcotic Laws, 1964).

CODEINE

Codeine is milder than the drugs discussed above in its power to induce sleep and relieve pain. It is widely used as an ingredient in cough medicines. It is manufactured as an odorless white crystal or crystalline powder and is used as a tablet or in solution. Generally, throughout the United States, preparations containing not more than one grain of codeine per ounce can be sold over the counter, but the pharmacist must record the name of the purchaser. In some states preparations will bear a label with these words, "Contains Codeine (Opium derivation) WARNING—may be habit-forming. Do not give to children except upon advice of a physician."

Narcotics addicts will sometimes resort to the use of codeine when deprived of their regular supply of heroin. It is not widely used because of its mild effects, but it is still very addicting.[11]

SYNTHETIC NARCOTICS

Synthetic narcotics differ from the opiates in that they are made synthetically in the laboratory, starting with coal-tar or petroleum products, which, before chemical conversion, have no narcotic properties. Some of the more commonly known synthetic narcotics are Demerol, methadone, Dromoran, and Amytal.

The likelihood of addiction with synthetic narcotics is less than that with morphine or heroin, but all produce addiction and strong withdrawal symptoms in the addict when the drug is abruptly withdrawn. The use of synthetically produced narcotics, such as Demerol or Seconal, is limited mostly to the medical and paramedical professions, where they are available, rather than on the illegal market.

Some of the opiate derivatives and their compounds are now produced synthetically, because of the high cost of the natural production of opium. The more common synthetic compounds are Dionin, Dilaudid, Percodan, Nucodan, Perco-barb, and Nalline.

BARBITURATES

A variety of drugs can produce a state of depression of the central nervous system resembling normal sleep. These drugs are referred to as hypnotics. In small doses many can produce drowsiness; when used in this manner they are known as sedatives. The most important hypnotics are the barbiturates, which have the ability to induce sleep, but are

[11] J. D. Williams, *op. cit.*

either completely devoid of any ability to relieve pain or possess this property to a very minor degree.

Several hundred barbituric compounds have been synthesized and tested; approximately 20 of them have been found to possess properties satisfactory for medical use. The barbiturates induce sleep promptly and, because of their action on the cerebral cortex, are especially effective in treating conditions of worry, muscular twitching, tremors, and convulsions. The compounds differ chiefly in the duration of their effect. The hypnotic effects of barbital and phenobarbital may last as long as 8 hours; those of sodium pentothal, used as a surgical anesthetic, as little as 20 minutes.

On the illegal market, barbiturates are known as "goof-balls." The individual names of separate barbiturates commonly found are shown in Fig. 4.6.

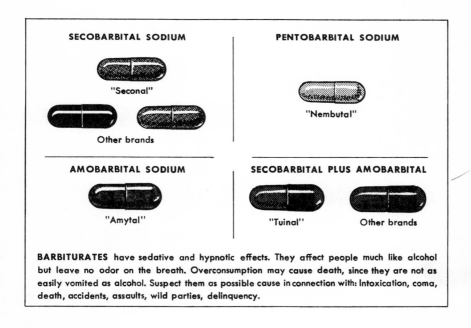

SECOBARBITAL SODIUM

"Seconal"

Other brands

PENTOBARBITAL SODIUM

"Nembutal"

AMOBARBITAL SODIUM

"Amytal"

SECOBARBITAL PLUS AMOBARBITAL

"Tuinal"   Other brands

BARBITURATES have sedative and hypnotic effects. They affect people much like alcohol but leave no odor on the breath. Overconsumption may cause death, since they are not as easily vomited as alcohol. Suspect them as possible cause in connection with: Intoxication, coma, death, accidents, assaults, wild parties, delinquency.

Fig. 4.6 Barbiturate drugs, actual size. (California State Bureau of Narcotic Enforcement.)

Barbiturates are usually taken orally ("dropped"); however, addicts have been known to dissolve the compound and inject it hypodermically. Sometimes they are "dropped" with alcohol and sometimes with benzedrine or dexedrine (amphetamines) to overcome the depressing effects of the barbiturates.

A person under the influence of barbiturates acts like one who has had enough alcohol to show signs of it. How much of the drug is necessary to produce the degree of intoxication observed depends mostly on how accustomed to the drug the person is. Addicts keep taking more and more, and in time they get to amounts that would kill anybody who had not grown accustomed to the drug gradually. Whenever a person acts as if he has had a little or a great deal to drink, but there is no odor of alcohol, it is possible that he has been using barbiturates. Sometimes when barbiturates and alcohol are taken together, they produce what looks like an ordinary "drunk" but the "drunk" takes much longer to sober up. The person who gets drunk on barbiturates follows about the same course as the person who takes a drink and keeps on until he passes out. A small amount makes him feel relaxed, sociable, and good-humored, but he loses alertness and is slow to react. After taking more, he becomes sluggish, gloomy, maybe quarrelsome. His tongue becomes "thick," he staggers about for awhile, and then gradually he slumps into a deep sleep; or, if he has had a large amount of the drug, he may suddenly collapse into a coma. In a coma, he may die unless he receives medical attention promptly. Barbiturates are more dangerous than alcohol because they are not vomited, and all the drug that is taken into the stomach will be absorbed unless the stomach is pumped. Even when there is no sign of life from a person in a coma, a doctor should be called at once, because some cases have been revived.

Those who become addicted to barbiturates must have them to prevent going into withdrawal. Without the drug they will have seizures that resemble epileptic convulsions and which very often are severe enough to cause death. Sudden withdrawal from barbiturates without medical attention often results in death.

BROMIDES

The bromides exert a sedative effect on the central nervous system. They were widely utilized in medicine and by the general public in the past. But with a growing recognition of the dangers of chronic bromide intoxication, the cumulative action of the drugs, and the development of much more effective sedatives, the modern physician finds few uses for bromides. They are still important to a health study, however, because of the problems of bromide intoxication and poisoning.

The administration of sodium bromide or other bromide salts produces sedation, drowsiness, and sleep. Chronic administration of bromide tends to produce mental depression, confusion, and lethargy. Many individuals in this condition may be suspected of suffering from emotional conditions; in fact, some individuals have been admitted to mental hospitals when the toxic nature of the symptoms were not recognized. In bromide intoxication, various skin lesions, intestinal disturbances, and destruction of the membranes of the eyes and respiratory passages are common.

Bromides, although capable of inducing psychogenic dependence, are rarely abused, and neither tolerance nor physical dependence is induced in the user at any dosage level. This drug is not addicting, but it is highly dangerous because of its extreme toxicity.[12]

CHLORAL HYDRATE AND PARALDEHYDE

Both chloral hydrate and paraldehyde are effective hypnotics whose popularity has been decreased considerably, largely because the barbiturates are now much more convenient to administer. Both chloral hydrate and paraldehyde have a disagreeable taste and must be taken in special solutions to disguise their unpleasant properties. Addiction to these two hypnotics is very uncommon.

Chloral hydrate, when taken orally, tends to cause some stomach irritation but induces rapid and refreshing sleep. The toxicity is low, but with the simultaneous administration of alcohol, it is increased. Chloral hydrate is the basis of so-called "knockout drops." The lethal dose of this drug is highly variable.

Paraldehyde is an odorous liquid. Oral administration, usually over shaved ice or in some cold drink, induces rapid sleep in most persons. Paraldehyde is seldom used as an ordinary hypnotic. Its disagreeable and characteristic odor is noticeable to others for many hours following ingestion of the drug. It is used in hospitalized patients in the management of delirium tremens, withdrawal illness, and convulsions.[13]

ALCOHOL

Alcohol is a truly addictive drug. The sudden withdrawal of alcohol in the addict produces serious disturbances. These may vary from craving, anxiety, and tremors to the full-blown picture of delirium tremens, which is found in the most severe cases of alcoholism. Although some psychiatrists believe that delirium tremens is an acute toxic psychosis (alcoholic psychosis), other experts in the field regard it as a form of withdrawal syndrome.

Further information and discussion of alcohol and alcoholism will be found in Chapter 5.

12 H. N. Wright and M. Montag, *Pharmacology and Therapeutics*, 7th ed., Philadelphia, Saunders, 1959.
13 *Ibid.*

TRANQUILIZERS

The essential difference between older hypnotics and the newer tranquilizers is that the newer compounds can suppress anxiety, diminish abnormal behavior, and calm an individual at dose levels that do not result in a profound hypnotic effect.

The introduction of these drugs has had a great impact on psychiatry and medicine in general. It must be recognized that they are drugs which do not cure emotional and mental illnesses nor eliminate the cause of anxiety, but they have facilitated the management of various conditions. Some of the most universally used compounds are Equanil, Atarax, Librium, and Valium. The list of these drugs is still growing.

Tranquilizers, in themselves, are not commonly used illegally, because they do not produce an euphoric effect. Any addiction would be from increased dosage over a long period of time. Some addiction to these drugs has been recorded, but dosages recommended by a physician may be maintained for extremely long periods of time without adverse effects. When large doses are taken for long periods, a sudden withdrawal may result in muscular twitching, convulsions, and other physiological changes.

The deliberate or accidental taking of overdoses of tranquilizers is now as common as former overdoses of barbiturates. Suicidal attempts with meprobamate (Miltown or Equanil) are not uncommon; but, since the drug does not cause the same intensity of central nervous system depression as do other drugs, these attempts are rarely successful. In the United States, in 10 years only 8 suicidal deaths were reported with compounds containing this tranquilizer.

STIMULANTS

The action of stimulants is directly opposite to that of the hypnotics and narcotics in that they are used to produce energy or wakefulness. As a group they are not physically addicting, but the user does show psychological dependence and psychotoxic effects during their administration.

COCAINE

In criminal law cocaine is classified as a narcotic, although its general effect is stimulating rather than depressing. In the medical sense cocaine has a depressing effect only locally, when used as a local anesthetic; the systemic effect to the body is to stimulate and induce excitement.

The cocaine is extracted from the leaves of the coca shrub (*Erythroxylon coca*). This plant is a native of Peru and Bolivia, where the leaves have been habitually chewed by the natives for over 400 years. Cocaine is processed into an odorless, white, fluffy, fine crystalline powder, similar to snow in appearance. Consequently, on the criminal market it is commonly referred to as "snow." It is usually sold in the same type of containers as heroin. However, the price is much higher because of its scarcity.

Cocaine is taken by sniffing into the nostrils, rarely by hypodermic injection. Sniffing is the most popular method because the rate of absorption is slower, the effects last longer, and the drug's intensity is tempered. Advanced narcotics addicts mix cocaine and heroin for hypodermic use. This type of a shot is called a "speed-ball."

Under the influence of cocaine, the user presents dilated pupils (see Fig. 4.2) which will not react to light. He has a twitching of the nerves and a tendency to rub the nose and grit the teeth. He is very talkative and will not listen; he is flighty and excitable and finds it hard to focus his attention. The first general effects of use of cocaine are pleasure; fatigue disappears and the user feels strong and superior. At this time the user may have auditory and visual delusions and hallucinations. These last only a short time and are followed by depression and nervous apprehension, which are only relieved by his taking another dose. Prolonged use of cocaine causes deterioration of the nervous system, which brings about tremors, sleeplessness, and general emaciation. The last stage of cocaine addiction leads to a state of delirium in which the user develops what is known as "Bull horrors" or "seeing Steve."

This powerful drug is harsher than morphine, and its attack upon the mentality and physique is swifter and stronger. It is habit-forming but not addicting. The withdrawal symptoms found in narcotics addiction are not encountered with cocaine.

AMPHETAMINES

The two most widely used amphetamines are benzedrine and dexedrine. On the illegal market they are known as "bennies," "dexies," or "pep" pills (Fig. 4.7). These are central nervous system stimulants.

Medicinal doses taken by mouth tend to keep an individual awake, decrease the feeling of fatigue, and decrease the appetite. Higher or prolonged use produces hallucinations, feelings of elation and superiority, excitement, and relief from fatigue. As their effects wear off, the user feels weak, depressed, and restless. The physical appearance of someone under the influence of amphetamines greatly corresponds to that of a user of cocaine.

Amphetamines make a person active; if he keeps taking more, he can keep going for hours or even days without sleep or rest. Consequently, these drugs are misused by individuals who want to work or play harder or longer than their normal capacity allows. Also, persons who feel that the drugs make them more lively, talkative, and self-confident become highly habituated to the amphetamines. The stim-

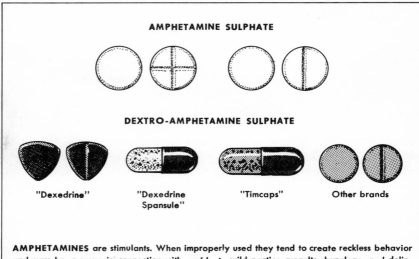

AMPHETAMINE SULPHATE

DEXTRO-AMPHETAMINE SULPHATE

"Dexedrine"   "Dexedrine   "Timcaps"   Other brands
                      Spansule"

AMPHETAMINES are stimulants. When improperly used they tend to create reckless behavior and may be a cause in connection with accidents, wild parties, assaults, burglary, and delinquency. They are less dangerous than barbiturates to the persons consuming them.

Fig. 4.7 Amphetamine drugs, actual size. There are many other brands of amphetamine sulfate available in white or colored tablets and time disintegration capsules. (California State Bureau of Narcotic Enforcement.)

ulating effect of amphetamines is sometimes relied upon by criminals to increase their "nerve." Barbiturate addicts will often take amphetamines and barbiturates together because the amphetamines will counteract the hypnotic action of the barbiturates. Possibly the greatest danger from amphetamines is the effect they have on automobile drivers. When many of these drugs are taken at one time, or if they are used over too long a period without rest or sleep, they may produce hallucinations in which a person thinks he sees something that really is not there. He may even "black out" suddenly while driving at high speed.

Amphetamines do not create energy in the body, but whatever energy is stored is released by the drugs' suppressing the feeling of fatigue and the need for sleep. They decrease the appetite, cutting down the normal intake of food. This lack of food, sleep, and rest can ruin the physical health of a long-time user. Figure 4.8 clearly illustrates this point. These are three photographs of the same individual taken 6 months apart. His physical deterioration is evident.

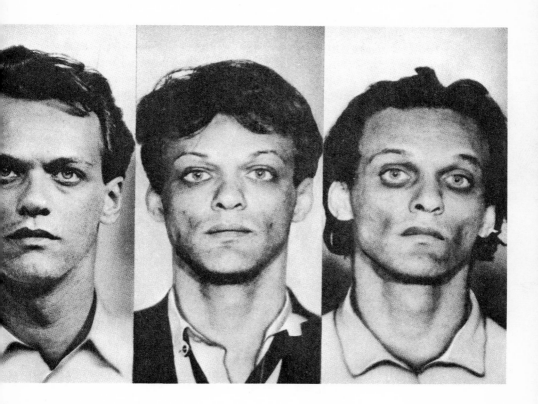

Fig. 4.8 Physical characteristics of an amphetamine user. (From *Chicago's American*.)

A strong psychological habituation may occur with these drugs. But since the body does not develop a tolerance, there are no true withdrawal symptoms, and thus physical addiction does not occur.

MARIJUANA

Marijuana is a highly unpredictable drug consisting of the dried leaves and flowering tops of the hemp plant (*Cannabis sativa*). Many varieties of this plant are grown throughout the world. The leaves and flowering tops secrete an amber-colored resin containing the substance *cannabine,* or *cannabinol,* which is believed to be the substance causing the intoxication. Cannabis is known under many names throughout the world. The word *marijuana,* or *marihuana,* is a Mexican word of uncertain derivation. Other names include Indian hemp, Canadian hemp, kif, hashish, bhang, charas, ganja, Indian hay, and loco ("crazy") weed.

This plant attains a height of from 3 to 16 feet. The flowers are irregular clusters of seed of a light yellowish-green. The leaves are compound, of from 5 to 11 (always an uneven number) leaflets or lobes extending from 2 to 6 inches from the center diagonally to the edges. The two outer lobes are always very small compared with the others. The leaf is deep green on the upper side and lighter green on the lower edge. The live green plant has a peculiar odor, is sticky to the touch, and is covered with fine hairs that are barely visible to the naked eye. The stalks and stems are used in the textile industry for the manufacture of rope, twine, mats, bags, and certain grades of coarse paper.

Most of the marijuana sold in the United States is grown in Mexico, although it grows wild in the United States and has been cultivated illegally on roofs, in backyards, between rows of corn, and in many other places. Marijuana is sold in bulk "tins" (old tobacco cans) or as cigarettes. The cigarettes are usually rolled in brown wheat-straw paper, ordinarily utilizing a double thickness to prevent the sharp edges of the plant from cutting through the paper. The ends of the cigarette are folded to prevent losing the marijuana when it is being carried. When smoked, the material burns faster and brighter than an ordinary cigarette, a difference easily discernible to an observer at night. Burning marijuana has the smell of burning hay or weeds.

The chief causes of the use of marijuana are curiosity and a desire to escape from an unpleasant environment. The majority of users are adolescents. Adolescent use is particularly dangerous, because after awhile the "kicks" from marijuana are not as great as they were in the beginning and then the user looks for something stronger, "graduating" to heroin, morphine, or barbiturates. Marijuana has been called the stepping stone to addiction.

Marijuana is an excitant or stimulating drug. It disrupts the brain functions and distorts the mind. It attacks the central nervous system and violently affects the mentality and the five physical senses. Time, space, and distance are obliterated, and hallucinations occur. This drug used with alcohol intensifies its violent properties. It gives a feeling of exaltation and physical power. Marijuana, like cocaine, has been known to be the immediate and direct cause of many violent crimes. A person under the influence of marijuana is very dangerous. The great danger of this drug is its unpredictable release of the user's inhibitions, accompanied by a diminution or loss of moral sense. The user is very often dangerous to handle or control, has no fear, and feels no pain.

Physical reactions usually appear approximately one-half hour after smoking the drug; they include quickening of the pulse, rapid heart beat, muscular twitchings, and dilation of the pupils of the eyes (see Fig. 4.2). The individual may be violent, happy, morose, stuporous, or "high." He has intense emotions, ranging from laughter to weeping, and not infrequently an intense fear, often of impending death. There is strong euphoria accompanied by hallucinations. There is an intense desire for activity, which finds expression in fantastic motions, dancing, running, and jumping. It is during this stage that most of the users' crimes are committed. The phases of stimulation and hallucination later give way to a period of indescribable calm and contentment. This period passes into one of drowsiness and finally into sleep. The sleep lasts for several hours; then the individual awakens feeling refreshed, with a clear memory of the experiences through which he has passed.

Marijuana is not an addicting drug. It creates a strong psychological dependence but no physiological dependence. When the user is deprived of the drug, there are no withdrawal symptoms; at most, he will feel a mere craving much like that of a tobacco user.

SOLVENTS

The deliberate inhalation of solvent vapors from plastic or airplane cement to induce sensations of euphoria and exhilaration has become a source of major concern to physicians, school authorities, and law enforcement officials. "Glue-sniffing," as it is popularly called, results in effects which vary from an early state of mild intoxication to disorientation and coma if exposure to the vapors is prolonged.

Several dangerous solvents are used in the manufacture of these cements. The most common and most deadly are isoamyl acetate and ethyl acetate. Other dangerous solvents used are benzine, toluene, and carbon tetrachloride. High concentrations of these solvents are also found in cleaning fluids, paints, and thinners. Prolonged inhalation of any of them may cause death.

In the initial stage of inhalation, prior to addiction, a few whiffs of the vapors will produce a "jag"; but tolerance to the solvents develops very rapidly, and then the user "takes" the contents of many tubes in order to experience the desired effect. The immediate effect is one of pleasant exhilaration, euphoria, and excitement, closely simulating the early stages of alcohol intoxication. The individual acts "drunk" and exhibits disorientation and slurred speech. This period of intoxication lasts 30 to 45 minutes after inhalation. Drowsiness, stupor, and unconsciousness may then ensue. The person may remain unresponsive for periods of as long as an hour or more.

An addicted glue-sniffer's breath often has an unpleasant odor and he may experience excessive oral secretions. These secretions result from the vapor's irritation of the mucous membranes of the nose and mouth and require frequent expectoration. The sniffer suffers from insomnia, nausea, and weight loss.

The toxic effects of these solvents have been carefully observed. They include irritation of mucous membrane, skin, and the respiratory tract; excitation and depression of the central nervous system; cellular injury to the heart, liver, and kidneys; and bone marrow depression, which results in anemia, leukopenia (reduction of the number of white blood cells), and thrombocytopenia (decrease in the number of blood platelets). There have also been reports of mental deterioration, acute liver damage, and death following kidney failure.

The strong psychological dependence, the psychotoxic effects (during administration), strong tolerance, and the necessity to increase the dose would seem to categorize the solvents as addicting drugs. But upon withdrawal of the solvents from a user there are few severe withdrawal symptoms. Consequently, some individuals classify them as habituating drugs.

HALLUCINOGENS

Hallucinogenic, or *psychotomimetic,* drugs are drugs capable of turning a normal person temporarily into a psychotic. The first recognized hallucinogens were mescaline, a drug obtained from the cactus peyote (*Lophophora williamsii*); psilocybine, extracted from a vision-producing mushroom (*Psilocybe mexicana*); and a synthetic drug based on lysergic acid, a chemical derived from ergot, a black fungus that grows on rye and wheat, known as LSD (lysergic acid diethylamide). Since that time a number of other hallucinogenic drugs have been extracted or synthesized and tested. Two of the more common are DMT (dimethyltryptamine) and CI-395 (phencyclidine). LSD, mescaline, and DMT are all chemically related and usually administered in tablet or liquid form. CI-395 is administered intravenously.

The strongest of all of the hallucinogens is LSD; it is 100 times more potent than psilocybine and 7000 times stronger than mescaline. The effects of LSD last 8 to 12 hours; of psilocybine, 4 to 6 hours; of DMT, about 1 hour.

LSD

LSD is a tasteless, colorless, and odorless drug. Although no true addiction to LSD has been recorded, it can be definitely stated that habituation to its psychological effects does occur. Individuals with access to large supplies have taken the drug many times and have had great difficulty in breaking themselves of the habit. Under clinical conditions toxic or prolonged psychological complications from its use have been rare. But LSD is an extremely dangerous drug; severe physical damage, including death, has occurred to those who have illegally purchased and administered LSD without supervision.

LSD dilates the pupils, raises the systolic blood pressure, and increases the strength of the reflexes. It stimulates the brain's sensory centers, at the same time blocking the inhibiting mechanisms. LSD produces visual hallucinations in all ranges of color, intensifies hearing, increases the sensitivity to feel texture, and may produce a tingling feeling and a numbness of the hands and feet. Changes in taste and smell are infrequently reported; when they do occur, they are enhanced. Subjects often report cross-overs of sensation; for example, they may hear colors or smell music.

Under clinical conditions, the side effects of LSD seem to be physical discomfort—nausea, vomiting, aches, and pains. Anxiety and panic occur during the subject's struggle to maintain control of the situation and fear frequently occurs because of his distorted time perception.

At the present time illegal commerce in LSD, mescaline, and psilocybine is concentrated in the larger cities and on some university campuses. LSD is peddled in pills and ampules, and on paper or sugar cubes onto which a small amount of the drug (in liquid form) has been dropped. Because of the extremely disturbed reactions of those who have used it illegally, this drug may either have been contaminated or been mixed with other substances. Since the legal production and distribution of LSD is closely controlled, very little, if any, is going into the illegal market. Illegal supplies are being produced in Mexico and other foreign countries, and in basement laboratories in the United States. California and Nevada were leaders in outlawing LSD and other psychotomimetic drugs. These laws are modeled after their state laws pertaining to the possession and selling of heroin.

The hallucinogenic drugs have been used by psychologists as research tools into some of the emotional conditions affecting man. LSD especially has been used experimentally in the treatment of alcoholism with mixed results. Some researchers have found it to be a useful tool while others seem to think the results are not lasting or may lead to further emotional dysorganization.

MESCALINE

Mescaline comes from the button-like leaves of a small cactus plant, peyote (*Lophophora williamsii*), shown in Fig. 4.9. The normal growth area of this cactus is the watershed of the Rio Grande River. The

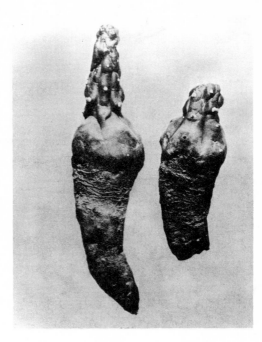

Fig. 4.9 Peyote (*Lophophora williamsii*). (California State Bureau of Narcotic Enforcement.)

button-like leaves may be dried and later chewed, or boiled and the broth drunk. Buttons which have been chewed and swallowed produce intoxication lasting from 12 to 18 hours.

Its physiological effects include increased pulse rate, elevated blood pressure, muscle twitching, and profuse sweating. The psychic reactions that occur are visual hallucinations, in which the person "sees" beautiful colors in fantastic geometric patterns. Feelings of depersonalization are common, and toxic psychosis may develop.

The use of mescaline is almost entirely culturally determined, being legally restricted in North America to certain Indian tribes in the West, Southwest, and Mexico. Peyote is ritualistically chewed about an hour before important religious festivals. Mescaline is a hallucinogen legally listed as a narcotic and therefore has state laws restricting its cultivation and use.

SUMMARY

I. Drug Abuse
   A. When abused, drugs become man's worst enemies.

B. *The History of Narcotics Addiction in the United States* is shown in Fig. 4.1.

II. Drug Habituation (drug abuse)—the use of drugs for purposes other than those intended in medicine.

III. Medical Definition of Drug Addiction
    A. Drugs which evoke:
        1. Psychological dependence—an uncontrollable compulsion to experience the drug's euphoric effects at any cost.
        2. Tolerance—a survival mechanism permitting body cells to be exposed to toxic substances without producing damage.
        3. Physical dependence—successive larger and larger doses are necessary to achieve the euphoric effects desired.
        4. Sudden withdrawal of drugs produces withdrawal illness or abstinence syndrome.

IV. Legal Definition of Addiction
    A. Based upon the illicit or illegal possession of a narcotic or dangerous drug.
        1. Narcotics, as defined by federal laws, are
            a. Opium and coca leaves or their derivatives.
            b. Marijuana or peyote (mescaline).
            c. Specific synthetic drugs.
        2. Dangerous drugs are declared and listed by the federal Pure Food and Drugs Administration.

V. Legal Control of Narcotics and Dangerous Drugs
    A. Federal control of narcotics:
        1. First federal law (1909) prohibited the importation of opium, except for medicinal purposes.
        2. First effective law—Harrison Narcotic Act (1914).
        3. Narcotic Drugs Import and Export Act (1922), an extensive revision of the Harrison Act.
        4. Marijuana Tax Act (1937) is now part of the Internal Revenue Code.
        5. Opium Poppy Control Act (1942) prohibits the cultivation of the opium poppy except under license from the federal government.
        6. Federal statutory penalties are set forth in the Narcotics Control Act (Bogg's Act, 1956).
    B. Federal and state control of dangerous drugs:
        1. Federal Food, Drug and Cosmetic Act (1938) established dispensing procedures for drugs considered unsafe for self-medication.
        2. Durham-Humphrey Amendment (1951) strengthened and clarified controls and distribution of dangerous drugs.
    C. Control of narcotics by states:
        1. Model uniform state narcotics law submitted to states in 1932.
        2. In recent years heavier penalties have been enacted by several states.

VI. Economic Aspects of Drug Abuse
    A. Principal sources of illicit narcotics are
        1. Opium and heroin—Communist China, Italy, Mexico.
        2. Cocaine—Peru and Bolivia, through Cuba.
        3. Marijuana—Mexico.
        4. Legally manufactured drugs are diverted into the illicit market many ways.

B. Prices of illicit narcotics and dangerous drugs depend upon the supply and demand.

VII. Public Health Aspects of Drug Abuse. Two distinct philosophies with respect to the abuse of drugs:
    A. One sees the drug offender as a criminal first and a drug offender second.
    B. Other views the drug user as a sick person who must be protected from himself and be prevented from spreading his disease to others.

VIII. Social Aspects of Drug Abuse
    A. Relatives and friends are invaluable in the task of stamping out the drug traffic.
    B. Approval or disapproval of his social group to the drug taker's initial experience is important.
    C. Advanced knowledge of the properties of drugs and the social reactions to their use can influence the course of an individual's addiction.

IX. Medical Aspects of Drug Abuse
    A. Physical aspects of narcotics addiction.
        1. Recognition of an addict is extremely difficult.
        2. The eyes develop a sluggish or "frozen" reaction to light.
        3. Long-term addicts are often pale and malnourished, and suffer from constipation.
    B. Treatment for narcotics addiction.
        1. The only known cure is abstinence.
        2. Legal commitment for drug addiction
            a. Two federal treatment centers: Lexington, Kentucky, and Fort Worth, Texas.
            b. States show universal lack of proper treatment facilities.
        3. Civil commitment for drug addiction—a legal mechanism utilized in lieu of a criminal commitment to control addicts and potential addicts.

X. Effects of Narcotics and Other Drugs
    A. Depressant drugs produce analgesia, sedation, hypnosis, and euphoria.
        1. Opium
            a. Juice obtained by cutting the unripe capsule of the Oriental poppy (*Papaver somniferum*).
            b. Seldom used in the United States.
            c. American addicts use its derivatives—heroin, morphine, or codeine.
        2. Morphine, the chief derivative of opium.
        3. Heroin
            a. Produced from morphine.
            b. Considered the most dangerous of the narcotic drugs.
        4. Codeine—not widely used as a narcotic because of its mild effects.
        5. Synthetic narcotics—produced synthetically in the laboratory.
        6. Barbiturates—a variety of drugs which can produce artificial sleep. Sudden removal forces an addict into withdrawal-producing seizures resembling epileptic convulsions, often severe enough to cause death.
            a. hypnotics.
            b. sedatives.
            c. sleeping pills.

7. Bromides—central nervous system sedatives. Drug is not addicting, but is highly dangerous because of its extreme toxicity.
8. Chloral hydrate and paraldehyde.
   a. Addiction is very uncommon.
   b. Used in hospitals in the management of:
      (1) delirium tremens.
      (2) withdrawal illness.
      (3) convulsions.
9. Alcohol, see Chapter 5.
10. Tranquilizers
   a. Compounds that can suppress anxiety, diminish abnormal behavior, and calm individuals at dose levels that do not produce sleep.
   b. Not commonly used illegally.
   c. Do not produce sleep.
   d. Deaths from overdoses are rare.
B. Stimulants are used to produce energy or wakefulness. As a group are not physically addicting, but user shows psychological dependence and psychotoxic effects during their administration.
   1. Cocaine
      a. Its systemic effect to the body is to stimulate and induce excitement.
      b. Habit-forming but not addicting.
   2. Amphetamines—central nervous system stimulants.
      a. Produce feelings of:
         (1) elation.
         (2) excitement.
         (3) relief from fatigue.
         (4) hallucinations.
      b. Two most widely used are:
         (1) benzedrine.
         (2) dexedrine
   3. Marijuana is a highly unpredictable drug consisting of dried leaves and flowering tops of the hemp plant (*Cannabis sativa*).
      a. Greatest danger is its unpredictable release of the users' inhibitions, accompanied by a loss of moral sense.
      b. User may be difficult to handle or control, has no fear, and feels no pain.
      c. Not an addicting drug, but does create a strong psychological dependence in the user.
C. Solvents
   1. Abuse results from deliberate inhalation of solvent vapors from plastic or airplane cement to induce:
      a. euphoria.
      b. exhilaration.
   2. "Glue-sniffing" is the popular term for use of solvents.
   3. Produces:
      a. strong psychological dependence.
      b. psychotoxic effects during administration.
      c. rapid development of tolerance.
      d. necessity to increase the dose.
   4. These are classified by some as addicting drugs and by others as habituating.

D. Hallucinogens
  1. Drugs capable of turning a normal person, temporarily, into a psychotic.
  2. Two most common are:
     a. LSD (lysergic acid diethylamide)—a tasteless, odorless drug derived from ergot, a black fungus that grows on rye and wheat.
     b. Mescaline—comes from the button-like leaves of a small cactus plant, peyote (*Lophophora williamsii*).

Glossary

. If you cannot find the word you wish in this glossary, check the index for text and glossary references.

abdomen (ab dō′mən, ab′ də mən) (L. possibly from *abdere,* to hide). The area between the diaphragm and the pelvis; the *belly.*

abstinence syndrome (ab′sti nəns sin′drōm) (G. *abstinere,* to abstain; G. *syndrome,* concurrence). A set of symptoms which occur together resulting from withdrawal of alcohol, depressants, and opiates.

addict (ad′ikt) (L. *addicere,* to consent). To form a habit, as for the use of a drug or alcohol.

amphetamine (am fet′ə mēn). A central nervous system stimulant.

anesthetic (an əs thet′ik) (G. *anaisthesia,* insensibility). Agent that produces insensibility to pain or touch.

barbiturates (bahr bit′yoor it) (L. *barbatus,* bearded; G. *ourikos,* pertaining to urine). Drugs used in medicine as hypnotic and sedative drugs.

Benzedrine (ben′zə drēn). A trade name for an amphetamine.

benzene (ben′zēn). Colorless liquid used as a solvent for fats, resins, and other substances.

bromide (brō′mīd) (G. *bromos,* starch). Central nervous system depressant.

carbon tetrachloride (kahr′bən tetrə klōr′īd). Colorless, clear, heavy liquid with a characteristic odor. Used in fire extinguishers, as a cleaning agent, and for exterminating destructive insects.

chloral hydrate (klōr′əl hī′drāt). Narcotic drug used as a sedative, hypnotic, and anticonvulsant.

cocaine (kō′kān) (Quechua, *coca, cuca,* a South American plant). Drug used in medicine as a narcotic or local anesthetic; a stimulant to the central nervous system.

codeine (kō′dēn) (G. *kodeia,* poppy head). Analgesic, hypnotic sedative derived from opium; effects resemble those of morphine, but it is less narcotic than morphine.

coma (kō′mə) (G. *koma,* lethargy). An abnormal deep stupor.

delirium tremens (də lēr′ē əm trē′mənz) (L. *de-,* off; *lira,* track, thus, "off the track"; *tremere,* to shake). A psychic disorder involving hallucinations, both visual and auditory, delusions, incoherence, anxiety, and trembling; found in habitual users of alcoholic beverages and some drugs.

Demerol (dem′ə rol). An analgesic producing effects similar to those of morphine; it is addicting.

dependence (də pend′əns) (L. *de,* from away; *pendere,* to hang). The total psycho-physical state of an addict in which the usual or increasing doses of the drug are required to prevent the onset of withdrawal symptoms.

Dexedrine (dek'sə drēn). A central nervous system stimulant, one of the amphetamines (a trade name).

disorientation (dis or ē en tā'shən) (L. *dis-*, free of, undo; Fr. *orienter*, to face the east). A state of mental confusion.

dosage (dō'sij) (G. *dosis*, a portion). Amount of a medicinal preparation to be taken at one time.

epileptic (ep i lep'tik) (G. *epilepsia*, seizure). A person affected with epilepsy; a disturbance showing generalized convulsions.

euphoric (yoo for'ik) (G. *eu*, well; *pherein*, to bear). Characterized by a feeling of well-being; in psychiatry, exhibiting an abnormal or exaggerated sense of well-being.

hallucinogen (hə loo'si nə jen). An agent producing hallucinations; examples of hallucinogenic drugs are LSD, mescaline, and DMT.

intoxication (in tok si kā'shən) (L. *in-*, intensive; G. *toxikon*, poison). State of being poisoned; condition produced by excessive use of alcohol.

intravenous (in tra vē'nəs) (L. *intra*, within; *vena*, vein). Into a vein, as an intravenous injection.

irritability (ir i tə bil'i tē) *(L. irritare*, to tease). The ability to respond to stimuli.

lactose (lak'tōs) (L. *lac*, milk). Milk sugar.

leukopenia (loo kə pē'nē ə). Reduction of the number of *leukocytes* (white blood cells) in the blood.

marijuana (mar i wahn'ə) (Am. Sp. *marihuana*). A Mexican name for a poisonous hemp. It is not physiologically addicting, but can create psychological dependence.

medicinal (mə dis'i nəl) (L. *medicinalis*). Having healing qualities.

mescaline (mes'kə lin) (Sp. *mexrialli*, to drink). A poisonous oil extracted from peyote (*Lophophora williamsii*). It produces an intoxication with delusions of color and music.

morphine (mor'fēn) (G. *Morpheus*, god of sleep). A widely used analgesic and sedative.

nausea (naw'zē ə, naw'zhə) (G. *nausia*, seasickness). Inclination to vomit.

opiate (ō'pē it) (G. *opion*, poppy juice). A drug containing or derived from opium, a narcotic.

opium (ō'pē əm) (L. fr. G. *opion*, poppy juice). A narcotic drug consisting of the dried juice of the opium poppy (*Papaver somniferum*).

paraldehyde (pə ral'də hīd). A hypnotic, having prompt action as a sedative.

peyote (pā ō'tē) (Sp. *pejote*, caterpillar; refers to the downy center of the button). A common name for the cactus *Lophophora williamsii*.

phenobarbital (fē'nō bahr'bi tol). Drug used as a hypnotic in nervous insomnia and states of nervous excitement and as a sedative in epilepsy.

psychogenic (sī kō jen'ik) (G. *psyche*, mind, soul; *genesis*, to produce). Originating in the mind, as a disease.

sedative (sed'ə tiv) (L. *sedativus*, calming). A remedy that allays excitement; quieting.

solvent (sol'vənt) (L. *solvens*, to dissolve). Dissolving, producing a solution.

stimulant (stim'yoo lənt) (L. *stimulus*, a goad). Any agent temporarily increasing functional activity as coffee, tea, cocaine, benzedrine, dexedrine, etc.

subcutaneous (sub kyoo tā′nē əs) (L. *sub,* under; *cutis,* skin). Under the skin, as a subcutaneous injection into the tissues.

synthetic narcotic (sin thet′ik nahr kot′ik) (G. *synthetikos,* placed together; *narkotikos,* benumbing). An artificially produced drug inducing stupor or sleep.

tachycardia (tak ə kahr′dē ə) (G. *tachys,* swift; *kardia,* heart). Abnormal rapidity of heart action; usually, pulse rate of above 100 per minute.

thrombocytopenia (throm′bō sī tə pē′nē ə). Decrease in the number of blood platelets.

tolerance (tol′ər əns) (L. *tolerantia,* tolerance). Increasing resistance to the usual effects of a drug.

tourniquet (tur′ni-kit) (Fr., a turning). Any constrictor used to make pressure over a blood vessel and to control the flow of blood.

toxicity (tok sis′i tē) (G. *toxikon,* poison). The quality of being poisonous.

tranquilizer (tran′kwi līz ər) (L. *trans,* across, through; *quies,* calm, rest). A drug that acts on the emotional state of overactive and disturbed patients.

withdrawal illness (with draw′əl il′nis). The symptoms of insomnia, restlessness, distress, vomiting, and collapse which follow the sudden withdrawal of a drug on which an addict has become dependent.

CHAPTER 5

ALCOHOL ABUSE

PHYSIOLOGICAL EFFECTS
OF ALCOHOL

PROBLEMS RESULTING
FROM ALCOHOL

NATURE AND EXTENT OF
ALCOHOLISM

PHASES OF ALCOHOLISM

TREATMENT OF ALCOHOLISM

SUMMARY

PHYSIOLOGICAL EFFECTS OF ALCOHOL

In Chapter 4 alcohol was mentioned as one of the habit-forming drugs. It is the most widely used and abused of such drugs, especially in the United States. For that reason all of Chapter 5 will be devoted to a discussion of alcohol and alcoholism.

NATURE OF ALCOHOLIC BEVERAGES

Although many chemical compounds are classified as alcohols, the only alcohol of importance in alcoholic beverages is ethyl alcohol, also called ethanol or grain alcohol. Chemically similar, but highly toxic to humans, are methyl alcohol (wood alcohol) and isopropyl alcohol (used in rubbing alcohol). Ethyl alcohol has numerous industrial and household uses; for these purposes it is usually denatured (made toxic through the addition of poisonous substances). Ethyl alcohol in beverages is always a product of the fermentation of sugar by yeast. The type of beverage resulting depends upon the source of sugar—usually grapes, other fruit, or grains. The mixture resulting from this fermentation may be consumed directly, as in beer and wine, or after distillation, as in whisky, gin, and brandy. Since ethyl alcohol is essentially the only alcohol in alcoholic beverages, the unmodified word "alcohol" used in this chapter will indicate ethyl alcohol.

The alcohol content of American beer is commonly 4 to 5 percent by volume, wines range from 12 to 21 percent alcohol, and distilled liquors range from 40 to 50 percent alcohol. The term *proof* as used in the United States indicates a figure of twice the percent of alcohol. For example, 100 proof indicates 50 percent alcohol.

Alcohol is among those substances most rapidly absorbed into the blood stream, because no digestion is necessary and absorption may take place directly through the stomach wall. This absorption is most rapid when the stomach is empty; it may be retarded by the presence of food.

If judged as foods, alcoholic beverages provide insignificant amounts of proteins and vitamins, but highly significant amounts of calories. Pure alcohol provides 7 calories per gram, approaching the energy content of a pure fat or oil, which contains 9 calories per gram. Many of the physical problems of chronic alcoholics are not the direct result of alcohol but the effects of malnutrition, since the alcoholic frequently neglects proper nutrition, deriving most of his energy requirements from alcohol.

EFFECT OF ALCOHOL ON THE BRAIN

The chief effect of alcohol on the brain is that of a narcotic or depressant. The feeling of stimulation following one or two drinks is actually an indirect result of the depression of the highest areas of the brain, those dealing with inhibition and judgment. The apparent stimulation that may result is actually the feeling of loss of inhibition. As the level of alcohol in the blood increases, progressively more primitive parts of the brain are affected, until, with extremely high concentrations, the respiratory and circulatory centers are depressed, resulting in death.

The degree of intoxication produced by a given amount of alcohol varies considerably among humans. One factor is the body weight of the person in question. The blood alcohol level produced by a fixed amount of alcohol is in approximate inverse proportion to the body weight, and it is this blood alcohol level that determines the degree of intoxication. In effect, the lighter person becomes more intoxicated by the same amount of alcohol.

But even with people at the same blood alcohol level, there are differences in degrees of intoxication. It has been demonstrated that a tolerance for alcohol develops in the frequent heavy drinker, resulting in a lower degree of intoxication than that reached by the moderate or occasional drinker. In most states, a driver is considered legally intoxicated when his blood alcohol level exceeds 0.15 percent. In numerous experiments, however, it has been shown that even the most regular drinker becomes a dangerous driver at a lower blood alcohol level; thus many authorities now feel that the level of alcohol in the blood for legal intoxication should be lowered to 0.10 percent.

EFFECT OF ALCOHOL ON OTHER ORGANS

In addition to its effect upon the brain, alcohol affects other parts of the body. One easily noticed effect is the dilation of the small blood vessels in the skin. As a result, the face and neck become flushed (red) and the person feels warm. The internal body temperature is not changed, however. The total effect of alcohol upon the circulatory system is not significant.

The problems of coordination experienced by the intoxicated person do not reflect any effect of alcohol upon the muscles themselves, but rather its depressant effect upon the nerves controlling the muscles.

Contrary to popular belief, alcohol has only slight direct effect on the digestive processes. When a drink before or with a meal seems to improve the digestion, it does so indirectly through relieving the nervous tension which may interfere with digestion. Indirectly, however, because he neglects proper nutrition, the heavy drinker may develop such medical problems as gastritis or cirrhosis of the liver.

Another widely held misconception is that alcohol serves as a sexual stimulant. Some persons do become more sexually active under the influence of alcohol, but this effect is also indirect. The actual effect of the alcohol is to eliminate the normal inhibitions or judgment.

ELIMINATION OF ALCOHOL BY THE BODY

Although small amounts of alcohol are lost from the body with the breath, sweat, and urine, over 90 percent of the alcohol taken into the body is disposed of by oxidation to carbon dioxide and water. This oxidation takes place through several steps, the first of which occurs almost exclusively in the liver. Although the remaining steps take place rapidly in various body tissues, it is the liver which governs the rate of the total process, since the second step cannot proceed until the liver completes the first step.

Although the rate of alcohol oxidation varies among individuals, it is remarkably constant for any single individual. This rate remains constant whether the blood alcohol level is high or low. The average person can oxidize each hour the amount of alcohol contained in one-half to one ounce of whisky or six to twelve ounces of beer. This information has practical application in that a person can estimate how long he should wait before driving after drinking. A waiting period of one hour per drink consumed is adequate for most individuals.

PROBLEMS RESULTING FROM ALCOHOL

ALCOHOL AND SOCIETY

The relationship between alcohol and society is complex, each influencing the other. Many social problems, such as divorce, unemployment, and accidents are unquestionably aggravated by drinking. On the other hand, drinking may be a response to a pre-existing social problem. Thus we find that the intricate interaction between alcohol and society often leads to "vicious circle" situations in which drinking results from a problem, then intensifies that same problem or creates another. But all men experience problems at some time, and the choice of alcohol as a means of relief for tension and frustration may be influenced by an environment in which social drinking is common.

Much of the effect of alcohol upon society is intangible, but there are certain readily apparent costs which may be measured in terms of dollars spent, homes broken, or lives lost.

ALCOHOL AND THE FAMILY

The place of alcohol in a family will be influenced by the religious, ethnic, and social affiliations of that family. So long as the drinking practices of the family are in accord with those of the larger social groups to which the family belongs, drinking is usually not associated with family problems.

When drinking does become associated with family problems, it is of prime importance to attempt to determine whether the drinking is the *cause* of the family problem or a *symptom* of a deeper family or personal problem. In the past, the former explanation was automatically accepted, with drinking being held responsible for family poverty, divorce, child neglect, juvenile delinquency, and most family problems. Today, drinking is recognized as one symptom of a deeper emotional problem. However, a circle often develops in which personal and family problems lead to drinking, which leads to deeper family problems, which lead to the eventual destruction of the family unit.

ALCOHOL AND CRIME

The police consume considerable time and effort handling excessive drinkers. Many of these people are charged only with being drunk in a public place or with being drunk and disorderly. But many others have become involved in much more serious offenses, such as assault, murder, or felony traffic violations. It must be emphasized that a person need not be an alcoholic or even a regular drinker to become involved in serious trouble as a result of drinking. Many serious crimes and fatal traffic accidents have resulted from a single isolated occasion of drinking.

A very high percentage of prison inmates are imprisoned as a direct or indirect result of alcohol. Alcoholics and intoxicated persons are more likely to become involved in crimes against people than they are in crimes against property. Alcohol seldom plays a part in organized crime-for-profit, since in this highly efficient realm there is little room for the bungling that might result from drinking. The alcohol-related crime is likely to be an impulsive aggression against another person, without motive of profit.

ALCOHOL AND DRIVING

Alcohol is believed to be a contributing factor in 25 to 50 percent of all fatal traffic accidents. Although not listed as the actual cause of the accident in many of these cases, alcohol is thought to be responsible for many accidents blamed on "high speed" or "failure to negotiate a curve." Few people realize that the driving performance of every driver begins to deteriorate with the very first drink. No amount of alcohol ever results in an improvement of driving practices. After as little as one drink, a driver may begin to take chances he might not otherwise risk. In addition to the deterioration of judgment, alcohol impairs vision and lengthens the time required for muscular reaction. Under today's driving conditions of high speed and crowded roads, there is absolutely no margin for alcohol-induced error.

ALCOHOL AND SEXUAL BEHAVIOR

Although not a sexual stimulant, alcohol taken into the body can often lead to sexual behavior which gives cause for later regret. For example, venereal disease is often contracted by drinkers whose judgment before drinking would lead them to greater selectivity in sexual partners. Unplanned pregnancy, for both married and single women, is another common result of alcohol-induced carelessness in sexual behavior.

ALCOHOL AND ECONOMICS

The abuse of alcohol places an enormous economic burden upon many families and upon society in general. The family of the heavy drinker must bear the high cost of the liquor itself, plus the often greater burden of alcohol-caused unemployment, accidents, and illness. The cost of alcohol abuse to society is so great that every wage earner and taxpayer must pay a share. Among the many tolls placed upon society are loss of productivity; accidents and crime; maintenance of jails, prisons, and hospitals for alcoholics; and welfare payments to families destitute as a result of heavy drinking.

NATURE AND EXTENT OF ALCOHOLISM

Several definitions of alcoholism exist. Some are of a highly restrictive nature; others, of a more general nature. An example of a relatively restrictive definition is that of M. E. Chafetz and H. W. Demone, who view alcoholism as

> . . . a chronic behavioral disorder manifested by undue preoccupation with alcohol to the detriment of physical and mental health, by a loss of control when drinking has begun, although it may not be carried to the point of intoxication and by a self-destructive attitude in dealing with relationships and life situations.[1]

An example of a more general definition of alcoholism is that of O. Diethelm. He considers an alcoholic to be an individual who

> . . . uses alcohol to such an extent that it interferes with a successful life (including physical, personality, and social aspects) and is either not able to recognize this effect or is not able to control his alcohol consumption, although he knows its disastrous results.[2]

Since there is no established system for reporting the incidence of alcoholism in the United States, any figures given for the prevalence of alcoholism are, of necessity, estimates. Since much alcoholism escapes medical or legal detection, and there are various definitions of "alcoholism," it is natural that a wide range occurs among published estimates of the extent of alcoholism in the United States. A fair estimate may be that of Keller and Efron, who believe that 4.5 percent (about one in twenty) of the adults in the United States are alcoholics. This estimate

[1] M. E. Chafetz and H. W. Demone, Jr., *Alcoholism and Society*, New York, Oxford, 1962.
[2] O. Diethelm, *Etiology of Chronic Alcoholism*, Springfield, Ill., Charles C Thomas, 1955.

has remained relatively constant for many years. It is also estimated that about 70 percent of the adults in the United States are users of alcoholic beverages, and of those adults who do use alcoholic beverages, about one in every fourteen is an alcoholic.

THEORIES ON CAUSE OF ALCOHOLISM

Many theories regarding the cause of alcoholism have been proposed, but none has yet gained widespread acceptance. Some theories relate alcoholism to physiological causes; others, to psychological or sociological factors. Among physiological causes that have been proposed are nutritional deficiencies, blood chloride levels, allergic reactions resulting in a craving for alcohol, disturbed glandular functions, and hereditary metabolic defects. Psychological causes proposed include oral craving, repressed homosexual traits, pleasure fixation, unconscious urges to destroy oneself or to dominate, feelings of inferiority or insecurity, and numerous other theories. Often cited as evidence that sociological factors exist in alcoholism are the cultural patterns of Orthodox Jews and native Italians, among whom drinking is almost universal but alcoholism very low. With these groups, alcoholic beverages are an integral part of their religious and social traditions. In summary, no single theory of causation has been adequately proven; in fact, there probably is no single cause of alcoholism. More likely, alcoholism is the result of many complex factors acting together.

The concept of alcoholism as a disease or illness is widely accepted today and is well within the medical definition of disease. It is best to think of the alcoholic as a sick person rather than as a weak or sinful person. Although there have been many attempts to describe "the" alcoholic personality type, alcoholics with any type of personality can be found.

PHASES OF ALCOHOLISM

Since at least one in twenty of those reading these lines will become an alcoholic, it is important for every person to be able to recognize the early signs and symptoms of alcoholism. Hopefully, if a person someday noticed these symptoms in himself, he might have the good judgment to cease drinking before he reaches more advanced stages of alcoholism.

SIMILARITIES AMONG ALCOHOLICS

An extensive research project in which the late Dr. E. M. Jellinek surveyed over 2000 alcoholics revealed that most alcoholics pass through definite progressive stages with characteristic symptoms. This progression is graphically represented in Fig. 5.1. On this graph, time proceeds from left to right. There can be no fixed scale of months or years, since some alcoholics make the entire progression in a matter of months and others may take many years to reach the same point. Dr.

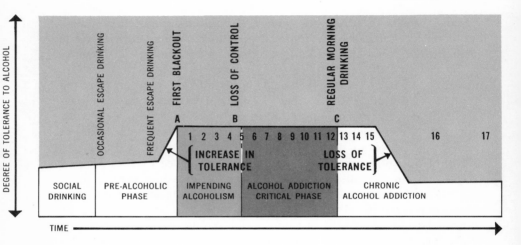

Fig. 5.1 The phases of alcoholism. (Reproduced by permission from the *Quarterly Journal of Studies on Alcohol*, Vol. 13, 1952. Copyright 1952 by Journal of Studies on Alcohol, Inc., New Brunswick, N.J.)

Jellinek points out that the development of alcoholism in women is frequently more rapid than in men, with the stages less clear-cut. The line on the graph indicates the amount of alcohol required to reach a given degree of intoxication.

The pre-alcoholic phase begins when the individual occasionally drinks for the specific purpose of release from tensions. About 20 percent of all drinkers fall into this category. In the person destined for alcoholism, this escape drinking gradually becomes more and more frequent.

After a period of frequent drinking, a person develops increased tolerance for alcohol; that is, he must drink more to receive the same effect. At about this same time (indicated on the graph by A), he may reach his first blackout. A blackout is a period of temporary amnesia occurring when a person is drinking. In contrast to passing out, which results in unconsciousness, a person in a blackout walks, talks, drives, and does all the usual things, but he will have absolutely no recollection of anything that took place during his blackout. Anyone who drinks too much will pass out, but only the alcoholic or near-alcoholic blacks out.

At point **B** on the graph, the second major milestone of alcoholism, loss of control occurs. This means the loss of the ability to drink in a controlled fashion. It does not mean that the individual is forced to start drinking, but when he does start, he cannot stop and must continue to drink until he becomes intoxicated or sick. This period of drinking may last for a few hours or become a binge, lasting for days or weeks. This individual, now in the alcoholic phase, can choose when he starts drinking but not when he stops.

OTHER SIGNS OF ALCOHOLISM

Many other progressive drinking patterns are characteristic of the alcoholic. Some of these are given below and indicated in Fig. 5.1 in their most typical sequence.

1. *Secret drinking.* The alcoholic often "sneaks" his drinks.

2. *A preoccupation with alcohol.* For example, when the alcoholic is invited to a party, he is more interested in what drinks will be served than in who will be attending the party. The social aspects of the event are secondary to the drinks available.

3. *Gulping of the first two drinks.* The alcoholic is eager to achieve the effect of his drinks, since he drinks for effect.

4. *Guilt feelings about drinking.* As the alcoholic begins to realize, perhaps subconsciously, that his drinking habits are not normal, he develops vague feelings of guilt, which lead to several of the following symptoms. For example, he

　　a. *Avoids talking about alcohol.* When the college instructor hears his students bragging about their drinking escapades, he is usually not alarmed, because he knows that the person who is eager to talk about drinking is seldom a problem drinker. The alcoholic will, in contrast, try to change the subject if drinking comes up in a conversation, because he fears that he will be singled out for criticism about his drinking habits.

　　b. *Rationalizes his drinking behavior.* The alcoholic always has a "reason" for drinking. It never occurs to the normal drinker to need a reason. For the alcoholic, happiness or sadness are both good reasons for drinking. He drinks to celebrate or to drown his sorrows. These rationalizations are needed primarily for his own ego and only secondarily as alibis to his family and associates.

　　c. *Has grandiose behavior.* The alcoholic often goes through very extravagant and generous periods, during which he may spend money he cannot really afford to spend in that way. The purpose of such display is not so much to impress others as it is to convince himself that he is really not so bad as he had imagined. This is, of course, part of the rationalization system which influences every aspect of the life of the alcoholic.

    d. *Has persistent remorse.*   Often the guilt feelings of the alcoholic lead to periods of persistent remorse, which have the unfortunate effect of leading to still more drinking.

    5. *Periods of total abstinence.*   As a result of social pressures or his own concern, the alcoholic often goes "on the wagon." For several weeks or months he does not touch a drink; then he usually resumes drinking with renewed vigor because he is satisfied that he *can* still live without alcohol. Hence the often-repeated reassurance, "I can take it or leave it," becomes the theme song of the alcoholic.

    6. *Changing drinking patterns.*   In an attempt to drink in a normal, controlled manner, the alcoholic frequently varies his drinking pattern, trying different types of liquor, different mixers, or different times or places. He feels that there must be some way in which he can drink without loss of control.

    7. *Behavior becomes alcohol-centered.*   Instead of worrying about how his drinking is affecting his activities, he avoids activities which might interfere with his drinking. This engrossment results in a great loss of outside interests, with the alcoholic becoming increasingly egocentric.

    8. *Change in habits of family.*   The family of the alcoholic may either withdraw into the home for fear of embarrassment or, in contrast, may become very active in outside activities as a means of escape from the home environment.

    9. *Unreasonable resentments.*   The alcoholic often builds up tremendous resentments and self-pity, brooding for long periods over some minor or imaginary injustice he has suffered.

    10. *Hiding bottles.*   The alcoholic often takes elaborate precautions against the possibility of running out of liquor.

    11. *Neglect of proper nutrition.*   Since the chronic alcoholic is little interested in food, he may suffer from serious malnutrition, which may actually cause more physical damage than the toxic effect of alcohol does.

    12. *Decrease in sexual drive.*   As a result of his poor physical and emotional condition, the alcoholic may suffer a decrease in sexual drive. This decrease in turn leads to alcoholic jealousy, in which the alcoholic accuses his spouse of extramarital affairs. The marriage which has survived to this point is often shattered by such jealousy.

    13. *Regular early-day drinking.*   Having heard that morning drinking is characteristic of the alcoholic, he avoids this practice as long as possible, but eventually a degree of physical dependence is reached which makes the "eye opener" a very necessary part of the morning ritual. Without it he suffers from "the shakes." This dependence indicates chronic alcohol addiction (C on Fig. 5.1).

14. *Prolonged periods of intoxication.* Another result of the addiction aspect of alcoholism occurs when the alcoholic finds himself intoxicated in the morning on a working day and continues in that condition for several days. Each such "bender" lasts until the alcoholic is too sick to continue drinking.

15. *Loss of tolerance.* After a long term of heavy drinking, the alcoholic loses the tolerance to alcohol he previously had acquired. This loss is possibly connected with a decrease in the ability of the liver to oxidize alcohol. Following this loss of tolerance, he becomes intoxicated on far less liquor than ever before and stays intoxicated much longer. He is able to remain intoxicated at all times with only a moderate total consumption of alcohol.

16. *Mental impairment.* In the later stages of alcoholism, the thought processes are clouded with or without the presence of alcohol. With the absence of alcohol, vague fears and tremors develop; even simple mechanical acts such as winding a watch become impossible. The early alcoholic could choose when he started drinking, although not when he stopped; the fully addicted alcoholic must have alcohol constantly. Delirium tremens, commonly called the "D.T.s," may result, with the alcoholic experiencing hallucinations and great excitement and anxiety. Intensive medical treatment is required in such cases.

17. *Failure of the rationalization system.* Eventually the elaborate system of rationalization which has sustained the alcoholic for several years breaks down and he admits defeat. Although he continues to drink, he is now readily accessible to treatment and willing to try anything to regain sobriety. Fortunately, it is not necessary for the alcoholic to reach this stage before he can be helped. The alcoholic can be successfully treated at any stage *if he really wants to stop drinking.*

TREATMENT OF ALCOHOLISM

MEDICAL THERAPY

Many drugs have been investigated in the treatment of alcoholics, with variable success. Among early drugs used with limited success were the stimulant Benzedrine and the hormone ACTH. Of greater value have been the tranquilizing drugs, which sometimes are effective in decreasing such symptoms as anxiety, tremor, and restlessness common in the alcoholic.

Alcoholics characteristically suffer severe nutritional deficiencies, especially of vitamin B_1 (thiamine). The deficiency of thiamine interferes with the function of the nervous system, producing serious physical symptoms and progressive clouding of the consciousness. To overcome these symptoms, massive doses of thiamine are commonly administered during the early rehabilitation of the alcoholic.

An approach of widespread popular interest is use of the drug Antabuse. If a person drinks an alcoholic beverage after taking Antabuse tablets, he becomes violently ill, suffering flushed skin, difficult breathing, and nausea. As in all other types of current therapy, the alcoholic must want to stop drinking or he will not take the necessary daily dose of Antabuse. However, this drug does prevent him from impulsively taking a drink, since three to seven days after the last dose of Antabuse are required before he can drink without illness.

PSYCHOTHERAPY

The success of psychotherapy in treating alcoholics is variable, depending upon the nature of the alcoholic and the skill and experience of the psychiatrist in handling alcoholics. As in other psychotherapy, the approach may be either a superficial emotional reinforcement of the patient, or a deep exploration of the subconscious mind to uncover underlying emotional conflicts that may be contributing to his alcoholism.

GOVERNMENT PROGRAMS FOR THE ALCOHOLIC

There are still very few effective government facilities for the treatment of alcoholics. With the widespread acceptance of alcoholism as a public health problem and realization that the alcoholic can often be helped, some government programs for the prevention and treatment of alcoholism have been formed. Some examples today include outpatient clinics, city and county general hospitals willing to admit the alcoholic, and specialized state hospitals for alcoholics. Such programs are usually more successful when they are nonpunitive and voluntary.

Some major business concerns now have psychiatric programs designed to help their employees who have drinking problems.

ALCOHOLICS ANONYMOUS

The most successful approach to the problem of alcoholism to date has probably been the fellowship of Alcoholics Anonymous, often called A.A. Alcoholics Anonymous is a loosely organized group of individuals whose sole purpose is to help its members stay sober. Today, there are over 200,000 members of A.A., belonging to over 10,000 groups ranging in size from only two or three members to over one hundred. In a large city there may be groups meeting every night of the week.

The approach taken by A.A. is that of group therapy, in which members find a deep personal, emotional, and spiritual experience through association with other sober alcoholics. At a typical A.A. meeting, several members may stand and relate their stories of trouble and misery during their drinking years. The new member, at first usually defensive and skeptical, hears experiences similar to his own and finds that he can identify strongly with a person who has just stood and made the statement "I am an alcoholic." The new member learns to think of alcoholism as an illness and finds encouragement in seeing alcoholics who have remained sober for years. The new member takes an important step when he admits his alcoholism. He can now feel a part of A.A., finding himself eager to help others still suffering the agonies he so recently felt himself.

It must be emphasized that A.A. does not *cure* the alcoholic, but rather *controls* his illness, much as insulin does not cure diabetes, but does enable the diabetic to live a normal life. There have been numerous cases of individuals becoming overconfident after several or many years in A.A. and attempting social drinking, with disastrous results often within a matter of weeks. A.A. firmly believes that no alcoholic can ever return to social drinking.

Also, it must be stressed that A.A. cannot help the alcoholic who does not fulfill three essential qualifications:

1. A sincere desire to stop drinking.
2. A willingness to admit that he, by himself, is unable to solve his problem—that he must have help.
3. The ability to be honest with himself.

SUMMARY

I. Physiological Effects of Alcohol
  A. Nature of alcoholic beverages
    1. All contain ethyl alcohol.
    2. Alcohol consumed is rapidly absorbed into the blood.
    3. Alcohol has little food value, but does contain high amounts of calories.
  B. Effect upon the brain and other organs
    1. Narcotic, sedative, or depressant effect.
    2. Apparent feeling of stimulation due to loss of inhibition.
    3. Degree of intoxication depends upon:
      a. given amount of alcohol consumed.
      b. body weight.
      c. degree of tolerance for alcohol.
    4. Produces dilation of blood vessels.
    5. Has little direct effect on digestive system.
  C. Elimination of alcohol
    1. Primarily through oxidation to carbon dioxide and water.
    2. Rate of oxidation determined by liver.

II. Problems Resulting from Alcohol
  A. Alcohol and society

1. Many social problems caused or aggravated by drinking.
2. Drinking affected by social patterns and problems.
B. Alcohol and family
  1. Role influenced by:
    a. religious affiliation.
    b. ethnic affiliation.
    c. social affiliation.
  2. Problem drinking may be:
    a. cause of family problems
    b. symptom of deeper family or personal problems.
C. Alcohol and crime
  1. Considerable police time and effort spent handling excessive drinkers.
  2. Offender need not be regular drinker; many serious crimes and fatal accidents result from a single isolated occasion of drinking.
D. Alcohol and driving
  1. Alcohol is contributing factor in 25 to 50 percent of all fatal accidents.
  2. Driving performance deteriorates with the first drink.
E. Alcohol and sexual behavior—common results of alcohol-induced carelessness:
  1. venereal diseases.
  2. unplanned pregnancies.
F. Alcohol and economics
  1. Family bears cost of:
    a. dollars spent or lost.
    b. unemployment.
    c. accidents.
    d. illness.
    e. homes broken.
    f. lives lost.
  2. Societal costs are:
    a. loss of productivity.
    b. accidents.
    c. crime.
    d. welfare payments to families of alcoholics.

III. Nature and Extent of Alcoholism
  A. Several definitions of alcoholism exist
    1. Restrictive definitions based upon the concept of loss of control and inability to stop at a predetermined number of drinks.
    2. More general definition is that of a person whose drinking interferes with a successful life.
  B. Estimates of incidence of alcoholism varies with definition followed, complicated by the unknown incidence of undetected alcoholism.
    1. A fair estimate may be that one in twenty adults in the United States is an alcoholic.
    2. Excluding total abstainers, about one in fourteen adults is an alcoholic.
  C. Theories on cause of alcoholism
    1. Alcoholism is result of many complex factors acting together.
    2. Alcoholism is a disease.

IV. Phases of Alcoholism
  A. Most alcoholics pass through definite progressive stages.
  B. Time required may vary from a few months to many years.

   C. Early symptoms include:
      1. Blacking out (temporary amnesia).
      2. Loss of control—inability to stop at a predetermined number of drinks.

V. Treatment of Alcoholism
   A. Medical therapy—use of drugs which decrease the desire to drink and which produce illness if a person drinks.
   B. Psychotherapy—depends upon the nature of the alcoholic and the experience of the psychiatrist.
   C. Government programs for the alcoholic—more successful when non-punitive and voluntary.
   D. Alcoholics Anonymous
      1. The most successful approach to control of alcoholism to date.
      2. Approach is group therapy.
      3. Not a cure, but a control.
      4. Cannot help the alcoholic who does not desire to stop drinking.

Glossary

If you cannot find the word you wish in this glossary, check the index for text and glossary references.

amnesia (am nē′zē ə, or am nē′zhə) (Gr. *amnesia,* forgetfulness).   Inability to recall past experiences.

blackout (blak′out).   A period of temporary amnesia occurring while drinking, usually associated with alcoholism.

denatured (dē nā′churd).   Having its nature changed; rendered unfit for human consumption, as denatured alcohol.

CHAPTER 6

FOODS AND DIGESTIVE SYSTEM

ENERGY RELATIONSHIPS

TYPES OF FOODS

THE DIGESTIVE SYSTEM

ASSIMILATION OF FOODS

PATHOLOGICAL CONDITIONS ASSOCIATED WITH DIGESTION

SUMMARY

ENERGY RELATIONSHIPS

The human body acts as a very efficient energy conversion machine. Energy (defined as the capacity to do work) exists in two basic forms: *potential energy,* such as is found in a sugar cube or a rock perched on the edge of a cliff; and *kinetic energy,* active forms of energy such as heat, motion, light, and electricity. The human body converts potential energy from foods into kinetic energy in the forms of heat and work (movement). This energy conversion takes place through a complex system of *enzymes,* protein substances which cause a chemical reaction to take place, but are not themselves used in the reaction. The normal human body contains some 200,000 different enzymes, most of which are within the cells. If only one enzyme is missing, the results may be serious or even fatal.

THE CALORIE

The traditional unit for expressing the energy content of food is the *large calorie* or *kilocalorie,* abbreviated as C. One kilocalorie is the amount of energy required to raise 1 kilogram (2.2 pounds) of water by 1° centigrade.

METABOLISM

The term *metabolism* is used to refer to the total series of chemical reactions which make up the process of life. Metabolism includes both energy-releasing reactions (catabolism) and reactions in which tissues or products such as enzymes and hormones are produced (anabolism). Anabolism reactions use up energy.

A person uses a considerable amount of energy just staying alive. Such basic functions as breathing, heartbeat, and glandular secretion all require energy. This unavoidable energy expenditure is called the basal metabolic rate (BMR) which is measured while the person is awake, but reclining and completely relaxed. The basal metabolic rate is markedly influenced by the degree of secretion by the thyroid gland of the hormone *thyroxin.* An abnormally high thyroxin level results in loss of weight, nervousness, and possibly protruding eyeballs due to excess fat in the eye sockets. A low thyroxin level results in a person's being overweight and physically and perhaps mentally sluggish. Extreme thyroid deficiency in the child results in *cretinism* —a chronic condition characterized by physical and mental retardation.

The number of calories required for basal metabolism varies with weight, sex, and stature as well as thyroid level. The basal metabolic rate is highest in childhood and drops gradually throughout life, requiring a gradual adjustment in eating habits in order to avoid excess weight gain. The basal metabolic rate of females is typically lower than that of males. The average adult utilizes some 1500 to 1800 calories per day for his basal metabolism. An approximation of the number of calories needed for the basal metabolism of the average individual may be obtained by allowing one calorie per hour (24 per day) for each kilogram (2.2 pounds) of body weight. For example, an adult male of average stature weighing 154 pounds (70 kilograms) would require 1680 calories per day (24×70) for basal metabolism.

TOTAL ENERGY REQUIREMENTS

In addition to the energy needed for basal metabolism, a widely varying quantity of energy is needed for everyday activities. The sedentary or inactive person may utilize as little as 500 additional calories, whereas a large man doing heavy manual labor may need several thousand additional calories. Thus the total energy requirement may range from slightly more than the energy needed for basal metabolism to more than double that amount.

TYPES OF FOODS

In addition to their obvious function as sources of energy, foods are necessary for several other important body requirements. Foods must supply materials for growth and replacement of worn or damaged cells, as well as for the manufacture of cellular products such as enzymes and hormones. Other materials (vitamins) are needed in minute amounts for various functions in the body. Some vitamins form a part of vital body chemicals; others act as regulatory agents. Although the hundreds of substances we consume as foods may show little similarity, the actual nourishing materials they contain fall into only six classes: Organic[1] food substances yielding energy, (1) carbohydrates, (2) fats, (3) proteins; organic food substances, not yielding energy, (4) vitamins; inorganic food substances not yielding energy, (5) minerals, (6) water.

CARBOHYDRATES

The carbohydrates in the diet consist of the sugars and starches. For the majority of people in the world today, the carbohydrates are the most important source of energy. Foods high in carbohydrates include rice, corn, and other grains; potatoes; and any sweet food.

Carbohydrates consist of one or more simple sugar units, called saccharides. Each simple sugar molecule, called a monosaccharide, contains six carbon atoms plus hydrogen and oxygen atoms. The simple sugars glucose (dextrose) and fructose are found in many fruits and in honey.

Those carbohydrates consisting of two simple sugar units are called disaccharides. Examples of disaccharides are sucrose, which is table sugar (cane and beet sugars are identical); maltose, produced by germinating grains; and lactose, found only in milk.

The starches are among the polysaccharides, consisting of long chains of simple sugar units. One polysaccharide, cellulose, although present in most of our foods from plant sources, is not available for conversion into energy by humans, since we lack the digestive enzymes necessary for its breakdown. Cellulose is, however, useful in stimulating intes-

[1] The word *organic*, so often misused by "health food" salesmen, indicates a substance based upon a chain of carbon atoms. See Chapter 12 for further discussion.

tinal activity through its addition of bulk or roughage to the diet.

It actually matters little whether carbohydrates are consumed as monosaccharides, disaccharides, or polysaccharides, since the process of digestion reduces them all to their monosaccharide components before there is absorption into the blood. Those monosaccharides other than glucose are further converted by the liver into glucose, which is the only carbohydrate used as a source of energy by the cells of the tissues. The liver and muscle tissues store some carbohydrate in the form of glycogen, an animal starch which is available for rapid conversion into glucose when energy is needed.

The primary function of carbohydrates in the body is to supply energy. Each gram of carbohydrate consumed yields 4.1 calories of energy. Table 6.1 compares the energy value of the several basic food

TABLE 6.1   **ENERGY VALUES OF FOODS**

Food Type	Calories, per gram	Calories, per pound
Carbohydrates	4.1	1860
Fats	9.3	4220
Proteins	4.1	1860

groups. If the diet is low in carbohydrates, fats or proteins will be converted into glucose as a source of energy. If there is a surplus of carbohydrates in the diet, they are quite readily converted into human fats and stored in the adipose tissues for possible future use.

FATS

Fats are abundant in such foods as meat, whole milk, cheese, nuts, and olives. Some food products, such as butter, margarine, oils, and shortenings, are almost pure fat. The oils are fats of low melting points, being liquid at room temperature.

The fats have the highest available energy content of any known foods, yielding 9.3 calories per gram, over twice as much energy as carbohydrates. In addition to being used as a source of energy, fats serve several other functions in the body. They serve as the body's reservoir for the long-term storage of energy. Fats are important in the membranes of all cells and in the nerve sheaths. Small quantities of fats in the diet appear to be necessary for the absorption into the blood of the fat-soluble vitamins.

A fat molecule is the result of the union of one glycerol molecule with three fatty acid molecules; through digestion it is broken down into its components. The human body is able to produce most of the fatty acids through conversion of carbohydrates, but is unable to manufacture several of the necessary unsaturated fatty acids. Fatty acids the body needs but is unable to produce itself are referred to as essential fatty acids and must be obtained through food. Fortunately, they are widely distributed in foods in abundant quantities and fat deficiency is almost unknown in the United States.

PROTEINS

Of the three groups of energy-yielding foods, the proteins are the most complex in structure and the most essential to life. Protein molecules are chains of *amino acids,* organic compounds containing nitrogen, hydrogen, carbon, and oxygen. Some contain sulphur, but all contain NH_2 (amino group) and $COOH$ (carboxyl group). Through digestion, proteins are broken down into their component amino acids before absorption into the blood. Thousands of different proteins occur in foods, the type being determined by the sequence of the amino acids. No specific protein is an absolute necessity in the human diet, since the amino acids are separated during digestion and later rearranged by the body cells into human forms of protein. Among the 20 commonly occurring amino acids, only eight, the essential amino acids, must be present in the human diet. The remaining amino acids can be produced within the body. The absence from the diet of any one of the essential amino acids would have the same effect as a total protein deficiency, since it is impossible to synthesize a protein molecule if any of its component amino acids is missing.

Proteins are classified as complete if all eight essential amino acids are present in significant quantities. A protein low in one or more essential amino acids is said to be incomplete. Most proteins from animal sources are complete, but many plant proteins are incomplete. A vegetarian might, however, plan his diet so that several incomplete proteins complement each other to yield all the essential amino acids.

Since almost every tissue and secreted product required for growth and maintenance of the human body is based upon amino acids, proteins are of prime importance in the diet. Also of importance is the availability of amino acids as energy sources. Such utilization takes place when the diet is high in protein but low in fats and carbohydrates. The amino acids are first converted into carbohydrates by removal of the amino group (NH_2), a process called *deamination.* As sources of energy, the proteins yield 4.1 calories per gram, equivalent to that of the carbohydrates.

VITAMINS

Vitamins are organic (carbon-based) compounds needed in minute amounts for proper functioning of the body. Many vitamins are believed to function much like enzymes; they enable a chemical reaction to take place, but are not themselves incorporated into the product of the reaction. Vitamins are not energy sources in that they yield no calories. The major properties of the vitamins are summarized in Table 6.2.

It is important to recognize the difference between recommended daily allowance (R.D.A.), given in the table, and minimum daily requirement (M.D.R.). The recommended daily allowance is the amount of a nutrient needed to insure optimum health; the minimum daily requirement is the amount necessary to prevent a definite deficiency disease. To compare vitamin preparation formulas, we must know which standard the manufacturer has stated. The solubility of a vitamin, whether water or fat soluble, is important in that it influences the source of the vitamin, its absorption into the body, and its fate within the body. In general the fat-soluble vitamins are more persistent in the body, with possible toxic effects in overdoses. Unlike the carbohydrates, fats, and proteins, the vitamins have no underlying chemical similarity other than their all being organic compounds.

The complete absence of a given vitamin from the diet is referred to as *avitaminosis,* a condition rare in the United States today. However, many Americans suffer from *hypovitaminosis,* the diet falling below the optimum quantity of one or more vitamins. Such individuals are not seriously ill, but lack the health and vitality to enjoy life to its fullest.

MINERALS

In contrast to the complex organic structure of the vitamins, the minerals are usually consumed as rather simple inorganic compounds. Once in the body, however, the minerals may be incorporated into some very complex organic compounds. Some of these compounds are vital parts of cells, bones, teeth, and blood; others are equally important to secreted products, such as hormones.

As many as thirteen minerals are now believed by some authorities to be required for optimum human health. Minerals which are believed to be essential and which are almost never deficient in the American diet include sodium, potassium, chlorine, copper, sulfur, zinc, manganese, and magnesium. Those minerals which are more likely to be deficient in the diet are discussed in Table 6.3.

WATER

No other chemical compound serves the body in so many distinct and vital functions as does water. The body weight of man is over 50 percent water and many of his tissues contain 70 to 90 percent of this

TABLE 6.2   **VITAMINS**

Vitamin	Rich Sources	Properties
Fat-Soluble Vitamins		
Vitamin A	Cheese, green and yellow vegetables, butter, eggs, milk, fish liver oils. Carotene in vegetables converted to vitamin A by liver.	Lost through oxidation during long cooking in open kettle. Overdose possible.
Vitamin D	Beef, butter, eggs, milk, fish liver oils. Produced in the skin upon exposure to ultraviolet rays in sunlight. No plant source.	One of the most stable vitamins. Large doses may cause calcium deposits, poor bone growth in children, congenital defects.
Vitamin E	Widely distributed in foods. Abundant in vegetable oils and wheat germ.	Lost through oxidation during long cooking in open kettle. Overdose not known.
Vitamin K	Eggs, liver, cabbage, spinach, tomatoes. Produced by bacteria of intestine.	Destroyed by light and alkali. Absorption from intestine into blood depends upon normal fat absorption.
Water-Soluble Vitamins		
Vitamin B_1 (Thiamine)	Meat, whole grains, liver, yeast, nuts, eggs, bran, soybeans, potatoes.	Not destroyed by cooking, but being water-soluble, may dissolve in cooking water. Not stored in body; daily supply needed.
Vitamin B_2 (Riboflavin)	Milk, cheese, liver, beef, eggs, fish.	Not destroyed by cooking acid foods. Unstable to light and alkali.
Niacin (Nicotinic acid)	Bran, eggs, yeast, liver and kidney, fish, whole wheat, potatoes, tomatoes. Can be synthesized from amino acid tryptophan.	Not destroyed by cooking, but may dissolve extensively in cooking water.

TABLE 6.2 (Continued)

Function	Deficiency Symptoms	Recommended Daily Allowance
Necessary for growth, tooth structure, night vision, healthy skin.	Slow growth, poor teeth and gums, night blindness, dry skin and eyes (lack of tears).	5000–8000 units for adult. 1500–5000 units for child.
Necessary for metabolism of calcium and phosphorus. Essential for normal bone and tooth development.	Rickets. Poor tooth and bone structure. Soft bones.	400 units.
Not definitely known for humans.	Not definitely known for humans.	Not established.
Necessary for blood clotting.	Slow blood clotting, anemia.	Not established. Often given to pregnant women and newborn infants since newborns lack bacteria which normally produce an adequate supply.
Necessary for carbohydrate metabolism, normal nerve function. Promotes growth.	Beriberi. Slow growth, poor nerve function, nervousness, fatigue, heart disease.	0.8 to 1.6 mg for adult. 0.4 to 1.4 mg for child.
Essential for metabolism in all cells.	Fatigue, sore skin and lips, bloodshot eyes, anemia.	1.2 to 2.0 mg for adult. 0.6 to 2.0 mg for child.
Necessary for growth, metabolism, normal skin.	Pellagra. Sore mouth, skin rash, indigestion, diarrhea, headache, mental disturbances.	13 to 20 mg for adult. 6 to 22 mg for child.

TABLE 6.2 (Continued)

Vitamin	Rich Sources	Properties
Vitamin B6 (Pyridoxine)	Meat, liver, yeast, whole grains, fish, vegetables.	Stable except to light.
Vitamin B12 (Cyanocobalamin)	Meat, liver, eggs, milk, yeast.	Unstable to acid, alkali, light.
Vitamin C (Ascorbic acid)	Citrus fruits, tomatoes, potatoes, cabbage, green peppers, broccoli.	Least stable of the vitamins. Destroyed by heat, alkali, air. Dissolves in cooking water.

substance. The importance of water to the body is so great that a loss of only 10 percent of its water results in death.

The great solvent properties of water make it the medium in which all the chemical reactions of metabolism take place. Digestion, absorption, and secretion can take place only in a water medium. Water moistens the surfaces of the lungs to make possible gas diffusion. Water is important in uniformly distributing heat throughout the body and in eliminating excess heat through evaporation. It is the vehicle for transport of many vital substances through the body. It serves as a cushion of the brain and spinal cord. Water takes part in many of the chemical reactions of the body, such as digestion.

The daily water requirement depends greatly upon the environmental temperature and the degree of activity. The moderately active person on a cool day might lose only $2\frac{1}{2}$ quarts of water through the four channels of loss—kidneys, lungs, skin, and digestive tract. The same person working vigorously on a hot day might lose several times as much water.

In addition to the water contained in liquids, the average person consumes a considerable amount of water as a part of the solid foods he eats. Many fruits and vegetables are from 80 to 95 percent water; even a seemingly dry piece of bread is 30 to 35 percent water. Other water is produced through metabolism, being one of the end products of the breakdown of carbohydrates to yield energy.

Although thirst is usually an accurate indicator of water needs, it is usually agreed that a water intake slightly in excess of that dictated by thirst is advantageous for good kidney health.

TABLE 6.2 (Continued)

Function	Deficiency Symptoms	Recommended Daily Allowance
Functions in amino acid metabolism.	Dermatitis. Deficiency rare.	Not established.
Necessary for production of red blood cells and growth.	Pernicious anemia.	Not established.
Essential for cellular metabolism. Necessary for teeth, gums, bones, blood vessels.	Scurvy. Poor teeth, weak bones, sore and bleeding gums, easy bruising, poor wound healing.	70 to 100 mg for adult. 30 to 80 mg for child.

NOTE: Several other water-soluble vitamins are believed to be essential to human nutrition, but are not as well understood as the above vitamins and their deficiency is less common.

THE DIGESTIVE SYSTEM

Cells require that their nutrients be presented to them already dissolved in the tissue fluid which surrounds them. The problem facing the body is to break down complex foods into molecules small enough to pass through tissues so that they can enter the blood stream or lymphatic system and be delivered in a soluble form to the various cells which make up the body. This activity is known as *digestion*—the breaking down of insoluble complex food materials into simple soluble, absorbable forms. The passage of substances through the mucous membrane lining the stomach and small intestine into the blood and lymph is known as *absorption*.

ANATOMY AND PHYSIOLOGY OF THE DIGESTIVE SYSTEM

The general design of the human digestive tract (also called the alimentary canal or gastrointestinal tract) is a long muscular tube (up to 25 feet in length) which begins at the mouth and ends at the anus. At these sites its mucous membrane lining becomes continuous with the skin. The digestive tube consists of the mouth, pharynx, esophagus, stomach, small intestine, and large intestine (Fig. 6.1). The wall of the digestive tube takes its general form in the lower part of the esophagus and extends as such to the lower end of the large intestine. Throughout this length it is generally composed of an inner lining, the mucous

TABLE 6.3 **MINERALS**

Mineral	Rich Sources	Characteristics
Calcium	Dairy products, leafy vegetables.	Element most likely to be deficient in diet. Lack of vitamin D prevents use of calcium.
Phosphorus	Milk, liver, meat, beans, whole grains, cottage cheese, broccoli.	Most functions of any mineral in body. Diet adequate in calcium will usually contain sufficient phosphorus.
Iron	Liver, meat, shellfish, egg yolk, legumes, dried fruits.	Very little iron in milk; infant or child must have other source.
Iodine	Iodized salt.	Soil and water in some areas of U.S. very low in iodine. Only mineral in which deficiency in soil is reflected in deficiency in diet.
Fluorine	Drinking water in some areas of U.S.	Excess causes mottling of teeth.

membrane, two or three layers of muscle, and an outer serous membrane.

The over-all function of the digestive system is digestion and absorption. This digestive action involves the splitting of large complex molecules of food substances—such as carbohydrates, fats, and proteins—into smaller and simpler soluble and absorbable molecules. This process involves the action of many enzymes and several specific areas of the di-

TABLE 6.3 (Continued)

Function	Deficiency Symptoms	Recommended Daily Allowance
Building material for bones and teeth. Necessary for blood clotting and nerve function.	Rickets. Poor bone and tooth structure. Stunted growth. Cramps, twitching, and other symptoms of increased nerve irritability.	0.8–1.0 grams for adult, 0.8–1.4 grams for child, up to 2 grams during pregnancy and nursing.
Essential in cell metabolism. Building material for bones and teeth. Serves as buffer to maintain proper pH of blood. Important in many enzyme systems including energy release.	Poorly developed teeth and bones, stunted growth, rickets, weakness, loss of weight.	1.5 grams for adult, 1.0 gram for child. Ratio of phosphorus to calcium should be 1.5:1 for adult and 1:1 for child.
Ingredient of hemoglobin, the oxygen-carrying pigment in red blood cells. Necessary for enzymes of cellular respiration.	Anemia (low oxygen-carrying capacity of blood).	10–15 mg for adult, 8–15 mg for child.
Basis of thyroid hormone.	Low metabolic rate. Goiter.	0.15–0.30 mg.
Strengthens bones and teeth.	Tooth decay.	1 part per million in drinking water.

gestive tract: salivary digestion occurs in the mouth; gastric digestion, in the stomach; and intestinal digestion, in the small intestine. In the last section of the digestive tube (the large intestine) no digestion takes place, but water is absorbed, bacteria flourish, and the unabsorbed solid residue is excreted as feces. This complex process is shown as a continuous flow-chart of digestion in Fig. 6.2.

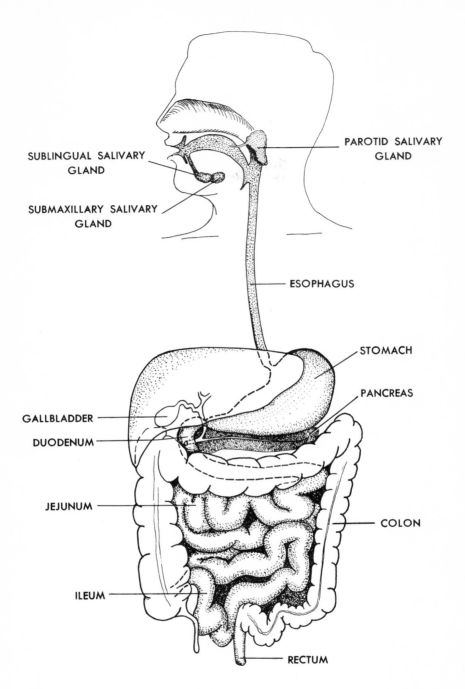

SUBLINGUAL SALIVARY GLAND

SUBMAXILLARY SALIVARY GLAND

PAROTID SALIVARY GLAND

ESOPHAGUS

STOMACH

PANCREAS

GALLBLADDER

DUODENUM

JEJUNUM

COLON

ILEUM

RECTUM

Fig. 6.1 General plan of digestive system.

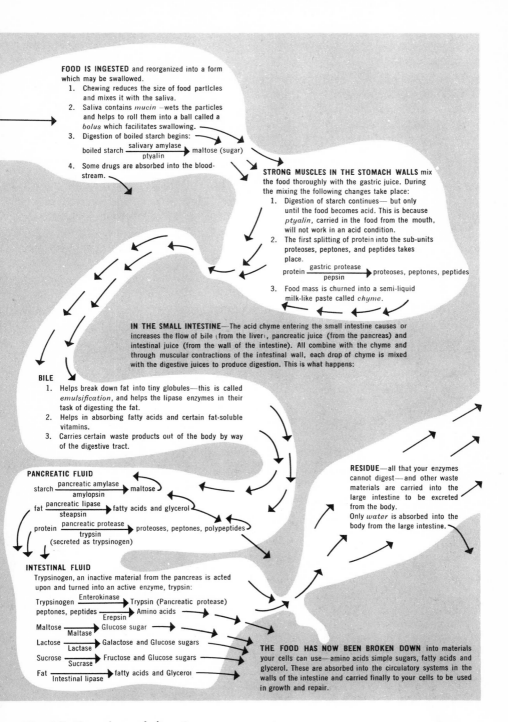

Fig. 6.2 Flow chart of digestion.

ACCESSORY STRUCTURES OF THE DIGESTIVE SYSTEM

Several glands located outside the digestive tract are of importance in the digestive process. These glands originate as outgrowths of the digestive tract during its embryonic development and are connected by ducts to its wall. These structures include the *salivary glands,* the *liver,* and the *pancreas.* Each produces secretions which function in the digestive process; therefore, each is considered an accessory structure of the digestive tract and thus part of the digestive system.

SALIVARY GLANDS

There are three pairs of salivary glands, named according to their location. They are the parotid, the submaxillary or mandibular, and the sublingual (see Fig. 6.1). These glands secrete a fluid known as *saliva.*

LIVER AND GALLBLADDER

The liver is one of the largest organs in the body. It is a dark chocolate brown and is situated mainly on the right side of the abdomen, lying under and protected by the lower ribs. The liver is in contact with the undersurface of the dome of the diaphragm.

The liver is the great chemical laboratory of the body. It is the seat of the fundamental processes concerned in the metabolism of carbohydrates, proteins, and fats (explained elsewhere in this chapter).

The digestive function of the liver is to secrete bile, which passes on into the intestine after storage in the gallbladder. The gallbladder lies in a depression at the edge of the front surface of the liver. When it is full, its size and shape resemble that of an elongated pear (see Fig. 6.1). Bile salts, secreted by the liver, are concentrated in the gallbladder; a precipitation of these bile salts leads to the formation of gallstones. Because the gallbladder is not a vital organ, its removal is often resorted to when gallstones form.

The duct from the gallbladder is joined by the duct from the pancreas just as it enters the duodenum, slightly below the pylorus of the stomach. A sphincter valve guards the common entrance of this duct, except during a meal, at which time the sphincter relaxes and bile is squirted into the intestine when the gallbladder contracts.

PANCREAS

The pancreas is the single most important source of digestive enzymes in the digestive system. It is the second-largest gland connected to the digestive tube. A soft, pink-white organ, this gland extends from the middle portion of the duodenum transversely across the abdomen to the spleen. In the adult it is approximately six inches in length and about one inch in width. The pancreas secretes digestive juices into the duodenum by way of the pancreatic duct.

Besides producing pancreatic juice, certain cells arranged within the pancreas in definite groups called the *islets of Langerhans* manufacture an endocrine hormone, *insulin*. This hormone plays an important role in the control of carbohydrate metabolism of the body. (The function of the islets of Langerhans and their relationship with diabetes will be considered in Chapter 17.)

Thus, the pancreas functions as both an *exocrine* (with duct) and *endocrine* (ductless) gland.

SALIVARY DIGESTION

The oral cavity commences at the lips and continues into the pharynx. The cavity of the mouth is bounded on the sides by the cheeks, its roof is the palate, and the greater part of its floor is formed by the tongue. The mouth contains the teeth, which reduce food to smaller pieces and thoroughly mix it with the saliva by the action of mastication (chewing) so that it may be swallowed as a premoistened, soft, round bolus (lump) of material. It also acts as a receiver for the ducts of the salivary glands (see Fig. 6.1); these glands produce saliva, a viscous, colorless liquid that contains water, salts, proteins, mucin, and an enzyme known as salivary amylase (ptyalin).

The enzyme *amylase* functions to change cooked starch and glycogen (animal starch) to maltose sugar. The food remains in the mouth too short a time for the digestion of starch to proceed very far. However, the action of amylase is still maintained even after the food is swallowed; then the acid gastric juices of the stomach penetrate the food mass and stop its digestive function.

The *mucin* contained in saliva lubricates the food and thus assists swallowing. In addition, saliva functions as a solvent for certain constituents of food, thus serving the sense of taste. One can taste only materials which are in solution. Saliva also aids in keeping the mouth and teeth clean.

Continuing on from the mouth is the *pharynx*, which also opens into the nasal cavity. The nose and mouth are separated from one another by the *hard palate*, which has a pliable extension called the *soft palate*. The soft palate projects backwards and reaches almost to the back wall of the pharynx. When a person swallows, the soft palate elevates, preventing the possibility of foods being pushed up into the nasal cavity.

At its lower end the pharynx is continuous with the first part of the

TABLE 6.4 **PRINCIPAL DIGESTIVE**

Enzyme	Gland	Where Found
Salivary amylase (ptyalin)	Salivary glands	Saliva, mouth
Gastric protease (pepsin)	Stomach	Gastric juice, stomach
Rennin	Stomach	Gastric juice, stomach
Gastric lipase	Stomach	Gastric juice, stomach
Pancreatic protease (trypsin)	Pancreas	Pancreatic juice, small intestine
Pancreatic amylase (amylopsin)	Pancreas	Pancreatic juice, small intestine
Pancreatic lipase (steapsin)	Pancreas	Pancreatic juice, small intestine
Enterokinase	Intestine	Intestinal juice, small intestine
Erepsin	Intestine	Intestinal juice, small intestine
Maltase	Intestine	Intestinal juice, small intestine
Lactase	Intestine	Intestinal juice, small intestine
Sucrase	Intestine	Intestinal juice, small intestine
Intestinal lipase	Intestine	Intestinal juice, small intestine

air passage, the *larynx* (see Fig. 6.1). Consequently, the pharynx is a tube common to both the respiratory and digestive systems, and both food and air flow through this section.

Behind the entrance of the larynx the pharyngeal tube becomes the esophagus, a collapsed, muscular tube having a total length of approximately ten inches (see Fig. 6.1). It is positioned in the midline of the body with its upper two inches in the neck and lower eight inches in the chest cavity (thorax). The esophagus transports foodstuffs from the pharynx to the stomach.

After leaving the mouth, the food is carried through the lower pharynx and esophagus by wavelike contractions of the muscles, a process called *peristalsis*. The only secretion produced in these areas is *mucus*, a viscous liquid which coats the bolus of food, making it slippery.

ENZYMES IN MAN

Substance Changed	Products Formed
Boiled starch	Maltose
Protein	Proteoses and peptones
Casein (milk)	Insoluble paracasein (curd)
Fat	Fatty acids and glycerol
Proteins	Proteoses, peptones, and polypeptides
Starch	Maltose
Fats	Fatty acids and glycerol
Trypsinogen	Trypsin
Peptones and peptides	Amino acids
Maltose sugar	Glucose sugar
Lactose sugar	Galactose and glucose sugars
Sucrose sugar	Fructose and glucose sugars
Fat	Fatty acids and glycerol

GASTRIC DIGESTION

The stomach (see Fig. 6.1) is an expanded portion of the digestive tube having an average capacity of about one quart. It is usually the shape of the letter J and lies partly to the right of the midline of the body at about the level of the navel. The shape of the stomach and the position of its lower part changes from time to time according to the degree to which it is filled with food. The opening of the esophagus into the stomach is called the *cardiac orifice*. The rounded upper part of the stomach is called the *fundus*. The middle or main part is known as the *body*. The lower portion, corresponding to the hook of the J, is called the *pyloric* portion. The opening through which the food passes from this part into the intestine is called the *pyloric orifice,* or *pylorus*. The pyloric orifice is formed by a very powerful *sphincter,* a valve created by the enlargement of the normal circular musculature of the digestive tube. This valve controls movements of fluids or semifluids into the small intestine.

Waves of contraction begin as shallow ripples near the cardiac orifice and become deeper and stronger as they move toward the pyloric orifice. These muscular waves tend to mix and churn the food. Within two to five hours after a person has eaten, his stomach has reduced the food to a partially digested state. This partially liquified material, consisting of food and digestive enzymes, is called *chyme.* As the stomach completes its phase of digestion, its wavelike action squirts food out through the pyloric orifice into the *duodenum.*

The wall of the stomach is composed of three muscular layers. Food entering through the cardiac orifice undergoes a thorough churning and mixing with the digestive juices, which are secreted by glands lining the walls of the stomach. Normal gastric digestive juice is a thin, light yellow fluid which is weakly acid in infants and children but increases its concentration until it is very acid in adults. The acid condition is due to the presence of *hydrochloric acid.* In addition, gastric juice contains various salts and enzymes, gastric protease (pepsin), rennin, and gastric lipase (Table 6.4). The major function of the hydrochloric acid is to provide a medium in which the pepsin can act most satisfactorily.

Pepsin is an enzyme in gastric juice that specifically acts on proteins to break their long, complex chain formation into shorter fragments, called *proteoses* and *peptones.* These fragments are later broken down into amino acids by the proteolytic (protein-splitting) enzymes of the pancreatic and intestinal juices. Pepsin works best in the acid medium provided by the gastric contents; its activity is stopped in the alkaline environment of the intestine.

The fact that the stomach wall, itself a protein, is not digested by pepsin or irritated by the high concentration of hydrochloric acid is attributed to the buffering action of the mucus secreted in the stomach and to the presence of antienzymes in the cells of this mucous membrane.

Rennin is an enzyme that coagulates protein; its main function in gastric digestion is the curdling of milk. The specific action of rennin is to convert the soluble casein of milk into its insoluble form, paracasein. *Paracasein* is precipitated to form milk curd, which is then digested by pepsin or other proteolytic enzymes found in the small intestine.

It is not certain whether rennin is present in the gastric juice of adults, but since the action of this enzyme requires a less acid environment than is found in the adult stomach, if it is present, it must be almost inactive.

Gastric lipase is a fat-splitting enzyme that has limited action at the normal acidity of the adult stomach. Its optimum activity is in solutions with concentrations of low acid. Thus it may function importantly as a fat-splitting enzyme in the stomachs of young children, where gastric acidity is lower than that in adults.

Gastric juice also contains an *intrinsic factor*. This acts on certain components of food, such as vitamin B_{12}, to form an antianemic factor necessary for the normal development of red blood cells in the body.

The pyloric orifice of the stomach leads into the small intestine (see Fig. 6.1), a tube about 23 feet long, which is divided into three portions—the duodenum, the jejunum, and the ileum.

INTESTINAL DIGESTION IN THE DUODENUM

The *duodenum* is the shortest section of the small intestine, being only about ten inches in length. It is relatively thick walled, and its mucous membrane is thrown into deep folds which possess large duodenal digestive glands. These glands produce the largest portion of the *intestinal digestive juice*. The bile duct from the gallbladder and the pancreatic duct from the pancreas open into the duodenum. Through these ducts the *bile* secreted by the liver (via the gallbladder) and the *pancreatic juices* are added to the intestinal digestive juices.

BILE

Bile is not an enzyme but contains many salts, fatlike substances, and pigments. The bile pigments are derived from the hemoglobin of the red blood cells. In the spleen, dying red blood cells are decomposed; the iron is removed, stored in the spleen or liver, and used later from time to time for the manufacture of new hemoglobin. The remaining part of the hemoglobin molecule is passed on to the liver cells, where it is excreted in the bile as a waste product. These pigments produce the color present in feces.

The fatlike substances in bile are lecithin and cholesterol. They are of interest because their concentration in relation to the concentration of the bile salts is an important factor in the production of gallstones. This relationship is discussed more completely later in this chapter.

The bile salts are the active constituents of bile. Bile contains no enzymes which act upon the food, but the bile salts act as wetting agents, lowering the surface tension of the fatty film surrounding fat particles in food. This process is termed *emulsification*. It enables the fats to undergo division into smaller globules and form a fine emulsion, which facilitates closer contact between the lipase enzymes and the fat particles. The digestive action of the enzymes is increased many times by this close contact.

PANCREATIC JUICE

The pancreatic juice is a colorless fluid with a strong alkaline reaction. The major enzymes found in pancreatic juice are:

1. *Pancreatic protease (trypsin).* Pancreatic protease acts to split proteins into proteoses, peptones, polypeptides, and some free amino acids. Thus its action is similar to that of pepsin in the stomach. Trypsin is secreted in the pancreas as an inactive form known as trypsinogen, which keeps the enzyme from digesting the pancreatic ducts conveying it into the small intestine. When the trypsinogen reaches the intestine, it is activated and changed into trypsin by enterokinase, an enzyme secreted from the mucous lining of the intestine.

2. *Pancreatic amylase (amylopsin).* Amylopsin is an enzyme similar to salivary amylase in the mouth, except that the pancreatic form possesses a greater digestive power than that found in saliva and readily digests starch into maltose.

3. *Pancreatic lipase (steapsin).* Steapsin is a secretion of the pancreas. It is the most important fat-splitting enzyme in the digestive tract, capable of splitting the neutral fats in the diet into fatty acids and glycerol.

INTESTINAL JUICE

The *intestinal juice* has a definite alkaline reaction and contains a large number of enzymes that complete the digestive process. The most important of these enzymes are:

1. *Erepsin.* Erepsin is a very powerful enzyme that attacks partially digested fragments of the protein molecule after their initial digestion by the trypsin of the pancreatic juice or the pepsin of the stomach. Erepsin separates the individual amino acids from one another and so carries the digestion of protein to its final stage.

2. *Maltase.* Maltase acts on the maltose sugar produced by the digestive actions of the amylase enzymes of the mouth and the pancreatic juice. Maltase splits this sugar into two glucose molecules, which then may be readily absorbed across the walls of the small intestine into the blood stream.

3. *Lactase.* Lactase is specific in splitting each molecule of milk sugar (lactose) into one molecule of glucose and one molecule of galactose sugar. These simple sugars are thus in a form which may be absorbed into circulation.

4. *Sucrase.* Sucrase acts upon table sugar (sucrose), breaking the molecule into its readily absorbable constituent molecules—glucose and fructose. No digestion of this sugar occurs until it reaches the intestine

and comes into physical contact with the sucrase enzyme of the intestinal juice.

5. *Intestinal lipase.* This enzyme splits the molecules of neutral fat in the diet into its constituent forms capable of being absorbed into the lymphatics—glycerol and fatty acid.

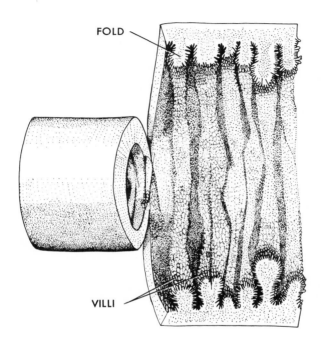

FOLD

VILLI

Fig. 6.3 Small intestine showing folds and villi.

DIGESTION IN THE JEJUNUM AND ILEUM

The final actions of digestion are accomplished in the small intestine; however, most of the liquified food leaving the duodenum is in a form which is readily *absorbable* by the remaining sections of the small intestine.

The remaining 22 feet of the small intestine is made up of the *jejunum* (the upper two fifths) and the *ileum* (the lower three fifths). There is no given line of distinction between these two, and the division is arbitrary. These sections show a heightened degree of peristalsis, the muscular action of the digestive tube which moves its contents. The lumen, the channel within the tube, gradually decreases from a diameter of nearly two inches at the upper end of the duodenum to one inch at the lower end of the ileum. The area of mucous membrane lining the inner surface of this portion is greatly increased by deep folds (Fig. 6.3). These folds are lined with *villi*—microscopic fingerlike projections extending into the lumen. The enormous number of villi give a nubby appearance to the interior surface, which is velvety to the touch. Each villus contains an *arteriole,* a *venule,* and a lymph vessel called a *lacteal.* At the base of the villi are the openings of glands which secrete intestinal digestive enzymes.

ASSIMILATION OF FOODS

ABSORPTION IN THE SMALL INTESTINE

The process of digestion breaks proteins into amino acids; carbohydrates into simple sugars such as glucose, galactose, and fructose; and fats into fatty acids and glycerol. Nearly all of the ingested food, if properly digested, is absorbed in the course of its passage through the approximately 23 feet of small intestine; little is excreted in the feces. The absorption of certain drugs occurs through the mucous membranes of the mouth, and small amounts of water, salts, glucose, and alcohol can be transferred through the stomach mucous membrane into the blood stream, but the absorption of most materials is through the small intestine. The villi (Fig. 6.3) are the structures responsible for the absorption of digested food materials from the lumen of the small intestine into the vessels of the circulatory and lymphatic systems.

Other significant materials which are absorbed in the small intestine are cholesterol and related substances, vitamins, water, and salts. The absorption of cholesterol takes place mainly in the upper small intestine of man. It is incompletely absorbed (only 40 to 60 percent), in contrast to dietary fat (normally 95 percent absorbed). Dietary cholesterol is absorbed mainly by the lacteals into the thoracic duct of the lymphatic system. Related plant sterols are not absorbed from the intestine, with the exception of ergosterol, which is absorbed after it has been converted to vitamin D. The fat-soluble vitamins A and D are absorbed along with dietary fats. Vitamin K is absorbed only when bile salts are present. Thus in cases where bile is not secreted (such as after removal of the gallbladder) into the intestinal tract, vitamin K is not absorbed. A lack of vitamin K in the body produces an increase in clotting time and a tendency in such persons to hemorrhage. The water-soluble vitamins— C, B, and the others—are readily absorbable through the intestine. Water is mainly absorbed across the mucous membrane by osmosis. Salts and metallic ions are actively transported across the intestinal lining. Some vitamins enhance this process. The absorption of iron salts through the intestinal lining appears to be regulated by the amount of iron stored in the body. When iron stores are depleted, iron absorption increases; absorption decreases when the iron content of the body is above normal.

ABSORPTION IN THE LARGE INTESTINE (COLON)

The small intestine opens into the first part of the large intestine, the *cecum* (Fig. 6.4). The entrance into the large intestine is guarded by a

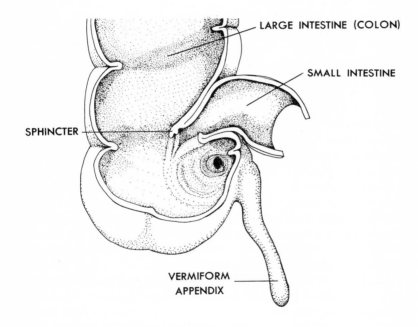

Fig. 6.4 Cecum, showing the ileocecal sphincter and appendix.

sphincter which prevents the backflow of the cecal contents into the ileum. Opening into the cecum is a blind sac, the *vermiform appendix* (Fig. 6.4), ranging in length from two to eight inches. If the appendix becomes infected, it must be removed surgically or it will become a menace to the body of the individual.

The large intestine extends up the right side of the abdomen from the cecum as the *ascending colon,* across the abdomen beneath the stomach as the *transverse colon,* and down the left side of the abdomen as the *descending colon.* After making an **S** curve called the *sigmoid* *colon,* the large intestine terminates as the *rectum* (see Fig. 6.1). The rectum is about six inches long and opens to the exterior of the body through the *anus.* Two sphincter valves regulate the anal orifice—the *internal sphincter,* which is a thickening of the involuntary smooth muscle lining the rectum; and the *external sphincter,* a ring of skeletal muscle under voluntary or conscious control. The retention of the rectal contents is controlled by the external sphincter. This muscle is constantly active and contracted except during evacuation of the waste product, the *feces.*

Though no digestive enzymes are secreted by the large intestine, bacteria present break any unabsorbed amino acids into simpler compounds and gases, many of which have strong odors and may be toxic. The odor of feces is due mainly to this process. The color of the fecal material is caused by the action of bacteria on the bile pigments. As well as these effects, the bacterial action of the intestine performs an important function in nutrition. It synthesizes vitamin K and certain vitamins of the vitamin B complex, which are then absorbed into the blood stream.

One of the principal functions of the large intestine is the absorption of water. Material entering into the cecum is fluid, but by the time the undigested wastes have reached the lower portion of the descending and sigmoid colon their consistency is that of paste, owing to loss of water. Little if any digestible food remains in the feces. In other words, almost all the protein, fat, and carbohydrate that is eaten is absorbed; the food residue of the feces consists almost entirely of indigestible substances. Vegetable material, since its framework is composed of indigestible cellulose, contributes more bulk to the feces than do other foods. This indigestible material, or "roughage" as it is commonly called, serves a useful purpose in that it acts as a mechanical stimulus, increasing the mobility of the ingested material as well as the secretions of the intestinal wall. Fecal material consists of bacteria (about 9 percent), solids (mainly nitrogenous wastes), and minerals excreted into the large intestine from the blood, together with loose epithelial cells and white blood cells shed from the intestinal lining. This waste material accumulates in the lower portion of the intestinal tract, which serves as a storehouse for the feces awaiting *defecation.*

PATHOLOGICAL CONDITIONS ASSOCIATED WITH DIGESTION

The digestive system is one of the largest organ systems in the body and its diseases are of great importance. In addition to infectious diseases and parasitism (to be discussed elsewhere in this book), many significant pathological conditions are directly related to the structures and functions of, and the foods ingested into, the digestive system. The sequence of the digestive tube, beginning at the mouth and ending at the anus, will be used to order the pathological conditions of, or those resulting from, the digestive system.

THE MOUTH

The most important physical change that foods undergo is that of mastication (chewing). Four outstanding benefits are derived from thorough mastication.

1. The food is broken up into small particles, enabling the digestive juices to work quickly and thoroughly upon them. Many cases of chronic indigestion have been traced to faulty mastication due to bad teeth.
2. Proper mixing of saliva and food is facilitated by proper mastication.
3. The taste of food is enhanced and thus increased pleasure is derived from eating. This greater pleasure causes a greater flow of saliva and gastric juice and thereby favors digestion.
4. Thorough chewing increases the blood flow to all the structures of the mouth. In children such increased blood flow, in conjunction with many other factors such as heredity, nutrition, and proper tooth eruption, helps to strengthen and increase the size of the jaw-bones and thereby give sufficient room for the proper placement of the teeth.

STRUCTURE OF THE TEETH

Man has two sets of teeth, a temporary and a permanent set. In man the temporary, deciduous teeth (commonly called "milk" teeth) for each lateral half of each jaw consist of two incisors, one canine, and two molars. They begin to erupt at about the sixth or eighth month (lower central incisors) and continue erupting to the twenty-fourth month (second molars). The permanent teeth later begin to erupt and gradually replace and supplement the temporary teeth. This process begins during the fifth or sixth year (first molars) and continues until the seventeenth or even the twenty-fifth year (third molars, or "wisdom teeth"). This permanent set of teeth, shown in Fig. 6.5, includes two incisors, one canine or cuspid, two bicuspids or premolars, and three molars for each lateral half of each jaw. The total number of teeth contained in the adult mouth is 32.

A tooth is composed of an inner structure known as the *dentin* (Fig. 6.6), a soft bonelike material that forms the frame and substance of the tooth. The part of the dentin projecting beyond the jawbone is known as the *crown* (Fig. 6.6), which is covered with an exceedingly hard material, the *enamel.* The section of the dentin embedded into the bone is known as the *root;* it is surrounded by a layer of *cementum* (Fig. 6.6). The cemento-enamel junction is termed the *neck* (Fig. 6.6) of the tooth. Inside the dentin is a cavity containing *tooth pulp,* consisting of a form of connective tissue; blood vessels; and nerves, which enter the tooth through the opening (foramen) at the apex of the root. The root, surrounded by the *periodontal membrane,* is situated in an *alveolar socket* in the bone of the jaw. This periodontal (also "periodental") membrane, made up of thousands of tiny fibers, attaches the root to the

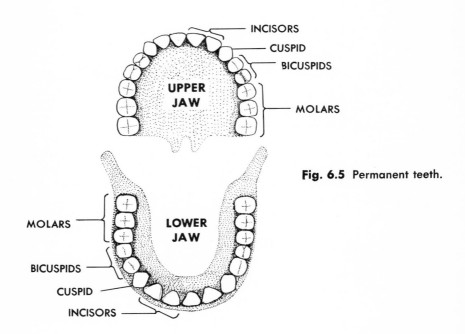

Fig. 6.5 Permanent teeth.

alveolar socket. It helps to support the tooth in its socket, acts as a cushion by taking up the shock of chewing, and allows for some movement of the teeth. This movement is best illustrated in the field of orthodontia (straightening of teeth), where constant, gentle pressure is applied to move the teeth in the direction desired.

PREVENTIVE DENTAL CARE

People may minimize the amount of trouble they may have with their teeth by caring for their teeth from birth to adolescence. Barring physical illness or accident, if a child's teeth are properly cared for from infancy up to his fifteenth year, a foundation is laid which will minimize dental trouble in his adult years. Also, personal habits will have been produced in him which will insure continued care of his teeth throughout life.

At age 3 each child should begin visits to the dentist and serious dental care (see Appendix C, Suggested Lifetime Preventive Medical Schedule). Up to this time the most important care is that of general body welfare—good nourishment, plenty of milk, and sufficient vitamins

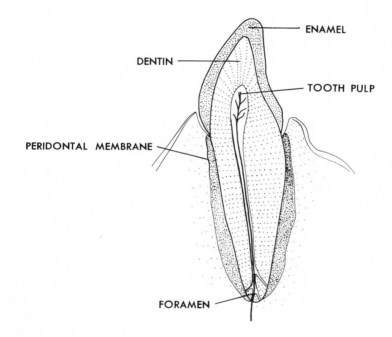

ENAMEL

DENTIN

TOOTH PULP

PERIDONTAL MEMBRANE

FORAMEN

Fig. 6.6 Longitudinal section of an incisor tooth in the alveolar socket.

and minerals. The rearing of a healthy child helps to develop healthy teeth.

After the first visit to a dentist, at age 3, and any additional visits necessary to fill whatever cavities may exist, the child should be taken to the dentist's office regularly every six months. At these appointments his teeth should be cleaned, checked, and any decay taken care of.

DENTAL CARIES (TOOTH DECAY)

Tooth decay and the common cold are the most frequent diseases of man. In dental caries the insoluble calcium salts of the hard structures of the teeth (enamel and dentin) are transformed into soluble materials by chemical action; these soluble materials are washed away and a *cavity* forms. This destruction is generally attributed to acids formed by bacterial decomposition of food lodged upon and between the teeth. Bacteria (*Lactobacillus* and others) are always present in the mouth. The presence of food residue, other than during meals, is determined by the brushing habits of the individual. In addition to adequate oral hygiene, the reduction in the diet of fermentable carbohydrates, especially sugar, on which acid-forming bacilli flourish, will help to reduce the conditions required for tooth decay. Whether a tooth can withstand the attacks of these acids depends upon its physical and chemical structure, as determined by heredity and diet. Some teeth are so excellent in their makeup that no external aid is required for their preservation; others are of such poor quality that no help can save them.

Calcification of the permanent teeth is a postnatal phenomenon. Therefore, during infancy and childhood the diet should be well fortified by foods rich in calcium, phosphorus, and vitamins A, C, and D. These materials can best be obtained from milk, egg yolk, cod liver oil, and citrus and fruit juices. Experimental results in lower animals seem to indicate that the susceptibility to caries in other mammals is influenced by the calcium, phosphorus, and vitamin content of the food. But adequate diet in itself seems to be no guarantee against tooth decay, and caries may be absent in people who subsist on an insufficient diet.

Cavities expose the dentin, causing the nerves (dental pulp) to register sensitivity to sweets and to temperature (hot and cold). Pulpitis (inflammation of the dental pulp) will occur when the decay of the dentin goes deeper and comes closer to the pulp cavity containing the nerves of the tooth. Once the carie has eroded the harder enamel, the erosion of the softer dentin usually takes place very quickly.

FLUORIDATION OF THE TEETH

The element fluorine plays an important role in the construction and preservation of teeth. It has been found that when drinking water containing 1.8 parts of fluorine per million parts of water is used, 25 percent of children from 12 to 14 years old are completely free from caries, and in children having caries the incidence is significantly reduced. An excess of fluorine, however, more than 2 parts per million parts of water, produces teeth which are stained with a brown or chalky substance that cannot be brushed away. This condition is now termed "mottled enamel." The resistance of mottled teeth to tooth decay was the discovery that prompted research on the prevention of dental decay by fluoridation. As a result, it is now known that a concentration of 1 part of fluorine per million parts of drinking water will greatly benefit the enamel of growing children without mottling or otherwise endangering the teeth or health of the individual. Also, children who have used fluoridated water will retain its benefits for life.

Some researchers explain this finding by postulating that fluoride renders the tooth enamel more resistant; others think it has a restraining influence on enzymes and bacteria.

Fluoride solutions are now widely used in another way to prevent caries in young people. Solutions of sodium fluoride or stannous fluoride are applied directly to the teeth by the dentist (topical application). This manner of using fluorides has resulted in an average 40 percent reduction in tooth decay. Topical application is of great value to young people showing high tooth decay and to rural families where fluoridation of the water supply is not practicable; there are even indications that such application in adults may reduce their tooth decay.

APICAL TOOTH INFECTIONS

Apical infections may be acute or chronic and usually involve the peridontal membrane, tooth cementum, and bone in the area of the apex of the tooth. These infections are called *abscesses* and are usually caused by dental caries that have extended into the pulp cavity, causing pulpitis. These infections extend down through the root canal and apical foramen of the tooth into the underlying tissues. An abscess may also be caused by trauma to the tooth or by a localization of pathogenic organisms in the apex area of the tooth. The acute and chronic abscesses show different symptoms and signs.

The acute abscess may develop a local swelling of the *gingiva* (gums) opposite the apex of the root, known as a *gum boil*. In severe cases, or if the gum boil goes untreated, these infections can become the most dangerous type of infection found in the mouth. A swelling around the eyes and a puffing of the lips may occur. The swelling may extend into the cranial cavity and to the structures forming the floor of the mouth, causing extreme tissue destruction and serious consequences to the individual.

The chronic abscess forms lesions that are ordinarily symptomless, usually being discovered only by x-ray examination. They may become apparent to the individual by pain caused when adjacent teeth are depressed upon the abscess during chewing. All symptoms or signs of an abscess require immediate treatment by a dentist. There are various treatments—draining of the gum boil, cleaning out of the root canal of the tooth and disinfecting the area aiding in bone repair, or extraction of the tooth.

MALOCCLUSION

There are several types of malocclusion (irregular teeth) (Fig. 6.7). One is what appears to be protruding upper incisors, commonly referred to as "buck teeth"; another is a protruding lower jaw, which gives the youngster an appearance of pugnacity; another type is that in which the palate is inherently narrowed to cause crowding or protrusion of the cuspid teeth; in still another type, the lower teeth bite up into the palate

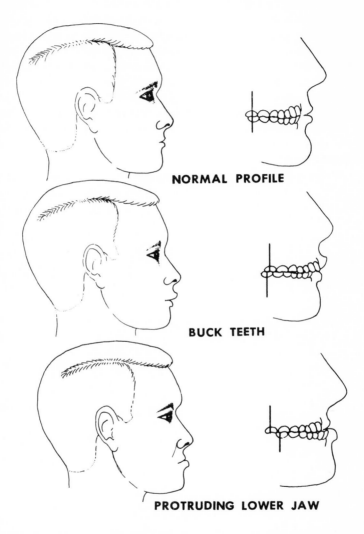

NORMAL PROFILE

BUCK TEETH

PROTRUDING LOWER JAW

Fig. 6.7 Normal occlusion and malocclusion using the six-year molar as guide.

rather than into the tongue (lingual) surfaces of the teeth. Many other types and variations of malocclusion may be recognized only by a dentist. The correction of malocclusion and the realignment of teeth is accomplished by a specialist known as an orthodontist.

Not all teeth that look crooked need orthodontic treatment. As the teeth erupt at various ages, the combination of large with small teeth in the same mouth, the development of the jaws, and the usual space between the central incisors all give the youngster an awkward appearance and may frighten the mother. Under such circumstances neighbors and friends are *not* the people to go to for advice. They will confuse parents with all kinds of misinformation or smatterings of some other person's experience, and the result will be bewilderment. One's dentist is the person to be consulted in such instances. If the child has been brought to him regularly for care, he will have noticed irregularities long before the parent does.

The guide the orthodontist uses to determine the type of irregularity he has to contend with is the relationship of the upper six-year molars to the lower six-year molars (Fig. 6.7). These teeth are called "the keys to the dental arch."

Generally speaking, orthodontic treatment should begin as soon as an undesirable condition is noticed or as soon as the child is old enough to give the orthodontist the required cooperation. Excellent results have been obtained by those orthodontists who make it a rule, almost without exception, to begin treatment when the child is about 12. The primary thing for the parent to consider, regardless of the age at which orthodontic treatment is begun, is that it is a long process, sometimes taking several years, and that it requires regular cooperation by the youngster.

PROSTHETIC DEVICES

Prosthetic dentistry is the art of dental replacements. This is the phase of dentistry which deals with tooth replacement, restorations, crowns, bridgework, and dentures. American dentistry has developed with remarkable speed in the matter of correcting tooth deformities after they have occurred. Nowhere in the world has restorative dentistry been so energetically and seriously practiced as in the United States. Americans needing prosthetic devices and restorations may be assured that they will have the best.

PERIODONTAL DISEASES

Periodontal diseases are those showing inflammation or degeneration, or both, of the gingiva (gum tissues) and the underlying structures (periosteum, bone, and tooth cementum) surrounding the teeth. For a more complete identification of these diseases, their symptoms, manifestations, treatment, and prevention the reader is referred to Appendix A, Diseases of Man, in this book.

1. *Gingivitis.* Gingivitis is an inflammation of the gums characterized by congested, red, and swollen gingiva. It is usually painless, but the

gums tend to bleed easily on pressure. The inflammation may be acute or chronic and generalized throughout the mouth or confined to certain areas. The causes of gingivitis are usually traced to local factors such as poor oral hygiene; malocclusion of the teeth; an accumulation of calculus, also called tartar—a hard, crustlike material on the teeth at or slightly below the gum margin and neck region; or faulty dental restorations. General systemic conditions which may cause gingivitis are lack of specific vitamins (usually vitamins B and C) in the diet; allergic reactions; disturbances of the endocrine system of the body, such as diabetes or those of pregnancy and menstruation; and drug toxicity—chronic poisoning, alcoholism, or drug addiction. Gingivitis may be the first sign of an underlying systemic disorder, such as leukemia.

In the treatment of gingivitis, factors contributing to the condition should be eliminated as soon as possible by a dentist or physician. A thorough cleaning of the teeth under the direction of a dentist is the only manner by which accumulated calculus may be removed. Also, malocclusion and faulty dental restorations should be remedied. Systemic factors, such as drug toxicity, diabetes, and chronic infections should be corrected as completely as possible. In the treatment of inflammation of the gingiva, a dentist may prescribe vitamins, antibiotics, or the topical application of ointments; in severe cases a portion of the gums may be removed surgically (gingivectomy) to facilitate drainage and healing. More extensive removal is often used in treating periodontitis (pyorrhea).

2. *Vincent's angina.* Vincent's angina is a severe form of gingivitis which received special study during World War I because of its prevalence among soldiers (hence its common name, "trench mouth"). It may affect the mucous membranes of the mouth and pharynx and is due to one or two specific bacteria (*Borrelia vincenti* and *Bacteroides fusiformis*). The symptoms are the same as those for general gingivitis, but are usually more widespread. Treatment was a serious problem before the advent of antibiotics, but penicillin now offers a rapid and effective means of curing this disease. Usually within 24 hours all symptoms of fever, pain, body discomfort, and foul breath will invariably clear up. However, as the condition clears, the patient should be given instructions in the correct method of brushing teeth. All dental conditions must be alleviated, and frequent gargles and mouth washes must be used to cleanse and heal the ulcers. The tars present in tobacco appear to seal the disease organisms into the sores and prolong the condition; consequently, the elimination of tobacco is necessary to effect a cure.

This is an infectious disease that is passed on through dishes, drinking glasses, or personal articles which come in contact with the mouth. Infected individuals should be warned against kissing or letting associates use anything that might have been contaminated by the mouth.

3. *Periodontitis (pyorrhea).* Periodontitis is characterized by inflam-

matory tissue changes, resorption of the bone around the teeth, and recession of the gingiva severe enough to cause loosening or loss of the teeth. In periodontitis the changes are usually due to local irritation caused by calcareous deposits on the teeth, improperly contoured restorations, or incorrectly designed prosthetic devices. In addition, malocclusion may result in foods being impacted between the teeth, causing pockets to form and giving rise to bacterial growths which may aggravate or cause the condition.

The bleeding of gums while brushing the teeth, separation of gingiva from the teeth, loose or shifting teeth, and persistent "bad breath" are symptoms and signs which should cause a person to seek early consultations with a dentist. If not treated, this condition may continue until extreme bone resorption may cause the teeth to fall out.

Local irritative factors should be corrected or eliminated at the beginning of the treatment if the teeth are to be saved. In advanced conditions the diseased gingival tissue may be surgically removed to produce an environment in which tartar cannot deposit, or the teeth may have to be extracted.

GASTROINTESTINAL DISORDERS

INDIGESTION

Common causes of indigestion are eating too much or too rapidly; inadequate mastication, often as a result of teeth's being lost prematurely and not replaced, malocclusion, or neglected dental caries which make chewing painful; eating during emotional upsets; and swallowing large amounts of air. Other factors are excessive smoking, constipation, ingestion of poorly cooked foods or foods high in fat content, and eating certain kinds of foods.

The major symptoms of indigestion are nausea, heartburn, and flatulence. Nausea may be produced by any condition that increases the tension upon the walls of the lower end of the esophagus, stomach, or duodenum. Distention of any part of the esophagus may result in what is usually called "heartburn." Flatulence, an excessive accumulation of gas in the stomach or intestine, may be produced by any of the conditions listed in the previous paragraph; it is a common symptom of indigestion.

A physician should be consulted whenever indigestion is severe enough to produce pain or excessive discomfort. Generally speaking, common indigestion may be alleviated by eating a balanced diet; allowing an hour for eating the meal; thoroughly chewing the food without haste; and, whenever possible, eating the meal in a pleasant, quiet, relaxed environment. Following a meal the individual should avoid excitement or exercise. Smoking immediately before a meal may cause indigestion.

PEPTIC ULCER

A peptic ulcer is an open sore (lesion) produced by an erosion of the mucous membrane in one of four places—the lower end of the esophagus, the stomach (gastric ulcer), the duodenum (duodenal ulcer), or the junction of the duodenum and jejunum. The exact causes of peptic ulcers are unknown. Emotional tensions seem to play an important part in the mechanism of ulcer formation by producing an oversecretion of the acid in gastric juice.

Pain is the outstanding symptom of a peptic ulcer. It has four distinctive characteristics: (1) it seems to always appear in the same area; (2) it recurs periodically, with long periods of absence of pain; (3) it may become chronic; (4) the pain is related to the digestive cycle—usually is absent before breakfast, appears during the day from one to four hours after mealtime, and often is sufficiently severe at night to awaken the individual. The pain is relieved by food and antacids and aggravated by alcohol and spices. Such symptoms may last for a few days, a few weeks, or several months and may leave and reappear during periods of emotional tension.

If an ulcer is not properly treated by a physician, complications such as the following may occur: perforations or holes in the walls of the intestinal tract, which can cause death within a few hours; massive hemorrhaging of the intestinal wall, causing the vomiting of blood; and partial to complete obstruction of the outlet of the stomach.

All treatment of peptic ulcer should be by a physician. Generally, the individual requires mental and physical rest and improvement of his diet.

APPENDICITIS

Appendicitis is an inflammation of the vermiform appendix (see Fig. 6.4). The inflammation results from obstruction and from the infection of the wall of the appendix by the numerous bacteria present in the intestine.

Typically, appendicitis is heralded by pain in the umbilical region, sometimes accompanied by nausea and vomiting. After several hours, the pain shifts to the lower right portion of the abdomen, is continuous, may be dull or severe, and is accompanied by coughing or sneezing.

Early diagnosis and treatment of appendicitis is imperative. Because it is safer to operate than to permit an inflammation to proceed to rupture, surgery is common. The operative mortality in early appendicitis is extremely low—in many hospitals, less than 1 percent. But once the disease has progressed to rupture, the prognosis becomes very grave. The use of a laxative, cathartic, purgative, or application of heat can cause early rupture of the appendix in the abdominal cavity, with death as a possible outcome.

CONSTIPATION

Constipation is the difficult or infrequent passage of feces in which large quantities of very dry, hard feces accumulate in the descending colon.

There are two general types of constipation. One is the *irritable colon,* in which the evacuating mechanisms of the colon are impaired. Numerous factors produce this condition, but chronic cases may usually be traced to long-standing faulty bowel habits. In children who fail to defecate, the muscles controlling the process become progressively less active over a period of time. Early establishment of regular bowel habits in children is important. Adults who are tense, anxious, and hurried; have long-standing habits such as rapid and irregular eating; have food allergies; or overuse laxatives may suffer periodically from constipation.

A second type of constipation is called *inactive colon;* it is commonly found in elderly invalids or in people confined to bed as the result of illness. In these people feces accumulate because the colon does not respond to the usual nerve stimuli prompting defecation. These people often lack normal eating and physical activity.

Imaginary constipation is common in people who are excessively bowel conscious and harbor fear that their bowel movements are abnormal. This fear promotes the use of laxatives, suppositories, and enemas, with the result that a normal colon becomes irritated, sensitive, and impaired, causing real constipation. Daily bowel movements are not essential for everyone. No real harm comes from the bowel that has not moved for a period up to four days. The bowel itself must be given a chance to work, and laxatives or enemas taken more frequently than once every three days may cause constipation.

Megacolon is an abnormally large colon, congenital or acquired, usually found in children. This is a disorder of the nervous network controlling the large intestine. Because of this disorder, the sigmoid colon remains contracted instead of relaxing when peristalsis in the transverse and descending colon attempts to fill the rectum. Bowel movements occur infrequently and never evacuate the colon completely. The abdomen enlarges, and the disease usually becomes noticeable within the first year.

HEMORRHOIDS (PILES)

Hemorrhoids is a very common condition in which there is dilation of the veins in the mucous membranes of the anal canal and rectum. It may be further complicated by congestion, inflammation, and even bleeding if left untreated. These blood vessels appear as small, rounded, purplish tumors covered with skin. They are soft and seldom produce pain except during defecation. The condition is classified as internal if the lesions appear within the mucous membrane of the anal canal before its junction with the skin. External hemorrhoids are lesions which appear below this junction and external to the anal canal (outside the rectum). Lesions may appear in both areas simultaneously.

The individual suffering from hemorrhoids should always consult a physician as soon as possible; patent medicines may cause severe, irreparable damage. If not treated, hemorrhoids may become inflamed, break, and bleed profusely. External hemorrhoids appear and disappear suddenly at times, but without proper treatment they will reappear. Internal hemorrhoids bleed very easily and cause a feeling of anal fullness.

SUMMARY

  I. Energy Relationships
      A. Energy—ability to do work; exists in two forms:
          1. potential energy.
          2. kinetic energy.
      B. Calorie (kilocalorie)—amount of energy required to raise one kilogram (2.2 pounds) of water by 1° centigrade.
      C. Metabolism—total series of chemical reactions which make up the process of life.
      D. Total energy requirements—the widely varying quantities of energy needed for everyday activities.

 II. Types of Foods
      A. Organic food substances
          1. Substances yielding energy
              a. carbohydrates—sugars and starches.
              b. fats.
              c. proteins.
          2. Substances not yielding energy are vitamins.
      B. Inorganic food substances not yielding energy
          1. minerals.
          2. water.

III. The Digestive System
      A. Digestion is the process of breaking down insoluble complex food materials into simple soluble, absorbable forms.
      B. Absorption is the passage of substances through the mucous lining of the stomach and small intestine into the blood and lymph.
      C. The digestive system is a long muscular tube which begins at the mouth and ends at the anus. It consists of:
          1. Mouth (salivary digestion)
              a. Acts as receiver for food and ducts of the salivary glands, which produce *saliva*.

      b. Contains teeth, which function to reduce food into smaller pieces and thoroughly mix it with saliva.

   2. Pharynx, palate, and esophagus

      a. Pharynx—a downward extension of the mouth, continuous with the esophagus.

      b. Palate—the roof of the mouth; its soft extension (soft palate) elevates and prevents the possibility of foods being pushed up into the nasal cavity when a person swallows.

      c. Esophagus—a collapsed, muscular tube leading into the stomach.

   3. Stomach (gastric digestion)—food entering the stomach from the esophagus undergoes a thorough churning and mixing with the digestive juices. Upon completion of this phase of digestion, the stomach's wavelike action (peristalsis) squirts *chyme* out through the pyloric orifice into the small intestine.

   4. Small intestine (intestinal digestion)—chyme passed into the small intestine is mixed with *bile* from the liver, *pancreatic juice* produced by the pancreas, and secretions from glands of the mucous lining of the intestine (*intestinal juice*).

IV. Assimilation of Foods

  A. The absorption of certain drugs occurs through the mucous membranes of the *mouth;* and small amounts of water, salts, glucose, and alcohol can be transferred to the blood through the *stomach walls*; but the absorption of most materials is from the *small intestine*.

  B. The principal function of the large intestine (colon) is absorption of water, leaving an undigested waste material in with the consistency of paste, *feces*.

V. Pathological Conditions Associated with Digestion

  A. The mouth

   1. Teeth produce the most important physical change to food through *mastication* (chewing).

   2. Preventive dental care—care of the teeth in adolescence is a guide to minimizing adult dental troubles.

   3. Dental caries (tooth decay)—the most frequent disease of man. Fluoridation helps in the prevention of tooth decay.

   4. Apical tooth infections (abscesses)—caused by dental caries which have extended into the pulp cavity, causing pulpitis; these extend down through the root canal and apical foramen of the tooth into the underlying tissues.

   5. Malocclusion—the incorrect or irregular alignment of the teeth.

   6. Prosthetic devices—tooth replacement, restorations, crowns, bridgework, and dentures.

   7. Periodontal diseases—diseases showing inflammation or degeneration, or both, of the gingiva, or soft tissues, and the underlying structures surrounding the teeth:

      a. gingivitis—an inflammation of the gums (gingiva).

      b. Vincent's angina infection (trench mouth)—severe form of gingivitis caused by specific bacteria.

      c. periodontitis (pyorrhea)—an inflammatory tissue change, resorption of the bone around the teeth, and recession of the gingiva severe enough to cause loosening or loss of the teeth.

  B. Gastrointestinal disorders

   1. Indigestion—characterized by nausea, heartburn, and flatulence.

2. Peptic ulcer—an open sore (lesion) produced by an erosion of the
   mucous membrane in one of four places:
   a. lower end of the esophagus.
   b. stomach (gastric ulcer).
   c. duodenum (duodenal ulcer).
   d. junction of the duodenum and jejunum.
3. Appendicitis—inflammation of the vermiform appendix.
4. Constipation—difficult or infrequent passage of feces, causing large
   quantities of very dry, hard feces to accumulate in the descending
   colon caused by: ·
   a. irritable colon.
   b. inactive colon.
   c. megacolon—an abnormally large colon; a disorder of the nervous
      network controlling the large intestine.
5. Hemorrhoids (piles)—dilation of the veins in the mucous membranes of the anal canal and rectum.

Glossary

If you cannot find the word you wish in this glossary, check the index for
text and glossary references.

abscess (ab′ses) (L. *abscessus,* from *ab,* away; *cedere,* to go). A localized collection of pus in a cavity formed by the disintegration of tissues.

absorption (ab sorp′shən) (L. *absorptio,* from *absorbere,* to suck in). The
taking up of a liquid or gas through the mucous membrane, skin, or other
vessels.

alveolar socket (al vē′ə lər sok′it) (L. *alveolaris,* a cavity). The socket of a
tooth.

amino acid (ə mē′nō as′id). One of about 33 different organic compounds containing the amino (NH_2) group and the carboxyl (COOH) group; are the
building blocks of protein and the end products of protein digestion.

amylopsin (am i lop′sin) (fr G. *amylon,* starch). A pancreatic enzyme which
changes starch into maltose.

anabolism (ə nab′ə lizum) (G. *anabole,* a building up). The building up of
the body substance; constructive metabolism.

avitaminosis (ā vī′tə mi nō′sis) (G. *a-,* without; L. *vita,* life). Condition due to
a lack or deficiency of vitamins.

bile (bīl) (L. *bilis,* bile). The yellow or greenish fluid secreted by the liver;
used in the digestion of fats.

bolus (bō′ləs) (G. *bolos,* lump). A mass of food ready to be swallowed or a
mass passing along the intestines.

calorie (kal′ə rē) (L. *calor,* heat). The calorie used in the study of metabolism
is the *large* calorie or *kilocalorie,* and is the amount of heat required to
raise 1 kilogram of water from 15 to 16° C.

carbohydrate (kahr′bō hī′drāt) (L. *carbo,* coal; G. *hydro,* water or liquid). A
group of compounds containing carbon, hydrogen, and oxygen, and including the sugars, starches, and celluloses.

cardiac orifice (kahr′dē ak or′i fis) (G. *kardia,* heart; L. *orificium,* opening,
mouth). The opening between the esophagus and the stomach.

caries (kair'ēz) (L. rottenness). Disease of the calcified external portions of the teeth, causing their disintegration and the formation of cavities.

catabolism (kə tab'ə lizm) (G. *katabole,* a throwing down). Destructive metabolism. Any destructive process by which complex substances are converted by living cells into more simple compounds.

cathartic (kə thahr'tik) (G. *kathartikos,* a cleansing agent). A medicine that quickens and increases evacuation from the bowels.

cecum (sē'kəm) (L. *calcum,* blind). The intestinal pouch into which the ileum, colon, and vermiform appendix open.

cementum (sə men'təm) (L. *caementum,* rough, unhewn stone). The layer of bony tissue covering the root of a tooth.

cholesterol (kə les'tə rol) (G. *chole,* bile, anger; *stereos,* solid). A white, fatty, crystalline substance, tasteless and odorless. Found in bile, blood, gallstones, egg yolk, etc.

chyme (kīm) (G. *chymos,* juice). The semifluid, creamy material produced by gastric digestion of food.

cretinism (krē'tən izm) (Fr. *cretin,* dwarf; G. *ismos,* condition). A condition due to congenital lack of thyroid secretion; characterized by physical and mental arrested development.

crown (kroun) (L. *corona,* a crown). The portion of a tooth which is covered with enamel.

deamination (dē am i nā'shən) (L. *de,* without; *amine,* from ammonia). Removal of the amino group (NH_2).

defecation (def ə kā'shən) (L. *defaecare,* to deprive of dregs). The discharge of fecal material from the bowel.

dentin (den'tin) (L. *dens,* tooth). The chief substance or tissue of the teeth which surrounds the tooth pulp and is covered by enamel.

digestion (di jes'chən) (L. *digestio,* from *dis-,* apart; *gerere,* to carry). The process of converting food into materials able to be absorbed and assimilated.

duodenum (doo ə dē'nəm, doo od'ə nəm) (L. *duodeni,* twelve). The first 10 to 12 inches of small intestine.

emulsification (i mul si fi kā'shən). Conversion into an emulsion, a preparation of one liquid distributed in globules, throughout a second liquid.

enamel (i nam'əl) (AF. *enameler, enamayller,* to coat with enamel). The white, calcareous, very hard substance that covers and protects the softer layers of the tooth.

endocrine (en'də krin) (G. *endon,* within; *krinein,* to separate). Pertaining to internal secretion; glands that produce such internal secretions.

enema (en'ə mə) (G. *enema,* send in). Injection of a liquid into the rectum.

enterokinase (en tə rō kī'nās) (G. *enteron,* intestine; *kinesis,* motion). An enzyme of the intestinal juice which activates trypsinogen into trpysin.

enzyme (en'zīm) (G. *en,* in; *zyme,* leaven). A complex organic compound that accelerates or catalyzes chemical change.

erepsin (i rep'sin) (G. *ereptesthai,* to feed on). An enzyme of the intestinal juice, capable of decomposing proteoses and peptones to produce amino acids.

esophagus (i sof'ə gəs) (G. *oisen,* to carry; *phagema,* food). A canal extending from the pharynx to the stomach.

exocrine (ek'sə krin) (G. *exo*, outside; *krinein*, to separate). To secrete externally, as glands that discharge their secretion through a duct.

fat (fat) (AS. *faett*, firm). Whitish, animal or plant substance, also called *adipose* tissue.

feces (fē'sēz) (L. *faeces*, refuse). The discharge from the intestine, consisting chiefly of food residues, bacteria, and intestinal excretions.

flatulence (flat'yə ləns) (L. *flatulentia*, a blowing). Distention of the stomach or intestines with air or gases.

fluoridation (floor i dā'shən). Treatment with fluorides, specifically, addition of fluoride to water to reduce the incidence of dental caries.

fundus (fun'dəs) (L. *fundi*, the bottom). The base or part of a hollow organ remotest from its mouth.

gallbladder (gawl'blad ər) (AS. *gealla*, bile; AS. *blaedre*, a sac). The pear-shaped reservoir for the bile on the under surface of the liver.

gallstone (gawl' stōn). A concretion formed in the gallbladder or bile duct.

gastric digestion (gas'trik di jes'chən) (G. *gaster*, stomach). That part of digestion which takes place in the stomach.

gingiva (jin jī'və) (L. *gingiva*, gums). The gums. The tissue which covers the alveolar processes of the upper and lower jaws and surrounds the necks of the teeth.

gingivitis (jin ji vī'tis) (L. *gingiva*, the gums; G. *-itis*, inflammation). Inflammation of the gums.

globule (glob'yool) (L. *globulus*, a small globe). Any small spherical mass of material.

glycerol (glis'ə rol) (G. *glykys*, sweet). A clear, colorless, syrupy liquid compounded of various fats and oils.

glycogen (glī'kə jən) (G. *glykys*, sweet; *gennan*, to produce). An animal starch that can be stored in the body for rapid conversion to glucose.

heartburn (hahrt'burn). A burning sensation in the esophagus, a symptom of indigestion.

hemorrhoids (hem'ə roidz) (G. *haimorrhois*, from *haima*, blood). A swelling of the veins in the mucous membranes of the anal canal and rectum.

hypovitaminosis (hī'pō vī'tə mi nō'sis) (G. *hypo*, under; L. *vita*, life; *osis*, a condition of). A condition due to a deficiency of one or more essential vitamins.

ileum (il'ē əm) (L. *ilium*, groin). The last division of the small intestine; the part between the jejunum and large intestine.

indigestion (in di jes'chən). Lack or failure of digestion.

insulin (in'sə lin) (L. *insula*, island; *in*, ending indicating a chemical compound). A protein hormone formed by the islets of Langerhans in the pancreas and secreted into the blood, where it regulates carbohydrate (sugar) metabolism.

jejunum (ji joo'nəm) (L. *jejuno*, "empty"). That portion of the small intestine which extends from the duodenum to the ileum.

kinetic energy (ki net'ik en'ər jē) (G. *kinetikos*, from *kinetos*, movable). Energy engaged in producing work or motion.

lactase (lak'tās) (L. *lac*, milk; *-ase*, enzyme). An intestinal enzyme that splits lactose into glucose and galactose.

lacteals (lak'tē əl[z]) (L. *lacteus*, milky). The intestinal lymphatics that take up fats.

lactose (lak'tōs) (L. *lactis,* milk).   A sugar obtained from milk.

larynx (lar'inks) (G. *larynx,* larynx).   The structure situated at the top of the trachea and below the root of the tongue. It is the organ of voice.

laxative (lak'sə tiv) (L. *laxare,* to unloose).   A medicine causing defecation.

lecithin (les'i thin) (G. *lekithos,* yolk of egg).   A colorless, compound found in animal tissue, especially nerve tissue, semen, yolk of egg, and in smaller amounts in the bile and blood.

lipase (lī'pās, lip'ās) (G. *lipos,* fat; *-ase,* enzyme).   A fat-splitting enzyme.

lumen (loo'mən) (L. *lumen,* light).   The cavity or channel within a tube or tubular organ.

malocclusion (mal ə kloo'zhən) (L. *malum,* ill; *occlusio,* to close).   Failure of the jaws to close properly, as a result of poor placement of the teeth.

maltase (mawl'tās) (L. *malt,* grain; *-ase,* enzyme).   An enzyme which breaks down maltose into dextrose.

maltose (mawl'tōs) (L. *malt,* grain).   A sugar obtained from starch.

mastication (mas ti kā'shən) (L. *masticare,* to chew).   The chewing of food.

metabolism (me tab'ə lizm) (G. *metaballein,* to change).   The sum of all the physical and chemical processes of the body.

mineral (min'ə rəl) (L. *minerale,* mineral).   An inorganic element or compound occurring in nature.

mucin (myoo'sin) (L. *mucus,* mucus).   The chief constituent of mucus.

mucous membrane (myoo'kəs mem'brān) (L. *mucosus,* pertaining to mucus; *membrana,* membrane).   The lining membrane of the body cavities and canals which are connected with the outside.

mucus (myoo'kəs) (L. *mucus,* mucus).   The viscid, slippery secretion produced by mucous membranes which it moistens and protects.

nausea (naw'zē ə, naw'zhə) (G. *nausia,* seasickness).   An uncomfortable sensation related to the alimentary system, with a desire to vomit.

orthodontia (or thə don'shə) (G. *orthos,* straight; *odous,* tooth).   The branch of dentistry which deals with the prevention and correction of irregularities of the teeth and malocclusion.

osmosis (os mō'sis) (G. *osmos,* impulsion).   Passage of a solvent from a lesser to a greater concentration through a membrane which is permeable to the solvent.

palate (pal'ət) (L. *palatum,* palate).   The roof of the mouth.

pancreas (pan'krē əs) (G. *pan,* all; *kreas,* flesh).   A large gland located behind the stomach; its secretion (pancreatic juice) is used in digestion.

pepsin (pep'sin) (G. *pepsis,* digestion).   The chief enzyme of gastric juice which acts upon proteins (protease).

peptic ulcer (pep'tik ul'sər) (G. *peptikos,* pertaining to digestion; L. *ulcus,* ulcer).   An open lesion occurring in the lower esophagus, stomach, or duodenum.

peptone (pep'tōn) (G. *pepton,* digesting).   The product derived by the first step of protein digestion.

perforation (pur fə rā'shən) (L. *perforare,* to pierce through).   Act of piercing through a part.

periodontal membrane (per ē ə don'təl mem'brān) (G. *peri,* around; *odous,* tooth; L. *membrana,* membrane).   The tissue that connects the cementum of a tooth to the surrounding structures.

periodontitis (per ē ə don tī'tis) (G. *peri,* around; *odous,* tooth; *-itis,* inflammation). Inflammatory reaction of peridontal tissues.

peristalsis (per i stal'sis) (G. *peri,* around; *stalsis,* contraction). Progressive wavelike contractions by which muscles of the alimentary canal propel their contents.

pharynx (far'inks) (G. *pharynx,* pharynx). The part of the digestive canal between the cavity of the mouth and the esophagus.

polypeptides (pol'ē pep'tīdz) (G. *poly,* many; *peptein,* to digest). A union of three or more amino acids.

potential energy (pə ten'shəl en'ər jē) (L. *potentia,* power). Existing energy, ready for action but not yet active.

prosthetics (pros thet'iks) (G. "a putting to"). A branch of surgery involved with replacement of an absent part of the body by an artificial one, for example, dentures.

protein (prō'tēn, prō'tē in) (G. *protos,* first). Any of a class of complex organic combinations of amino acids which are essential constituents of all living cells.

proteose (prō'tē ōs) (G. *protos,* first; L. *-ose,* full of). Any of a class of intermediate soluble protein derivatives formed by digestion.

ptyalin (tī'ə lin) (G. *ptyalon,* spittle). An enzyme occurring in the saliva which converts starch into maltose and dextrose.

purgative (pur'gə tiv) (L. *purgare,* to cleanse). Cathartic, causing evacuations from the bowels (defecation).

pylorus (pī lor'əs) (G. *pyloros,* from *pyle,* gate; *ouros,* guard). The opening between the stomach and the duodenum.

pyorrhea (pī ə rē'ə) (G. *pyo,* pus; *rhoia,* flow). A discharge of pus; pus-filled inflammation of the sockets of the teeth.

rectum (rek'təm) (L. "straight"). The last few inches of the large intestine, terminating in the anus.

rennin (ren'in) (ME. from *rennen,* to run). A gastric enzyme that coagulates milk.

saliva (sə lī'və) (L. *saliva,* saliva). The first digestive secretion, emitted from the salivary glands into the mouth.

salivary glands (sal'i ver ē gland[z]) (L. *saliva,* saliva; *glans,* acorn). The three pairs of glands which secrete saliva.

serous membrane (sē'rəs mem'brān) (L. *serum,* whey). A membrane lining a serous cavity, for example, pleural, peritoneal, and pericardial.

sigmoid (colon) (sig'moid) (G. *sigmoeides,* shaped like the letter S). The lower part of the descending colon, shaped like the letter S.

sphincter (sfingk'tər) (G. *sphinkter,* binder). A ringlike muscle which closes a natural opening.

steapsin (stē ap'sin) (G. *stear,* fat; *pepis,* digestion). An enzyme present in pancreatic juice that digests fats (lipase).

sublingual gland (sub ling'gwəl) (L. *sub,* under; *lingua,* tongue). Salivary gland in floor of mouth.

submaxillary gland (sub mak'si ler ē) (L. *sub,* under; *maxilla,* the jaw). Salivary gland in floor of mouth.

sucrase (soo'krās) (Fr. *sucre,* sugar). An enzyme in intestinal juice that begins digestion of sugar (amylase).

sucrose (soo'krōs) (Fr. *sucre,* sugar).   A sugar; chiefly derived from sugarcane and sugar beets.

suppository (sə poz'i tor ē) (L. *suppositorium,* that which is placed underneath).   A medicated preparation for introduction into rectum, vagina, or urethra.

tartar (tahr'tər) (G. *tartaron,* dregs).   Material deposited on the teeth; consists of lime.

thyroid gland (thī'roid) (G. *thyreos,* shield; *eidos,* form).   A hormonal gland of internal secretion (endocrine) in the neck.

thyroxin (thī rok'sin) (G. *thyreos,* shield).   The principal hormone secreted by the thyroid gland; has a profound influence on growth.

tooth pulp.   Inner portion of the tooth which contains the connective tissue, capillaries, lymph vessels, and nerve endings.

trypsin (trip'sin) (G. *tripsis,* a rubbing).   An enzyme in the pancreatic juice (protease).

trypsinogen (trip sin'ə jən) (G. *tripsis,* a rubbing; *gennan,* to produce).   The proenzyme or inactive form of trypsin.

vermiform appendix (vur'mi form ə pen'diks) (L. *vermis,* worm; *forma,* shape; *appendere,* to hang upon).   A worm-shaped process projecting from the cecum.

Vincent's angina (vin'sənts an jī'nə).   Painful ulcerative disease of the gingiva which may affect the tonsils and pharynx, commonly called "trench mouth."

villi (vil'ī) (L. *villus,* tuft of hair).   Short, fingerlike projections found on certain membranous surfaces, mainly in the digestive system.

vitamin (vī'tə min) (L. *vita,* life).   A general term for a number of organic substances that are necessary for the normal functioning of the body.

CHAPTER 7

DIET AND
WEIGHT
CONTROL

DETERMINING DESIRABLE WEIGHT

OVERWEIGHT AND OBESITY

UNDERWEIGHT

FOOD FADS AND FALLACIES

MEAL PLANNING

SUMMARY

Although much of the world today is faced with very real problems of malnutrition due to too little food, the average American is preoccupied with the consequences of overeating. The degree of this concern is reflected in the fact that one out of every four Americans tries to reduce his weight to some extent every year. Not only are these 50 million Americans a reflection of the importance we attach to proper weight, but also they are a frank commentary on the failure most people encounter in their attempts to reach and maintain a satisfactory weight. Obesity is not a new health problem. Benjamin Franklin made a sage comment on the matter when he mused, "I have seen few die of hunger; of eating, a hundred thousand."

Some people, desiring to resemble as closely as possible the slender image chosen by the clothing designers, are very "weight-conscious." Medical and nutritional authorities, however, are alarmed by the problem of weight control for an entirely different reason. Studies show that people who are overweight are almost twice as likely to have heart trouble (the number one cause of death) as people with normal weight. Evidence is mounting that overweight increases the chances of a person's encountering other breakdowns in health. Life insurance companies have been very interested in these statistics. Inasmuch as a shorter life span means an earlier payment of death benefits, these companies are interested in people's living as long as possible.

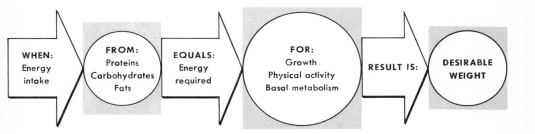

Fig. 7.1 Achieving a desirable weight.

DETERMINING DESIRABLE WEIGHT

To determine the ideal weight for an individual is difficult, if not impossible. Body weight varies with sex, age, height, skeletal structure, rate of basal metabolism, and endocrine peculiarities. Since the so-called "ideal" or "average" individual does not exist, it is neither realistic nor possible to suggest an "ideal weight" that could be applied to all adults. Consequently, in trying to arrive at a reasonable weight recommendation for adults, the Food and Nutrition Board of the National Research Council has had to take a number of factors into consideration. Life insurance actuarial tables have indicated that the most favorable health expectation is associated with the weight normally achieved at age 25. It is accordingly recommended that the desirable weight for this age is a proper weight to maintain throughout adult life. Maximum body development in either sex is usually attained several years earlier than 25 years—at 18 years of age in the female and at 20 years of age in the male. In Table 7.1 adjustments in recommended weights are made for sex, height, and body build. An individual with a smaller-than-average frame would be expected to weigh somewhat less than the weight recommended for his given height, whereas an individual with a larger-than-average frame would usually weigh more. The adjustments on the table provide for this variation. A general ideal to keep in mind for maintaining a desirable weight is summarized in Fig. 7.1.

OVERWEIGHT AND OBESITY

The terms *overweight* and *obesity* are generally considered synonymous. Actually, they represent somewhat different things. Overweight is defined as any weight in excess of the weight recommended for a given person according to the Desirable Weight table. The cause of the excess weight does not matter. Although probably due to excess fat, it may also be due to an excessively muscular physique or a heavy skeletal framework. Obesity is defined as an excessive deposition of fat beyond what is considered normal for a given age, sex, and build. An obese person may or may not be overweight. He can be the desirable weight

TABLE 7.1   **DESIRABLE WEIGHTS FOR HEIGHT**

Height[a] in inches	Weight in Pounds Men	Women
60		109 ± 9[b]
62		115 ± 9
64	133 ± 11	122 ± 10
66	142 ± 12	129 ± 10
68	151 ± 14	136 ± 10
70	159 ± 14	144 ± 11
72	167 ± 15	152 ± 12
74	175 ± 15	

[a] Heights and weights are without shoes and other clothing.
[b] Desirable weight for a small-framed woman at this height would be approximately 109 lb. minus 9 lb., or a total of 100 lb.; for an average-framed woman, 109 lb.; for a large-framed woman 109 lb. plus 9 lb., or a total of 118 lb.
SOURCE: Food and Nutrition Board, National Research Council.

and yet be obese because his amount of body fat in relation to his muscle mass might be greater than normal. The problem is that there is no easy way to measure body fat in relation to the person's total weight. Generally speaking, however, total body weight, as measured on the scales, can be a fairly good reflection of the presence or absence of excess body fat. In further discussion in this text no distinction will be made between the terms overweight and obesity.

In the United States approximately 20 percent of the population weigh more than they should.[1] Further studies point out that 23 percent of male college freshmen and almost 36 percent of female college freshmen are overweight.[2] The problem generally increases with age. As a

[1] F. J. Stare, *Eating for Good Health*, Garden City, N.Y., Doubleday, 1964, p. 106.
[2] S. Grollman, *The Human Body*, New York, Macmillan, 1964, p. 460.

person ages his basal metabolic rate drops, but he tends to eat as much as he did when he was younger. Three out of five American men in their 50s are considered overweight.

CAUSES OF OVERWEIGHT

In general, overweight is the result either of faulty metabolism or of faulty regulation of the diet.

Fat cells in adipose tissue (fat deposit of the body) are in a continual state of flux. Within these cells fatty acids are continually being built up for storage and broken down for metabolism. Each individual has a unique metabolic rate. Some use this stored food faster or slower than others and, accordingly, have a higher or lower rate of metabolism. These differences in rate occur in response to specific hormone and enzyme activities in the body. They are influenced by inherited or developmental differences; they can be altered by disease in the pituitary or thyroid gland. A faulty metabolism can reflect itself in either overweight or underweight.

Far more often overweight is the result of failure on the part of the person to regulate his food intake. A person's appetite is influenced by various factors, some of which are physiological. These include the concentration of blood sugar, the temperature of the blood, the amount of active fat available, and the concentration of the amino acids in the blood. These physiological factors affect the appetite centers in the brain.

Other factors also can affect a person's eating habits. Some of these contribute to overweight more than others. Some of these factors are:

1. *Home environment.* Some individuals have come from homes where meals are rich and where excessive eating is common. Others are accustomed to heavy between-meal eating, particularly of sweets such as soft drinks, candy, ice cream, and pastries. Still others have been accustomed to too little exercise as a result of easily available transportation, lack of organized sports, modern conveniences, and laziness.

2. *Poverty.* Some families because of limited finances buy cheap foods which tend to be high in carbohydrates—sugars and starches.

3. *Occupation.* Housewives who are often around food sometimes become habitual samplers and nibblers. The same holds true for people who work in such food industries as candy shops, restaurants, and bakeries.

4. *Emotional factors.* Some people find eating a pleasant break from a monotonous routine. Others find it a satisfying compensation for domestic troubles, financial problems, illness in the family, social upsets, anxiety over school work or a pending business deal.

5. *Age and disease.* As a person grows older, his dietary needs change, but he may have difficulty in diminishing long-established eat-

ing patterns. Disabilities may reduce the previous amount of activity and make a change in earlier eating habits necessary.

Regardless of the underlying causes of obesity, the basic problem is simply one of taking in more calories than are needed for one's total activities—basic metabolism, heat loss, work, and exercise. Unused calories from any source are stored in the body as fat, each pound of stored fat representing about 3500 calories. We either use the calories or we store them, regardless of where they come from. The more stored calories, the greater the degree of obesity (Fig. 7.2).

EFFECTS OF OVERWEIGHT

There are various reasons why overweight is undesirable. Life insurance records show that overweight individuals, for several reasons,

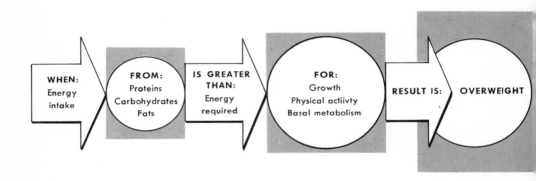

Fig. 7.2 Process of becoming overweight.

are poorer risks than those who have normal weight. First of all, their life expectancy is less. The danger of death increases in direct proportion to the amount of overweight. The principal killers of overweight persons are heart and artery diseases, diabetes, cirrhosis of the liver, gallstones, digestive system diseases, and certain forms of cancer. In addition, other painful conditions are common—varicose veins, gout, high blood pressure, pulmonary emphysema, nephritis, and toxemia in pregnancy. The carrying of extra pounds wears down tissue in joints such as the ankles, knees, and hips (as in *osteoarthritis*). With every pound of added fat tissue, there is also added an additional three fourths of a mile of blood vessels, all of which places added stress on the heart and blood vessels. Excess fat complicates all surgery and increases surgical risk. The same is true in the delivery of a child. It is work to carry around body weight that is not needed, giving the overweight person "that tired feeling." Fat accumulating around internal vital organs tends to crowd them. The individual is less agile, has more balancing problems, and moves more slowly; he tends to have more physical accidents than a person of normal weight. Thus overweight leads not only to an unpleasant appearance, but also to a shortened life. It is an unfavorable factor in a number of diseases.

REDUCING

The problem of reducing weight is a personal one. An overweight person must *want* to lose weight badly enough to go through the rigors of ignoring the sight and smell of appealing food within his reach. He must have intention plus will-power. Motivation can be created in various ways. Young people may be strongly motivated by the desire for a pleasing appearance. Older people may require other reasons, such as the advice of a doctor or the prospect of living longer and possibly avoiding certain bodily disorders.

The next thing the overweight person must do is to admit that his obesity in all likelihood was caused by overnutrition—that his intake of food has exceeded his output of energy. If intake is reduced to equal the output, a person should be successful in "holding his own." The overweight person needs to go one step further; intake must be reduced to the point where it will be less than output. Accordingly, as the body uses more energy than is being taken in, body fat will be reduced and weight will diminish. This assumption is the basis for most reducing programs.

How can this reversal be achieved? One of several methods or combinations of them may be followed. First of all, food intake can be cut by going on a reducing diet. Second, the body's use of calories can be increased through increased exercise or through taking prescribed drugs which speed up body metabolism. The best choice combines reduced food intake and increased exercise to improve muscle tone and body regulation mechanisms. Third, a method recommended by physicians only in very extreme cases, is *lipectomy*. This is a surgical removal of layers of excessive fat from those parts of the body that are easily accessible and which tend to receive the largest accumulations of stored fat. Such removal would usually be done from the abdomen, breasts, arms, or legs. Lipectomy is a beginning in severe cases; it needs to be followed by the first or second plan if the patient is to reach and maintain desirable body weight.

REDUCING DIETS

Today we find suggestions on every hand for losing weight. These range all the way from the "miracle diets" that will take off 10 pounds in two weeks; through the oils, tablets, seeds, juices, extracts, and high fat or protein diets; through the prepared formulas one can buy in the form of cookies or prepared drinks; to simply eating less of whatever food one normally chooses to eat. Some of these have value and some are considered medically dangerous. Although it is not our intention to enumerate the many products advertised to help lose weight, a few general statements are necessary.

The basic problem is in readjusting the regular diet. Whatever is taken or done to accomplish weight loss must be viewed in terms of the total picture. Although various aids may be helpful temporarily, one does not want to use them the rest of his life, and besides, some of them are expensive. At best they may be aids to help the overweight person change his eating habits. They are not magical in solving the problem. There just is no easy way to lose weight.

Generally, no reducing diet is decidedly better than another. Any one of them faithfully followed should help a person to lose weight successfully. Several guidelines should be observed in deciding upon which reducing diet to follow. The following should be considered:

1. *See a physician.*   Let him decide whether or not it is safe to lose weight, how much weight to lose, and how long the reduction should take.

2. *Choose a practical diet.*   The problem of dieting will be life-long. Therefore a person should choose a type of reducing diet he will be able to follow without undue regimentation. It should be compatible with the eating habits he is accustomed to and likes. It is not necessary to stop eating the foods he cherishes, but he may have to cut out some things or govern the amount he eats. This regulation is not only true for *losing* extra pounds, but also for *maintaining* a desirable weight. Unless he can successfully readjust his old diet that allowed him to become fat, he will likely end up with the old overweight problem all over again, and all the discomfort of reducing will have been in vain.

3. *Reduce the calories taken in.*   Some studies indicate that calorie reduction can best be done by limiting the carbohydrate intake; some, by reducing fats eaten; and others, by limiting protein intake. Regardless of the method, calories *do* count (even if one refuses to count them). Many kinds of food that don't look "rich" (high in calories) are actually abundant in them. The same could be said for certain drinks. Table 7.2 is a listing of the calories in some favorite foods and drinks, based on a usual restaurant serving.

4. *Plan a diet.*   A reducing diet should contain all the basic food groups—meat, milk, vegetables and fruits, and cereals. During the reducing period the body will still be functioning. It will need not only proteins, minerals, and vitamins, but also limited calories. Generally, a reducing diet should provide at least 1200–1800 calories a day. Some commercial reducing formulas allow a minimum of 900 calories per

TABLE 7.2 CALORIES IN SOME FAVORITE FOODS AND DRINKS

Breakfast	Calories	Drinks	Calories
1 scrambled egg	110	Whole milk, 1 cup	160
2 slices fried bacon	100	Nonfat milk, 1 cup	90
Ham, slice, lean and fat	245	Malted milk, 1 cup	280
1 wheat pancake	60	Cocoa, 1 cup	235
1 waffle	210	Orange juice, frozen,	
Grapefruit, ½ whole	55	1 cup diluted	110
Cantaloupe, ½ melon	60	Apple juice, 1 cup	120
Corn flakes, 1 oz.	110	Grape juice, canned, 1 cup	165
Oatmeal, 1 cup	130	Yoghurt, 1 cup	120
White bread, 1 slice	60	Cola drink, 1 cup	95
Butter, 1 pat	50	Ginger ale, 1 cup	70
Jam, 1 tablespoon	55	Beer, 1 cup	100

Lunch or Dinner		Snacks	
Tomato soup, 1 cup	90	Cheddar cheese, 1-inch cube	70
Spaghetti, meat balls and		Bologna, 1 slice	85
tomato sauce, 1 cup	335	Peanut butter, 1 tablespoon	95
Pork chop, 1 slice lean	130	Peanuts, roasted, 1 cup	840
Roast beef, 1 slice lean	125	10 potato chips	115
Hamburger, meat only, 3 oz.	245	Raisins, dried, 1 cup	460
1 frankfurter, cooked	155	1 apple	70
Chicken, ½ breast	155	1 banana	85
Mashed potatoes, buttered,		1 orange, navel	60
1 cup	185	1 peach	35
Pizza, 1 section	185	Watermelon, 1 wedge	115
Cottage cheese, creamed,		Popcorn, 1 cup	65
1 cup	240	2 graham crackers	55
Custard, 1 cup	285	1 doughnut, cake type	125
Angelfood cake, 1 section	110	Candy, milk chocolate, 1 oz.	150
Iced chocolate cake,		Marshmallows, 1 oz.	90
1 section	445	Pretzels, 5 small sticks	20
Apple pie, 1 section	345	1 fig bar	55
Ice cream, 1 cup	285	1 cookie, 3-inch	120
Sherbet, orange, 1 cup	260		
Corn starch pudding, 1 cup	275		

SOURCE: *Nutritive Value of Foods*, Home and Garden Bulletin No. 72, rev. September 1964, Washington, D.C., U.S. Department of Agriculture.

TABLE 7.3 A 1200 CALORIE PER DAY DIET PATTERN

Breakfast
  Fruit—1 medium serving, fresh, frozen, or canned
  Egg—1, poached or boiled
  Toast—1 slice with 1 teaspoon butter or margarine

      or

  Cereal—½ cup with ¼ cup milk, no sugar
  Coffee or tea—no cream or sugar

Mid-Morning snack
  Nonfat milk or buttermilk—1 glass

Luncheon
  Meat or cheese—1 3-oz. portion
  Vegetable—1 medium serving; may be raw, as a salad such as lettuce and
    tomato, or cooked; use lemon or vinegar for seasoning rather than butter
    or salad dressings
  Fruit—1 medium serving, fresh or unsweetened canned
  Bread—1 slice
  Butter or margarine—1 teaspoon or 1 pat
  Tea or coffee—no cream or sugar

Mid-Afternoon
  Iced tea, lemonade, or a soft drink

Dinner
  Bouillon or consommé or vegetable-juice cocktail—1 serving
  Meat—1 3-oz. portion
  Potato or a substitute for potato—1 small serving of mashed or baked potato,
    steamed rice, corn, lima beans, or macaroni; or 1 slice bread
  Vegetable—1 serving, raw, as a salad, or cooked; one vegetable a day should
    be a green, leafy one
  Butter or margarine—1 teaspoon, for potato
  Fruit—1 medium serving, fresh or unsweetened canned
  Tea or coffee—no cream or sugar

Evening or Bedtime
  Nonfat milk, buttermilk, soft drink, or glass of beer
  Crackers or pretzels—2

day. This minimum is acceptable when such products are supplemented by certain nutrients such as vitamins and minerals. Table 7.3 suggests a pattern for a 1200 calorie per day reducing diet. Generally, however, a person should not try to account for all calories in foods eaten, because it is almost impossible to do an accurate job of counting calories. The calorie charts do not and could not list all foods. In addition, such counting unnecessarily regiments eating so that many people give up the whole idea of weight reduction as impossible.

5. *Know what the goal is.*   To lose one pound of stored fat in a week a person will have to reduce his calorie intake by at least 3500 calories a week, or 500 calories a day. To lose two pounds a week, a person should reduce his intake by 1000 calories a day. Nutritionists suggest that a good reducing regimen should work toward a loss of one to two pounds of weight a week. A more rapid rate of loss may result in deficiencies in essential dietary elements and, therefore, is less likely to result in a permanent improvement in eating habits. The reducer should weigh himself daily on a good bathroom scale. He should do it at the same time each day and under similar conditions. He should consider each pound lost a reduction of 3500 calories of stored fat. (A "crash" diet claiming to take off 10 pounds in two weeks would mean a calorie reduction of 2500 calories a day, which is more calories than most women normally get. Such a reducing suggestion represents starvation and is therefore preposterous.)

6. *Graph the progress.*   A person gains weight gradually; ideally, he should lose it the same way. Because gradual reducing programs can be discouraging, a person might lose sight of his initial goal. A good psychological crutch to use in keeping track of progress is a simple graph set up at the beginning of the program. A person should program his weight loss according to how many pounds he needs to lose. He should aim at one to two pounds of weight loss per week, then construct a graph. The graph shown in Fig. 7.3 is set up on the basis of one pound of weight loss per week. A straight line can be drawn from where one's weight is when he began to diet to where he wants it to be when he finishes. Weight is measured each morning. A dot is put at the point where his weight is each day. The line of dots will tell him how close he is to his plan of weight loss on any particular day during the reducing time. The idea is not to allow his weight to stray too far from the suggested weight in any given week. The graph will serve as a daily reminder of progress. This method has been used with success as a help during a reducing regimen.

7. *Exercise regularly.*   A reasonable program of regular physical exercise helps a person resist weight gain through expenditure of energy. In addition it improves muscle tone and contributes toward a general feeling of well-being, both physical and mental. However, a person must be careful not to look upon physical exercise as a substitute for controlled calorie

intake. Only about 100 calories are used by walking a mile. More vigorous sports activities such as tennis or active swimming use up as many as 1000 calories an hour. Too strenuous an exercise, however, is apt to result in an increased appetite. Moderate and regular periods of exercise will help to use up stored energy without increasing the appetite.

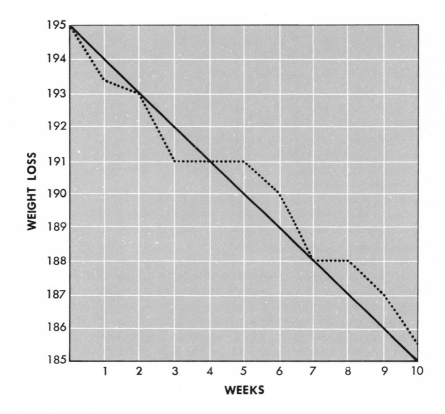

Fig. 7.3 A reducing graph.

As a person becomes older, his calorie requirements decline. The National Research Council suggests that an individual's calorie allowance should be reduced by 5 percent per decade between the ages of 35 and 55 and an additional 8 percent per decade between the ages of 55 and 75. A further reduction of 10 percent is recommended for people 75 and older.

As the American "way of life" becomes less strenuous, the calorie requirements for the average American decrease as well. The National Research Council has found that it takes fewer calories today to maintain an adult at the desirable age 25 weight than it did a decade ago.

Consequently, the Recommended Dietary Allowances of the Food and Nutrition Board of the National Research Council have been reduced. It becomes important for an adult to be guided in his diet by his weight, rather than by his eating habits he may have learned before life became quite as automated and leisurely as it is in this country today.

PHARMACEUTICAL AIDS

Another approach in the management of overweight has been through the use of drugs. Viewed by some physicians as a controversial method of weight reduction, drugs nonetheless have been found to assist some individuals in achieving a negative caloric balance, according to a report by the Council on Drugs of the American Medical Association. Different compounds, affecting the body in different ways, have been used. Generally, these drugs serve to decrease or distract the appetite, increase metabolism, tranquilize the body, or speed up loss of body fluids. Most of these drugs are potentially dangerous and should never be used unless medically prescribed. Any of them may have undesirable side effects. At best, they are aids in restricting caloric intake. They cannot be considered an easy road to reducing.

REDUCING DON'TS

In addition to certain specific reducing dangers already pointed out in the text, several general things should be mentioned.

1. Don't blame overweight problems on inheritance. Although there are surely a few cases of faulty heredity which tend to make overweight more of a problem for some people than others, most cases can be traced to either a personal or a cultural problem. Even though an overweight problem can be traced to a physical problem of some kind, many physical problems can be successfully treated. Be careful not to misconstrue faulty home practice in matters of overeating as being a hereditary problem.

2. Don't be tempted by "crash" diets. Any diet plan which claims to take off any number of pounds in a short period of time should be carefully scrutinized. It may be a case of misleading advertising, or it may be a case where drugs are being used which can cause organic damage to the body. Seeing a physician before going on any reducing diet should give one ample protection against such plans.

3. Don't follow the food fads. Some such diets are not palatable, others are monotonous, and many of them turn out to be expensive. Balanced nutrition calls for a variety of foods. A diet purporting to succeed with a single food could well result in malnutrition. Good nutrition for the body is not to be considered a luxury, but a basic essential. Don't be convinced that a so-called "perfect" food should be substituted

for the wide variety of appealing and nutritious foods available at reasonable cost in our grocery stores today.

UNDERWEIGHT

The underweight person is the exception in the United States today. Fortunately for him, our culture, both medically and socially, considers a lighter weight more desirable today than it did in the past. Unless there is a case of malnutrition, the underweight person today should feel increasingly comfortable socially. As recommended daily dietary

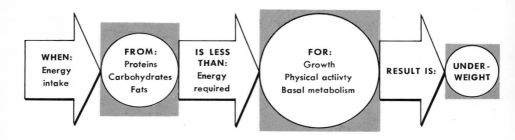

Fig. 7.4 Process of becoming underweight.

allowances become less, the individual who once was considered to be underweight comes closer to what is now held to be a normal weight.

An individual may be underweight for various reasons, including malnutrition, disease, endocrine disorders, lack of appetite, overactivity, or nervousness. Underweight frequently is the result of faulty nutrition. Symptoms may include anemia, chronic digestive disturbances, low resistance to disease, and mental and physical slowness. In severe forms, malnutrition can lead to various deficiency diseases brought on by inadequate amounts of vitamins or minerals. In selected cases malnutrition may result from the inability of the body to digest or use certain foods it needs. This inability may be due to faulty enzyme action. In any case, malnutrition can lead to additional problems—increased susceptibility to diseases (such as tuberculosis), injury to certain body organs (such as the heart or kidneys), or, in severe cases, death (Fig. 7.4).

WAYS TO GAIN WEIGHT

In order to gain weight, a person must raise his caloric intake above his energy needs by including more high-calorie foods in his daily diet. He should consider increasing his intake of butter, eggs, and cream or cream products (malted milks, milk shakes, ice cream) and replacing low-calorie foods with high-calorie ones. The appetite may be increased by selecting particularly appetizing foods. If there is a low limit to the amount of food a person eats during normal meals, he may be able to increase his food intake by eating more frequently, including an extra meal or a snack at bedtime.

If underweight is being caused by some emotional problem—brought on by unpleasant working conditions, family problems, worry—the underweight person should try to change the situation or remove himself from it. If underweight is due to physical ailments such as infected body organs (tonsils, teeth), the use of drugs, or physical limitations (such as eyes which need correction or defective ears), the family physician should be consulted.

FOOD FADS AND FALLACIES

The United States Department of Agriculture estimates that over 10 million Americans waste in excess of $500 million a year on quack diets, fake pills, and other products of modern "medicine men." Although the food faddist may be sincere in his beliefs about food and is honestly concerned about his health, he frequently turns into a disciple attempting to convert his friends to his particular beliefs regarding food. He finds it easier to believe the bizarre and spectacular claims of a quack than the more moderate, but realistic, statements of proper authorities.

All kinds of food faddism may be found, for example, for molasses, yoghurt, oysters, cottage cheese, wheat germ, or seaweed extracts. Some people feel that fish is a brain food or that carrots will make hair curly. Some warn against drinking milk and eating acid fruits together, because the acid will curdle milk in the stomach (curdling occurs

Product	False Cures Claimed for Product
Honey and vinegar	Constipation, high blood pressure, asthma, tooth decay, corns, and pyelitis
Wheat germ oil	Arthritis, gallstones, gangrene, cirrhosis of the liver, epilepsy, shingles, and ulcers
Carrot juice	Varicose veins, gout, cystitis, Addison's disease

naturally as a result of the normal activity of stomach acids), or against eating ice cream with rhubarb or buttermilk with cabbage. A few warn against drinking milk entirely for fear of cancer, constipation, or indigestion.

Food faddism can be serious and dangerous for several reasons. It is usually a waste of money, it tends to give the faddist a false sense of security, and it may keep him from seeing a doctor in time. The federal courts have forced some producers of certain quack products to either relabel their products or destroy them.

Food faddism may involve substances which are harmful or which can lead to malnutrition because they have replaced too much of the normal diet. It also tends to undermine public confidence in the scientific study and practice of nutrition.

FORMS OF FADDISM

Although food faddism is practiced in many forms today, we will discuss only a few forms that have large followings and particularly vocal supporters.

NATURAL FOODS

The follower of the "natural food" fad implies or states that all foods should be eaten in their natural states. He may cook, wash, or treat his food, but not process it specially. He is convinced that the processing of foods into white flour and milled and enriched cereals, the canning of fruit and vegetables, and the pasteurizing of milk destroys their nutritive value and makes them unfit for human consumption. He advocates using raw sugar instead of refined sugar, sea salt for regular table salt, lemon juice for vinegar, and whole grains instead of enriched bread. Although there is no harm in eating natural foods, most nutritionists are convinced that processing foods does not destroy their value.

RAW FOODS

Raw food faddists contend that raw foods are best, since cooking or heating of natural foods destroys much of their nutritive value; they also are opposed to the pasteurization of milk. Pasteurization, while protecting the consumer against certain bacteria, *does not* destroy the nutritive value of the milk. And vegetables and other foods if properly cooked retain most of their nutritive value. In addition, cooking makes them more palatable and more easily digested.

A new line put forth by raw food faddists is that "liquified vegetables" have marvelous properties. They contend that by drinking vegetable juices or purees the consumer will be cured of rheumatism and indigestion, relieved of high blood pressure and gallbladder ailments, and improved in his complexion. Although there is certainly nothing wrong with vegetable juice, it has no more nutritive value than the vegetable it came from. Usually, the promoter of the fad is also selling juicing devices at a favorable profit.

MIRACLE FOODS AND FOOD SUPPLEMENTS

Some special foods, along with special food combinations, are supposed to have unique nutritive and therapeutic value. They are supposed to cure "subclinical deficiencies," "hidden hunger," and "that tired feeling." They are special supplements that have "miracle ingredients" or that remedy "devitalized food." The list includes blackstrap molasses, wheat germ, yeast, honey and vinegar, sunflower seeds, alfalfa extract, and kelp. One of them, royal jelly ("the miracle food of the queen bee"), was purported to have the ability to beautify the face and bring back the "joy of life," not to mention being beneficial for cataracts, drunkenness, and other unwanted conditions. One minor sidelight—it was available at $140 an ounce.

It is easy to see how a sufferer from painful arthritis, high blood pressure, gallstones, ulcers, or any of many other conditions might be tempted to believe that his condition was due to a lack of essential nutrients and that this lack could be supplied by some miracle food or supplement available at a special price. It is important to scrutinize carefully all claims of "miracle substances" that purport to cure these ancient diseases and to recognize that modern medicine and nutrition sciences are the surest road to any kind of remedy that is or will be available to treat and prevent disease.

SOURCES OF RELIABLE INFORMATION

Where can a person obtain reliable information on foods and nutrition? He may check with his personal physician or nurse or write the Council on Drugs and Nutrition of the American Medical Association. Occasionally there are articles dealing with nutrition in *Today's Health,* the *American Journal of Nursing,* and *Science News Letter. Nutrition Reviews* is a professional nutritional journal containing technical reports of research being conducted in nutrition. Publications such as *Food: The Yearbook of Agriculture* (1959) or *Nutritive Value of Foods* (Home and Garden Bulletin No. 72) are available from the U.S. Department of Agriculture, and such a publication as *Recommended Dietary Allowances* (1964) is available from the National Research Council. Material dealing with proper nutrition is also generally available from State Departments of Agriculture or state universities. Many libraries have books containing good information on this subject.

MEAL PLANNING

The preceding chapter and sections within this chapter have emphasized the importance of adequate intake of various foods for maintenance of good nutrition and health. The next problem then is the proper correlation of this information for the planning of a satisfactory daily diet. Meal planning is not a mere counting of calories or grams of protein. It is impossible to obtain good nutrition without the daily inclusion of the necessary nutrients; it is impractical to consider feeding from the standpoint of essentials alone. Such factors as digestibility, palatability, and economy determine whether or not the food supplied will be eaten.

A good way to keep away from stereotyped meals is to include in the meal plan at least one different food or one new recipe each week. This innovation should give satisfaction to the homemaker who is preparing the meal and also extend the tastes of the children and the family. Foreign foods may suggest new combinations for menus, as will recipes from neighbors, recipe books, food articles in magazines and newspapers, and food advertisements.

THE FIVE BASIC FOOD GROUPS

Foods may be grouped according to the nutrients they provide. They have traditionally been divided for this purpose into four groups —dairy foods, meats, fruits and vegetables, and bread and cereals. The authors of *Health Science* have chosen to separate the fruits and vegetables, thus creating the *five* basic food groups. It is felt that this change will give added insurance of adequate amounts of vitamin C and other vitamins and minerals.

Even though this guide is general, it is specific in that it stresses foods of pre-eminent value—those foods that when left out of the diet cause deficiencies.

GROUP 1: DAIRY FOODS

This group includes milk, cheese, ice cream, and other foods made with milk, such as soups, beverages, desserts, and sauces. Milk and its many products are our main source of calcium; they also contribute protein, riboflavin, and vitamins A and D. Butter and cream products supply flavorful fat and vitamins A and D, but they do not contain the protein, riboflavin, and calcium of milk. Skim milk and buttermilk supply all the nutrients of whole milk except vitamins A and D and fat, which have been removed together. The nutritional value of cereals and breads are enhanced when they are combined with the protein of dairy foods. Thus traditional combinations of cereal and milk or macaroni and cheese provide good nutrition. Table 7.4 lists the daily minimums advisable for the family.

TABLE 7.4 DAILY FOOD GUIDE

Food Groups	Number of Servings Per Person Per Day	
Group 1		
Dairy Foods	**Milk**	
	Children	3 to 4 cups
	Teen-agers	4 or more cups
	Adults	2 or more cups
	Pregnant women (latter part of pregnancy)	1 quart
	Nursing women	1½ quart
	Alternate Dairy Products	
	1-inch cube cheddar or processed type cheese	⅔ cup milk
	½ cup of cottage cheese	⅓ cup milk
	2 tablespoons cream cheese	1 tablespoon milk
	½ cup ice cream	¼ cup milk
Group 2		
Meat, Fish, Poultry, and Eggs	**Main group**	
	Beef, veal, lamb, pork, variety meats, poultry, eggs, fish, and shellfish	2 or more servings
	Alternates	
	Lentils, peanuts, peanut butter, dry beans, dry peas, and nuts	2 servings occasionally as an alternate
	Servings	
	Lean, cooked meat (without bone, fat, or gristle)	2 to 3 ounces (1 serving)
	2 eggs	1 serving
	1 cup cooked dry beans, dry peas, or lentils	1 serving
	4 tablespoons peanut butter	1 serving
Group 3		
Vegetables	**2 or more servings**—including 1 serving at least every other day of a *dark-green* or *deep-yellow* vegetable for vitamin A (listed in Appendix B).	

TABLE 7.4 **DAILY FOOD GUIDE (Continued)**

Food Groups	Number of Servings Per Person Per Day
Group 4	
Fruits	**2 or more servings per day** including 1 serving each day of a *citrus fruit* or other good source of vitamin C (Appendix B).
Group 5	
Breads and Cereals	**4 or more servings per day**
	5 slices of bread — 4 servings
	3 slices of bread and ½ cup of cooked cereal — 4 servings
	1 ounce of ready-to-eat cereal — 1 serving
	½ to ¾ cup of cooked cereal (including corn-meal, grits, macaroni, noodles, rice, and spaghetti—1 serving
Additional Foods	**Fats and oils**—throughout the week as desired (if not covered by dairy products group)
	Miscellaneous foods—coffee, tea, cocoa, chocolate, salt, pepper, other seasonings, and flavorings. No quantities are suggested for these items.
	Fish-liver oil, or some other source of vitamin D if it is not included in the milk for small children and adults who have little opportunity for being in sunshine.

SOURCE: Prepared from *A Guide to Eating Food,* Yearbook of Agriculture, Washington, D.C., U.S. Dept. of Agriculture, 1959, pp. 267–270.

GROUP 2: MEAT, FISH, POULTRY, AND EGGS

The meat group includes all foods which supply nutrients similar to those in meat—fish, poultry, and eggs, as well as dried beans, nuts, and peanut butter. These last three items contain some incomplete proteins and are best consumed with cheese, meat, milk, or eggs to make their proteins complete and useful to the body. For example, a peanut butter sandwich could be eaten with a glass of milk, or pork and beans with cheese. Foods in the meat group are rich sources of protein. Eggs and meat, especially liver, are important sources of iron, B vitamins, and vitamin A. Pork is an especially good source of vitamin B_1 (thiamine). Dried beans, peas, and nuts are good sources of thiamine and iron.

Any one of the foods in the meat group has great potentialities for injecting variety into family meals. The daily minimums for the family are listed in Table 7.4.

GROUP 3: VEGETABLES

Vegetables are important sources of minerals and vitamins when prepared correctly. Overcooking or cooking at high temperatures or in large amounts of water decreases the amounts of water-soluble vitamins present in this group. They also supply the needed bulk and roughage and give a variety of interesting colors and flavors to daily meals. The recommended two or more servings a day are easy to plan in the form of cooked or raw vegetables and salads. A dark-green, leafy vegetable, or a deep-yellow fruit or vegetable should be eaten daily for vitamin A. Because water will absorb the nutrients, vitamins, and flavors of vegetables, it is nutritionally sound to use the water in which vegetables have been cooked to make soups, gravies, and sauces.

GROUP 4: FRUITS

Two servings of fruit each day is the recommendation. At least one of these should be a citrus fruit or tomato or other food high in vitamin C. Since vitamin C is not stored by the body, it is needed every day. Fruits are easily included in the diet as fresh, frozen, or canned whole fruits or juices, fruit desserts, or snacks. Fruits and vegetables and their juices supply approximately the same nutrients whether they are fresh, frozen, or canned. Children should be encouraged to enjoy fruits in place of other sweets for desserts and snacks.

GROUP 5: BREADS AND CEREALS

This group contains a wide variety of foods, including breads; cereals, both cooked and ready to eat; cornmeal; grits; rice; spaghetti; macaroni; noodles; and all baked products made with whole grain or enriched flours (see Appendix B). The foods in this group are the body's most valuable sources of carbohydrate energy; they also provide thiamine, riboflavin, niacin, and iron. A combination of bread or cereal and protein from the dairy or meat group makes the most satisfying meal and will delay hunger longer than any other combination of nutrients.

The Basic Five Food groups, used daily in recommended amounts as shown in Table 7.4 will supply all the essential nutrients except vitamin D. This vitamin is obtained in sufficient amounts by a person's direct exposure to sunlight and from fish-liver oils and milk to which vitamin D has been added. Vitamin D should be supplemented in the diets of infants, children, expectant mothers, nursing mothers, and adults who work inside and receive little exposure to sunlight.

There are no foods which in themselves are nutritional necessities. Any one food may be high in a variety of nutrients or it may make no essential contribution to the diet. No food is actually bad or harmful, except perhaps when illness forces strict dietary regulation. No food is especially beneficial; people who believe certain foods possess unusual curative or cosmetic properties have been badly misled. In the long run, more benefits come from eating a well-balanced diet regularly than from consuming any one food, tonic, or dietary supplement.

SIMPLE NUTRITION FOR STUDENTS

Studies have shown that many Americans of college age are suffering from nutritional deficiencies.[3] If a person tires easily, or if his physical appearance, as indicated by the luster of his hair and the texture of the skin, is not what it should be, this person could be suffering from a nutritional deficiency. The only person able to tell an individual specifically what he is deficient in is a physician. But the average individual should first check his over-all diet by writing down everything eaten in seven days and comparing this list with the recommended nutritional amounts needed by the body, shown in Table 7.4. If his over-all nutrition is not what it should be, this person should put himself on a Two-Week Demonstration Diet. If such a course is followed for two weeks, the person may see a marked improvement in his energy and appearance; if not, he should consult a physician for an extensive examination of his specific body needs.

SIMPLE TWO-WEEK DEMONSTRATION DIET

When students are attending college, especially if they are living away from home, their time is limited. They do not have time to plan meals days ahead. Consequently, the authors have secured a simple-nutrition plan which will provide an adequate diet without lengthy planning. This diet is known as the "four-five-five plan."

The four-five-five plan stresses adequate amounts of every substance known to be nutritionally necessary by putting emphasis on the five basic food groups. One simple way to incorporate the preceding requirements into a diet and have it come out correct each day is to count these groups after each meal, as shown in Fig. 7.5. Whenever the person is about to order something to eat, he should think back to the last

[3] F. J. Stare, *Eating for Good Health*, Garden City, N.Y., Doubleday, 1964, p. 64.

meal or snack and count off which of the groups were covered by that snack and which should be covered by this meal.

After breakfast (or midmorning snack if the morning meal is split) he should be able to count off four groups. After lunch, or a midafternoon snack, he should count off all five. After dinner, he should count off all five once more. Without the advance menu planning assumed by the Basic Five and other popular plans of nutrition instruction (almost impossible for most college students), he can still achieve a sound

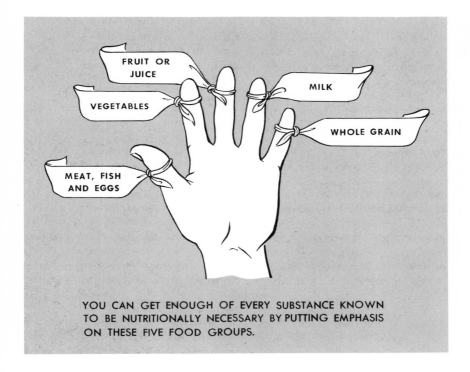

Fig. 7.5 Count 4-5-5 diet.

nutrition by this portion-counting technique, counting four-five-five every day to keep energy and resistance to illness at a well-nourished peak.

There is no need to worry about proportions with this scheme because the average individual will eat the amount that satisfies his hunger; this will probably be more than enough in total amount of food consumed. The main nutritional problem with college students is in the lack of *variety* of foods needed for a proper nutritional diet.

APPLYING THE BASIC FIVE IN FAMILY MEALS

A person cannot trust chance or a spur-of-the-moment selecting of foods to consistently provide good meals. A plan is needed. This "planning" may not involve writing down menus and keeping tedious records, but the results should be good nutritious meals, achieved through an informal, relaxed approach to the job of menu-making as a pleasurable task.

Most families tend to buy by the week to take advantage of lower sale and bulk prices (the economy of buying will be discussed later) and the changing needs and desires of the family; thus, a plan should usually be made by the week. Unless the planning is done on a weekly or longer basis, a balanced diet is difficult to maintain.

The basis of the plan is the selection of the amount of food needed for the family from each of the food groups. The local food advertisements and Appendix B of this book used together can become a habit for the homemaker's planning of meals containing the correct amounts of the basic five food groups.

Planning should include all the meals and between-meal items eaten at home and elsewhere. Planning for extra items, or at least being aware of them, makes it easier for the family to pick the foods that are best for them. It must be a cooperative family effort or it will not work. Such planning for a family group may become fairly complex unless one adheres to certain basic rules.

STEP 1: THE MENUS

The first step is to decide which foods and amounts of foods are needed to make a nutritionally adequate and pleasant diet for each person in the family. A sensible rule to follow is to select foods which give the most nutritional value for the calories present. Each person in the family will have different caloric needs (explained in the preceding chapter). A tense, active, underweight youngster needs additional food allowances; a placid, less energetic individual needs a smaller caloric intake. A man doing heavy outdoor labor or a college athlete may need as many as 3000 to 3500 or more calories daily; he can eat all the essential foods plus a number of extra high-calorie foods to fill his great energy requirement. Other people must budget their calories more strictly. A homemaker, a business person, or a coed who does not exert a great deal of physical effort may need only 1600 to 2500 calories a day. *But the lower the calorie requirement, the greater is the need to find satisfaction and variety in the essential foods.*

STEP 2: BUDGETING THE FOOD BILL

Apportioning money for meals eaten at home or away is not a problem that is limited to any one income group. Considering the large percentage of family income that goes for food, it is amazing how often it is spent with little or no thought.

Careful planning of the family meals will make shopping easier and more economical. A shopping list, made according to the meal plan for a week, will be a real help in buying the right foods in the right amounts. The fact that changes will be made during shopping need not detract from the value of the list. Flexibility and substitution are badges of an informed shopper; but without a list, a person's purchasing is likely to be unorganized and expensive.

The smart shopper will make careful preparation before starting to the market. In addition to thoughtful meal planning, she will read the food advertisements before making her shopping list. The advertisements will provide tips on seasons, supply, price, grades, and brands. With this background information, combined with the shopping list, the shopper is alerted to particular items to watch for in the store.

The following are suggestions for economy that have been found to be valuable in lowering the food bill:

1. Plan menus for, at the very least, one week at a time to meet the nutritional needs of the family. These menus should be sufficiently flexible so that advantage can be taken of sales and leftover food.

2. Select the most economical method of marketing. Weekly shopping will cut down shopping time and the time and expense of travel. Of course, milk and other highly perishable items must be obtained more frequently. In-between buying can usually be tied in with other trips to avoid extra costs. It is very uneconomical to drive a car on a special trip to buy a loaf of bread; the trip will probably cost more than the bread. Home delivery may be more economical.

3. Know what constitutes a good purchase. A knowledge of cuts of meat, for example, will help to determine when a cheap cut is a wise selection or when the waste is so great that it becomes false economy.

4. Be familiar with the grades and brands of foods, and know what grades can be used for the meal planned. For example, broken pieces of canned fruit may be just as satisfactory in fruit salad as the more expensive perfect whole fruit or canned whole fruit. The less highly advertised product is often as good as one with a well-known brand name. Reading labels and comparing prices are important in careful shopping. Great variations occur in brands, style of pack, ingredients, size and weight, and the number of servings obtainable from canned, frozen, or packaged food. Substituting one food for another, one variety

TABLE 7.6 SUGGESTED METHODS AND TIMES FOR STORING COMMON FOODS

Method of Storage and Food	Maximum Time in Days
In the refrigerator (38°–40°F.)	
Steaks, chops, roasts[a]	3
Freshly ground meat[a]	2
Liver, heart, other variety meats[a]	2
Table-ready meats—frankfurters, bologna, liver sausage, etc.[a]	7
Fish[a]	2
Chicken[a]	2
Turkey[a]	3
Eggs—large end up and covered	14
Milk—covered	5
Cheese	
Cottage—covered	7
Cream—covered	7
Cheddar—tightly wrapped	until used
Processed—tightly wrapped	until used
Butter—tightly wrapped or covered	14
Margarine, lard, oil—tightly covered container	until used
Fresh fruits—lightly covered	7
Fresh vegetables—in hydrator	7
In the freezing compartment or ice trays of the refrigerator (15°–25°F.)	
All fruits, juices, vegetables, meats, and other items purchased in the frozen state	up to 2 weeks
In the home freezer or compartment at (0°F.)	
Meats and frozen foods bought on special sale	up to 3 months
Bread supply	1 to 2 weeks
In unrefrigerated storage at room temperature (70°F.)	
Potatoes, onions, bananas, hydrogenated cooking oils and fats, staples such as flour, sugar, coffee, etc.	until used

[a] Wrap loosely and store in coldest part of refrigerator. Signs of deterioration are drying, discoloration, slickness, and off odor.

SOURCE: Lola T. Dudgeon, *Buying Food for Your Family,* Food Marketing Leaflet 13 (revised September 1960), p. 3 (New York State College of Agriculture and Home Economics, Cornell University, Ithaca, N.Y.). Reprinted from Carton E. Wright, *Food Buying: Marketing Information for Consumers,* New York, The Macmillan Company, 1962.

TABLE 7.7 STORAGE-LIFE RECOMMENDATIONS FOR HOME-FROZEN FOODS AT 0°F.

Food	Maximum Storage Period (Months)
Fruit	8 to 12
Vegetables	8 to 12
French-fried potatoes	2 to 6
Meats	
Beef	6 to 12
Lamb and veal	6 to 9
Pork	3 to 6
Sausage and ground meat	1 to 3
Cooked meat—not covered with gravy or other sauces	1
Meat sandwiches	1
Poultry	
Chicken	6 to 12
Turkeys	3 to 6
Giblets	3
Cooked poultry meat	1
Cooked poultry dishes	3 to 6
Precooked combination dishes	2 to 6
Baked goods	
Cakes	
Prebaked	4 to 9
Batter	3 to 4
Fruit pies, baked or unbaked	3 to 4
Pie shells, baked or unbaked	1½ to 2
Cookies	6 to 12
Yeast breads and rolls	
Prebaked	3 to 9
Dough	1 to 1½

SOURCE: *Food, the Yearbook of Agriculture,* 1959, Washington, D.C., U.S. Department of Agriculture.

for another, or one can or package for another within the shopping plan can save money.

5. Buy foods that are in season and in abundance on the market, since their cost should be less. Meats, for example, go up and down in price from year to year and season to season. The choice, more expensive, quick-cooking cuts vary more in price than those in less demand. It pays to watch for pork bargains in the late fall and beef bargains in late

winter. That is when prices are usually lowest for the year. If the family eats more of the expensive cuts in the low-price season, it can balance them off by using more of the less expensive cuts in the high-price season. Very pronounced seasonal price changes occur with fresh fruits and vegetables. Prices tend to be lowest for the year when individual produce items can be secured from local producing areas. Substitution of one fresh fruit or vegetable for another with the ups and downs of supplies and prices offers a real opportunity for savings with little or no sacrifice in quality, nutritive value, or variety.

6. Buy foods in bulk if they are sold under sanitary conditions since they are less expensive than boxed products.

7. Buy foods in quantities if there is adequate storage space and if the food can be used without waste through spoilage. The time to fill the freezer is when prices are low. With poultry and fish, whether for immediate use or for stocking the freezer, money can be saved by taking advantage of low seasonal prices. When fresh vegetables and fruits are in season, canned and frozen counterparts decline in price; this is the time to buy quantities for use during the off-season. It pays to stock up when there are bargains.

8. Compare weights and prices of packaged and canned goods.

9. Buy less expensive forms of food whenever possible. Margarine fortified with vitamin A is a good substitute for butter. Lard, suet, and vegetable oils are less expensive than hydrogenated fats and olive oil. Bread is more economical than fancy rolls. Color and grade of eggs do not affect their food value. In some places canned or powdered milk is more economical than fresh milk.

10. Store foods properly after their purchase to avoid loss of vitamin values and to prevent spoilage. Suggested storage methods and times for different kinds of food are shown in Table 7.6. Newly purchased food should always be placed so that the older food will be used first.

Canned or frozen foods purchased by the case may provide real savings if there is space to store them. With canned foods it is a question of space. If one has a freezer, frozen foods can be stored for the periods of time shown in Table 7.7. The only question is the cost of the freezer—does it more than offset the savings on the food stored in it? The combined ice tray–freezer compartment of the refrigerator will usually remain at 15° to 24°F.; frozen foods can be kept at this temperature for a few days, but they cannot be kept for long periods of time as in a separate freezing compartment of a refrigerator or in a freezer. Most refrigerators maintain a temperature of 38° to 42°F. This is fine for keeping refrigerated foods for a few days, but not for longer periods of time.

11. Do not let pride and prejudice dictate the buying habits of the family. Food misconceptions are frequently passed along in family lines; they are difficult to dissipate.

TABLE 7.8 PROBLEMS THAT OCCUR IN FREEZING FOODS

Food	Problem	Solution
Potatoes, cooked	Loss of texture	Do not add to stews or other cooked dishes before freezing; add when reheating
Rice, noodles, and macaroni, cooked	Loss of texture	Freeze only if in sauce or gravy, or add when reheating dish
Creamed soups	Separate or curdle	Add milk or cream when reheating
Creamed foods	Become rancid	Use as little fat as possible; reheat at very low temperature
Chicken dishes, cooked	Meat separates or shreds	Freeze when chicken is partially cooked
Poultry or meat cut in small pieces, cooked	Loss of flavor	Cover with sauce or gravy before freezing
Fatty meats, cooked	Become rancid	Cut away excess fat before freezing
Rich sauces	Curdle, separate, or become runny	When reheating, mix almost constantly until very smooth
Garlic	Develops off-flavor	Add when reheating

Some foods cannot be frozen. The following is a list of the general foods affected and the problems:

Food	Problem
Raw clams	Lose texture, become tough
Hard-cooked eggs	Become tough and rubbery
Milk custard	Curdles
Mayonnaise	Curdles
Salad greens	Lose crisp texture

MEAL-PLANNING PROBLEMS OF WORKING WIVES

When both adult members of a family work outside the home, the meals served are often not adequate although the expenses for feeding the family may be extremely high. The ideas in this section have been found helpful in bringing better nutrition to such a working family, releasing the working wife from excessive weekly meal preparation, and lowering the family's food costs.

The main problem with general meal planning during the working week is the daily time involved in preparation of the meals. Tired adults do not consistently prepare planned nutritious meals. The key to such a preparation is precooked frozen meals.

During hours of relaxation the wife may plan the following week's meals. With the aids established in previous sections of this chapter, she can make out a menu and shopping list. After she has completed the shopping, one free morning of the weekend may be set aside to prepare and freeze the following week's meals. After this an average of one-half hour each night is needed to thaw, warm, and prepare the previously cooked meal and produce a delicious, well-planned, nutritious meal.

Instructions found in booklets which are given to an individual with purchase of a new freezer have been found to be valuable for organized weekly planned frozen meals. Not all foods freeze equally well; some of the problems that occur in freezing precooked foods are found in Table 7.8. Also—and this is vitally important with meat and fish dishes—the additional cooking time necessary to reheat the frozen dish must be calculated in the original cooking time. For example, it generally takes about one-half hour to reheat the average dish, so this time must be subtracted from the original cooking time wherever possible. If it normally takes one and one-half hours to cook a given dish for immediate consumption, the original cooking time should not be one and one-half hours but one hour when it is to be frozen, or the reheated dish will be overcooked.

As another timesaver, the homemaker will find it almost as easy to prepare enough of a given dish for several additional meals. When the dish is one-half hour from completion, she should remove all but what is required for that evening's meal and freeze the balance in portions suitable for one meal.

Too much stress cannot be placed upon the proper protection of foods to be frozen. Whether the food is raw or cooked, it must be wrapped so that as much air as possible is excluded from the package. Pointers on packaging of food for freezing are explained in Table 7.9.

Specific instructions are set forth in individual recipes; the following are the *basic* rules:

TABLE 7.9 POINTERS ON PACKAGING FOODS

Food	Method of Packaging
Egg whites	Freeze each egg white in individual ice cube trays, wrap, and seal. Larger numbers can be frozen in covered containers (label with the number of egg whites). Remove and thaw four hours before using.
Egg yolks	Stir lightly and add 1 teaspoon of salt for each cup of yolks and freeze. One tablespoon of sugar may be added instead of the salt, but then they can only be used for sweet dishes.
Whole eggs	Follow the above instructions for yolks.
Broths and stocks	Freeze in ice-cube trays; then remove and wrap, seal, label, and return to freezer. A cube added to soup or stew is a marvelous supplement.
Stews and casseroles	Line a casserole with foil; freeze stew in it; then lift out. Wrap, seal, label, and return to freezer. Heat in original casserole when ready to use.
Herbs	Chives, dill, parsley, and all herbs may be frozen ready for use. Wash and dry thoroughly; then chop. Pack into small freezer containers, or wrap in foil, Saran, or freezer paper. Use from the frozen state without thawing.

1. For storage longer than one week, food should be placed in a moisture-vaporproof wrap. When foods are frozen quickly, they should be covered with foil or plastic wrap first. After quick-freezing, they should be overwrapped and returned to the freezer for storage. When thawing, foods should be kept wrapped unless otherwise specified in the recipe.
2. Undercook foods by approximately one-half hour (this is the average length of time required to reheat in most cases).
3. Cool as quickly as possible by placing the pot or dish in ice water, over ice, or in the refrigerator.
4. Skim as much fat as possible from the dish (this may be re-added when reheating).
5. Do not overfill containers; leave about one inch at the top to allow for expansion.
6. Label each package with the name, number of servings, and date (for example, "Roast duck with cherry sauce, 4, October 8").
7. Place freshly prepared dishes in the back of the freezer and bring older ones gradually to the top and front so they will not be overlooked.
8. Do not keep foods longer than the time specified under the individual categories.

These ideas and suggestions, when worked into the over-all picture of meal planning, may very readily offer a substantial nutritional basis for any family.

FOOD STANDARDS AND GRADES

More foods are being processed, packaged, or prepared in such a way as to make it difficult to know what actually goes into a product in terms of quality, quantity, condition, or cleanliness. Thus, it has become important over the years to establish standards for certain foods.

Several federal agencies have authority to establish standards for foods in interstate commerce. Some standards are mandatory—they must be met unless the product is clearly labeled with a *substandard* legend, including the reason it is substandard. Other standards are optional; the manufacturer or distributor can decide whether or not to label products according to these voluntary standards. If he chooses to use such standards, the product so labeled must comply with them.

The basic types of standards are *identity standards, quality standards, fill of container standards*—all established and administered by the U.S. Food and Drug Administration—and *grade standards,* which were established and are administered by the U.S. Department of Agriculture and the U.S. Department of the Interior (Bureau of Commercial Fisheries).

IDENTITY STANDARDS

Identity standards describe the nature and character of a given product or specify the kinds and amounts of various ingredients that must or may go into a product. Such standards are *mandatory*; they have been established for about 200 products. An example is the standard of identity for fruit preserves and jellies. This standard requires not less than 45 parts of fruit or fruit juice to each 55 parts of sugar. Substandard or low-fruit jam can be legally marketed, but the label on such foods must be clearly marked "Imitation."

After a standard of identity has been established for a food product, such as mayonnaise, catsup, or mustard, only the name of the food and any optional ingredients added (such as mustard *and* horseradish) must be listed on the label. For this reason the labels of some foods do not have a complete list of ingredients.

QUALITY STANDARDS

Quality standards are mandatory. They apply chiefly to canned fruits and vegetables and describe the condition of the ingredients which go into the product. Canned foods falling below standard in appearance must be labeled "Substandard," "Below Standard in Quality," or

"Good Food—Not High Grade" with the reason, such as "excess peeling." These foods are wholesome and entirely suitable for some uses, particularly in prepared dishes where the original appearance and texture of the food is lost.

FILL OF CONTAINER STANDARDS

Some standards regulate the quantity of food in the container. In general, standards of fill require packages to contain the maximum quantity of food that can be sealed in the container and processed without damaging the food. These standards apply mainly to products that may shake down or settle after filling or those which are made up of a number of units or pieces packed in a liquid. For example, a canner is not allowed to half-fill a can with peas and fill the rest with water. Fill of container standards apply only to food such as canned fruits and vegetables, tomato products, and shellfish.

GRADE STANDARDS

Grading standards have been established for many agricultural and fishery products. The U.S. Department of Agriculture establishes the grade standards for agricultural products; grades for fish and sea food products are established by the Bureau of Fisheries, U.S. Department of the Interior.

The standards of grading are based primarily on quality and appearance, not on food value. Federal and state grading systems exist for foods which represent more than half of the nation's food bill—milk, butter, cheese, meat, poultry, and fresh, canned, and frozen fruits and vegetables. Most of these systems of grading are optional or voluntary and may or may not be followed; a few are mandatory.

The food shopper may find federal or state grade marks on many of the foods seen in the market. If the foods are graded, the grade marks will be apparent. If the grade marks are not there, the food is probably not graded. The ungraded foods may be just as good as those with grade labels, but the purchaser must depend on a personal judgment of quality. As a reference for the shopper, a list of U.S. grades is shown in Table 7.10.

Meat grades depend on the appearance of the food, including the color of the meat and fat, the amount and distribution of the fat, and the conformation or build of the live animal. These grades, to the homemaker, can be clues to appropriate uses for the meat.

Top grades of meat come from well-fed animals; they have more fat and consequently can be aged to develop more flavor than lower grades. More cuts of top-grade meat are suited for oven roasting and broiling than are lower grade cuts. The lower grades, with a higher proportion of lean meat to bone, give more economical meat and, with skillful cooking to increase flavor, are tender, tasty, and nutritious. Ground meat, stewing meat, and pot roasts are among the popular cuts from lower grades of meat.

There are eight official government grades of beef, as shown in Table 7.10. The first five may be found in retail stores; the last three— ordinarily used in processed, pre-cooked, and canned meat products— are rarely sold in retail stores. U.S. Prime (top grade) is used mainly by restaurants and is rarely found in retail stores. If the beef has been federally graded, it will carry one of the U.S. grade stamps, in the shape of a shield, as shown in Fig. 7.6.

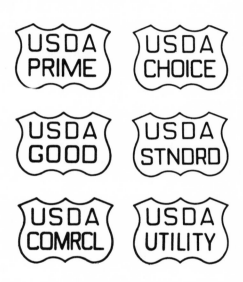

Fig. 7.6 Federal grade marks for beef. (U.S. Department of Agriculture.)

Veal, calf, lamb, and mutton are also federally graded and carry the shielded grade mark similar to that for beef. In addition, the kind of meat will be indicated by stamping on the surface of the animal. Such stamping will be *veal, calf, yearling mutton,* or *mutton.* For veal, if the animal was under three months old, the stamp will read "veal"; if over three months old, it will read "calf."

Poultry grades are based on appearance and freedom from skin cuts, tears, bruises, broken bones, and pinfeathers. The federal grades for ready-to-cook poultry, found in Table 7.10, are voluntary. The grade marks may not be used unless the poultry has first been inspected for wholesomeness and has been processed in an approved plant under prescribed sanitary conditions. The grade marks are shown in Figs. 7.7 and 7.8.

The federal inspection mark in Fig. 7.7 is used on tags or packages to show that poultry and poultry products so marked have been processed under sanitary conditions and found to be clean and healthy. The round mark is used only on poultry and poultry products inspected under the compulsory inspection law.

Eggs are graded by quality and according to weight ' classes. The federal grades are often adopted by states as their official grades. The grades shown in Table 7.10 are based on interior quality and condition of the shell. There are six separate U.S. weight classes for eggs, based on the weight of a dozen eggs. They are Jumbo, 30 ounces; Extra Large, 27 ounces; Large, 24 ounces; Medium, 21 ounces; Small, 18 ounces; and

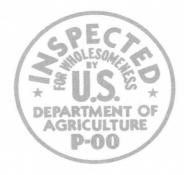

Fig. 7.7 Federal compulsory inspection mark for poultry. (U.S. Department of Agriculture.)

Peewee, 15 ounces. The grade letters indicate quality only; the weight classes indicate size only. Grade AA eggs will have the same quality whether they are Large, Medium, or Peewee. The color of the shell determines neither size nor quality. Cracked eggs should be avoided as they may harbor *Salmonella* bacteria, which cause intestinal infections. The usual sizes of eggs seen in retail stores are Extra Large, Large, Medium, and Small. All grade qualities AA through C may be found in the markets.

Of *dairy products,* butter is the item most commonly sold by federal grade, although cheese and nonfat dry milk also have federal grades. The U.S. grades of cheese and nonfat dry milk are shown in Table 7.10. The "score" legend need not appear on the grade label.

Many states have butter grades which usually conform to the federal grades. Unless the prefix "U.S." appears on the grade label, the butter has not been certified by a federal grader. (This is true of all federal grade marks.) Many butter distributors will use the letters or the score on their packages without the federal or state designation. In these

TABLE 7.10   U.S. GRADES

Product	First Grade	Second Grade
Beef	USDA Prime	USDA Choice
Veal	USDA Prime	USDA Choice
Calf	USDA Prime	USDA Choice
Lamb	USDA Prime	USDA Choice
Yearling mutton	USDA Prime	USDA Choice
Mutton		USDA Choice
Butter	U.S. Grade AA (U.S. 93 Score)	U.S. Grade A (U.S. 92 Score)
Cheddar cheese	U.S. Grade AA	U.S. Grade A
Swiss cheese	U.S. Grade A	U.S. Grade B
Nonfat dry milk	U.S. Extra Grade	U.S. Standard Grade
Cottage cheese		No grades—may
Poultry	U.S. Grade A	U.S. Grade B
Eggs	Fresh Fancy Quality U.S. Grade AA	U.S. Grade A
Milled rice	U.S. No. 1	U.S. No. 2
Brown rice	U.S. No. 1	U.S. No. 2
Dried beans	U.S. Choice Handpicked U.S. No. 1	U.S. No. 1 Handpicked U.S. No. 2
Dried peas	U.S. No. 1	U.S. No. 2
Processed fruits and vegetables (and related products)c	U.S. Grade A (Fancy)	U.S. Grade B (Choice or Ext. Std.)

a Three lowest grades are USDA Utility, Cutter, and Canner.
b Lowest grade is USDA Cull.
c Grades used for these products are usually as listed here, but there are some exceptions.

cases, the buyer must depend on the distributor's statement as to the quality of the butter.

Whole milk and other dairy products are not covered under federal grade inspection and usually are controlled locally by the county, city, or state.

AT A GLANCE

Third Grade	Fourth Grade	Fifth Grade
USDA Good	USDA Standard	USDA Commercial[a]
USDA Good	USDA Standard	USDA Utility[b]
USDA Good	USDA Standard	USDA Utility[b]
USDA Good	USDA Utility	USDA Cull
USDA Good	USDA Utility	USDA Cull
USDA Good	USDA Utility	USDA Cull
U.S. Grade B		
(U.S. 90 Score)		
U.S. Grade B	U.S. Grade C	
U.S. Grade C	U.S. Grade D	

be marked USDA "Quality Approved"
U.S. Grade C
| U.S. Grade B | U.S. Grade C | |

U.S. No. 3	U.S. No. 4	U.S. No. 5
U.S. No. 3	U.S. No. 4	
U.S. No. 2	U.S. No. 3	
Handpicked	Handpicked	
U.S. No. 3		
U.S. No. 3		
U.S. Grade C		
(Standard)		

Federal standards and grades exist for a large number of *fresh and processed fruits and vegetables*. Most of these are wholesale grades for use by growers and shippers, but they may be used in advertising or in the market. Also, some strictly consumer grades are optional. Their use might spread if more consumers knew the grades and sought this kind of information.

Commonly, the wholesale grades for fresh fruits and vegetables fol-

TABLE 7.10   U.S. GRADES

Product	Consumer Grades First Grade	Second Grade
Beet greens	U.S. Grade A	
Potatoes	U.S. Grade A Large	U.S. Grade B Large
	U.S. Grade A Medium to Large	U.S. Grade B Medium to Large
	U.S. Grade A Medium	U.S. Grade B Medium
	U.S. Grade A Small	U.S. Grade B Small
Brussels sprouts	U.S. Grade A	U.S. Grade B
Carrots	U.S. Grade A	U.S. Grade B
Corn (husked, on the cob)	U.S. Grade A	U.S. Grade B
Cranberries	U.S. Grade A	
Kale	U.S. Grade A	U.S. Grade B
Parsnips	U.S. Grade A	U.S. Grade B
Spinach leaves	U.S. Grade A	U.S. Grade B
Tomatoes	U.S. Grade A	U.S. Grade B
Turnips	U.S. Grade A	U.S. Grade B
Celery	U.S. Grade AA	U.S. Grade A (3rd Grade— U.S. Grade B)
Apples	None	None

d Partial listing of commodities for which there are wholesale grades, to show how these grades compare with consumer grades.

e Same as U.S. No. 1 except for color.

f Same as U.S. No. 1 except for color, maturity, and size.

g Same as U.S. No. 1 except for hail injury.

	Wholesale Grades[d]		
First Grade	Second Grade	Third Grade	Fourth Grade
U.S. No. 1			
U.S. Fancy	U.S. No. 1	U.S. Commercial	U.S. No. 2
U.S. No. 1	U.S. No. 2		
(Topped carrots) U.S. Extra No. 1	U.S. No. 1	U.S. No. 2	
(Green corn) U.S. Fancy	U.S. No. 1	U.S. No. 2	
U.S. No. 1	U.S. Commercial		
U.S. No. 1	U.S. No. 2		
U.S. Extra No. 1	U.S. No. 1	U.S. Commercial	
U.S. No. 1	U.S. Combination	U.S. No. 2	
(Topped turnips) U.S. No. 1	U.S. No. 2		U.S. No. 3
U.S. Extra No. 1	U.S. No. 1	U.S. No. 2	
U.S. Extra Fancy	U.S. Fancy	U.S. No. 1	U.S. Utility
		U.S. No. 1 Cookers[e]	
		U.S. No. 1 Early[f]	
		U.S. Hail Grade[g]	

SOURCE: *Shopper's Guide to U.S. Grades for Food, Home and Garden,* Bulletin No. 58, revised January 1961. Washington: U. S. Department of Agriculture. Reprinted with permission of The Macmillan Company from C. E. Wright, *Food Buying.* Copyright © 1962 by C. E. Wright.

low the numbering pattern shown in Table 7.10. Consumer grades for fresh fruits and vegetables use letters for quality and further designations of words or numbers to show size.

Among the factors that determine the grade into which fruits and vegetables may fall are size, color, and freedom from defects. Workmanship in peeling and cutting fruits and vegetables for canning and freezing also affects the grades of these items.

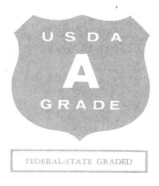

Fig. 7.8 Federal grade mark for poultry in conjunction with federal-state grading programs. (U.S. Department of Agriculture.)

Fruit and vegetable grades can help a discriminating shopper choose them with specific uses in mind. Top grades of fruits and vegetables are attractive when the plan is to use them whole or in large pieces. The lower grades, which may be smaller, less perfect in shape, and have more blemishes are very satisfactory in many cooked dishes. The commercially canned products usually use such grades or lower. Some defects just mar appearance; others cause waste.

Fish and sea food products carry seals for inspection and grade authorized by the U.S. Department of the Interior. Use of a shield on frozen fishery products indicates that the product was prepared, according to approved specifications, from wholesome raw fish or sea food in a plant where a trained government inspector was continuously present.

SIGNS, SEALS, AND GRADE MARKS

Many food products bear seals or statements of approval, from either government or private agencies. The seals have meaning only if what they stand for is known.

The grade marks for food which has been federally graded usually appear in the form of a *shield*. Unless the number or letter grades are official U.S. or state grades, the consumer may be fooled. "Grade A" may be a meaningless term unless it has the letters "U.S." in front of it. Many foods are sold as "choice," "1st quality," "top grade," and so on, when the term has no connection with grade at all. Private brands are only as meaningful as one's understanding of them. The shopper should not be confused by meaningless designs or words. He should look for official government sponsorship (federal, state, or local); it is the best guide to true meaning.

SUMMARY

   I. Determining Desirable Weight
     A. Determination of ideal weight for an individual is difficult.
     B. Factors to consider include:
       1. sex.
       2. age.
       3. height.
       4. body build.

  II. Overweight and Obesity
     A. Terms have different meanings.
       1. Overweight—any weight in excess of the weight recommended for a given person by the Desirable Weight Table.
       2. Obesity—excessive deposition of fat beyond what is considered normal.
       3. Usage of either term in the text implies a condition of overweight due to obesity.
     B. Causes of overweight.
       1. Faulty metabolism is occasional cause of overweight.
       2. Faulty regulation of diet is the more common cause of overweight.
     C. Effects of overweight—life expectancy is lessened.
     D. Reducing—success depends upon adequate motivation.

 III. Underweight—many factors may be responsible.

 IV. Food Fads and Fallacies
     A. Natural foods.
     B. Raw foods.
     C. Miracle foods.
     D. Food supplements.

  V. Meal Planning
     A. Five basic food groups:
       1. Dairy foods—milk, cheese, ice cream, and other foods made from milk.
       2. Meat, fish, poultry, and eggs.
       3. Vegetables—dark-green or deep-yellow.
       4. Fruits—fresh, frozen, or canned.
       5. Breads and cereals.
     B. Simple nutrition for students:
       Four-five-five plan devised for college students stresses the basic five groups:
       1. Breakfast and midmorning snack should together include items from four groups.

2. Lunch and midafternoon snack should together include items from five groups.

3. Dinner and the evening snack should together include items from five groups.

C. Applying the basic five in family meals:
   1. Menus.
   2. Budgeting the food bill.

D. Meal-planning problems of working wives.

E. Food Standards and Grades:
   1. Identity standards have been established for about 200 products which need not have ingredients listed on label.
   2. Quality standards are mandatory and must be met or labeled as substandard.
   3. Fill of container standards do not apply to all foods.
   4. Grade standards—most are optional, a few mandatory.
      a. Meat grades—based upon the appearance of the food.
      b. Poultry grades—based on appearance and freedom from blemishes.
      c. Eggs—graded by quality and put into weight classes.
      d. Dairy products—most covered by state or local, rather than federal, inspection.
      e. Fruit and vegetable grades—primarily used in wholesale transactions.
      f. Fish and sea food products—graded under standards of the U.S. Department of the Interior.
   5. Signs, seals, and grade marks:
      a. Many products bear seals of approval, from either government or private agencies.
      b. Private seals or grades may have little significance.

Glossary

If you cannot find the word you wish in this glossary, check the index for text and glossary references.

diet (dī′ət) (G. *diaita,* way of living).   The customary allowance of food and drink taken by a person from day to day.

lipectomy (li pek′tə mē) (G. *lipos,* fat; *ektome,* excision).   Cutting out of fatty tissue from fatty areas of the body.

malnutrition (mal nyoo trish′ən) (L. *malus,* bad; *nutritio,* to nourish).   Any disorder of nutrition.

minimum daily requirements.   The amounts of each nutrient which are regarded as necessary in the diet for the prevention of deficiency diseases.

nutrient (nyoo′trē ənt) (L. *nutriens,* nourishment).   A substance which provides nourishment to the body.

nutrition (nyoo trish′ən) (L. *nutritio,* to nourish).   The process of assimilating food into the body for nourishment.

obesity (ō bē′si tē) (L. *obesus,* that has eaten itself fat).   An increase in body weight beyond skeletal and physical requirements, as the result of an excessive accumulation of fat.

osteoarthritis (os′tē ō ahr thrī′tis) (G. *osteon,* bone; *arthron,* joint; *itis,* inflammation).   A chronic joint disease which is degenerative.

overweight (ō'vər wāt').   An excess of more than 10 percent above the desirable weight.

recommended daily allowances.   The amounts of nutrients which are considered adequate for the maintenance of good nutrition in healthy persons in the United States.

underweight (un'dər wāt').   A deficiency of more than 10 percent under the desirable weight.

CHAPTER 8

SUCCESS IN MARRIAGE

FACTORS TO CONSIDER
BEFORE MARRIAGE

PREMARITAL SEXUAL
ADJUSTMENT

BEGINNING MARRIAGE

DIVORCE

SUMMARY

Marriage has been used to regulate the relations between the two sexes in all parts of the world. Ancient in its origin, marriage has been revered and considered as essential to the conduct and perpetuation of civilization.

As times have changed, the attitudes of people toward social practices and reasons for conforming to them have also changed. Our reasons for marriage today are somewhat different from what they were 100 years ago. The man on the frontier selected a "help-mate" who could share the chores, keep house, and raise strong children. The pioneer woman looked for a man who could provide for her and their children. As the social structure changed, considerations in the choosing of a partner also changed. A young person today looks upon the romantic appeal of the other sex as an important factor in the proper selection. Since each new generation lives in a somewhat different world from the preceding generation, old questions must be given new answers, particularly the question of marriage. In the following discussion the authors attempt to deal with some present considerations for achieving a successful and enduring marriage.

FACTORS TO CONSIDER BEFORE MARRIAGE

A marriage becomes the sum of the personal characteristics both individuals bring into it. Desirable or undesirable, many of these remain unchanged after marriage; although the marriage relationship will change a person to some degree, it will not alter his basic personality traits. Therefore, before the marriage contract is signed, each prospective partner should take a long, careful look at the traits of the other.

PERSONAL TRAITS

The following personal traits can be considered important to a marriage.

PERSONALITY

Reasonable ability to adjust to surrounding conditions should be a must. A balanced person should accept other people for what they are and expect to be so accepted by others. He should recognize that, since he is human, he has limitations and not spend his life agonizing over capacities that he neither has nor can develop. Although temperaments differ, a person should look at the brighter side of issues and attempt to improve situations whenever possible. He should have honest concern for the needs of other people and a desire to do things that bring pleasure to them. He should show some degree of responsibility for social conventions and ethics, with some sense of balance between the two extremes of license and prohibition. In life—and certainly in marriage—a sense of humor is a great asset.

HEREDITARY TRAITS

Each person is the carrier of a line of traits passed on to him through each of his parents. Each person's genetic make-up is strictly the result of fate, depending upon the interactions of his inherited genes. Many of these traits are desirable. Most individuals, however, are the carriers of some unfavorable genes, which often are hidden and go unrecognized.

Occasionally some express themselves in a person's physical development.

Some of these unfavorable genes are known to lead to abnormal congenital development. Others tend to show up only during the years of childhood, youth, or adulthood. It is wise to consider the type of children that may be produced from a marriage. Their genetic make-up will be determined by both partners' germ plasm. Adverse genetic traits must be considered in terms of passing them on to one's children. In any marriage some risk of passing along defective genes exists, even when both parents appear to be normal.

Some individuals come from families in which congenital defects have been known to occur, but are themselves normal. Such a person may nonetheless be a carrier of undesirable hidden genes. It may be reasonable to marry such a person, although such a couple may need to consider more carefully the consequences of producing children with possible congenital defects. If there is any question regarding the probability of transmitting defective genes, it would be wise to seek genetic counseling from a physician. Any decision to marry and not have children or to marry and have children should be based upon such advice.

INFATUATION OR LOVE?

The distinction between feelings of infatuation and feelings of love is not always clear, although to the observant person infatuation has some detectable characteristics. Infatuation is frequently associated with immaturity, a "puppy love" dress rehearsal for mature love. It is a kind of substitute for love until a person has the capacity to love someone deeply and fully. It tends to involve physical attraction rather than attraction to an entire personality. Tending to be unrealistic, infatuated partners want to idealize each other as the "dream mate"— the fantasied ideal that is perfect in every respect ("love is blind"). Infatuation is often immediate ("love at first sight"), whereas love develops over time. Often infatuation wears off quickly. On the other hand, it may also develop into mature love.

A person truly in love tends to be concerned with the loved one's happiness and well-being; he is tender, protecting, and loyal. Love stimulates a person to strive for worthy ideals and goals which he wants to share with another. He will overlook neither the faults nor the strengths of the other person but will take the loved one for what she is and what her potentialities suggest she may become. (This applies to a woman's reactions to the man she loves, too, of course.) Love nurtures affections that grow with time, feelings which each knows are good and which will give balance and meaning to life.

DIFFERENCE IN BACKGROUND

All marriages involve two people possessing certain differences. We expect these differences because each has his own personality and family background. Sometimes the differences are minor; at other times they are considerable and obvious and may have a significant bearing on the marriage. Differences may involve age, race, economic status, family background, education, intelligence, religion, or previous marital status. It is important for any couple approaching marriage to attempt a critical, objective look at major differences. Most marriages can be successful if the couple is willing to work out the special problems involved.

Here are several kinds of differences and some of the problems to which they may lead.

1. *Age.*   Where there are wide differences in age, one must examine why he wants to marry a person considerably younger or older than himself. He ought to be sure that his desire to marry this person is not *simply* a desire for immediate economic security, an inability to find a partner more nearly his own age, or a feeling of flattery at getting the attention of a more mature or more youthful person. The younger partner should look into the reasons why the older partner is not already married, asking the following questions: Does he have personality or emotional problems? Is he an undesirable choice? Have unavoidable circumstances hindered him from an earlier marriage? The older a person gets, the more inflexible he becomes and the harder it is for him to adapt to another person. The problem of finding common friends with similar ages and interests may also be encountered.

2. *Race.*   Racial differences can be one of the more difficult problems to be faced in marriage. Although no biological barrier exists, segments of society show resentment toward some interracial marriages. A few states still prohibit the issuance of marriage licenses to a racially mixed couple. Although a new social emancipation of Negroes is taking place, social patterns change slowly and painfully. An interracial couple approaching marriage should prepare to face certain unique problems, including the finding of friends who will accept both partners, the social acceptance of future children, and the possibility of local prejudice affecting housing and employment. However, an increasing number of racial intermarriages is helping to break down these barriers.

3. *Economic status.*   Fortunately, wide differences in economic levels are not as common in this country as they used to be. However, there are still situations where such distinctions exist. In circumstances where two people in love are faced with wide economic differences, the easier solution is that in which the man has the greater wealth, as the posi-

tion of economic inferiority is generally easier for a wife to accept. But such a wife should not expect luxuries beyond what her husband wants to or can provide. The less wealthy partner should be prepared to adjust to his mate's higher social level, including the mate's cultural tastes and activities. This adjustment may not be enjoyable, particularly when the old ways were considered desirable. Where the wife is distinctly the richer, there should be a settling of financial arrangements before marriage. Such a wife may not wish to turn all of her financial rights and privileges over to the management of her husband. Each partner must be sure that he can accept a mate from a profession or occupation having less pay and perhaps less social status.

4. *Family background.*   College students away from home, detached from the family, may not reflect the full nature of their backgrounds nor see such reflections in their colleagues. Yet when these individuals leave college and move back into their home communities or on to other places, their background may have a bearing on their manners, attitudes toward their marriage partner, treatment of other people, kinds of food they desire, recreation they seek, and use of their leisure time.

There are superior individuals who have come from poor backgrounds and some disappointing persons have come from very good backgrounds. Nevertheless our family backgrounds tend to be a pattern of life for many of us, and we do not move into new patterns easily or quickly.

5. *Educational differences.*   Even with more educational opportunities open to young people today, a disparity in educational background is far from rare. Along with more education frequently goes an improvement in reading tastes, personal goals, and social sophistication. A better educated partner may become impatient with his mate if there is lack of interest in, or desire to learn about, the other's field of interest and training. The one with better training may be able to help raise the other one culturally. On the other hand, he may be dragged down to the lesser cultural level.

6. *Intelligence.*   The emphasis on glamor today causes some young people to overlook other human attributes, such as intelligence. In marriages in which there is too wide a contrast in intellectual ability, it is possible for the two partners to grow apart. Not only may the more intelligent partner long for stimulating expression with some other person, but also the less intelligent person may develop definite feelings of inferiority. Either of these roads may lead to loneliness. If such partners find appeal in each other, marital success may be attained. But if success is to be achieved, each partner must recognize the other's strong points and allow the other to excel in his way. Those parts of their lives in which there is the greatest common ground must be stressed.

7. *Religion.*   Young people who are not yet faced with deeply per-

plexing problems may give insufficient thought to the value of religion. They may tend to disregard religious background as an important consideration in the selection of a mate. Religious practice, however, affects a person's basic beliefs, attitudes, treatment of certain days, and sometimes the kinds of food he eats. As young people mature, experience adult responsibilities, and learn to know both joy and sorrow, they often find strength from religious worship and experience.

Religion can serve to unite a marriage and bring forward the finest kinds of attitudes, particularly if it is an interest shared by husband and wife. On the other hand, marriage partners observing widely different and conflicting religious practices might find it difficult to adjust to each other. A study of over 12,000 young people between the ages of 16 and 24 conducted in Maryland by the American Council on Education supports this statement. Regarding the marital status of the young people's parents, the study indicated that where both parents were Jewish, there was a 4.5 percent rate of separation; where both were Catholics, a 6.4 percent rate of separation; where both were Protestants, a 6.8 percent rate of separation; where the parents were of mixed religions, there was 15.2 percent rate of separation; and where the parents held *no* religious affiliation, a 16.7 percent rate of separation.

For instance, the disparity in tenets between most Protestant denominations and the Roman Catholic Church are such that a marriage involving partners from such different faiths, where each remains faithful to his religion, may be difficult. First of all, in a mixed marriage the Catholic church requires an *antenuptial agreement,* which must be signed by the Catholic partner before the wedding can be conducted in a Catholic church. Then, to be valid in the eyes of the Church, the wedding must be conducted by a priest. Following marriage, the couple is expected, according to the antenuptial agreement, to follow the dictates of the church on matters of birth control, sterilization, artificial insemination, the rearing of children, and divorce. Any non-Catholic contemplating marriage with a Catholic should give these requirements careful consideration.

The situation is somewhat different between Jewish and non-Jewish people in this country. Although many rabbis will not officiate at the marriage of a Jew to a non-Jew, the wedding is nevertheless considered valid by Jews. One problem to be faced in such marriages may be the prejudice of one of the religious groups, which may be extended to the partner who is not of that group, and may even be extended to the children of the mixed marriage.

As the study referred to earlier suggests, conflict may also be encountered in a marriage between a religious and a nonreligious person. Potentially the difference here could be wider than that between those of two different faiths.

It is therefore wise for a couple to come to a mutually agreeable decision regarding religious loyalties as soon as they begin to talk of marriage.

8. *Previous marital status.*   One out of every five or six marriages today involves a person who has been married before. The chances of a young person's falling in love with a divorced or widowed individual are not remote. Marrying a person who has been divorced or widowed will not be the same as marrying one who has never been married before. A past marital experience affects the attitudes a person brings to a second marriage. These effects may be memories of a happy marriage. They could just as well, however, be the effects of marital disappointment. If the previously married person can now make the proper selection of a mate and can earnestly work at making necessary new adjustments, the new marriage can turn out to be desirable and happy.

In some marriages, problems that were causes of trouble in the first marriage reappear. Before marrying an individual who was previously married, the other partner should ask several questions. Has the divorced or widowed person recovered sufficiently from the first loss to now make a wise choice, or is he desperate? If his first partner is still living, what are his attitudes toward that former partner? What are the chances of that former partner's coming between the new partners? Can the new mate consent to live in a home previously occupied by the former partner? Are the real causes for the divorce, rather than simply the legal reasons, known to the new mate? Is there any assurance that the same circumstances will not recur? Has the one seeking remarriage been divorced more than once? Is divorce a way of life for him?

If one partner has had children from a former marriage and has custody of those children, a prospective spouse should want to be assured of acceptance by them. Also, of course, one's attitude toward being a stepparent should be explored as honestly as possible. Often grandparents have a close interest in their grandchildren, and this association should be explored to ferret out any roadblocks to a successful marriage. In the event there are children produced by the second marriage in addition to children present from the first one, the new parents must make every effort to avoid actions of partiality toward one set of children.

A good aid for a young person making a thoughtful selection of a marriage partner would be to sit down and list all of the qualities he considers desirable in a partner. Out of this list he should select the ten most essential qualities for his ideal. He should then grade the person being considered as a mate. This criterion should give some indication of the partner's general acceptability, as well as the kind of counterbalancing traits needed to make the marriage succeed. He should not expect to find an individual who has *all* of the ideals he is looking for. A happy marriage results when two imperfect people work toward the same goal, each making the necessary adjustments.

PREMARITAL SEXUAL ADJUSTMENT

Love is a personal relationship between people. In courtship and marriage the human body becomes an instrument in the expression of love. As the feelings of two individuals deepen, physical contacts—the kiss and the embrace—become meaningful kinds of expression. Desire for sexual expression accompanies the development of such affection. However, lest we forget, love also requires the development of other values. These include respect and admiration for the other person, concern for his welfare, and an interest in helping him develop all his abilities to their fullest.

CHANGING STANDARDS

American society today is not unanimous in what it considers right or wrong on matters of sexual conduct. Today, as in the past, individual codes range from license to prohibition. Yet there has been a distinct easing in the general attitude over the past fifty years. Most people today consider sex wholesome and a source of pleasure. Some feel that our attitudes toward it are *too* permissive.

Today, as always, couples must decide on their own course of conduct. Old questions must be reanswered. How intimate should we become? What about petting? Is it right to "go all the way"? Are petting and premarital sexual intercourse the only sex outlets?

PETTING

There are various degrees of sexual involvement. To simplify definitions, this text will consider petting as including all relations beyond kissing, but short of sexual intercourse.

Although it is easy to generalize about petting, much depends upon the stage of courtship the couple is in, their individual attitudes and backgrounds, and the frequency and intensity of the indulgence. Petting serves as a transitional step in courtship between immature and mature sexual attitudes. It both serves as an outlet for sexual energies and stimulates further sexual desire. Petting is cumulative; consequently, intensive petting may arouse the couple physically to the point where they find it difficult to stop short of sexual intercourse.

Although courtship petting may be pleasurable, it should not be practiced to the exclusion of other pursuits—cultural, intellectual, or social. It should not cause the couple to neglect other activities which would help them to learn to know each other as whole people.

Couples can control petting by avoiding situations of boredom, by adhering to an agreed upon standard of conduct, and by engaging in other mutually interesting activities. In courtship, petting must be placed in proper perspective—a pleasurable step toward a more mature love.

PREMARITAL SEX RELATIONS

Premarital sexual intercourse is a subject of considerable interest among young people today. In this country much has been studied and written concerning it. Our knowledge on the extent of this practice is fragmentary at best.

Sexual activity is an integral part of human behavior. Sexual actions, however, carry with them certain consequences and responsibilities. Strong sex drives are necessary for human survival. Society expects a person to master and control his expression of sex impulses. The manner in which a person expresses his sex life is important to his family, his friends, and surely to his sex partner.

Marriage involves the deepest kind of human values. Hopefully, a person entering marriage has not promiscuously shared himself with persons other than his marriage partner-to-be. A marriage in which the partners have reserved the deepest sexual expression for each other knows a unique sense of exclusiveness. This is reflected in our feelings that our spouses are ours to pet and fondle, and not the property of everyone else. Marriage involves a kind of possessiveness which develops from the days of dating and engagement.

The highest interests of marriage are not served to the degree that one individual wants to use another sexually only for personal satisfaction. Such exploitation is selfish and shows little concern for the feelings of the other person. It may also place the female partner in unnecessary jeopardy of pregnancy. Premarital sexual intercourse may be engaged in to satisfy a person's own sex drives, even at the expense of the other person's enjoyment.

Premarital sexual relations must be viewed in terms of an individual's and a couple's long-range goals in life. Although a couple engaging in such relations may intend to be married, situations may arise in which the couple breaks off the romance. Then their premarital sexual relations are changed from an introduction to marriage into merely a sexual episode. The following are some considerations a couple may give thought to on the matter of premarital sexual relations.

PSYCHOLOGICAL CONSIDERATIONS

1. Does the future husband or wife want to accept a spouse who has had sexual intercourse with someone else? Sometimes two people in accepting each other have to recognize this fact with regret.

2. Premarital sexual relations may leave the male physically and emotionally satisfied, while the girl may be left unsatisfied and frustrated. This feeling may lead her to thinking that she is desired simply for her physical qualities, rather than for her personal qualities.

3. Sometimes a woman feels a special attachment to the man with whom she first had sexual intercourse. If this man is her husband, the feeling strengthens their marriage. If he is now some other woman's husband, the feeling may leave the woman unhappy and disturbed.

4. Fear of discovery may drive couples to seek less than ideal places for the experience—making for haste, apprehension, and emotional strain.

5. The individuals involved may be considered promiscuous. Word often spreads, much to the displeasure of both partners. Kinsey[1] found that women who have had premarital sexual intercourse are almost twice as likely to have extramarital sexual intercourse as are women who have not had premarital sexual intercourse. The partner of a formerly promiscuous person surely would have to wonder if the new relationship was strong enough to prevent future promiscuity.

PHYSICAL CONSIDERATIONS

1. There *is* the possibility of contracting venereal disease. Each year in the United States over 100,000 cases of syphilis and over 200,000 cases of gonorrhea are reported to the public health agencies. However, a survey of physicians conducted by the American Medical Association indicates that less than 10 percent of all diagnosed venereal disease cases are reported. About 50 percent of all cases have been shown to occur in the 15 to 24 year age group. It is difficult for a woman to detect whether the man she is having sexual intercourse with has also had intercourse with some infected person (see Chapter 18).

2. There is always the clear possibility of pregnancy. Although a number of contraceptive devices are now available, many unplanned pregnancies still occur, even among married couples. The use of a contraceptive device does not insure against a pregnancy. Also, intercourse under the influence of sudden passion or alcohol is apt to involve inadequate contraceptive protection (see Chapter 9). Where conditions for sexual intercourse are less than ideal, the risk is likely to be greater than usual. Premarital pregnancy leads to one of the following consequences:

(a) *Abortion* (see Chapter 9).

(b) *Illegitimacy*. The prospect of rearing a child out of wedlock is not pleasant to most women. Whether the mother keeps the child or gives it up for adoption will depend largely upon her social background.

[1] Alfred C. Kinsey, Wardell B. Pomeroy, Clyde E. Martin, and Paul H. Gebhard, *Sexual Behavior in the Human Female*, Philadelphia, W. B. Saunders, 1953, p. 427.

(c) *Forced marriage.* Although many couples confronted with unexpected pregnancies dream of an eventual marriage, some of them have not yet made a firm decision. If they marry out of necessity, one of them may later question whether he would have married the same person under different circumstances. Thus, there may be resentment on the part of one partner or both. Premature marriage can also terminate educational programs and thrust the man into a job before he has adequate training and earning potential. The divorce rate for premaritally pregnant couples is higher than that for other couples.

Although the woman involved in premarital sexual intercourse runs the risk of pregnancy, the man also assumes some risk, notably:

(a) *Accusation of forcible rape.* It is not uncommon for a woman, for one of several reasons, to claim rape. Although it is usually her word against his, convictions are not unusual. Even when the charge is dismissed (as it more often is), being the defendant in such a case is not pleasant.

(b) *Accusation of statutory rape.* Each state has its own minimum age of consent, often 18 years, below which a girl must have parental consent to have sexual intercourse. Even though a well-developed, underage girl may lie about her age and entice a man into intercourse, he is still liable for prosecution for statutory rape. Statutory rape is considered a felony.

(c) *Accusation of paternity.* If a girl becomes pregnant, any man who has had intercourse with her during a given period of time may be the subject of a paternity suit. Unfortunately, blood tests do not always identify the true father. In fact, in some courts such information is not even admissible as evidence.

MASTURBATION

In the not-too-distant past masturbation was considered evil and was thought to lead to insanity, feeble-mindedness, shifty eyes, and acne. It is now generally considered a natural inclination for a human being from infancy to explore his body and to discover that his genital organs are particularly sensitive and that stimulation of them brings pleasure. There is no evidence to prove that masturbation is physically harmful. It is to be expected in normal wholesome sexuality in both the male and the female. Girls should be warned against inserting harmful objects into the vagina to induce self-stimulation; such objects may cause hemorrhage or infection.

The most important consideration is whether or not the practice represents a retreat from life, a kind of psychological placebo. Feelings of guilt from practicing self-stimulation can lead to fears and tensions. Parents should be careful not to lead the child to develop a sense of guilt over it nor to threaten the child with false consequences in order to suppress the act. They should not make an issue of it, recognize that it generally diminishes with maturity as the individual finds more satisfying sexual outlets, plan interesting activities that make the practice less necessary, refrain from punishing the child for it, and, by all means, keep the door of discussion open with the child.

ARE YOU READY FOR MARRIAGE?

Marriage involves not only finding the right person and learning to know that person, but also developing sufficient maturity to meet the responsibilities of marriage. Readiness for marriage should depend upon the following considerations:

EMOTIONAL MATURITY

The emotional demands of marriage are greater than those a couple experiences during courtship. Thus, a most crucial requirement for marriage is some degree of emotional maturity. With many people this develops with chronological maturity, but some remain adolescents emotionally, even though they are legally adults.

The truly mature person has learned how to establish and maintain personal relationships. More than simply recognizing the needs of others, he must be willing to assume some responsibility for meeting these needs. He strives for emotional stability. In spite of both good intentions and good planning, some situations turn into frustrating personal roadblocks. These the mature person will accept rationally and alter his plans as necessary. He will not be easily blocked in accomplishing his long-range goals.

A person should be free from emotional maladjustments such as excessive moodiness, suspiciousness, insecurity, and anxiety. Their constant presence can disrupt interpersonal relations and jeopardize a marriage. A person who is subject to such maladjustments should seek professional counsel.

CHRONOLOGICAL MATURITY

The recognition that chronological age is generally some indication of maturity is reflected in the state laws which set a minimum age for marriage. In most states 18 years for boys and 16 years for girls is the age below which marriage is illegal. Parental permission is usually required until the age of 21 years for boys and 18 years for girls, after which each of them is allowed to decide for himself. On a national scale the median age at the first marriage has been coming down. It is now slightly under 23 years for the male and a bit over 20 years for the female (Table 8.1).

TABLE 8.1 **MEDIAN AGE AT FIRST MARRIAGE, BY SEX:**
1920 TO 1964

Year	Male	Female
1920	24.6	21.2
1930	24.3	21.3
1940	24.3	21.5
1950	22.8	20.3
1951	22.9	20.4
1952	23.0	20.2
1953	22.8	20.2
1954	23.0	20.3
1955	22.6	20.2
1956	22.5	20.1
1957	22.6	20.3
1958	22.6	20.2
1959	22.5	20.2
1960	22.8	20.3
1961	22.8	20.3
1962	22.7	20.3
1963	22.8	20.5
1964	23.1	20.5
1965	22.8	20.6

SOURCE: Based on the U.S. Department of Commerce, Bureau of the Census, *Current Population Reports*, Series P-20, No. 144.

SOCIAL MATURITY

Most adolescents need a measure of adolescent living in order to attain social maturity. This includes adequate acquaintance with new partners through sufficient dating—sufficient not only in number but also in variety. Social curiosity should be satisfied to the point where the marriage partner does not later need to feel he missed something in adolescence and that he is therefore justified in trying to compensate through extramarital sprees.

Many young people desire a sufficient measure of single, independent life before marriage. They desire a respite between the bondage of childhood and the bondage of matrimony. Some find this freedom permanently satisfying; most appreciate it to a point, after which they are ready for marriage.

Most people learn how to be good husbands or wives naturally. As children and adolescents they have been able to observe their parents in the respective roles. If parents set good examples, the children have adequate preparation. If parents set poor examples, the children may grow up with a deficiency. Such faults may haunt the children or cause them to follow the same inadequate roles as their parents. Thus, children from unhappy homes may be poor marriage risks.

FINANCIAL RESOURCES

Although not of the same significance as the preceding personal factors, financial resources must be accurately assessed before marriage. The minimum amount of money a couple needs to live on is highly variable. Many young couples approach marriage without extensive financial resources. A couple must gauge finances in terms of both husband's and wife's earning ability, without depending too heavily on the wife's income (which will likely stop in case of pregnancy). Not infrequently, couples depend upon their parents' subsidizing them in some manner temporarily.

Two married students should be able to live together as cheaply as two unmarried students live separately. However, married students might find that parental financial support stops when they marry. Then, unless one of the partners is through with education and can work (and they are able to delay pregnancy), financing a student marriage can impose extra burdens on the couple.

PROPER TIMING

A couple should not feel rushed into marriage. Properly done, marriage requires time both for prior preparation and for adequate adjustment. More will be said regarding this in the discussion on the wedding. Early extended separations create problems that strain the fragile new relationship. If military service, travel, or other factors promise to create an extended absence, the couple may need to consider postponing the wedding. An extended absence before marriage may terminate the entire relationship if the friendship and affection are not substantial enough to warrant marriage. A marriage is best timed when it allows both advance preparation and at least a year of married relationship before an extensive separation.

The timing of marriage frequently perplexes college students. Although student marriages are essentially not different from any other marriage, the couple must give special thought to financial resources, available time, and the effect a pregnancy may have on their educational plans.

Unless they are able to manage time to their mutual satisfaction, the partners may find that with their study and work schedule their free time together is undesirably limited. In the event of parenthood, full-time educational programs become very hard to maintain for the father and often impossible for the mother. A study at Michigan State University, among couples with their first child, showed that only about one third of these definitely planned the first pregnancy.[2] If an educational program may place too much stress on them, couples are wise to postpone marriage plans until after their education is complete.

ENGAGEMENT

PURPOSES OF AN ENGAGEMENT

Engagement gives a couple some security before marriage. During this time they can test their reactions to the new relationship in a more intense and exclusive manner.

This should be a time of increasing intimacy, leading toward unrestricted expression in marriage. The partners need not feel that they must give full expression to all sexual tension, since this is one of the reasons they desire marriage. The problem of petting need not be an all-or-none matter. The couple should feel free to engage in it, yet recognize limits they have agreed upon. The criterion for deciding these limits should be that those things making for a happier, less strained, less feared relationship should be continued. Those that accomplish the opposite should be discontinued.

The attitude of "ownership" toward each other during engagement should be fair. On the one hand, engagement should represent good intentions, which will, if everything goes well, culminate in marriage. Marriage should represent the final mate selection for both of them. Yet during the engagement the two people need not seal themselves off from society. If, for example, one of them is away in school, either should be allowed the liberty to date. Such dating can relieve some of the strain of separation and also be a good test of a couple's devotion. If their love can withstand a minor test like this, the chances are better that it can withstand the tests of matrimony. Such dating should be limited to pleasure and convenience, without serious interest or petting, and should not be limited to one person.

Exactly how long engagement should last must be answered by each couple. The accepted duration should include sufficient time to plan for and announce the wedding. During this time questions to be considered might be: When and where will the wedding be held? Who will

[2] Shirley Poffenberger, Thomas Poffenberger, and Judson T. Landis, "Intent Toward Conception and the Pregnancy Experience," *American Sociological Review*, 17 (Oct. 1952), 616–620.

be invited to attend? Where should the honeymoon be, and how much money should be spent on it? Do the partners adequately understand sexual intercourse and reproduction? What are their attitudes toward the use of contraceptives? Where is the husband going to derive his income and how much will it be? Do they have any general plans regarding the use of their money? Where do they plan to live? Does the wife plan to work? Are they going to attempt to have children, and if so, when and how many?

Engagement need not be a time for confessing all of the sins of the past. Uncalled for confessions may only arouse basic suspicions and create doubts. However, anything that has a bearing on the future relationship should be shared before, *not after,* the wedding.

PREMARITAL SEX RELATIONS DURING ENGAGEMENT

The extent of premarital relations during engagement is a matter for each couple to decide. Caressing and expressing of affection is normal and is a helpful preparation for marriage. Sexual intercourse at this time, however, can be hazardous. Some couples question its advisability, set limits of love-making, and abstain. Others agree that it is desirable and engage in it without any apparent fear. Still others face the dilemma—they want to do it, yet they do not think they should and either reluctantly abstain or guiltily engage in sexual intercourse. It is wise for a couple, during their less emotional moments, to decide how far they want to go and then attempt to stick with this agreement.

To the person approaching marriage who is troubled over past premarital experiences, here are several suggestions. Although there may have been undesirable consequences, the marriage is far from doomed. Try to minimize the past and build on the future; what is done is done. The past cannot be changed; however, it should not be allowed to destroy self-confidence permanently. Counseling with a friend, psychologist, teacher, pastor, or marriage counsellor is often helpful.

BROKEN ENGAGEMENTS

Although any engagement may be broken, the less thoughtful ones are more likely to be. The same thing holds true for teen-age engagements. The engagement should never be expected to accomplish things dating could not.

Although broken engagements can be unpleasant, they are preferable to broken marriages. If the partnership is incompatible, it is better to admit it before marriage than after. After careful contemplation, if either party desires to break an engagement, it should be broken. But breaking an engagement can be expected to be unpleasant and painful. Once a person makes up his mind to break an engagement, he should act promptly and kindly. He should not allow the opinions of family or friends, the fact that wedding plans are under way, or embarrassment or pride to prevent him from carrying out his decision. He should disregard any threats the other person might make. The wishes of the other party should not be given in to out of pity or fear. In time both parties will get over the experience. No person should ever assume a "this-one-or-nobody" attitude. There are thousands of compatible, affectionate people in the world, any one of whom would make a good marriage partner. Establishing new social contacts may be easier for the boy than for the girl. Even so, there are many opportunities for social contacts today for girls who are conscious of social values and who are willing to gain new acquaintances.

MARRIAGE LAWS

Each of the states considers marriage an institution to be protected, and each state has established laws to prohibit certain types of people from entering into marriage. Although these laws vary somewhat from state to state and are changed periodically, there are certain similarities between them.

MINIMAL AGE FOR MARRIAGE

There is a trend among states to raise age requirements for marriage. Yet they have sought to provide flexibility in individual cases where an earlier marriage would be in the interest of public morals. Minimal requirements range from 14 to 17 years for girls, and 15 to 18 years of age for boys. In the majority of states the ages are 16 for girls and 18 for boys. Two thirds of the states allow an exception to the minimal laws in cases of pregnancy, the birth of a child, or in certain other special circumstances.

PARENTAL CONSENT

All states require parental consent for marriage if either partner is below a given age. Generally such consent is required if the age of the boy is below 21 or, for the girl, below 18.

PHYSICAL EXAMINATION AND BLOOD TEST

All but a few states require a medical examination of some kind which generally includes a blood test. In the majority of cases this is for venereal disease only. A minority of states also examines for one or more of the following: feeble-mindedness, uncontrolled epileptic attacks, infectious tuberculosis, chronic alcoholism, mental illness, and drug addiction. Although most states have statutes requiring some type of physical examinations, such tests are not always administered.

Approximately two thirds of the states stipulate that the examination must be given not longer than 30 days before the issuance of the marriage license. In a few cases it must have been within 10 days of the issuance of the license.

WAITING PERIOD

Considerable variation exists in how long prior to the wedding the couple must obtain the license for marriage. Most commonly it is 3 days, although it ranges from no waiting period requirement up to as long as 7 days. States that require no waiting period are common marriage sites for eloping couples.

Several states stipulate that the wedding must occur within a given number of days after the license is issued, although the great majority of states say nothing on this matter.

PROHIBITED MARRIAGES

All the states prohibit marriage between relatives closer than first cousins, such as with brothers, sisters, fathers, or mothers. More than half of them prohibit the marriage of first cousins, and a few, even of second cousins. All states prohibit a person who is already married to one living spouse to marry another (bigamy). Marriage of a person who is legally judged to be mentally ill is prohibited in all states. Other prohibitions in some states extend to feeble-mindedness, epilepsy, fraudulent representation by one partner as to his character, and lack of mutual consent. Three states allow only a clergyman to conduct the ceremony, although in all others either a clergyman or a civil official is approved. Most states require witnesses to the vows.

COMMON-LAW MARRIAGES

A common-law marriage is one in which both parties give mutual consent to cohabitation as husband and wife. Although definitions vary somewhat from state to state, generally the consenting parties must be competent to enter into a ceremonial marriage. In this type of marriage no license or ceremony is required; thus the marriage involves no records. Since states can have little or no control over such unions, an increasing number of states are declaring them "null and void." Fewer than one third of the states now recognize such marriages as legal.

PREMARITAL COUNSELING

Today increasing emphasis has been placed on premarital counseling to assist couples in making an adequate marital adjustment. The American Institute of Family Relations in Los Angeles and the Marriage Council of Philadelphia were among the earliest institutions involved in this effort. It has been found that probability of happiness in marriage can be predicted by examining background factors, personality traits, engagement relations, engagement adjustment, and other anticipated factors.

The counsellor may be a professional marriage counsellor, a religious leader, or a physician. Some marriage counsellors use temperament tests to indicate a person's suitability for marriage. If either member of the couple has inadequate knowledge of sexual intercourse and reproduction, he or she may be counseled by books or discussions. The counsellor should be prepared to discuss with them any fears or inhibitions they may have regarding normal sex life. He should question them regarding financial plans, housing, budgets, time schedules, and any other phase of marital life that may be a subject of adjustment.

There is an advantage in seeing more than one type of counsellor, each trained to deal with a different area of marital adjustment. Each prospective partner should have a thorough physical examination and one or more sessions with his family physician or gynecologist regarding capacity to bear children; kinds of contraceptives and their need and use; and questions on genetics, such as any evident abnormalities in himself or hereditary factors that may affect children. A growing number of medical schools, hospitals, and universities are providing genetic counseling. If possible, a religious leader should be consulted, not only regarding the particulars of the wedding ceremony, its symbolisms and the meanings behind it, but also regarding the couple's religious outlook. As time passes, a couple is often in need of further help in solving problems. Some couples have found it helpful to have the acquaintance of a religious leader whose counsel they can trust.

BEGINNING MARRIAGE

THE WEDDING

Marriage represents a new status, and in our culture the wedding, as a public pronouncement, is the accepted portal into it. This pronouncement generally includes the ceremony, expressions of consent by the couple, witnesses, sanctions by the state and often by the church, and records. It implies that the married couple is now free to assume all the rights and privileges of marriage within the cultural patterns.

Both the state and the church have interests in marriage. Since marriage is a recognized moral expression and the state seeks to safeguard morals, it establishes the couple's rights to legal property. It determines the legitimacy of children and the responsibility for their support. Children borne by a married mother are assumed to be the children of her husband. Through marriage the law seeks to protect individuals from sexual exploitation. It establishes the legality of contracts. Through marriage regulations, the state seeks to control the propagation of biological defects, such as feeble-mindedness.

THE CEREMONY

The particulars of the wedding ceremony are usually determined by the marriage partners and their families. The parents may play a small or large role in these decisions. Although many couples want their weddings to be something they and their friends will remember, no wedding should cast an unbearable financial burden on either the family or the couple.

The wedding is the portal to a new relationship and not an end in itself. Plans should be laid carefully so that in the "mad whirl of partying," which is typical of many weddings, the couple does not become so confused and fatigued that the setting for a good honeymoon adjustment is lost. Generally, the couple schedules the wedding to occur between the wife's menstrual periods. The rite may be a brief statement before a civil magistrate or an elaborate church ceremony. Many religious groups have typical ceremonial forms that are followed, some more symbolic than others. Regardless of the form chosen, the ceremony should fit the social and spiritual needs of the couple, affirming their aspirations and pledging their commitment in terms that are meaningful to them.

ELOPEMENT AND SECRET MARRIAGE

There is a distinction between a secret wedding, or elopement, and a secret marriage. An elopement is a kind of "runaway" wedding in which the fact of the marriage is publicized after the wedding. In a secret marriage both the fact of the wedding *and* the marriage are kept secret for an extended period. The two are different only in degree. Knowledge of the secret marriage is shared by the license issuer, officiant, and witness, and, in some cases, parents and selected friends. All types of secret marriages are more or less similar.

There may be valid reasons for secrecy. Parents may have an unjustified opposition to the marriage, in spite of the reasonable age and maturity of the couple. Domestic factors such as illness, recent death, or parental disharmony may upset wedding preparations so that an elopement may seem more desirable. Such cases are, however, uncommon.

There are arguments against secret marriages. The couple may be overly hasty because of fear or fact of pregnancy. They may be attempting to avoid normal publicity or the expenses and preparations of a wedding. The couple may be by-passing the testing functions of the engagement during which they further prepare themselves for marriage both mentally and socially. They deprive themselves of the satisfactions of marriage preparations (tiring though they are) which should be a life-long source of pleasant memories. Parents, friends, and in-laws, whose support is needed during married life, are often hurt or alienated. People question the secrecy. If the marriage is kept secret for a period of time, the couple faces strange circumstances in keeping it quiet, yet fulfilling their marriage. When the news is out, the enthusiasm of other people may not be as great as expected. If the wife becomes pregnant, the explaining or the attempt at it becomes awkward. In attempting to "escape" from an undesirable situation, the couple often jumps into a worse situation. Marriage is desirable and should be entered into openly and deliberately.

THE HONEYMOON

The honeymoon is a special period during which, in privacy and isolation, the couple takes the first steps in adjustment to shared living. It represents the culmination of months and years of expectations. Although not every couple can or does have a honeymoon, it can help greatly in the transition from single to married life. It should be well planned to allow for as easy an adjustment as possible. Ideally, it should allow the partners to concentrate on each other, sexually and socially, rather than on business, extended travel, or crowded schedules. The site chosen for the honeymoon should be a place both can enjoy and afford. The honeymoon should last long enough to allow for adjustment, yet not so long that it leads to boredom or an excessive amount of anxiety about setting up the new household. The time should be spent leisurely and unhurriedly.

Even though couples may be well informed on sexual anatomy and physiology, not all of them find complete sexual success at first. Time is required to break down fears and inhibitions. Each should be concerned that the other partner find as satisfactory an adjustment as possible. He should display attitudes of tenderness and patience. Marital adjustment takes time. A satisfying honeymoon built upon a concern for the other's wishes will be a long step toward good marital adjustment.

MARRIAGE ADJUSTMENTS

Marriage is a dynamic rather than a static process. Adjustments are called for as long as the marriage lasts. Each spouse has constantly changing needs, so that the adjustments called for by one spouse from the other will be altered with time. With problems go tensions; with adjustment comes relief from those tensions. Any couple contemplating marriage must be prepared to face certain problems. The relative success of a given marriage will depend upon the couple's ability to reduce sources of friction as much as possible. If too many of them go unresolved, the stage for marriage failure is being set.

Many factors may have a bearing upon the success of a marriage; the following constitute several important ones:

IN-LAWS

Marriage involves a new alignment of family loyalties. A married couple belongs to three families—the paternal (his), the maternal (hers), and the couple's (theirs). The strongest of the three must be that of the couple.

A threat can develop if either his or her family intrudes into the new family. Although any in-law can intrude, common offenders are the mother-in-law or the sister-in-law. Because women generally take more responsibility for interfamily relationships than men, women generally are involved in these frictions sooner than men.

Desirable interrelations come about when parents can freely recognize new in-laws. Parents should neither ignore young couples nor interfere in their affairs. The entire relationship needs the chance to grow to maturity not only with the young couple, but also with parents and other relatives as well.

INDIVIDUAL PERSONALITIES

Our personalities include everything about us—our thoughts, emotions, attitudes, habits, behavior, reactions to people and things, fears, and aspirations. The individual does not *possess* a personality—his personality *is* him. People around us see some parts of it; other parts are rarely, if ever, seen. Usually the more a person knows of another's personality, the better the adjustment made to him. There are usually valid reasons why a person does what he does. Often such reasons can be known. Frequently the more we delve into why a person acts and reacts in certain ways, the easier it is for us to accept him.

In marriage, when two people attempt to adjust to each other, for better or for worse, some rough spots are sure to be encountered. Here are several suggestions to temper the reactions of one partner to the other:

1. Behavior is affected by illness, hunger, fatigue, and emotions.
2. Marriage partners should honestly try to agree with each other on *some* things. Normally, however, a couple cannot be expected to agree on all matters.
3. A marriage partner should not expect to change his spouse into someone different from what that person was before marriage. After choosing, the partners should try to adjust to each other.
4. Where possible, a good partner should be positive rather than negative. He should give criticism *only* if it will help the other person attain his goals.
5. Nagging is rarely worth the time it takes. If a partner needs improving, more constructive methods should be used.
6. Suggestions should be given at the right moment, preferably when the other partner asks for them. Advice given when it is not wanted can be useless.

This is just a beginning. The intelligent couple finds many ways of smoothing out the sources of irritation and hurt in the marital relationship.

CONFLICT

To some extent, every marriage is a "mixed" marriage. Each spouse brings into marriage different wants and wishes. The couple must decide whether one gives in entirely ("peace at any price"), whether there will be compromise, or whether open conflict is the only solution. Conflict is not bad in itself and can even help to achieve compromise and relieve tension if done constructively. However, it must be kept within bounds and not be allowed to become destructive to the marriage.

SEXUAL LIFE

Sexual satisfaction is not the only aim of marriage. But sex appeal may draw a couple together. As each partner's body becomes more commonplace in marriage, sexual love becomes secondary to companionate love. Placing too high an expectation on sex can be disappointing. Sex must be viewed as only a part of marriage. On the other hand, a couple should not neglect working toward a satisfying sex adjustment.

FINANCES

It costs money not only to marry but also to exist after marriage. The material needs of a married couple go on and on—home, furnishings, car, personal items, children, vacations, and insurance. Unless the newlyweds are subsidized from outside by parents or relatives, their income must at least meet expenses. To the husband's income (regular and extra) often is added the wife's. Few (if any) individuals, single or married, *ever* have enough money. If the couple can live within its income, fine; but if their tastes are too expensive for their income, trouble may be in the making. Methods of handling money should be well considered. A family financial discussion should include a plan of where the available money is to go (not simply a record of where it went); how to handle the actual spending wisely, purchasing in terms of both quality and quantity; a reasonable insurance program, including hospitalization, life, automobile, and, if desired, educational and retirement; the discreet use of credit buying; and a good system for recording where the money went.

EXTRAMARITAL SEXUAL RELATIONS

Since sex is the most intimate aspect of marriage, extramarital intercourse is its most profound betrayal. Adultery is one of the leading grounds for divorce. Generally, the better the marriage and the more meaningful the interpersonal relationship, the less likely the extramarital interests. Where breakdown occurs, it may be due to erosion of those interpersonal relations, loss of pleasure from the marital sexual relation, immaturity, or inner conflicts.

Regardless of the cause, when a married person falls into extramarital interests and involvements, a couple should reflect over the marriage. If they cannot do so objectively, they should seek professional counseling.

HAVING CHILDREN

Over 80 percent of all marriages result in children. For many people, having children is an important achievement and fulfills the desire to establish a home. This feeling stems from the biological urge which relates itself to sexual relations; reproduction represents one of the great creative acts couples are capable of. It also represents a response to social pressure and perpetuates the kind of family relations many of us have found enjoyable, including grandparents, parents, and brothers and sisters.

RESPONSIBILITIES

The decision to have children carries with it the responsibility of providing for them in many ways. Children are expensive. Although it will vary somewhat with a family's income and level of living, the cost of supporting a child to college age is estimated to be about $20,000 today. A couple should plan the size of its family in terms of the income and desired standard of living of both. The child will have a need to love and be loved. He will need to acquire a sense of security from his parents and their family relations within the home. The kinds of religious values the parents want to see the child acquire will depend largely upon the role religion plays in the parents' lives. The cultural background the child acquires will depend upon the things he has seen and been exposed to in the home. In order to accomplish the goals they might have for the child, the parents must exercise discipline. It will be required both in matters of behavior and in the accomplishment of long-range goals. Since children have many kinds of needs, parents must be committed to supplying them for the many years of childhood and adolescence—and, in some cases, even longer.

Although a pregnancy is unplanned, the parents should readily accept the baby. Only the parents were responsible for his conception. To react against the situation by resenting the child, by abandoning it, or by one of the parents' either deserting the marriage or seeking a divorce is surely a demonstration of immaturity. The child has no choice either of the situation or of his parents. Parents should overlook any disappointment and give the child the type of home he deserves.

TIMING

If possible, the first pregnancy should come only after the couple has had sufficient time to make a reasonable marital adjustment. It may be wise for pregnancy to come before the couple becomes too attached to material possessions and set schedules. The optimum biological time for child-bearing is between the maternal ages of 20 and 35 years.

A teen-age mother is frequently still faced with problems of emotional and social immaturity that distract from her effectiveness as a well-balanced mother. On the other hand, if the mother is too old, the physical dangers of childbirth to both herself and the baby are increased.

There is no one best time of the year to have a child. But the couple should bear in mind that the child will be born approximately 9 months after conception. If planned, the birth should come when the couple wants it in terms of vacations, holidays, school, and work schedules. Although a physician can attempt to determine the approximate time of birth, his estimation is not always accurate. However, the delivery is generally within several weeks of his projected time.

SPACING

Biologically, human mothers are potentially capable of bearing more than one child per year. The rearing of children, however, places great demands upon parents. Today, through the intelligent use of contraceptives, the couple can space and plan the coming of children to match their desires and resources. There are several appropriate reasons for

TABLE 8.2 **SIZE OF FAMILY PER HOUSEHOLD, 1890 TO 1960**

Date	Population
1890	4.93
1900	4.76
1910	4.54
1920	4.34
1930	4.11
1940	3.77
1950	3.52
1960	3.38

SOURCE: Based on U.S. Department of Commerce, Bureau of the Census.

doing so. The couple should be ready financially for each child; the previous child should be old enough that the mother does not need to carry him around during the second pregnancy; sufficient time should be allowed for the mother to regain her vitality. The amount of spacing will depend upon the wishes of the couple. Many consider a 2- to 3-year spacing most convenient. One should not forget that children spaced too far apart can be a problem in that too wide an age spread between children makes it difficult for them to share common interests. A degree of companionship between children not only assists in their development, but also often makes it easier for the mother, since the children tend to entertain each other and thus require less directed entertainment by the parents.

The total number of children desired is a personal matter. Hopefully, the number should reflect the planned desires of the couple in terms of their religious feelings, financial and emotional capabilities, and social settings. Table 8.2 shows the decrease in the average number of persons per family since 1890.

CHILDLESS COUPLES

A couple may be childless either because of plan or because of its inability to have children. Today no couple need feel it must have children simply to fulfill a moral obligation to society. Indeed, the world's population is increasing at an unparalleled rate in spite of the common availability of effective contraceptives. There may be some very legitimate reasons for wanting to remain childless. Some people desire to devote full time to their professions and careers. Others recognize the instability of their marriages and feel that until they achieve satisfactory marital harmony, the proper emotional atmosphere for raising children is not present in the home. Generally, the coming of children does not remedy an already sick domestic situation. Even in a domestically tranquil home the birth and rearing of children places new and great pressures on the parents. If the marital bond is already bending under pressures, the coming of children will add to and intensify these pressures rather than reduce them. It may even precipitate disruption of the marriage. Another reason for not desiring children may be insufficient finances to properly provide for their needs. The decision to not have children should be a mutual one.

If the desires of the partners are exactly opposite with regard to this matter, the one wanting children should realize that a child may be highly resented if the other partner wants no children. Once a decision to remain childless has been reached, the couple should feel no sense of betrayal to the cause of marriage. Such a decision is fully justified on the part of any couple.

INVOLUNTARY CHILDLESSNESS

Approximately 10 percent of all marriages are childless in spite of repeated attempts at pregnancy. A couple approaching marriage should not take for granted that it will be possible to have children. For some, childlessness is difficult to accept.

A number of physical factors may be responsible for sterility; some can be changed with medical attention, others cannot. Sterility may be due to improperly formed sex organs, cervical obstructions, defective sperm, glandular deficiencies, or other causes. It may result from developmental disease or emotional causes. If such a condition is known before marriage, it is the responsibility of the sterile partner to inform the other one. It is important that if such a couple wants children, both partners seek the aid of a physician, a fertility clinic, or the Planned Parenthood Federation. If, after proper deliberation and consultation, a pregnancy is not forthcoming, and if the couple still desires children, they may consider either artificial insemination or adoption. Artificial insemination will be further discussed in Chapter 9.

ADOPTION

There are well over 100,000 adoptions in this country each year. In many localities the demand for adoptions is greater than the supply of children. The first step is filing with an adoption agency an application to adopt a child. The processing of the application requires time, sometimes months. Some state laws even require a one-year waiting period during which the home is thoroughly checked by a local welfare agency.

Although some adoptions are independently handled directly between natural and adoptive parents or their representatives, many states prohibit such independent adoptions. Such prohibition is based on cases where children have been given away without sufficient cause, where adoptive home life was not suitable, where babies were not properly matched to their adoptive parents, or where adoptive parents were not legally protected either in terminating an unacceptable adoption or where their exclusive guardianship over the child was questioned by the natural parents.

It is preferable in all cases to work through either a private state-licensed agency or a public welfare department. Such agencies collect all available facts regarding the child's background, race, intelligence, education, and health. The same is done with the prospective adoptive parents, plus information regarding their social and economic position, their emotional acceptability as parents, and their reputation among their friends. The agency often checks out their homes. After the application for adoption has been approved, the child is matched as closely to his adoptive parents as possible. After the child is left with the agency, he is often held for medical observation for a few days. If healthy, he is placed in an adoptive home on probation for several months or a year, during which time the legal adoption papers are drawn up. During this time most abnormalities are noticed, so that there is a slim chance of an undesirable abnormality's cropping up afterwards. Actually, there is little more chance of having an imperfect adoptive child this way than there would be of having an imperfect child of one's own.

Unique problems are faced in adoptions, none of which are unsolvable. The adoptive child fills an important emotional place in his adoptive parents' lives and they in his. If relations are well handled, the adoptive child–parent relationship should be just as satisfying as a natural situation.

DIVORCE

With some marriages it becomes apparent that because of unresolved marital conflicts there is no longer a basis for trying to continue the relationship.

MEANS OF BREAKING THE MARRIAGE

The relationship of marriage may be broken formally or informally. It may be broken informally by desertion, in which one partner simply disappears, or by separation, in which the couple has agreed to live separately or has been directed to do so by order of a court (a legal separation). Neither desertion nor separation constitutes a legal divorce. The marriage may be dissolved legally by means of an annulment if it can be established that some legal requirement for marriage was never met (due to fraud, deception, illegal age, bigamy, or some other violation). A valid marriage may be dissolved legally by means of a decree of divorce if it can be established that one or both partners violated the marriage rights of the other partner. A decree of divorce constitutes a cancellation of the marriage contract, after which both partners are again legally free to remarry. Grounds for divorce vary considerably from state to state.

INCIDENCE OF DIVORCE

The divorce rate has climbed rather sharply over the last 100 years. Just after the Civil War there was only 1 divorce in every 36 marriages. By 1900 it had risen to 1 in 12; by 1960, to 1 in about every 4 marriages (Fig. 8.1). Although divorce occurs among all groups of people in this country, it tends to occur more frequently in cities than in rural areas and more often among those of lower economic status than among those of higher status. It tends to increase with an increase in education up through high school graduates and is more frequent during the first 5 years of marriage than later. The incidence of divorce is related to the age of persons at the time of marriage. Marriages in which one or both parties were less than age 20 at the time of marriage are more likely to terminate in divorce. Any increases in divorce must, however, be qualified. Divorce is a symptom of marriage failure, not a cause. There are couples whose marriage has failed but who have not obtained a divorce for moral or religious reasons, fear of affecting the husband's professional standing, the presence of children in the home, property considerations, or fear of admitting failure.

The increase in divorce rates is a result of a number of factors. Generally, states now allow more grounds for divorce and courts are

growing more lenient in interpreting divorce laws. There is a decline
in religious authority, which to some previously served as a deterrent.
Women have higher status, greater independence, and freedom to be
self-supporting. The evolving criteria for success in marriage place
greater importance on love and companionship, without which a marriage today is more often considered to be a failure. Public opinion
toward divorce is increasingly liberal. Last, but surely not unimportant,

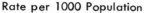

Rate per 1000 Population

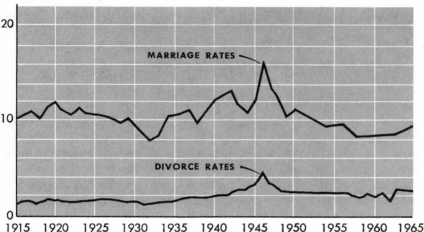

Fig. 8.1 Marriage and divorce rates since 1915. (U.S. Department of Health,
Education, and Welfare, Public Health Service.)

is the manner in which the press has treated divorce. Newspapers and
popular periodicals have added to the notoriety surrounding certain
domestic battles in the courts. Some of the time, but fortunately not
all of the time, the divorceé is pictured as being gay, free, and the
recipient of liberal alimony allotments. Actually, divorce is anything
but glamorous.

The majority of divorce decrees are awarded to women. There are
several reasons for this practice. Generally, women have access to more
legal grounds for divorce than men. The courts tend to be more sympathetic to the divorce suits of women and tend to award alimony more
readily to them. Yet, it is felt that women often encounter greater
difficulty in facing the public after divorce than do men. Our social
structure tends to allow the man to be more aggressive in seeking out a
new marriage partner.

There is considerable difference among the states as to what constitutes legal grounds for divorce. Grounds for absolute divorce include adultery, cruelty (physical or mental), desertion, nonsupport, alcoholism, impotency, insanity, pregnancy at marriage, bigamy, drug addiction, fraud, force or duress, felony conviction, and imprisonment. Since the legal grounds constitute narrow legal interpretations, individuals seeking divorce in a given state must show marital failure on the legally recognized grounds. Persons seeking divorce often go to extremes to establish complaints within these categories, even though the actual cause of failure was something entirely different. This practice is so frequent that marriage authorities believe the number of decrees awarded in certain categories tell very little of the true nature of marital conflicts among the couples involved.

EFFECTS OF DIVORCE UPON PARTNERS

Any couple contemplating divorce should not be oblivious to the consequences. Usually, all parties involved find it to be a painful experience, emotionally and socially; for some, it represents "jumping from the frying pan into the fire." Frequently, it does not solve the basic human problems. New problems are created for both the divorced persons and the children they have had. The divorced people may later feel they have been too hasty in seeking a decree. They may feel that if they had tried just a little harder to seek a solution, they might have been able to mediate the conflict. They may feel that someone they have loved and something they had pledged themselves to is broken and gone. They must now settle their anguish and resentment and repair their pride. The remarriage of either former spouse to a new spouse dashes all hopes for reinstatement. For some, the readjustment demanded is severe enough to call for the outside help of friends, the clergy, or psychiatrists.

EFFECTS OF DIVORCE UPON CHILDREN

Particularly bewildering is the effect of divorce upon children. They are in a no-man's land, being pulled in two directions. The best affection the divided parents can bestow is not comparable to the inherent security a youngster should feel in a warm home relationship. He is helpless in resolving his position with both his parents, sometimes feeling a loyalty to both of them. Any court battle over custody only aggravates the damage. Some children become so emotionally disturbed that their attitudes toward their school work and friends are noticeably affected. The world they should be accepting has collapsed. Unfortunately, the child is often aware of marital conflict even before the divorce. The decree only makes the damage permanent. As the child matures, it becomes necessary for him to achieve an outlook on the matter which does not warp *his* chances of achieving a successful marital adjustment. He must be convinced that his parents' problems do not reflect upon him. Most of all, he must learn from his parents' experiences and make every effort to avoid similar pitfalls.

DIVORCE PREVENTION

Surely marriage is supremely important and deserves our most constructive suggestions. Young people must be better educated for marriage. The availability and use of counseling services must be vastly improved. There must be a reemphasis on the moral values which relate so strongly to the privileges and obligations within the union of marriage. A stronger emphasis is needed on the adjustment of the individual to himself and other people in terms of emotional and intellectual values. Marriage is a biological convenience, not an experiment. It stands at the pinnacle of all social institutions. Its success determines the success with which we can creatively accomplish goals of all kinds and manage to live with each other effectively.

REMARRIAGE

Divorce need not terminate marital pleasure. Legally, it frees each spouse to pursue a new relationship. Although remarriages are common, their records of success are less than for first marriages. The divorce rate is higher among those remarried than among those married only once and goes higher the more times remarriage occurs. On the other hand, many find that a remarriage results in more happiness than the original marriage. Remarriages can turn out well if the new partners earnestly attempt to avoid the problems that destroyed the first marriage. If such adjustments are not made, however, the success of the second marriage may be no greater than that of the first.

SUMMARY

I. Factors to Consider Before Marriage
   A. Most important task is the reasoned selection of an appropriate partner.
   B. Personal traits:
      1. Personality.
      2. Hereditary traits.
      3. Infatuation or love?
      4. Differences in background.

II. Premarital Sexual Adjustment
   A. Changing standards have resulted in more leniency today toward the expression of feelings.
      1. Petting.

2. Premarital sex relations.
3. Masturbation.
B. Are you ready for marriage?
  1. Emotional maturity—the ability to establish and maintain personal relationships.
  2. Chronological maturity—should be at least sufficient to meet state minimal age laws.
  3. Social maturity.
  4. Financial resources must be adequate.
  5. Proper timing—adequate time allotted to provide for plans and adjustments.
C. Engagement
  1. Purposes are to give the couple:
    a. some security of choice while allowing them to further test their reactions with each other.
    b. opportunity for increased intimacy, leading toward unrestricted expression in marriage.
    c. sufficient time to plan and announce wedding.
    d. time to arrive at answers to problems such as:
      (1) finances.
      (2) employment.
      (3) honeymoon.
      (4) decisions about children and birth control.
      (5) housing.
  2. Premarital sex relations during engagement should:
    a. be a natural expression for each partner.
    b. not jeopardize a good adjustment following the wedding.
    c. be the decision of both partners.
  3. Broken engagements, although unpleasant, are preferable to broken marriage.
D. Marriage laws
  1. Minimal age for marriage varies, but is in the majority of states 16 for girls and 18 years for boys.
  2. Parental consent is required for marriage if a person is below a given age (often the legal age).
  3. Physical examination and blood test:
    a. required in most states prior to the issuance of a marriage license.
    b. generally given to detect venereal diseases.
  4. Waiting period is required in many states between the issuance of a marriage license and the wedding.
  5. Prohibited marriages:
    a. occur in all states.
    b. prevent the marriage of:
      (1) close blood relations.
      (2) bigamists.
      (3) mentally ill.
      (4) sometimes, racially mixed couples.
  6. Common-law marriages:
    a. require no license, ceremony, or records.
    b. are recognized in fewer than one third of the states.
E. Premarital counseling:
  1. Helps to predict the probable happiness of a marriage.
  2. May be done by:
    a. professional marriage counsellors.

   b. religious leaders.

   c. physicians and genetics authorities.

  3. Should include:

   a. thorough physical examination.

   b. explanation of use of contraceptives.

   c. discussion of any particular physical or religious problems.

   d. meanings and symbolisms behind the wedding ceremony.

III. Beginning Marriage

 A. The wedding serves to:

  1. pronounce publicly the fact of marriage.

  2. establish legal property rights.

  3. establish legitimacy of children and responsibility for their support.

  4. establish legality of contracts.

 B. The honeymoon is designed as a special period of privacy and isolation during which the first steps of adjustment to shared living are taken.

 C. Marriage adjustments are called for as long as the marriage lasts and may be made severe by:

  1. In-laws—should neither ignore nor interfere with the new couple.

  2. Individual personalities—for good interpersonal adjustments, both partners should try to:

   a. understand that behavior is affected by physical conditions.

   b. agree on *some* things.

   c. adjust to one another.

   d. show sufficient appreciation for one another.

   e. give only constructive criticism.

   f. eliminate nagging.

   g. give advice only when it is asked for.

  3. Conflict may achieve compromise and relieve tensions if kept within bounds.

  4. Sexual life can be a satisfying part of marriage if good adjustments are made.

  5. Finances should take into account a couple's tastes, yet should be consistent with their income, needs, and resources.

  6. Extramarital sexual relations are

   a. a most profound betrayal of a marriage.

   b. a leading ground for divorce.

 D. Having children

  1. Responsibilities of parents are the providing of:

   a. sufficient finances.

   b. cultural and social training.

   c. religious training.

   d. educational preparation.

  2. Timing—couple should allow for reasonable marital adjustments before having children.

  3. Spacing

   a. reasonable to space pregnancies.

   b. may be controlled by use of contraceptives.

  4. Childless couples need not feel they are neglecting to fulfill a moral obligation to society.

  5. Involuntary childlessness

   a. is common to about 10 percent of all marriages.

   b. may be due to physical factors which can be corrected by:

    (1) physician.

(2) fertility clinic.

(3) Planned Parenthood Federation

 6. Adoption:

  a. is a solution for parents unable to have children.

  b. is best handled through a private state-licensed agency or the public welfare department.

  c. an adopted child can be as well accepted by parents as a natural child.

IV. Divorce—may be resorted to when unresolved marital conflicts destroy the basis for companionship.

 A. Means of breaking the marriage:

  1. informally by desertion or separation.

  2. formally by annulment or divorce.

 B. Incidence of divorce:

  1. has climbed significantly over the past 100 years.

  2. due to a number of complex factors.

 C. Effects of divorce upon partners.

 D. Effects of divorce upon children.

 E. Divorce prevention.

 F. Remarriage.

Glossary

If you cannot find the word you wish in this glossary, check the index for text and glossary references.

abortion (ə bor'shən) (L. *abortio,* miscarriage).   The expulsion of the human fetus from the womb before the fifth or sixth month; expulsion after that time is termed a stillbirth.

age of consent.   The minimum legal age a person must have reached in order legally to give consent to sexual intercourse. (See **statutory rape.**)

annulment (ə nul'mənt) (L. *annullare,* to bring to nothing).   A legal dissolving of the marriage relation on grounds the marriage was not valid according to the laws of the state.

artificial insemination (ahr ti fish'əl in sem i nā'shən) (L. *inseminatus,* sown, from *in,* into and *semen,* seed).   The deposit of semen into a female by artificial means.

bigamy (big'ə mē) (L. *bi,* two; G. *gamos,* marriage).   Criminal offense of entering into a second marriage while a previous one is still legally in effect.

chromosomal mutation (krō'mə sō'məl myoo tā'shən) (G. *chromo,* color; *soma,* body; L. *mutare,* to change).   A sudden variation in some inheritable characteristic of an individual rising from an alteration in a chromosome.

common-law marriage.   A marriage not solemnized by religious or civil ceremony but effected by agreement to live together as husband and wife.

contraceptive (kon trə sep'tiv) (L. *contra,* against; *conceptus,* from *concipere,* to conceive).   A device for the prevention of the fertilization of the human ovum.

desertion (di zur'shən) (L. *desertus,* solitary, desert).   Act of abandoning a marriage partner.

divorce (di vors') (L. *dis,* apart; *vertere,* to turn).   A legal dissolving of the marriage relation.

illegitimate (il lə jit′i mit) (L. *in,* not; *legitimare,* to make lawful). Born to parents not married to each other.

masturbation (mas tər bā′shən) (L. *manus,* hand; *stuprare,* to rape). Self-excitation of one's genitals.

placebo (plə sē′bō) (L. *placebo,* I shall please). A medicine given merely to satisfy the patient and of no therapeutic value.

rape (rāp) (L. *rapere,* to seize). The crime of having sexual intercourse with a woman by force and without her consent.

separation (sep ə rā′shən). An arrangement by which a husband and wife live apart and separately by agreement.

statutory rape (stach′yoo tor ē rāp) (L. *statuere,* to set or ordain). Sexual intercourse, either voluntarily or forcibly, with an individual below the age of consent. (See **age of consent.**)

C H A P T E R 9

HUMAN
REPRODUCTION

Like almost all of the familiar plants and animals, human beings reproduce by a *sexual* process involving the fusion of specially produced sexual cells, the sperm and the egg. These mature sex cells are called *gametes*. The major biological importance of sexual reproduction is that it allows new genetic combinations each generation; throughout the course of evolution, this has been an important means of bringing together favorable mutations in the offspring. Even the most primitive plant and animal forms, which routinely reproduce by such *asexual* means as merely dividing into two smaller but similar halves, can also reproduce sexually.

Why such a basic and universal process should have become a source of prudery and embarrassment to many individuals is a matter of speculation. Perhaps the very fact that sexual intercourse is a source of great human pleasure has contributed to some of these attitudes about sex. If sex were still viewed in light of the concept that pleasure is evil, then some of the remaining puritanical attitudes about sex might be justified. But today's enlightened individual considers sex not only as important in reproduction, but also as a very legitimate and important source of pleasure in marriage. He gives his children a thorough and factual understanding of the reproductive processes; and, because he lives with well-adjusted, loving parents, the child gains a healthful attitude toward sex and the total relationship between man and wife.

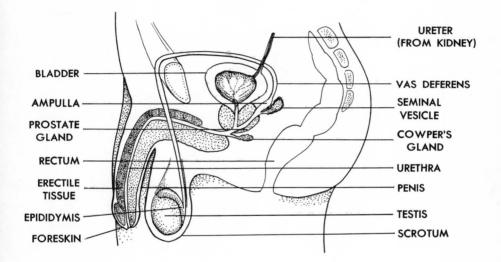

Fig. 9.1 Male reproductive system (side view).

HUMAN REPRODUCTIVE SYSTEMS

THE MALE REPRODUCTIVE SYSTEM (FIGS. 9.1 AND 9.2)

TESTIS

The primary reproductive organs of either sex are called the *gonads.* The gonads of the male consist of a pair of *testes,* often called *testicles* (Fig. 9.3). The testes serve a dual function, producing both *sperm* (the male *gametes*) and the male sex hormone *testosterone.* Human sperm cells (also called *spermatozoa*) are microscopically small, each measuring about 50 microns (thousandths of a millimeter) in length. Each sperm (Fig. 9.4) consists of a *head* containing the genetic material, *neck, middle piece,* and *tail,* with which it swims. Sperm cells secrete

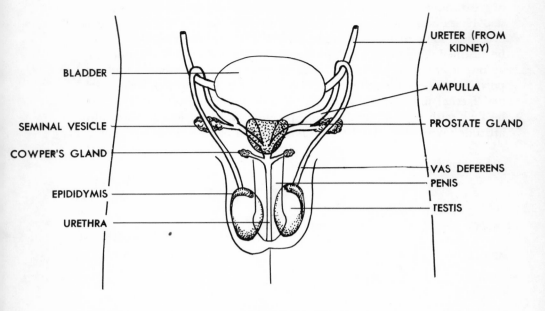

BLADDER

SEMINAL VESICLE

COWPER'S GLAND

EPIDIDYMIS

URETHRA

URETER (FROM KIDNEY)

AMPULLA

PROSTATE GLAND

VAS DEFERENS

PENIS

TESTIS

Fig. 9.2 Male reproductive system (front view).

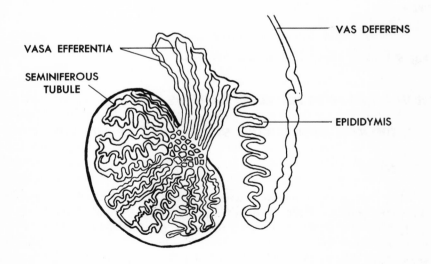

VASA EFFERENTIA

SEMINIFEROUS TUBULE

VAS DEFERENS

EPIDIDYMIS

Fig. 9.3 Structure of human testis.

the enzyme *hyaluronidase,* required for penetration of the egg. Although only one sperm will actually penetrate and fertilize an egg, many millions of sperm are required to secrete enough hyaluronidase for fertilization to occur. This important requirement will be discussed further in the discussion of fertility problems.

Each testis is composed of about 800 narrow, twisted tubes called *seminiferous tubules.* In the inner lining of each tubule the spermatozoa are produced by a special type of cell division (*meiosis,* also to be discussed later in this chapter). The production of sperm continues at a

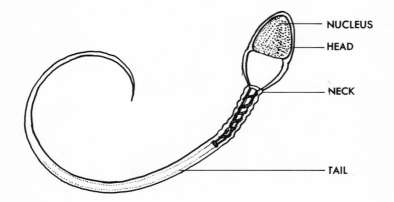

Fig. 9.4 Human sperm cell.

constant rate from puberty, the time of sexual maturity, often until a very advanced age. There is no definite cessation of sexual activity in the male, although the sexual processes do gradually decline with age.

Between the seminiferous tubules lie the *interstitial cells,* which produce testosterone. Testosterone production begins in adolescence in response to the production of *gonadotropic hormone* by the anterior lobe of the pituitary gland, located at the base of the brain. Testosterone stimulates the development of the male reproductive system and the secondary masculine characteristics, such as the beard, body hair, and muscle formation. The production of testosterone continues throughout life.

In the human being, as in most mammals, the production of spermatozoa cannot occur at the temperature found within the body cavity. For this reason the testes descend from the abdomen just prior to birth into the *scrotum,* a sac-like structure suspended at the base of the abdomen. The temperature within the scrotum is maintained at 3 to 4 degrees below body temperature by muscles within the scrotum, which draw the testes up tight against the body in response to cold (or fear), or relax, allowing the testes to fall away from the body in response to high temperature. Occasionally one or both of the testes may fail to descend into the scrotum, a condition which results in partial or total *sterility* caused by lack of sperm production, although the production of the hormone testosterone is not affected. An undescended testis can usually be corrected surgically, with resulting normal fertility.

EPIDIDYMIS

Attached to each testis is a long (18 to 20 feet), tightly coiled tube, the *epididymis.* The epididymis is a storage structure, holding the maturing sperm cells until they are discharged from the body. The sperm cells remain alive for 30 to 60 days, after which they die and disintegrate.

VAS DEFERENS

The vas deferens are small ducts carrying sperm upward from each epididymis into the abdomen. Constriction of the vas deferens is a common cause of sterility in the male. Surgical sterilization of the male usually consists of cutting and/or tying off each vas deferens. Near the end of each vas deferens is an enlarged section called the *ampulla,* which, like the epididymis, serves for storage of sperm.

FLUID-PRODUCING GLANDS

Sperm cells make up only a small portion of the male ejaculate, or *semen,* which is composed of sperm cells plus the fluid secretions of several glands. The most important fluid-producing glands are the *seminal vesicles,* one of which empties into the upper end of each vas deferens at the ampulla. The second source of fluid is the single *prostate gland.* The two vas deferens and the duct carrying urine from the urinary bladder unite within the prostate gland. The single duct, which now carries both semen and urine from the prostate to the tip of the penis, is called the *urethra.* Emptying by ducts into the urethra near the base of the penis are a pair of small *Cowper's glands.* In response to sexual stimulation the Cowper's glands produce a few drops of a clear lubricating fluid which prepares the urethra for ejaculation and is of some slight importance in lubricating intercourse.

EXTERNAL GENITALIA

The male organ of intercourse is the *penis,* adapted to deposit semen within the vagina of the female. In order for intercourse to occur, it is necessary for the penis to become hard and erect. *Erection* is made possible because the penis is made of a special spongy erectile tissue, highly supplied with blood vessels. In response to sexual stimulation, the veins carrying blood away from the penis are constricted, causing the spongy tissue to become engorged with blood. Thus it is the blood pressure of the male which is responsible for erection. The inability to attain erection is called *impotence* or *impotency;* it may be the result of either physical or psychological causes. Impotency, the inability to carry out sexual intercourse, must not be confused with *sterility,* a lack of sperm cells in the semen. A man can be totally sterile, yet fully potent.

SEXUAL INTERCOURSE

The climax of sexual intercourse in the male consists of *ejaculation,* accompanied by *orgasm*. Ejaculation is the expulsion of semen, brought about by muscular contractions of the ampullae, seminal vesicles, and urethra. Orgasm is the intensely pleasant sensation which accompanies ejaculation. The average male tends to come to orgasm more rapidly than the female, a problem which must be overcome by experience if the partners are to attain a mutually satisfactory relationship. Immediately after ejaculation, the male loses all sexual desires and the penis soon loses its erection. If the female has not yet reached orgasm, she may be frustrated and disappointed in her efforts.

NOCTURNAL EMISSIONS

A normal, virile male with limited sex experience may find periodic involuntary sexual release in nocturnal emissions, or "wet dreams." These are releases of seminal fluid and are usually accompanied by dreams relating to sex. They result from the natural accumulation of the fluid in the seminal vesicles. A normal occurrence, they are typically marked with pleasurable sensations.

THE FEMALE REPRODUCTIVE SYSTEM (FIGS. 9.5 AND 9.6)

OVARY

The primary reproductive organs or gonads of the female consist of a pair of *ovaries*. Unlike the testes, the ovaries do function at the internal abdominal temperature and are carried in the abdomen. But like the testes, the ovaries serve a dual function, producing both eggs and hormones. Both of these functions will be discussed in the section of this chapter covering the menstrual cycle.

FALLOPIAN TUBE

The duct which carries the egg from each ovary to the uterus is called the *fallopian tube* or *oviduct*. As may be seen in Fig. 9.6, the fallopian tube does not make a closed connection with the ovary, but is flared open near the ovary with numerous fingerlike projections called *fimbria*. The inner lining of the fallopian tube is covered with countless microscopic hairlike projections called *cilia*. When an egg bursts forth from the ovary (*ovulation*) it is caught by the fimbria and slowly carried down the oviduct by the cilia. One of the more common causes of sterility in the female is obstruction of the fallopian tube.

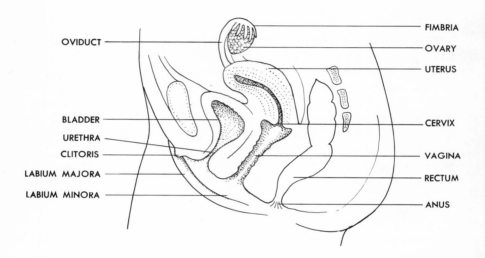

Fig. 9.5 Female reproductive system (side view).

UTERUS

The *uterus,* sometimes called the *womb,* is specialized for the growth and protection of the unborn child. The nonpregnant uterus is about the size and shape of a pear, with thick muscular walls. Its necklike portion, which extends down into the vagina, is called the *cervix,* which means *neck.* The inner lining of the uterus, heavily supplied with blood vessels, is the *endometrium;* it is shed with each menstrual period.

VAGINA

The *vagina* is the female organ of sexual intercourse and also the *birth canal.* It is a very flexible muscular tube, about 4 to 6 inches long, lined with mucous membrane. The vagina is provided with numerous small mucus-producing glands along with a pair of larger *Bartholin's glands,* all of which upon sexual arousal provide lubricating materials for intercourse. A few women produce insufficient lubricating material, requiring the use of additional lubricant for intercourse.

EXTERNAL GENITALIA

The opening of the vagina is surrounded by two pairs of *labia* (lips), also called *vulva,* the outer and larger *labia majora* and inner *labia*

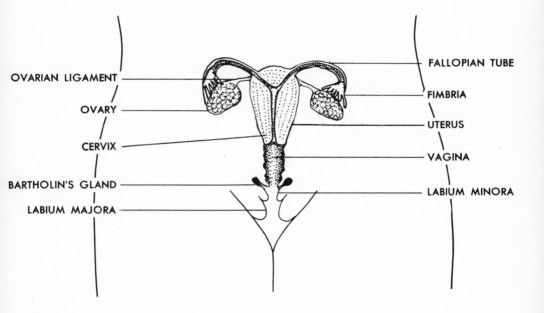

Fig. 9.6 Female reproductive system (front view).

minora. The external opening of the urethra lies forward of the vaginal opening, between the right and left labia minora, about halfway between the vaginal opening and the clitoris. Above the urethral opening, at the junction of the right and left labia majora, lies a small erectile structure, the *clitoris,* about the size of a pea. The clitoris, somewhat analogous to the male penis, is highly supplied with sensory nerve endings and erectile tissue and is the most intense center of sexual sensation in the female.

A partial membrane, the *hymen* ("maidenhead"), may be present across the opening of the vagina. The hymen varies greatly in size and thickness. In very rare cases the hymen completely covers the vagina and must be surgically broken to allow menstruation. In typical cases the hymen partially covers the vaginal opening and may or may not interfere with intercourse, depending upon its thickness. During a premarital examination, the physician can determine whether the hymen will present a barrier to intercourse and, if so, what preventive measures need to be taken. The presence or absence of the hymen should not be regarded as proof or lack of virginity, since the hymen sometimes survives intercourse or may be lost through physical examinations or treatment.

SEXUAL INTERCOURSE

The enlightened female expects to receive and does receive pleasure through intercourse at least equal to that of the male. For her to receive maximum pleasure, skill and consideration is required on the part of her husband. He must understand that the female is often more slowly aroused than the male, requires time prior to penetration to prevent pain, and often a longer duration of intercourse to achieve orgasm. Erotic response in the female can originate in almost any part of the body, especially the breasts; it is the husband's duty to find and stimulate responsive areas of the wife. The length of the penis does not influence the degree of pleasure in the female, since the nerve endings which respond during intercourse are most concentrated in the clitoris, abundant in the labia and lower vagina, but absent higher in the vagina.

Orgasm in the female involves no release of fluids, but consists of rhythmic contractions of the muscles of the vagina and highly pleasant diffuse sensations. Unlike the male, some females can achieve orgasm several times in rapid succession.

THE MENSTRUAL CYCLE

HORMONES OF REPRODUCTION

The human female reproductive system functions in a cyclic manner found only in man and some of the higher apes. The sexual cycle of the human female is referred to as the *menstrual cycle*. The menstrual cycle is under the control of the *anterior pituitary gland,* located at the base of the brain. The pituitary or "master" gland secretes hormones that stimulate the activity of other hormone-producing (endocrine) glands. The major hormones of the anterior pituitary and their effects are shown in Table 9.1.

Our knowledge of the last three pituitary hormones leads to our understanding of the menstrual cycle. In addition to the pituitary hormones, two types of hormones from the ovaries are important in the menstrual cycle. These ovarian hormones, referred to as *female sex hormones,* consist of the *estrogens* (actually six different hormones) and *progesterone*. The characteristics of the female sex hormones are summarized in Table 9.2.

TABLE 9.1 ANTERIOR PITUITARY HORMONES

Hormone	Effect
Somatotropic hormone (STH)	Stimulates growth of bones and muscles
Thyrotropic hormone (TSH)	Stimulates the thyroid gland to produce thyroxin
Adrenocorticotropic hormone (ACTH)	Stimulates adrenal cortex to produce its hormones
Follicle-stimulating hormone (FSH)[a]	*Ovary:* Stimulates growth of egg follicle and production of *estrogens*
	Testis: Promotes sperm production
Luteinizing hormone (LH), also called interstitial cell-stimulating hormone (ICSH) in male[a]	*Ovary:* Causes ovulation; causes a ruptured follicle to become *corpus luteum* and produce the hormone *progesterone*
	Testis: Stimulates production of the hormone *testosterone*
Luteotropic hormone (LTH), also called *prolactin*[a]	*Ovary:* Causes corpus luteum to secrete large amounts of both estrogens and progesterone during latter half of menstrual cycle
	Testis: Function unknown
	Breast: Promotes secretion of milk

[a] Called gonadotropic hormones, since they stimulate the ovaries or testes.

CONTROL OF THE MENSTRUAL CYCLE

With the widespread use of hormone products for the control of fertility and treatment of low fertility has come the necessity for the well-informed person to understand hormonal control of the menstrual cycle. The onset of sexual maturity (puberty) in the female is the result of the maturity of the ovaries and the increased production of gonadotropic hormones by the pituitary gland. The first menstrual period, called the *menarche,* usually occurs between ages 11 and 15 in the United States, the average age being about 13. Menarche occurs earlier in the United States than in most other countries, perhaps as a result of our moderate climate and good diet.

TABLE 9.2 **CHARACTERISTICS OF THE FEMALE SEX HORMONES**

Hormone	Source	Function
Estrogens	Ovary (egg follicle); placenta during pregnancy	Growth of the female sexual organs and promotion of secondary sexual characteristics of the female, such as breasts, hair distribution, voice, bone structure. Growth of the endometrium; inhibits production of FSH, increases production of LH.
Progesterone	Ovary (corpus luteum, the ruptured egg follicle); placenta during pregnancy	Primary function is to maintain endometrium of uterus for fertilized egg. Causes swelling of breasts, but not milk production. Causes salt and water retention in body. Inhibits production of LH.

Menstrual cycles take place, except during pregnancies, from puberty until their cessation at about the age of 45. The cause of this cessation, called *menopause* or *climacteric*, is not fully understood but seems to be due to a "burning out" of the ovaries rather than a change in the pituitary. At the time of sexual maturity, each ovary of the average woman contains about 30,000 to 40,000 immature *egg follicles*. During her reproductive years she will mature one egg follicle per menstrual cycle for a total lifetime production of about 400 mature eggs (*ova*). The remainder of the immature follicles gradually degenerate, until by the time a woman is 45 or 50, none remain to respond at a very high level to the gonadotropic hormones, since the production of estrogens by the ovaries drops to almost nothing. This loss of estrogens causes the characteristic complications of menopause, such as "hot flashes," irritability, anxiety, and fatigue. Such symptoms are often treated today through hormone therapy and also psychotherapy, since they are often partially psychosomatic in origin.

The events of the menstrual cycle are presented graphically in Figs. 9.7 and 9.8. The average menstrual cycle is 28 days in length, although there is great variation between different women and sometimes between different cycles in the same woman. Many physical and emotional factors can result in prolonged or irregular menstrual cycles. It is customary to refer to the first day of the menstrual period (menstruation) as day 1 of the menstrual cycle. *Menstruation* is the sloughing off or shedding of the endometrium. The usual duration of the menstrual period is 3 to 6 days, the average being 4 or 5 days.

During and following menstruation, the production of FSH by the pituitary reaches its highest level. Under the influence of FSH, one of the immature egg follicles (in either ovary) grows much larger, from a

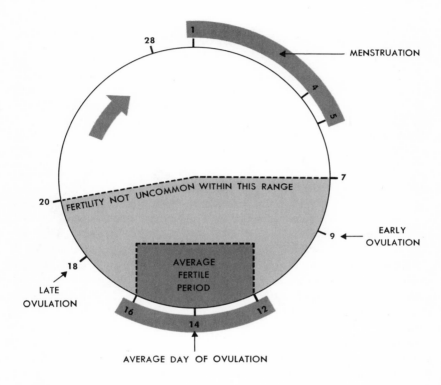

Fig. 9.7 Events of the typical menstrual cycle.

mere pinpoint to nearly one third inch in diameter. Inside, the fluid-filled follicle contains a maturing egg. The maturing follicle secretes much *estrogen,* which causes the endometrium of the uterus to thicken in preparation for the egg. The estrogen also feeds back to the pituitary gland, where it inhibits further secretion of FSH, but stimulates production of LH. When the LH level in the blood reaches a certain critical level, the mature follicle bursts (*ovulation*), expelling the egg into the abdominal cavity, where it is picked up by the fimbria of the fallopian tube. Ovulation occurs an average of 14 days after the beginning of menstruation, although it may commonly take place from the ninth to the eighteenth day; it is known in rare cases to take place outside these limits, even during menstruation. Following ovulation, the egg travels slowly down the fallopian tube, being carried by the cilia lining the tube. At this point the woman is fertile—capable of becoming pregnant. Although some reports differ, it is usually agreed that the egg remains viable (capable of being fertilized) for about 2 days.

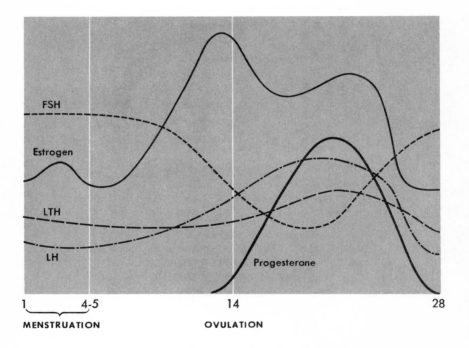

Fig. 9.8 Hormone levels during typical menstrual cycle.

The total trip down the fallopian tube takes about 6 days, so if the egg is to be fertilized, the sperm must meet it in the upper portion of the fallopian tube.

If the egg is not fertilized, it continues down the fallopian tube to the uterus, where it disintegrates. The human egg is about the size of the period after this sentence and forms no significant part of the menstrual flow. Following ovulation, the empty follicle, under the influence of LH, recloses to become the *corpus luteum.* Then under the direction of LH and LTH the corpus luteum produces the hormone *progesterone,* which serves to mature the endometrium and to prevent its sloughing off (menstruation). A reciprocal relationship exists between the levels of progesterone and LH and LTH similar to that between estrogen and FSH. As the level of progesterone in the blood increases, the production of LH and LTH is suppressed. As the level of LH and LTH in the blood drops, the corpus luteum degenerates, ceasing to produce progesterone; then menstruation occurs.

If the egg is fertilized, it continues down the fallopian tube, dividing and redividing into 2 cells, then 4, 8, 16, and so on, until by the time it reaches the uterus it consists of a hollow ball of cells resembling a tiny mulberry. Within 10 days after fertilization, the egg (now the *embryo*) *implants* itself into the endometrium of the uterus by digesting away the upper layers. Soon after implantation the embryo begins to produce a *gonadotropic hormone,* which functions much like the combination of LH and LTH in stimulating the corpus luteum to produce estrogen and progesterone. Rather than degenerating, the corpus luteum continues to grow and function for about the first 12 weeks of pregnancy. Its continued production of estrogen and progesterone causes the endometrium to continue growing, rather than degenerating as in menstruation. The sustained high level of estrogen and progesterone also prevents further egg follicle maturation and ovulation.

PREGNANCY

EMBRYOLOGY

A full-term human pregnancy usually lasts about 266 days after conception, or until about 280 days after the beginning of the last menstrual period. During the first 8 weeks of pregnancy, the developing child is called the *embryo;* beyond 8 weeks it is called the *fetus.* The study of the unborn child is the fascinating science of *embryology.* Today, very little mystery remains regarding this aspect of human life.

As previously mentioned, the fertilized egg *(zygote)* very quickly begins cell division by the process of *mitosis* (see Fig. 9.14) and becomes a multicelled *embryo* by the time it reaches the uterus. Unlike a bird egg, the human egg carries very little stored food. During the first 8 weeks of pregnancy, the embryo obtains most of its nutrition through digesting the surrounding endometrium by means of special *trophoblastic cells,* the same cells which have enabled the embryo to implant itself.

During the early weeks of pregnancy, the embryo surrounds itself with several membranes (Fig. 9.9), the most important being the *amnion,* the "bag of waters" which cushions the fetus, and the *chorion,* which interlocks with the endometrium to form the placenta. The *placenta* is the organ through which the fetus is nourished from 8 weeks of age until the termination of pregnancy. The fetus is attached to the placenta by the *umbilical cord,* which contains veins and arteries carrying blood to and from the placenta. It should be emphasized that no exchange

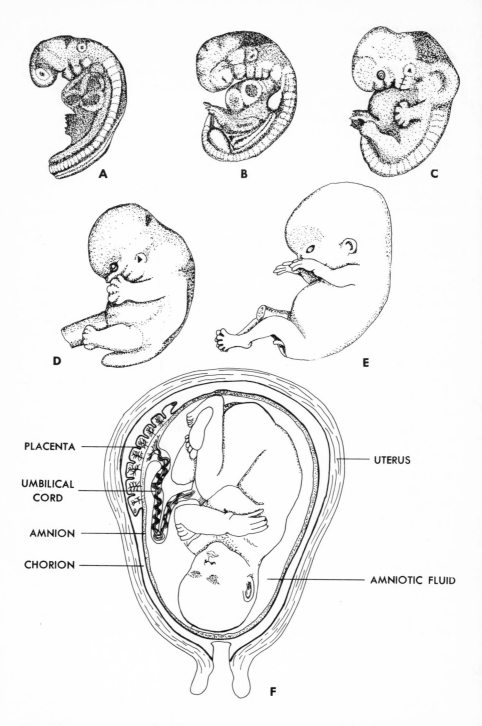

Fig. 9.9 Development of the human embryo. Approximate ages: (A) 25 days.
(B) 30 days. (C) 35 days. (D) 40 days. (E) 50 days.
(F) Full term.

or mixing of blood between the mother and child takes place in the placenta. All exchange of food and waste products between the mother and child takes place by means of diffusion through the membranes of the placenta.

During the latter part of pregnancy, the placenta serves as an extremely important source of the hormones *estrogen* and *progesterone*. By the end of pregnancy, the estrogen production reaches 50 to 60 times that of a nonpregnant woman, while the progesterone production increases tenfold. The higher levels of these hormones cause many changes in the body of the woman which better adapt her for pregnancy and childbirth. For example, the uterus and external genitalia enlarge, breasts enlarge, and pelvic ligaments relax. When pregnancy is full term, the placenta is a flat disc, about an inch thick and 6 to 9 inches in diameter. Following delivery of the child, the placenta is expelled as the *afterbirth*.

The pregnant woman has a great and understandable curiosity about the size and appearance of her child at the various stages of its development. Let us then briefly describe the embryo or fetus after each month of its development. Pregnancies are customarily measured in *lunar months,* four-week periods which correspond to menstrual cycles. It is also common to speak of the *three trimesters* of pregnancy, each consisting of 12 weeks. The month-by-month development proceeds as follows:

END OF FIRST LUNAR MONTH (4 WEEKS) (FIG. 9.9)

Embryo about 1/4 inch long, including tail (all young vertebrate embryos have tails); head very large in proportion to body, mouth and jaw present, but no eyes, ears, or nose; backbone formed, curved until head almost touches tail; small buds of arms and legs; heart formed and beating.

END OF SECOND LUNAR MONTH (8 WEEKS)

Embryo now unmistakably human, from this point on called a fetus. About 1 inch long; head large, face human, eyes, ears, nose visible; arms and legs more developed, webbed hands and feet present; tail starting to be absorbed.

END OF THIRD LUNAR MONTH (12 WEEKS)

Fetus now over 3 inches long, weight 1 ounce. Sex distinguishable; finger- and toenails appear; movements occur, but are too weak to be felt by mother.

END OF FOURTH LUNAR MONTH (16 WEEKS)

Length now 6½ inches, weight 4 ounces. Fine hair appears on body. Some women feel movements.

END OF FIFTH LUNAR MONTH (20 WEEKS)

Length 10 inches, weight 8 ounces. Mother definitely feels movement.

END OF SIXTH LUNAR MONTH (24 WEEKS)

Length 12 inches, weight 1½ pounds. Skin wrinkled and red; head large in proportion to body, eyebrows and lashes formed. If born, almost no chance for survival.

END OF SEVENTH LUNAR MONTH (28 WEEKS)

Length about 15 inches, weight about 2½ pounds. If born, chance of survival about 1 in 10.

END OF EIGHTH LUNAR MONTH (32 WEEKS)

Length about 16 inches, weight about 4 pounds. If born, good chance of survival.

END OF NINTH LUNAR MONTH (36 WEEKS)

Length about 18 inches, weight about 6 pounds. Now a fully mature infant, survival rate almost same as full term.

MIDDLE OF TENTH LUNAR MONTH (38 WEEKS)

Full-term infant. Average length about 20 inches, average weight 7 pounds if girl, 7½ if boy.

EARLY SIGNS OF PREGNANCY

CESSATION OF MENSTRUATION

In a healthy woman with a history of regular menstrual cycles, the cessation of menstruation is often the first sign of pregnancy. Even in a very regular woman, however, a delay of a few days in menstruation should not be automatically accepted as proof of pregnancy. Pregnancy should seldom be seriously considered before a delay of at least 10 days has occurred. Absence of menstruation may result from many conditions other than pregnancy. Emotional upset very commonly delays menstruation, especially when there is fear of pregnancy. Other influencing factors are change of climate, extreme cold, anemia, and hormone imbalance. By the time the second period has been missed, the chance of pregnancy is strong.

CHANGES IN THE BREASTS

The swelling of the breasts, normally occurring prior to each menstrual period, is exaggerated in early pregnancy. The breasts become larger and fuller and may have a heavy feeling as well as a throbbing or tingling sensation.

FREQUENT URINATION

Early in pregnancy, the enlarged uterus presses against the urinary bladder, giving the impression that the bladder is always full. As the pregnancy progresses, the uterus rises away from the bladder and this symptom disappears, to return during the last two months of the pregnancy when the head of the fetus presses against the bladder.

NAUSEA

About two thirds of all pregnant women experience some nausea or vomiting beginning about the time of the first missed period and lasting for 4 to 6 weeks. This is often called "morning sickness," but it may occur at any time of the day.

PREGNANCY TESTS

The married woman usually waits until about the time of the second missed menstrual period before visiting her physician. By that time he can usually diagnose pregnancy through visible changes in the skin, breasts, vagina, and uterus. If it is important to confirm pregnancy before this time, numerous pregnancy tests can diagnose pregnancy with a high degree of accuracy when the menstrual period has been delayed about 2 weeks. Most of the commonly used pregnancy tests depend upon the presence of the hormone *chorionic gonadotropin* in the urine or blood of the pregnant woman. The urine or blood is injected into a test animal (mouse, rabbit, frog, or toad); if the hormone is present, characteristic changes occur, depending on the type of animal.

In another type of test, oral tablets containing estrogen and progesterone are administered for 3 days, then discontinued. If menstruation does not occur within 15 days, there is a very strong possibility that pregnancy exists.

PRENATAL CARE

It is impossible to overemphasize the importance of proper care of the pregnant woman. She must be under the care of a qualified physician, and she must take excellent care of herself. The quality of prenatal care can influence not only the health and comfort of the woman, but also the future welfare of the child. The physician can detect many possible complications of pregnancy in their very early stages and can often prevent such complications from becoming a serious threat to the health of the mother or the child.

Between her routine visits to the physician, there are certain possible danger signs in pregnancy for which the woman should be alert. If *any* of the following symptoms appear, she should make an immediate report to her physician:

1. Vaginal bleeding, no matter how slight
2. Regular pains or contractions in abdomen
3. Sudden escape of water from vagina
4. Chills and fever
5. Extreme shortness of breath
6. Symptoms of toxemia:
    A. Severe continuous headache
    B. Dizzy spells
    C. Dimness or blurring of vision
    D. Persistent vomiting (in later part of pregnancy)
    E. Swelling of face, hands, ankles, fingers, feet
    F. Rapid gain in weight
    G. Reduced urine output

One of the most common complications of pregnancy is the condition known as *toxemia*. This is a condition which occurs only during pregnancy, seldom appearing before the last 3 months of pregnancy. About 7 percent of all pregnancies are complicated by toxemia. Although the word "toxemia" by derivation means "poison in the blood," no such poison has ever been isolated, and it is generally agreed today that none is involved. Toxemia is believed to be caused by an excessive retention of sodium by the kidneys, which leads in turn to an excessive retention of water throughout the body. This sodium retention is believed to be a result of the high hormone levels of late pregnancy. The pregnant woman is usually cautioned to limit her consumption of salt and salty foods. If the symptoms of toxemia appear (confirmed by *high blood pressure* and the presence of albumen in the urine), she is placed on a strictly sodium-free diet. This measure, along with plenty of rest, usually solves the problem of toxemia. If allowed to continue, toxemia leads to *eclampsia,* in which the woman goes into convulsions, coma, and may die. Fortunately, this condition never occurs when a woman is getting adequate prenatal care, since the physician detects toxemia in time to prevent eclampsia.

DIET IN PREGNANCY

In order to safeguard her own health as well as that of her child, the pregnant woman needs to pay careful attention to her diet. The one thing she must *not* do is to "eat for two." As indicated in Appendix B, the Recommended Daily Dietary Allowances, the pregnant woman needs significantly increased quantities of protein, vitamins, and minerals, but *only slightly increased* food energy (calories). She must greatly curtail her consumption of sweet, starchy, or fatty foods, concentrating on those foods which yield large amounts of proteins, vitamins, and minerals in proportion to their calorie value. She must be particularly careful to meet her daily 78-gram protein requirement. This protein requirement can be met through daily consumption of a quart of skim milk, one egg, and two average servings of lean meat. A quart of nonfat milk yields almost half the daily protein requirement, along with important calcium, yet is relatively low in calories.

Perhaps the biggest problem for the average pregnant woman is keeping her weight gain within her physician's allowance. The allowed gain has been dropping through the past few years, because physicians, as well as the general public, have become more weight conscious. The amount of weight the woman will be allowed to gain depends upon her weight at the beginning of the pregnancy. If her weight is ideal at that time, she may be allowed to gain 16 to 18 pounds. This weight gain is distributed as:

Baby	7 lb
Afterbirth	1 lb
Amniotic fluid	1½ lb
Increase in weight of uterus	2 lb
Increase in weight of circulating blood	1 lb
Increase in weight of breasts	1½ lb
Total	14 lb

The remainder of the weight gain is due to a deposit of fat, generally throughout the body, plus the extra fluid retained by the tissues. Therefore, a woman who gains 16 pounds should return to her original weight shortly after the delivery.

The underweight woman may be allowed several additional pounds weight gain; but the woman who enters into pregnancy while overweight may find herself placed on a strict reducing diet, and her total weight at the end of the pregnancy may be less than her original weight. The hazards of excess weight in pregnancy include difficult, prolonged labor and much greater chance of toxemia. Also, many women who gain excess weight in pregnancy never again lose that weight, growing heavier after each child. Yet many women after multiple pregnancies retain the figure of fashion models.

TERMINATIONS OF PREGNANCY

Since most pregnancies terminate in an uncomplicated, spontaneous delivery of a full-term infant, let us first consider such a delivery. Many women look forward to their first delivery with considerable apprehension or even with fear, yet, looking back at the same event, they can find nothing to justify such emotions. Perhaps it will be a young woman's first hospitalization, in which case she may fear the unknown world of the hospital. Some women worry about not getting to the hospital in time, although such cases are so rare that they receive much newspaper attention. Other women worry about the delivery itself; yet childbirth today has been refined to the point that it presents little hazard to either the mother or the child.

The word *labor* is used to describe the muscular contractions of the uterus through which the infant is expelled. Labor is divided into three rather distinct stages: (1) preparatory period, (2) birth of the baby, (3) delivery of the placenta (afterbirth).

FIRST STAGE

The preparatory stage lasts from the first labor pains until the baby is ready to be born, an average period of about 14 hours in first deliveries and about 8 hours for subsequent deliveries. Shorter or longer labors are not uncommon, nor are they abnormal. At first, the contractions are weak, infrequent (every 40 or 50 minutes), and irregular. Gradually they become more frequent, more regular, and stronger. When the contractions occur at 5- to 15-minute intervals and last for 30 seconds or longer, the physician will probably recommend that the woman go to the hospital, following a prearranged plan. Near the end of the first stage of labor, the cervix opens from a narrow slit into a wide passageway (Fig. 9.10).

SECOND STAGE

The second stage of labor begins with the dilation of the cervix and lasts until the baby is born, an average period of 1 to 2 hours in first deliveries and about ½ hour in subsequent births. If the "bag of waters" (amniotic membrane) has not broken late in the first stage of labor, it

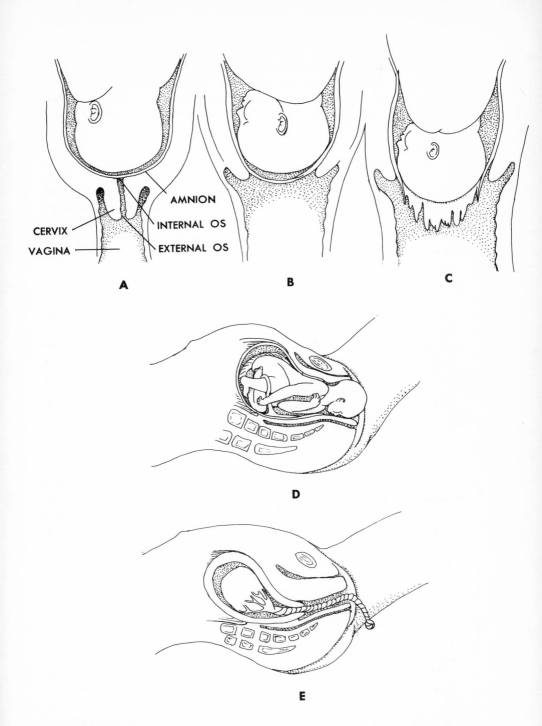

Fig. 9.10 Stages of normal delivery. (A) Cervix before dilation. (B) cervix fully dilated. (C) rupture of the amnion. (D) Birth of head. (E) delivery of placenta.

breaks early in the second. A small incision (*episiotomy*) is almost always made in the membrane extending back from the vagina toward the anus to prevent its tearing and to make delivery easier. Once the head of the infant appears, the remainder of the delivery is usually quite rapid.

THIRD STAGE

This final stage of labor consists of the expulsion of the afterbirth (placenta). It rarely lasts longer than 15 minutes and is accomplished with little or no pain. Following the birth of the child, the wall of the uterus greatly shrinks, causing the placenta to break loose. A few mild contractions of the uterus brings about its expulsion.

ANESTHESIA IN CHILDBIRTH

A wide variety of pain-relieving methods is available for childbirth. The actual choice of anesthetics will depend upon the nature of the woman, the ease of her labor, and the preferences of the physician. Many women are interested in so-called "natural childbirth," about which they have read so much in popular publications. There are many popular misconceptions about "natural childbirth." In the first place, it is not painless childbirth—not even the use of drugs insures a complete absence of pain. Second, it is not drugless childbirth—small amounts of anesthetics are used in almost every case.

Natural childbirth is based upon the fact that much (but not all) of the pain in childbirth is the result of fear and tension and that the fear and tension are the result of lack of understanding of the birth process. Thus, natural childbirth is in essence a matter of pre-education of the pregnant woman regarding all aspects of childbirth. Also usually involved are special exercises to strengthen the muscles that aid in delivery and practice in the relaxation which is so vital to an easy delivery.

INDUCED LABOR

Under special circumstances, labor is sometimes brought about or strengthened through the use of oral or injected drugs. Such a procedure might be followed in severe cases of toxemia, diabetes, Rh incompatibility (discussed later), or prolonged weak contractions. It must be emphasized that the drugs available for this purpose are effective only when the pregnancy is near full term; they are absolutely ineffective, and often dangerous, when used in an effort to produce abortion of an early pregnancy.

HYPNOSIS IN LABOR

Modern hypnosis, as practiced by qualified physicians, is today recognized by the American Medical Association, as well as the British Medical Association, as a safe and useful procedure in childbirth. Its use is not widespread, however, as much of the pain in childbirth is overcome by modern anesthetic methods, which are in general more reliable in their effectiveness than is hypnosis.

FORCEPS DELIVERY

Forceps delivery, often called *instrument delivery,* is frequently used in the late stages of a difficult or prolonged labor or in presentations other than the usual head-first one. The forceps is a large tonglike instrument with broad, flat grasping surfaces.

CAESAREAN DELIVERY

A caesarean section is a major surgical procedure in which the infant is delivered through an incision through the lower abdomen and uterine wall. This type of delivery is advisable only when some condition is present which prevents normal vaginal delivery, such as small bone structure, position of the child, or a heart condition in the woman. As a general rule (there are exceptions), one caesarean section limits a woman to this route for the delivery of all future children, owing to the scar left on the uterus. Although many women have had more than three caesarean deliveries, the physician usually advises that the fallopian tubes be tied off (*salpingectomy*) at the time of the third such delivery.

EXTRAUTERINE PREGNANCY

An extrauterine, or *ectopic,* pregnancy is one which develops outside the uterus. About 1 in 300 pregnancies is of this nature. The most common site of ectopic pregnancy is the fallopian tube, although some actually develop within the abdominal cavity. Tubal pregnancies tend to recur in the same woman, usually because of some condition which interferes with the travel of the fertilized egg down the tube. The usual early symptoms of pregnancy may or may not be present. Since the fallopian tube cannot stretch enough to accommodate the fetus, the pregnancy must be surgically aborted or the tube will rupture with severe internal hemorrhage.

PREMATURE DELIVERY

Premature delivery is the live birth of an infant before it is fully mature; its chance of survival is proportionate to its weight. After 28 weeks of pregnancy, at about 2½ pounds, the chance of survival is about 1 in 10. Any infant which weighs 5½ pounds or more is considered to be full term, and its chances of survival are almost the same as those for the 7-pound infant. The cause of the onset of labor, whether full term or premature, is not definitely known. Most labors that begin prematurely continue until the delivery of the baby, there being no sure method of stopping them.

SPONTANEOUS ABORTION

Although the word *abortion* is often associated only with criminal abortions, any termination of a pregnancy before there is any chance of survival of the infant (about 20 to 28 weeks) is properly referred to as abortion. The *spontaneous abortion* is more commonly called a *miscarriage*. It is believed that about 1 in every 10 pregnancies terminates in a spontaneous abortion. About 75 percent of these abortions occur during the second and third lunar months of pregnancy. Miscarriages are due to a variety of causes; most are entirely unavoidable, but some may be preventable. Most spontaneous abortions are due either to a defective sperm or egg, resulting in abnormalities of the developing fetus, or to a faulty intrauterine environment which may interfere with attachment of the placenta or nourishment of the fetus. Other causes may include physical shocks, such as falls or blows, acute infectious diseases which may be transmitted to the fetus, or a hormone imbalance which may lead to sloughing off of the endometrium. Hormone treatments can sometimes prevent the last problem.

THERAPEUTIC ABORTION

In addition to spontaneous abortions, there are intentionally *induced abortions*. These are designated as *therapeutic* or *criminal,* depending on the motive for the induction of the abortion. Although the laws relating to therapeutic abortion vary in the different states, they are fairly uniform in their intent to restrict abortion to those pregnancies in which the life of the woman is definitely threatened. Despite mounting pressure in many states for the liberalization of existing abortion laws to include pregnancies resulting from rape or incest or in which there is a great probability of defective offspring, there has been little inclination on the part of state legislators to make any change in current abortion laws. As a result, tremendous numbers of illegal abortions are performed, which is the subject of the following section of this chapter.

CRIMINAL ABORTION

It is estimated that 1 in every 5 pregnancies in the United States terminates in an illegal abortion, a total of about a million criminal abortions per year. Five to ten thousand women die each year as a direct result of inexpertly performed criminal abortions. In contrast to the public image of the abortionist's patron as a young unmarried girl, the majority of all abortions are performed on married women. The reasons why the unmarried girl seeks abortion are obvious; the married woman's reasons are much more varied. Married women obtaining illegal abortions are mostly in two age groups—16 to 25 and 40 to 50. The young married girl often finds herself urged to seek abortion by an immature, selfish husband who is unwilling to meet the responsibilities of fatherhood. The older woman, her children now young adults, cannot face the prospect of starting over again at her age with small children. Other factors which move the married woman to abortion include the potential psychological and economic effect of an additional child upon a family which already has too many children.

THE ABORTIONIST

The academic training and degree of skill of abortionists vary greatly. At the top of the scale is the occasional physician who performs illegal abortions, either for humanitarian reasons or for profit. Ethical physicians admit to occasionally performing technically illegal but morally justifiable abortions, such as when the chance of a defective offspring is unusually great or the mental health of the woman is gravely threatened by the pregnancy. The physician who routinely performs abortions for less valid reasons may be one who is unable to make a living through ethical practice.

Other abortionists, such as nurses, chiropractors, dentists, and midwives, have some degree of medical training but usually lack the ability to perform an abortion properly. In addition, the conditions under which such abortionists work are almost never adequate and many serious infections result, often leading to the death of the patient.

Still worse are the totally untrained abortionists. They include salesmen, housewives, prostitutes, barbers, and even unskilled laborers. A very great proportion of such abortionists possess less than a high school education. In these cases not only are the conditions horribly unsanitary, but also the abortionists usually have absolutely no knowledge of the female reproductive system or the standard methods of inducing abortion. Their methods very often result in fatal infections or permanent damage to the reproductive organs without even successfully aborting the pregnancy.

Some of the most dangerous of all abortion efforts are attempts at self-abortion. Desperate women will try methods which sicken even the most hardened observer. They try drugs of all kinds, douches of acid or caustic materials, wires, knitting needles, compressed air, screwdrivers, and countless other methods.[1] Self-induced abortions lead to the deaths of more women than any of the other types of abortions mentioned above. Numerous drugs have gained false reputations for producing abortion. Their reputations are perpetuated by the 10 percent of all pregnancies which terminate in spontaneous abortion and by the late menstrual period being mistaken for an induced abortion. *There is no drug known which will produce an abortion without grave danger to the life of the woman.*

In light of the very serious hazards associated with criminal abortion, it is obvious that any woman who submits to such a procedure does so at great risk to her own health and even her life. With the highly effective contraceptive methods available today, it is unfortunate that so many unwanted children are conceived. Yet when conception of an unwanted child does occur, it is far better for the woman to go through with the pregnancy than to risk her life with a criminal abortion.

FERTILITY PROBLEMS

LOW FERTILITY

Almost every married couple has some type of fertility problem. For about 90 percent of all couples, the problem is to control the excess fertility possessed by almost every species. Since almost every human born now lives to the age of sexual maturity and reproduction, it is no longer necessary to produce large numbers of offspring to insure the survival and reproduction of a few. On the other hand, for about 10 percent of married couples the frustrating problem of low fertility exists—difficulty in producing the desired number of children.

Sterility is an absolute term indicating total inability to produce a child. *Fertility* is a relative term indicating the ease with which children are produced. The man who produces sperm in low numbers or the woman who ovulates very infrequently exhibits a relatively *low fertility*, but is not sterile. The probable outcome of efforts to conceive a child at various levels of fertility is summarized below:

[1] J. E. Bates and E. S. Zawadski, *Criminal Abortion,* Springfield, Ill., Charles C Thomas, 1964, pp. 89–91.

Man and wife highly fertile	Prompt conception
Man and wife normally fertile	Conception within a few menstrual cycles
Fertility high in one, low in the other	Delay of several months likely
Fertility low in both man and wife	Conception after long delay or not at all
Either one or both sterile	Conception impossible

Among couples possessing low fertility, the cause is found in about one third to one half of the cases to lie in the male and in about one half to two thirds of the cases in the female. With a few couples, the cause lies in a specific incompatibility or interaction between the individuals involved, with the possibility of each's being normally fertile with another partner. For example, the wife may produce specific antibodies which destroy the sperm of the husband. In the more common case where a structural problem makes conception difficult in a woman, she might be able to conceive with a highly fertile man but unable to conceive with a man having a lower sperm production.

The most common cause of low fertility among males is a low sperm count in the semen. The average volume of semen in an ejaculation is about 3 or 4 cubic centimeters and the average sperm count is about 120 million in each cubic centimeter of semen. This means an average total of perhaps 400 million sperm per ejaculation. If the sperm count falls below about 40 or 50 million sperm per cubic centimeter, the male becomes less fertile than normal, his fertility decreasing progressively with any further diminishment in sperm count. A low sperm count is usually associated with a low level in the semen of the enzyme hyaluronidase, which is necessary for penetration of the egg. The sperm count can sometimes be raised and fertility improved through avoiding intercourse for about 2 weeks before ovulation is expected in the wife and then attempting to time intercourse to coincide with ovulation.

Low fertility in the female results from more diverse causes than in the male, being complicated by the relatively brief periods of fertility in the female. Sometimes the level of production of the pituitary gonadotropic hormones FSH and LH is so low that ovulation never occurs. Such cases may be treated through injection of gonadotropic hormones. Sometimes obstruction of the fallopian tubes prevents the egg from reaching the uterus or the sperm from reaching the egg. Occasionally the cervix of the uterus is so heavily plugged with mucus that the sperm cannot enter. In many cases the reason for the infertility of the female cannot be determined.

ARTIFICIAL INSEMINATION

Artificial insemination, the injection of semen by syringe into the vagina or cervix, is sometimes resorted to when infertility results from a low sperm count in the husband. Occasionally the semen of the husband is collected over a period of time and preserved through refrigeration until an adequate amount is obtained for fertilization.

In other cases, semen from a donor is used in artificial insemination. The identity of the donor should not be known to the couple. An effort is usually made to select a donor whose physical characteristics resemble the husband's. In addition to possible legal, moral, and religious objections to artificial insemination from a donor, there is a very great likelihood of psychological complications. The child may be distressed if told of his parenthood; the parents may feel anxiety in either case. The greatest psychological risk is probably taken by the husband. Unless he is blessed with an unusual degree of maturity and self-confidence, he may see the child as a constant reminder of his inadequacy or may become jealous of the biological father of the child. He may reject the child, feeling that it is more his wife's than his own. For most couples, adoption is probably wiser than donor artificial insemination.

CONTRACEPTION

All normally fertile married couples must use some method of contraception or birth control if they are to space their children as they desire and limit the total number of children produced. Indeed, a very high percentage of married couples, regardless of religion, *do* make use of contraceptive methods. With the availability of today's highly effective contraceptive methods, there is no medical justification for the conception of an unwanted child, with the resulting hardship and unhappiness for both the parents and the child. The goal of those active in family planning is that *every* child conceived be a *wanted child*.

HORMONAL CONTRACEPTION

Female oral contraceptive pills, now in use by many millions of women, are designed to prevent ovulation from occurring. Their function is based upon the hormonal control of the menstrual cycle. As discussed earlier in the chapter, the hormones FSH and LH from the pituitary gland are necessary for the maturity of an ovum (egg) and its consequent release from the ovary. To review further, the production of FSH is inhibited by the presence of estrogen and the production of LH is inhibited by the presence of progesterone. The earlier contraceptive pills contained synthetic forms of both estrogen and progesterone, creating a "false pregnancy" which prevented ovulation, but in many cases also caused such minor complications characteristic of early pregnancy as nausea, weight gain, and swelling and tenderness in the breasts. These side effects were minimized or eliminated with the production of pills of lower dosage and of sequential pills which provide estrogen and progesterone in the same sequence as in the natural menstrual cycle. These latter tablets give only estrogen for 15 days, then estrogen and progesterone for 5 or 6 days. Then there is a 7- or 8-day period of no pills during which menstruation takes place. Several other types of oral and injectable contraceptives for both men and women are also under development.

The oral contraceptives are generally 100 percent effective if the user follows the instructions exactly. An unplanned pregnancy can occur if only one pill is skipped, and other contraceptive methods should be used for the remainder of any cycle in which this happens. In addition to effectiveness, a major advantage of oral contraception is its detachment from the act of sexual intercourse, allowing a more spontaneous, uninhibited, and unencumbered sexual relationship. Another advantage is greater regularity in the menstrual cycles.

MECHANICAL CONTRACEPTION

Several types of devices are designed to mechanically prevent the spermatozoa from reaching the ovum. Prior to the development of hormonal contraceptives, such devices were the most effective contraceptives available and were most often prescribed by physicians. Even today, the popularity and use of mechanical contraception remains high. The most widely used mechanical devices are the rubber *condom* worn by the male and the rubber *diaphragm* worn by the female. If used *properly and carefully,* these devices are adequately effective for most married couples. The condom should be of high quality and must be handled carefully to prevent its tearing. Since the diaphragm must fit accurately into the vagina around the cervix of the uterus, its size must be determined by the measurements of a physician. Spermicidal creams or jellies are usually used with the diaphragm to form a tight seal around its edge and to hasten the death of the sperm cells.

CHEMICAL CONTRACEPTION

A variety of *spermicidal* (fatal to sperm) foams, creams, and jellies are available for the prevention of conception. Such products are inserted into the vagina prior to each intercourse. Their average effectiveness when used alone is believed to be somewhat less than that of the mechanical devices or pills, but is adequate for the purposes of many married couples. The effectiveness of the best of these products is about equal to that of the mechanical devices.

INTRAUTERINE CONTRACEPTIVE DEVICES

It has long been known that any type of foreign body in the uterus will prevent the implantation of the fertilized egg. This prevention may be caused by contractions of the uterine wall. A variety of plastic and stainless steel devices have been developed for use as intrauterine contraceptives. These devices are commonly called IUD's, IUCD's, or "coils." Such devices are inserted by a physician into the uterus and allowed to remain in place until a pregnancy is desired. The device is then removed by a physician. There is no residual effect on fertility after removal of the devices. The intrauterine devices have several advantages over oral contraceptives. Once they are inserted into the uterus, no further thought or effort is required by the user, nor is there any further cost except for periodic pelvic examinations which are desirable regardless of contraceptive method used. Disadvantages include the spontaneous expulsion of the device from the uterus of about 10 percent of those women fitted. Another 10 percent of the devices require removal due to side effects such as pain, bleeding, or infection. Among women retaining the devices, the contraceptive effectiveness is high, falling just below that of the oral contraceptives.

THE "RHYTHM" METHOD

One of the less effective methods of fertility control is the *rhythm method*. Actually not a true contraceptive method at all, this is a matter of *periodic abstinence* from sexual intercourse during that portion of each menstrual cycle when the wife is believed to be fertile. Were it possible to accurately predict the fertile period several days in advance, this method would be highly effective. Many efforts have been made to develop ways to predict ovulation, but none is totally successful. It is known that those sperm which reach the uterus live for about 2 days. It is also known that the egg remains capable of fertilization for about 2 days after ovulation. If the day of ovulation could be predicted, avoidance of intercourse for 2 days prior to ovulation would allow the death of all sperm in the female system and avoidance of intercourse for 2 or 3 more days following ovulation would allow for the death of the egg. But since ovulation is unpredictable and sometimes occurs as early as the ninth day or as late as the eighteenth day of the menstrual cycle, the period of abstinence must extend from the seventh day to the twentieth day to insure any degree of safety. Even then, the chance of unwanted pregnancy remains.

Since the body temperature rises a few tenths of a degree after ovulation, careful charting of body temperature for a few months aids some women in predicting ovulation. But since many physical and emotional conditions can influence the time of ovulation, this method is not highly reliable except in unusually "regular" women.

In addition to its unreliability, the rhythm method casts an air of uncertainty over the sexual relationship of a couple and the period of abstinence places a great emotional burden upon young and strongly sexed couples.

DOUCHES

Among the least effective contraceptive methods is the douche immediately following sexual intercourse. This consists of flushing the semen from the vagina with water or a solution of a special douching product. In addition to its low effectiveness, douching requires that the wife spring out of bed and douche immediately after the husband ejaculates—hardly a pleasant ending for the marital relationship.

WITHDRAWAL (COITUS INTERRUPTUS)

One of the oldest fertility control methods is the withdrawal of the penis from the vagina just before ejaculation so that the semen is deposited outside the vagina. The disadvantages of this method are numerous. Its effectiveness is low (though better than the rhythm method or the douche) and it greatly interferes with the enjoyment of intercourse by both husband and wife.

SURGICAL STERILIZATION

Though not technically considered a contraceptive method, surgical sterilization is a very positive and essentially 100 percent effective method of fertility control. Increasing numbers of married couples are turning to surgical sterilization of either the man or wife after they have produced a desired number of children. Sterilization of the male is a simple office procedure in which the vas deferens are clipped and/or tied off through a small incision at the base of the scrotum. This operation has no effect on either his desire or his ability to have intercourse. Ejaculation occurs as before, but the semen contains no sperm. There are published reports of occasional psychological effects of male sterilization, presumably due to an imagined loss of manliness. Sterilization of the female is more major, involving an abdominal incision through which the fallopian tubes are tied or removed. As in the male, there is no change in the sex life. It is to be stressed that sterilization of either the male or female is probably permanent. Those few specialists who do attempt to restore fertility after surgical sterilization report a maximum 50 percent rate of success.

CHOICE OF METHOD

The birth control method chosen should meet the approval of both partners as well as their physician. All pertinent medical, emotional, and religious factors must be taken into consideration. A maximum degree of protection is important early in marriage to delay the first pregnancy until the couple is sufficiently settled and financially ready for parenthood. Maximum protection again becomes important later in marriage after the desired number of children have been produced. During the intervening years of family growth, a couple may be satisfied with a less reliable method of contraception for the purpose of spacing their children.

Among couples using no contraceptive method, 80 to 90 percent of the wives will become pregnant within one year (the remaining couples are those of low fertility). Among those using the rhythm method, about 40 percent will become pregnant. Among those using chemical methods, perhaps 15 to 30 percent will become pregnant (variation between products). Among those using condoms or diaphragms, about 15 percent will become pregnant. From 2 to 4 percent of women using intrauterine devices will become pregnant. Virtually none of those properly using oral contraceptives will become pregnant, nor will any of those in which one member of the couple has been effectively sterilized. It must be emphasized that the effectiveness of any contraceptive method depends upon its being used (1) *properly*, (2) *carefully*, and (3) *consistently*.

FOR FURTHER INFORMATION

The best sources of family planning information include the private physician and organizations such as The Population Council, the National Committee on Maternal Health, and the Planned Parenthood Foundation of America, which have branches in most major cities. The public health departments of many states, counties, and cities offer aid in family planning. Other good sources of information include Guttmacher's *Planning Your Family*, the *Consumers Union Report on Family Planning*, and current articles in reliable periodicals.

HEREDITY

THE CELL

In order to understand the mechanisms of heredity, we need to consider briefly the basic structure of human cells and how cells divide. All human tissues are composed of cells, most of which are microscopic in size. By the time of birth, the single cell which was the fertilized egg has divided and redivided into *billions* of cells. Although these cells are differentiated (specialized) to serve specific functions, the genetic (hereditary) material contained in each is *identical*.

Figure 9.11 represents a typical unspecialized human cell, such as might be found in the early embryo. Every cell is surrounded by a *cell membrane*; everything inside the cell membrane is *protoplasm*. Within every cell is one *nucleus,* which contains the *chromosomes* and the *nucleolus.* All the cellular material outside the nucleus is called *cytoplasm.* Located in the cytoplasm are numerous tiny *ribosomes,* the site of protein synthesis. There are numerous other cellular structures, essential to life but not to our discussion of heredity.

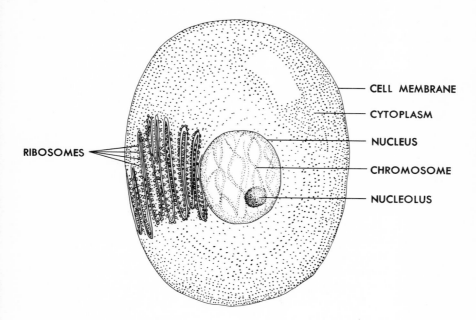

Fig. 9.11 An unspecialized cell, as in the early development of an embryo.

CHROMOSOMES

Within the nucleus of every cell are located the actual bearers of genetic information, the chromosomes. Every human body cell contains 23 pairs of chromosomes; every sperm or egg carries only 23 chromosomes—one member from each pair. Thus the fusion of the sperm with the egg creates a cell (the fertilized egg or *zygote*) carrying 23 *pairs* of chromosomes, one member of each pair having come from the sperm and the other from the egg. Every one of the billions of cells which will result from the normal fertilized egg will carry the identical 46 chromosomes.

THE GENETIC CODE

Every chromosome contains thousands of molecules of *deoxyribonucleic acid* (DNA), the chemical bearer of the information of heredity (genetic code). The insight into the structure and function of DNA is one of the high points of modern science. With this knowledge has come the exciting (and to many persons, frightening) possibility of man's control over human heredity and evolution. Each DNA molecule (Fig. 9.12) resembles a long, twisted ladder, the rungs of which are pairs of chemicals. The only two known pairs of these chemicals are *adenine*

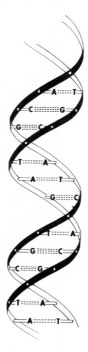

Fig. 9.12 DNA, the molecule of heredity. (W. G. Whaley *et al., Principles of Biology,* New York, Harper & Row, 1964.)

with *thymine* and *cytosine* with *guanine.* It is the sequence in which these "rungs" occur in the DNA molecule that determines the characteristics of every living thing. These rungs may be thought of as *letters,* which in sequence spell out the words of the "genetic code." There are only 4 known letters in the alphabet of the genetic code—adenine: thymine, thymine:adenine, cytosine:guanine, and guanine:cytosine.

But the thousands of such rungs or letters in a DNA molecule makes possible an almost infinite number of different arrangements. When we speak of genes, we are in fact speaking of the structure of DNA.

ACTION OF DNA

DNA has the ability, most unusual for a chemical molecule, of reproducing itself. Each time a cell divides, its DNA must first duplicate itself. It does this by "unzipping," with the two sides of the ladder unwinding and the rungs breaking in the center. Each half then reconstructs the original molecule by pulling the necessary parts from the surrounding materials. Thymine attracts adenine, adenine attracts thymine, cytosine attracts guanine, and guanine attracts cytosine. When this process is complete, the cell divides, as discussed below.

The way in which DNA is believed to function as a gene is shown in Fig. 9.13. DNA controls the characteristics of a living thing by controlling the synthesis of protein within each cell. The characteristics of any living thing are determined by the types of proteins it contains.

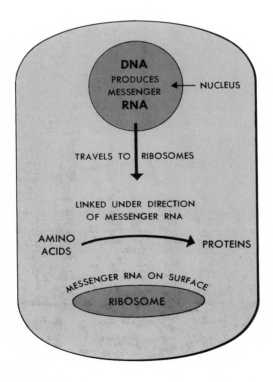

Fig. 9.13 Action of DNA in a typical cell.

The type of protein is determined by the sequence of the amino acids (see Chapter 6) it contains. DNA determines the sequence of the amino acids that make up each protein, thereby determining the characteristics of the individual. It is known that the manufacture of proteins takes place in the numerous *ribosomes* in the cytoplasm of the cell. A chemical messenger carries the genetic code from the DNA in the nucleus to the ribosomes in the cytoplasm. This messenger is called *messenger* RNA. RNA (ribonucleic acid) is similar to one half of a DNA molecule —as if the ladder were sawed in half lengthwise. The messenger RNA units attach themselves to the surface of the ribosomes. Other RNA units called *transfer* RNA transport single amino acids from other areas of the cell to the ribosome, where, with the aid of an enzyme, the messenger RNA arranges the amino acids into specific proteins. Many of these proteins are enzymes which will in turn enable vital chemical reactions to take place within the cell.

CELL DIVISION

Only two types of cell division are known to take place in the human body. One of these, *mitosis* (Fig. 9.14), is the more common type of cell division. All growth and replacement of cells takes place through mitosis. It is through mitosis that the fertilized egg divides into the billions of cells present at birth. The most important characteristic of mitosis is that it results in *two cells identical to the parent cell.*

The second type of cell division, *meiosis* (Fig. 9.15), takes place only in the ovary or testis in the production of eggs or sperms. Through the process of meiosis, which involves 2 cell divisions and results in 4 cells, the number of chromosomes in each cell is reduced from 23 pairs to 23 single chromosomes. Each sperm or egg gets one member of each pair. The most important characteristic of meiosis is the *random assortment* of chromosomes which takes place. When a man produces a sperm, for example, that sperm gets some chromosomes (maternal) that the man received from his mother and some chromosomes (paternal) that he received from his father. For each of the 23 pairs of chromosomes, a random assortment takes place—a given sperm being equally likely to receive a maternal or paternal chromosome. It is this random assortment of chromosomes that leads to the independent inheritance of characteristics which are determined by different chromosomes. This random assortment also means that every sperm or egg a man or woman produces receives a different combination of chromosomes. Thus a couple can produce many children, but never two with exactly the same combination of characteristics (except in the production of identical twins, in which case one fertilized egg divides to produce two genetically identical children).

MITOSIS

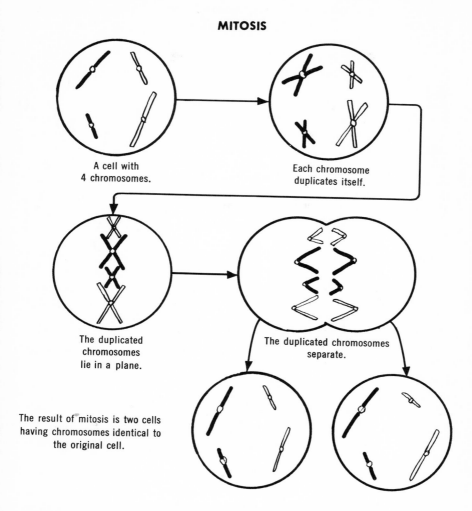

A cell with
4 chromosomes.

Each chromosome
duplicates itself.

The duplicated
chromosomes
lie in a plane.

The duplicated chromosomes
separate.

The result of mitosis is two cells
having chromosomes identical to
the original cell.

Fig. 9.14 Mitosis, cell division resulting in two genetically identical cells.

DOMINANCE AND RECESSIVENESS

Genes (DNA patterns) are often spoken of as being either *dominant* or *recessive*. For many characteristics there is a contrasting pair of dominant and recessive genes. If a child receives one dominant gene from either parent, he will exhibit the dominant characteristic. In order for the child to exhibit a recessive characteristic, the recessive gene must be received from each parent. Thus when a person does exhibit a recessive

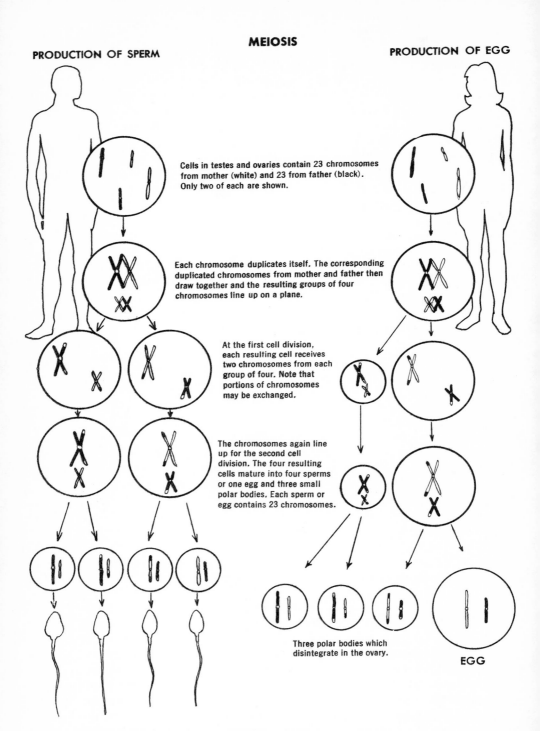

MEIOSIS

PRODUCTION OF SPERM

PRODUCTION OF EGG

Cells in testes and ovaries contain 23 chromosomes from mother (white) and 23 from father (black). Only two of each are shown.

Each chromosome duplicates itself. The corresponding duplicated chromosomes from mother and father then draw together and the resulting groups of four chromosomes line up on a plane.

At the first cell division, each resulting cell receives two chromosomes from each group of four. Note that portions of chromosomes may be exchanged.

The chromosomes again line up for the second cell division. The four resulting cells mature into four sperms or one egg and three small polar bodies. Each sperm or egg contains 23 chromosomes.

Three polar bodies which disintegrate in the ovary.

EGG

Fig. 9.15 Meiosis, the production of sperm or eggs.

characteristic, he is *homozygous* for that condition, meaning that he carries only the one type of gene. Every sperm or egg produced by that person will carry the recessive gene. A person showing a dominant condition may have received the dominant gene from each parent (he would be homozygous), *or* he may have received the dominant gene from one parent and the recessive gene from the other parent, a condition referred to as *heterozygous*. When dominance is complete, the appearance of the person is the same whether he is homozygous or heterozygous. For some hereditary characteristics, the heterozygous person presents an intermediate appearance—halfway between the homozygous dominant person and the homozygous recessive person. Such inheritance is called *incomplete dominance* or *intermediate* inheritance. For many human characteristics, not one but *several* pairs of genes help determine the appearance of the person. In such cases (examples are skin color, hair color, and stature) there are numerous intermediate conditions between the two extremes.

COMMON MISCONCEPTIONS ABOUT HEREDITY

It would be well at this point to clear up several common misconceptions about heredity. First of all, it is a common belief that recessive genes are always undesirable. A glance at the accompanying listing of human hereditary conditions (Table 9.3) will show that in many cases the recessive condition is the normal condition, the dominant being abnormal. For example, the gene producing 6 fingers on each hand is dominant over the gene for 5 fingers. Yet the possession of 5 fingers on each hand is considered by most of us to be the normal condition. The same example points out another common misconception—the idea that recessive genes occur less commonly than dominant genes. Obviously the recessive condition of 5 fingers per hand is much more common than the dominant in this case. The list of hereditary characteristics reveals many other similar cases.

GENES CAN CHANGE

In predicting the offspring from a particular mating, we assume a *stability* or lack of change in the genes (DNA), and 999,999 times out of 1 million we are correct in that assumption. But about once in every million cell divisions, an error is made in the self-duplication process of the DNA. If such an error is *stable* and is passed on with subsequent cell divisions, it is a *mutation*. With the change in DNA pattern a new gene has been produced. Mutations have a very important bearing upon the welfare of mankind. In the first place, mutations are the basis of *evolution*. That very small percentage of mutations which prove to be advantageous to the species are maintained through the ever occurring *natural selection*. Man has watched such a process taking place during the past few years as insects have become resistant to insecticides and bacteria to antibiotics. We also see mutations occurring in viruses, such as the often-changing flu viruses.

TABLE 9.3 SOME HEREDITARY TRAITS IN MAN

Dominant	Recessive
Eyes:	
Brown	Blue or gray
Green or hazel	Blue or gray
Normal	Color-blindness (sex-linked)
Nearsightedness	Normal
Farsightedness	Normal
Congenital cataract	Normal
Astigmatism	Normal
Nervous system:	
Huntington's chorea	Normal
Migraine headache	Normal
Normal	Phenylketonuria (PKU)
Hereditary tremor	Normal
Normal	Congenital deafness
Endocrine system:	
Normal	Diabetes mellitus
Circulatory system:	
Blood groups A, B, AB	Blood group O
Rh factor present (positive)	Rh factor absent (negative)
High blood pressure	Normal
Normal	Hemophilia (sex-linked)
Skin and hair:	
Normal pigmentation	Albinism
Dark hair	Light hair
Curly hair	Straight hair
Baldness (males)	Normal (males)
Normal (females)	Baldness (females)
Body structure:	
Six fingers each hand	Five fingers each hand
Webbed fingers or toes	Normal
Dwarfism	Normal
Stub fingers	Normal
Free ear lobes	Attached ear lobes

Mutations often seem to occur spontaneously, but they can be induced through exposure of cells to radiation or to certain chemicals.
It is *not* possible to produce mutations through physical change in an
organism. In breeds of dogs whose tails have been cut off for hundreds
of years, puppies are born today with tails not 1 micron shorter than
their ancestors of a hundred generations ago. Acquired characteristics
in human beings such as brain damage resulting from physical injury
are *not hereditary*. In considering the genetic desirability of a given
marriage, it is important to distinguish carefully between those characteristics which are hereditary and those which are acquired. There
are a growing number of *heredity clinics* available for those couples
concerned with the desirability of producing children when family
lines indicate possible hereditary defects. When there is a fair chance
of producing defective offspring, there can be strong arguments in
favor of adopting normal children, rather than taking the chance of
producing a defective child.

DETERMINATION OF SEX

The determination of the sex of an unborn child is quite a simple
matter. Of the 23 pairs of human chromosomes, one pair is called the
sex chromosomes. This is the only pair of human chromosomes in
which the two members are different in appearance. One is a fairly
large chromosome called the *X chromosome*. The other is a very small
Y chromosome. Females carry two X chromosomes in every cell; males
carry one X and one Y chromosome per cell. (Certain other combinations, such as XXX and XXY, are known to occur rarely, usually resulting in physical and mental abnormalities.)

During the production of eggs or sperm, the sex chromosomes, like
all other pairs of chromosomes, separate, each sperm or egg receiving
only one member of the pair. Since a female is XX, every egg she produces carries an X chromosome. A male, being XY, produces sperm
cells half of which carry an X chromosome and half of which carry a
Y. If an egg is fertilized by an X-bearing sperm, the child will be XX
and therefore female. If an egg is fertilized by a Y-bearing sperm, the
child will be XY and therefore male. Once the child is conceived, nothing that the mother, doctor, or anyone else can do will have any influence on the sex of the child.

SEX-LINKED HEREDITY

In addition to the sex of the child, certain other characteristics are
determined by the X chromosome. Such characteristics are said to be
sex-linked. The Y chromosome carries *no* corresponding genes. Sex-
linked recessive characteristics occur much more often in men than

in women. The reason for this frequency is that a male, with only one X chromosome, will exhibit the recessive characteristic if it is carried by his one X chromosome. But before a female will exhibit the sex-linked recessive, she must carry the gene on *each* of her two X chromosomes. The chance of receiving the same gene twice is, naturally, the *square* of the chance of receiving it once. If the chance in a male is 1 in 20, the chance in a female will be 1 in 400. The best-known examples of sex-linked characteristics are color-blindness and hemophilia (bleeder's disease).

Since a man transmits an X chromosome only to his daughters, a sex-linked characteristic is passed from a man to his daughter (who probably will be an unaffected "carrier") who in turn will pass the gene to half of her sons, who will be affected.

THE RH FACTOR IN PREGNANCY

One hereditary characteristic which occasionally complicates pregnancy is the *Rh factor.* This is a chemical substance which is usually present within the red blood cells (erythrocytes). If a person has this factor present in his red blood cells, then he is Rh *positive,* as are about 85 percent of Caucasoids, 92 percent of Negroids, and 99 percent of Orientals. If this substance is missing, then he is Rh *negative,* as are about 15 percent of Caucasoids.

The only set of circumstances under which the Rh factor can complicate pregnancy comes when an Rh negative woman, with an Rh positive husband, bears an Rh positive child. The Rh factor is inherited through a dominant gene, so a heterozygous positive man can father both positive and negative children. As diagrammed in Fig. 9.16, when a negative woman carries a positive child, small amounts of Rh factor diffuse across the placenta from the blood of the child into the blood of the mother. It is believed that the Rh substance involved is carried in the plasma of the blood, rather than in the cells, since no exchange of blood takes place in the placenta and the cells are too large to diffuse through the placental membranes.

Once the Rh factor enters the body of the mother, it acts as an *antigen* (see Chapter 15). The antigen stimulates her body to produce anti-Rh *antibodies* (also in Chapter 15), which will *destroy* red blood cells containing the Rh factor. This process has *no effect* upon the red cells of the mother, since they contain no Rh factor. But when the level of antibodies in the mother's blood becomes high enough, these antibodies diffuse back across the placenta into the blood of the child and destroy his red blood cells. This diffusion most commonly occurs with the second or third pregnancy. The result of this destruction is a type of anemia called *erythroblastosis fetalis,* in which the blood cannot carry sufficient oxygen for the infant. In extreme cases, this anemia may result in stillbirth, death following birth, or mental re-tardation. Such infants appear yellow (jaundiced), because of the by-products of the breakdown of the red blood cells. When tests indicate a dangerous level of antibodies has been reached, labor may be induced somewhat prematurely and the infant given blood transfusions. More recently, such transfusions have been performed upon infants still in the uterus, the first case of intrauterine therapy.

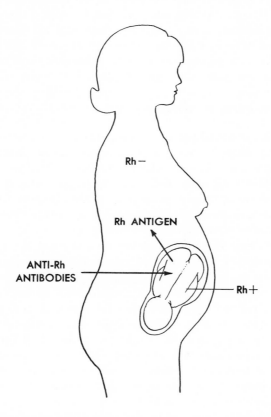

Fig. 9.16 Rh incompatibility in pregnancy.

OTHER BLOOD GROUPS

In addition to his Rh blood type, a person has a blood type from each of many other blood group series. Most of these series are inherited independently of each other, for the genes are carried by different chromosomes. (For a discussion of the best-known series of blood groups, the A-B-O series, see Chapter 13.) This series is inherited independently of the Rh series, so a person can have any combination of Rh and A-B-O blood types.

CONGENITAL ABNORMALITIES

Congenital abnormalities are abnormal conditions which are present at the time of birth. Such abnormalities remain a major problem in the United States today, 2 to 3 percent of all infants being born with *significant* defects in the formation of their bodies. Some of these deformities can be completely corrected through surgical procedures. Others result in lifelong debilities of varying degrees. Still others are so severe that they result in the death of the infant. Although other causes of infant mortality have yielded to medical research, congenital defects have remained a major cause of death during the first year of life. In addition, many spontaneous abortions are the result of abnormal development.

Most congenital abnormalities must still be thought of as unpreventable. Although it is often possible in retrospect to determine the cause of the abnormality, little can be done today to predict and prevent these unfortunate cases. Some malformations are genetically determined, some result from adverse intrauterine environmental conditions, and some are probably the result of a combination of the two causes. Many defects seem to be the result of an isolated accident in the complicated chain of events leading to a normal individual.

Some hereditary congenital defects arise when each parent is a carrier of the same recessive gene for the defect. Other defects of genetic origin arise as the result of an "accident" during the meiotic cell division leading to the sperm or egg. The egg or sperm resulting from such faulty cell division may deviate from the normal chromosome number of 23 and the resulting offspring show a corresponding deviation from the usual 46 chromosomes. Chromosome counts made of cells of living persons have revealed chromosome numbers ranging from 45 to 49. Individuals having other than 46 chromosomes are always abnormal. Their abnormalities usually include both physical malformities and mental retardation. A commonly occurring abnormality resulting from an extra chromosome is *mongolism*. The mongoloid person is characterized by short stature; broad, flat head; large tongue; slanting eyes; and very low mentality. The incidence of extra chromosomes increases markedly with the age of the mother. The risk of a mongoloid's being born to a woman in her twenties is about 1 in 3000. To a woman over 35, it is 1 in 300. To a woman over 40, it is 1 in 70, and over 45 it is 1 in 40. Fortunately, most women today bear their last child while still in their twenties. There is no known treatment for the child born with an abnormal chromosome number. Parents who have had one child with a chromosomal abnormality have an appreciable chance of producing more of such children in future pregnancies, because one of the parents may be carrying a chromosomal abnormality in the ovary or testis. The chance of a second defective child ranges from 1 percent to 33 percent, depending upon the maternal age and type of abnormality. Such parents should have genetic counsel before deciding upon another pregnancy.

Fully one fourth of all fetuses lost through miscarriage show abnormal chromosome numbers. In women having a history of repeated miscarriages of obviously defective fetuses, there is an increased chance that a full-term infant will also be defective. Naturally, when miscarriages have been due to a maternal factor such as a low progesterone level, no such increase in defective offspring occurs.

Environmental causes of congenital defects exert their greatest effect during the first 8 to 12 weeks of the life of an embryo. At this stage of development the body is undergoing rapid differentiation, with the formation of most organs taking place. Among the environmental factors which may seriously affect the embryo are excessive exposure to radiation, use of certain drugs by the mother, and exposure to disease agents. Virus diseases may have an especially severe effect upon the embryo. Many normally mild virus diseases, such as German measles, have been proven to cause serious defects when an embryo is infected during the first 3 months of pregnancy. Among bacterial diseases, syphilis has a very serious effect upon the fetus, up to 50 percent of children of infected mothers being either stillborn or physically or mentally defective.

Many congenital defects cannot be prevented, but as our knowledge of their causes increases, we also learn some precautions that can be taken. As previously shown, the first precaution is for the woman to complete her family while she is still young. (The age of the father has never been shown to influence congenital abnormalities.) Avoidance of extensive X-ray treatment during pregnancy is important. Drugs should be taken only when prescribed by a physician. The woman seeing a physician or dentist for any cause during early pregnancy should alert him to her condition, for knowledge of this might influence his choice of drugs or use of X ray. During the first 3 months of pregnancy, the woman should protect herself as much as possible from exposure to any diseases, even those as mild as the flu.

The birth of a defective child is accompanied by many emotional and social problems. The parents often have a feeling of guilt and either consciously or unconsciously express the feeling that they are at fault. They may feel that the defect is due to something they did or did not do during the pregnancy. Actually, according to our present knowledge, there are very few cases of congenital defects which can be classified as preventable. The birth of a handicapped child always imposes a strain upon the relationship between all the members of the family. The medical care, training, education, and social adjustment of the child may create a great financial and emotional burden. The parents should not hesitate to take advantage of the services of the government and voluntary agencies dealing with handicapped children. The attitude of the parents toward a moderately handicapped child will have a great influence upon the degree to which he develops the ability to live a normal life. If the parents treat the handicapped child the same as his brothers and sisters, minimizing his handicap, then his handicap will be minimized in the eyes of the other children and in his own attitude toward himself. If, on the other hand, the parents are unhappy or ashamed about a child, overprotect him, or keep him from contact with other children, he is apt to grow up feeling different and inferior and may be more restricted by an emotional handicap than by his physical one.

SUMMARY

I. Human Reproductive Systems
    A. Male reproductive system:
        1. Testis—produces both spermatozoa and testosterone.
        2. Scrotum—loose tissue covering testis.
        3. Epididymis—holds sperm cells while they mature.
        4. Vas deferens
           a. Small duct carrying sperm from the epididymis into the urethra.
           b. Near the upper end is an enlargement for the storage of mature sperm until ejaculation.
        5. Fluid-producing glands
           a. Seminal vesicles—most important source of fluid for the semen.
           b. Prostate gland.
           c. Cowper's glands.
        6. Penis—male organ of sexual intercourse.
    B. Female reproductive system:
        1. Ovary—produces both eggs (ova) and hormones.
        2. Fallopian tube (oviduct)—duct which carries eggs from the ovary to the uterus.
        3. Uterus—organ specialized for the growth and protection of the unborn child.
        4. Vagina
           a. Female organ of sexual intercourse.
           b. Produces lubricating materials upon sexual arousal.
        5. External genitalia
           a. Vulva—two pairs of labia surrounding the opening of the vagina.
           b. Clitoris—sensory erectile tissue lying at the forward junction of the labia.
           c. Hymen—membrane which may partially close the opening of the vagina.

II. Menstrual Cycle
    A. Hormones of reproduction:

1. Menstrual cycle is under control of pituitary gland.
2. Hormones stimulating the ovaries are:
   a. follicle-stimulating hormone (FSH).
   b. luteinizing hormone (LH).
   c. luteotropic hormone (LTH).
3. Two types of hormones from the ovaries are important in the menstrual cycle.
   a. estrogens.
   b. progesterone.
B. The menstrual cycle:
   1. Menarche—first menstrual period; usually occurs between the ages of 11 and 15.
   2. Menopause—cessation of the menstrual cycle at about age 45.
   3. Menstrual cycle lasts an average of 28 days and includes two important events:
      a. menstruation—occurring the first 4 or 5 days of the cycle.
      b. ovulation—occurring at about the midpoint of the cycle.

III. Pregnancy
   A. Embryology—full-term pregnancy lasts about 266 days from conception.
      1. During the first 8 weeks, developing child is called the embryo.
      2. Beyond 8 weeks, called fetus.
   B. Early signs of pregnancy:
      1. Cessation of menstruation—result of chorion-produced gonadotropic hormone which maintains production of progesterone by the corpus luteum.
      2. Changes in the breasts—become larger and fuller as a result of the continued high progesterone level.
      3. Frequent urination—enlarged uterus presses against the urinary bladder.
      4. Nausea—may begin at the time of the first missed period and last for 4 to 6 weeks.
      5. Pregnancy tests
         a. Most depend upon chorionic gonadotropin in the urine or blood of the pregnant woman.
         b. In other tests, estrogen and progesterone are administered for a few days in case the delay in menstruation is due to immaturity of the endometrium.
   C. Prenatal care (care of the pregnant woman):
      1. Of utmost importance to enable early detection of complications to pregnancy.
      2. Pregnant woman should know and be alert to the signs of possible complications.
   D. Diet in pregnancy:
      1. Pregnant woman needs significantly increased quantities of protein, vitamins, and minerals, but only slightly increased calories.
      2. Excess weight gain is very undesirable, leading to
         a. difficult, prolonged labor.
         b. greater chance of toxemia.
         c. often permanent obesity.
   E. Terminations of pregnancy:
      1. Most pregnancies terminate in a normal delivery of a full-term infant.

2. Premature delivery—live birth of an infant before it is fully mature, with weight being under 5½ pounds.

3. Abortion—any termination of pregnancy before there is any chance of survival of the infant.
   a. Spontaneous abortion, commonly called a miscarriage.
   b. Induced abortions:
      (1) therapeutic abortion—performed by a qualified physician and controlled by laws of the various states.
      (2) criminal abortions—those performed outside the restrictions of the laws.

IV. Criminal Abortion—estimated 1 in 5 pregnancies in the United States terminates in an illegal abortion.

V. Fertility Problems
   A. Low fertility—occurs in about 10 percent of all married couples.
      1. Cause may lie in either the man or the woman, or partially in each.
      2. Sterility—total inability to produce a child.
   B. Artificial insemination:
      1. Injection of semen by syringe into the cervix.
      2. Semen may be that of the husband or a donor.
   C. Contraception:
      1. Hormonal contraception
         a. Female oral contraceptives work through inhibition of the production of FSH and LH by means of synthetic estrogens and progesterones.
         b. Are essentially 100 percent effective if instructions are followed exactly.
      2. Mechanical contraception—several devices designed to prevent the spermatozoa from reaching the ovum.
      3. Chemical contraception—variety of spermicidal foams, creams, jellies of various degrees of effectiveness are available.
      4. Intrauterine contraceptive devices (IUD)
         a. A variety of plastic and stainless steel devices which can be inserted into the uterus.
         b. Effectiveness of such devices is very high.
      5. The "rhythm" method
         a. Periodic abstinence from sexual intercourse during the fertile period of the menstrual cycle.
         b. Is usually not highly effective.
      6. Douches—the least effective contraceptive method.
      7. Withdrawal ("coitus interruptus")
         a. Effectiveness is low.
         b. Interferes with enjoyment of intercourse.
      8. Surgical sterilization
         a. is usually permanent.
         b. does not affect sexual intercourse.
         c. is 100 percent effective in both male and female.

VI. Heredity
   A. Genetic material—identical in each cell of the body.
   B. Chromosomes contain the genetic information.
      1. Each sperm and egg contains 23 chromosomes.
      2. Each body cell contains 23 *pairs* of chromosomes.

C. Genetic code—chemical carrier of genetic information; *deoxyribo-nucleic acid* (DNA).

D. Action of DNA—controls the characteristics of a living thing by controlling the synthesis of protein within each cell.

E. Cell division:
   1. Mitosis results in two cells, each identical to the original.
   2. Meiosis
      a. takes place only in production of sperms and eggs.
      b. reduces the number of chromosomes from 23 pairs to 23 single chromosomes.

F. Dominance and recessiveness—shown in characteristics by contrasting pair of genes.
   1. If a child receives a dominant gene from either parent, he will exhibit the dominant characteristic.
   2. The recessive gene will not produce its characteristic if the opposing dominant gene is present.

G. Change in a DNA pattern is called a mutation.

H. Sex of child is determined by the sex chromosomes.

I. Sex-linked heredity—characteristics, other than sex, carried on the X chromosome.

J. The Rh factor in pregnancy—only Rh problem situation is an Rh negative woman carrying an Rh positive child.

VII. Congenital Abnormalities
   A. Abnormal conditions present at the time of birth.
   B. Some of genetic origin.
   C. Environmental pressures can produce abnormalities.
   D. Attitudes of the family toward the handicapped child will influence his chances for living the fullest possible life.

Glossary

If you cannot find the word you wish in this glossary, check the index for text and glossary references.

adrenocorticotropic hormone (ə drē'nō kor ti kō trop'ik hor'mōn) (G. *tropikis,* turning). A hormone from the anterior pituitary having a stimulating influence upon the adrenal cortex.

afterbirth (af'tər burth). The placenta and associated membranes, expelled from the uterus after the birth of a child.

amnion (am'nē ən) (G. *amnion,* lamb). The membrane which surrounds the embryo within the uterus, secreting amniotic fluid to form the "bag of water."

ampulla (am pul'ə) (L. *ampulla,* jug). A dilated section of a tubular structure.

Bartholin's glands (bahr'tə linz) (Casper Bartholin, Jr., Danish anatomist, 1655–1738). Small glands, one on each side of vaginal orifice, secreting part of lubricant for sexual intercourse.

cervix (sur'viks) (L. *cervix,* neck). The neck or any necklike part of an organ.

chorion (kor'ē on) (G. *chorion,* membrane). The outermost embryonic membrane, part of which unites with the endometrium to form the placenta.

chromosome (krō'mə sōm) (G. *chroma,* color; *soma,* body). Small bodies contained in the nucleus of every cell, carrying the DNA which determines the inherited characteristics of the organism.

cilia (sil′ē ə) (L. *cilium,* eyelash). Minute hairlike structures attached to the outer surface of a cell, capable of wavelike motion.

climacteric (klī mak′tər ik, klī mak ter′ik) (G. *klimakter,* rung of ladder). The physical and mental changes occurring at the termination of the reproductive years in the female.

clitoris (klit′ə ris, klī′tə ris) (G. *kleitoris*). Small erectile sensory structure located at forward juncture of vulva of female external genitalia.

copulation (kop yə lā′shən) (L. *copulatio*). Sexual intercourse.

corpus luteum (kor′pəs loo′tē əm) (L. *corpus,* body; *luteum,* yellow). The ovarian follicle after discharge of the ovum, persisting as a yellow mass which secretes the hormone progesterone.

Cowper's glands (kou′pərz, koo′pərz) (William Cowper, English surgeon, 1666– 1709). A pair of small glands located in the lower abdomen of the male, secreting a lubricating fluid into the urethra upon sexual arousal and contributing a small amount of fluid to the semen.

cytoplasm (sī′tə plazm) (G. *kytos,* cell; *plasma,* plasm). The protoplasm (living material) of a cell exclusive of that of the nucleus.

deoxyribonucleic acid (DNA) (dē ok si rī′bō nyoo klē′ik). The chemical bearer of hereditary traits, located in the chromosomes.

eclampsia (i klamp′sē ə) (G. *eklampein,* to shine). Convulsions and coma occurring during pregnancy following uncorrected toxemia.

ectopic pregnancy (ek top′ik) (G. *ektopos,* displaced). A pregnancy outside the uterus, usually in the fallopian tube or abdominal cavity.

ejaculation (i jak yə lā′shən) (L. *ejaculatio,* expulsion). The expulsion of the semen.

embryo (em′brē ō) (G. *embryon,* unborn young). The early developing stage of any organism; in the human, during the first 8 weeks.

embryology (em brē ol′ə jē). The science which deals with the development of the embryo.

endocrine gland (en′də krin) (G. *endon,* within; G. *krinein,* to separate). A gland secreting into the blood a substance (hormone) that acts elsewhere in the body.

endometrium (en dō mē′trē əm) (G. *endon,* within; *metra,* uterus). The mucous membrane lining the inside of the uterus.

epididymis (ep i did′i mis) (G. *epi,* on; *didymos,* testis). An oblong body attached to each testis, in which sperm cells mature and are stored.

episiotomy (ə pē′zē ot′ə mē) (G. *epision,* vulva; *tome,* cutting). Surgical cutting of the vulvar orifice to prevent tearing in childbirth.

erectile (i rek′til) (L. *erectio,* erect). Capable of erection.

erection (i rek′shən). The condition of becoming rigid and elevated.

erythroblastosis fetalis (i rith′rō blas tō′sis fi tal′is) (G. *erythro,* red; G. *blastos,* germ; L. *fetus,* unborn child). Destruction of the red blood cells of the fetus or newborn child, usually resulting from Rh incompatibility.

estrogens (es′trə jənz) (G. *oistros,* a strong desire). Female sex hormones, promoting female sexual development.

fallopian tube (fə lō′pē ən).The paired ducts carrying the ova from the ovary to the uterus. Also called oviducts.

fertility (fər til′i tē) (L. *fertilis,* fruitful). Ability to produce offspring.

fetus (fē′təs). The unborn child after 8 weeks of development.

fimbria (fim′brē ə) (L. *fimbria,* fringe). The fringelike upper end of the oviduct.

follicle stimulating hormone (FSH) (fol′i kl) (L. *follis,* bag). A gonadotropic hormone from the anterior pituitary, stimulating the maturation of the ovarian follicle and its production of estrogen.

gamete (gam′ēt) (G. *gamete,* wife). A mature egg or sperm.

gene (jēn) (G. *gennan,* to produce). A DNA pattern responsible for producing a given hereditary trait; occurs at a definite location on a particular chromosome.

gonad (gō′nad) (G. *gone,* seed). An ovary or testis.

gonadotropic hormone (gō nad ə trop′ik) (G. *tropos,* turning). A gonad-stimulating hormone.

graafian follicle (graf′ē ən fol′i kl) (Reijnier deGraaf, Dutch physician, 1641–1673). The maturing ovarian follicle, containing the ovum.

heterozygous (het ər ə zī′gəs) (G. *heteros,* other; G. *zygotos,* yolked together). Possessing different genes in regard to a given character.

homozygous (hō mə zī′gəs) (G. *homes,* same). Possessing an identical pair of genes in regard to a given character.

hyaluronidase (hī′ə loo ron′i dās). An enzyme that softens cell membranes. Necessary for fertilization of human egg. Also found in snake and spider venoms and produced by pathogenic bacteria.

hymen (hī′mən) (G. *hymen,* membrane). The membranous fold which may partially or wholly close the external opening of the vagina.

impotence (im′pə təns) (L. *in,* not; *potentia,* power). Lack of power; especially incapacity for sexual intercourse. May be physical or emotional in origin.

interstitial cells (in tər stish′əl) (L. *inter,* between; *sistere,* to set). Cells lying between the seminiferous tubules of the testes; secreting testosterone.

labia (lā′bē ə) (L. *labia,* lips). The liplike portions of the female external genitalia.

labor (lā′bər) (L. *labor,* work). The series of processes by which the baby and other products of conception are expelled from the body of the mother.

luteinizing hormone (LH) (loo′tē ə nī zing) (L. *luteus,* yellow; G. *izein,* cause to be). A hormone from the anterior pituitary which stimulates corpus luteum formation in the ovary and the secretion of testosterone by the testis.

luteotropic hormone (LTH) (loo′tē ə trop′ik) (G. *tropikos,* turning). A hormone (also called prolactin) from the anterior pituitary which stimulates progesterone secretion by the corpus luteum and causes the breasts to produce milk.

meiosis (mī ō′sis) (G. *meiosis,* diminution). A special type of cell division occurring during the production of sperms or eggs, by which the usual double set of chromosomes is reduced to a single set.

menarche (me nahr′kē) (G. *men,* month; *arche,* beginning). The beginning of the menstrual cycles.

menopause (men′ə pawz) (G. *pausis,* cessation). Cessation of menstruation, occurring usually between ages 45 and 50.

menstrual cycle (men′stroo əl sī′kl) (L. *menstruare,* to menstruate). The regularly recurring cycle of physiological events including ovulation and menstruation.

menstruation (men stroo ā′shən).   The cyclic uterine bleeding resulting from the degeneration of the endometrium.

mitosis (mī tō′sis) (G. *mitos,* thread; *osis,* process).   The most common type of cell division, resulting in two cells, each genetically identical to the original.

mongolism (mong′gə lizm).   A type of idiocy resulting from the presence of one extra chromosome in each body cell. Also called *Down's syndrome.*

mutation (myoo tā′shən) (L. *mutatio,* change).   A stable, transmissible change in a DNA pattern (gene).

nocturnal emission (nok tur′nəl i mish′ən) (L. *noctis,* night; *emittere,* to send out).   The discharge of semen (seminal fluid) by males during sleep. Commonly begins shortly after puberty.

nucleus (nyoo′klē əs) (L. *nucleus,* kernel).   A spheroid body within a cell, containing the chromosomes.

orgasm (or′gazm) (G. *orgasmos,* swelling).   The climax of sexual excitement in the male or female.

os (os) (L. *oris,* mouth or *ossis,* bone).   (1) a mouth or orifice, (2) a bone.

ovary (ō′və rē) (L. *ovarium,* ovary).   The female sex organ in which are formed ova and hormones.

oviduct (ō′vi dukt) (L. *ovi,* egg; *ductus,* duct).   The tube carrying ova from the ovary to the uterus; the *fallopian tube.*

ovulation (ov yoo lā′shən) (L. *ovum,* egg).   The discharge of the mature egg from the graafian follicle of the ovary.

ovum (ō′vəm).   An egg.

penis (pē′nis) *(L.* penis).   The male organ of copulation.

pituitary gland (pityoo′i ter ē) (L. *pituita,* phlegm).   An endocrine gland located at the base of the brain; secretes numerous hormones, many of which stimulate the function of other endocrine glands. Also called the *hypophysis.*

placenta (plə sen′tə) (L. *placenta,* a flat cake).   A disc-shaped organ within the uterus through which takes place the exchange of materials between maternal and fetal blood.

progesterone (prō jes′tə rōn) (L. *pro,* before; *gestatio,* pregnancy).   A hormone produced by the corpus luteum of the ovary (and by the placenta), promoting the maturity of the endometrium and the maintenance during pregnancy.

prostate gland (pros′tāt) (G. *pro,* before; *histanai,* to stand).   A gland in the male surrounding the neck of the bladder and the urethra.

protoplasm (prō′tə plazm) (G. *protos,* first; *plasm,* plasma).   The living material within any cell.

puberty (pyoo′bər tē) (L. *pubertas,* transition).   The age at which sexual maturity is reached.

ribosome (rī′bə sōm) (ribose; G. *soma,* body).   Microscopic bodies within a cell, the site of protein syntheses.

salpingectomy (sal pin jek′tə mē) (G. *salpinx,* tube; *ektome,* removed).   Surgical removal of an oviduct.

scrotum (skrō′təm) (L. *scrotum,* bag).   The sac which contains the testes and related structures.

semen (sē′mən) (L. *semen,* seed).   The product of the male reproductive organs, a mixture of spermatozoa and fluid secretions from the prostate and various other glands and cells.

seminal vesicle (sem'i nəl ves'i kl) (L. *vesicula,* small bladder). A gland located on each vas deferens, the primary source of the fluid portion of semen.

seminiferous tubule (sem i nif'ər əs) (L. *semen,* seed; *ferre,* to bear). The numerous small tubes in the testis, the site of sperm production.

sex-linked (seks'lingkt'). Hereditary traits transmitted by genes carried on the X chromosome.

somatotropic hormone (sō'mə tə trop'ik) (G. *soma,* body; *tropos,* a turning). A hormone from the anterior pituitary gland, having a stimulating effect on body growth.

spermatozoon (spur'mə tə zō'ən) (Plural of G. *spermatos,* seed; *zoon,* animal). The mature male germ cell; the *sperm cell.*

sterility (stə ril'i tē) (L. *sterilis,* unfruitful). The inability to produce young.

testis (tes'tis) (L. *testis,* testicle). The male gonad, producing spermatozoa and testosterone.

testosterone (tes tos'tə rōn). The male sex hormone, produced by the testes, inducing male secondary sex characteristics.

thyrotropic hormone (thī'rə trop'ik) (thyroid; G. *tropos,* turning). A hormone from the anterior pituitary having a stimulating influence on the thyroid gland.

toxemia (tok sē'mē ə) (G. *toxikon,* poison; *haima,* blood). A series of conditions occurring in pregnant women, including high blood pressure, excess fluid in the tissues, and albumin in the urine.

trimester (trī mes'tər) (L. *trimestris,* of 3 months). A period of 3 months.

trophoblastic cells (trof ə blast'ik) (G. *trophe,* nutrition; *blastos,* germ). A layer of cells attaching the fertilized ovum to the uterine wall and supplying nutrition to the embryo.

umbilical cord (um bil'i kəl) (L. *umbilicus,* navel). The flexible cord connecting the fetus and the placenta, containing the umbilical arteries and vein.

urethra (yoo rē'thrə) (G. *ourethra,* urinary canal). The duct carrying urine from the bladder to the exterior of the body, and in the male also carrying semen.

uterus (yoo'tə rəs) (L. *uterus,* womb). The hollow, muscular, pear-shaped organ of the female wherein develops the fetus.

vagina (və jī'nə) (L. *vagina,* sheath). The sheathlike structure in the female for the reception of the penis in copulation.

vas deferens (vas def'ər enz) (L. *vas,* duct; *deferens,* carrying away). The duct carrying spermatozoa from the testis to the prostate.

vulva (vul'və) (L. *vulva,* cover, wrapper). The external genital organs of the female.

zygote (zī'gōt) (G. *zygotos,* yolked together). The fertilized ovum.

CHAPTER 10

CHOOSING
MEDICAL
SERVICES

MODERN MEDICINE

CHOOSING A PHYSICIAN

PARAMEDICAL
PROFESSIONS

FACILITIES FOR
PATIENT CARE

SUMMARY

During the past century medicine has made unbelievable strides. Maladies that carried the fear of death for our grandparents—diphtheria, scarlet fever, poliomyelitis, pneumonia, and tuberculosis—are now controlled to the point that few of us give little, if any, thought to them today. A child born today can look forward to a life expectancy half again as long as his ancestors could have 50 years ago. More exciting yet, medical men believe that life expectancy may well be further increased. Medical problems that have so far gone unsolved now seem to be within reach of cure or prevention through the greatest research efforts that have ever been mounted. These medical advances do not come to us automatically. They come through proper medical counsel and care, availability of hospital services, and use of appropriate drugs.

MODERN MEDICINE

Scientific medicine is built upon careful observation and research. Disease represents the end of a chain of events. In order to unravel this chain and cure or prevent the disease, medical men must know the causative agent, its life history, and how it transmits or causes the disease process in man. New bits of needed information are constantly being found. It is now known that the frequent damager of children's hearts, rheumatic fever, can be generally prevented by controlling strep (streptococcic) throat with sulfa drugs and antibiotics. This information has already reduced the number of young people suffering from such heart involvements, and the chances are good that rheumatic fever can be largely controlled in the years ahead. Not too many years ago coronary thrombosis could not be recognized even by physicians. Today, physicians are not only diagnosing and treating it, but are even beginning to recognize likely candidates for heart attacks from among their patients before the attacks strike, thereby being able to practice preventive medicine. A continuing search for the causes of cancer, arthritis, emotional troubles, muscular dystrophy, and other diseases is being carried on.

But finding the answers to all diseases is not the only goal of modern medicine. Of significant concern also are the problems faced in getting needed information and good medical care to the public. The finding of a cure to a dreaded disease will mean little to the average citizen unless he can find a satisfactory answer to the question, "How do I get the best in modern medical care for my family and myself?"

AIMS OF MODERN MEDICINE

The hopes of medicine today can be expressed in four major objectives:

1. Good medical care must be available to *all* people. Economically depressed communities, both in this country and elsewhere, have the right to expect cures from their diseases and infirmities.

2. The *prevention* of disease must be given top attention. As much as possible the physician must replace concern over how to treat an existing condition with interest in an effective way to prevent its initial occurrence.

3. The needs of the whole man must be ministered to. Areas of medical specialization tend to treat parts of a man. Important as specialization is, man is still an integrated individual of interrelated systems. When one part becomes ill, the whole man to a degree is ill and therefore needs attention.

4. Research into unconquered diseases and better methods of treat-

ment must be pursued. Medicine can never stand still in terms of research if the best of medical care is ever to be attained.

These objectives have not yet been accomplished. The medical profession must remain alert to better ways of blocking problems standing
in their way.

PROBLEMS FACED BY TODAY'S PHYSICIAN

A major problem facing the medical profession today is the increasing shortage of physicians. In spite of the fact that there are more
medical schools today, the ratio of physicians to patients is slimmer
than it was 50 years ago. In 1909 there was a physician for every 568
persons; in a recent census there was one for every 709 persons. (These
statistics are for the United States. In some countries the ratio is much
more startling.) Worse yet, the available physicians are not always
distributed evenly in terms of the population. This physician-patient
ratio is often somewhat better in urban centers and somewhat poorer
in rural areas. Many physicians prefer to practice in urban locations
close to modern medical facilities where they can render the highest
type of medical care. However, this urban concentration reduces the
number of physicians available for rural practices, sometimes depriving
scattered, rural populations of adequate medical personnel. Another
problem is that not all physicians are available for general health care.
Actually, at present there is only one *general practitioner* available for
every 2000 persons, and only one *internist* (a specialist in internal medicine) available for every 14,000 persons. Compounding this dilemma is
the greater demand the American public is making on the physician.
Today the average American sees a physician five times a year, twice
as often as he did in 1930.

Perplexed by the flood of new medical findings, more and more physicians have felt the need to restrict their practice to specialized areas
of medicine, changing the traditional reliance upon a "family physician" for all medical services (Fig. 10.1). Patients have been confused
as to "what kind" of a physician to go to.

The image the public has of the medical profession has changed.
Rapid changes in medical practice have occurred and the public has
accepted certain new trends, but are skeptical of others. As therapy has
become more mechanized and organized the busy physician has not
always communicated sufficiently well with his patient. People have
become somewhat wary where they have not properly understood techniques being used.

Some patients who have not been referred to specialists by their
family physician or a general practitioner have been disappointed with
their own choices of specialists. Since the "miracle drugs" have been
found useful in treating many diseases, other individuals feel these have

Physicians (M.D. and D.O.) per 100,000 Population

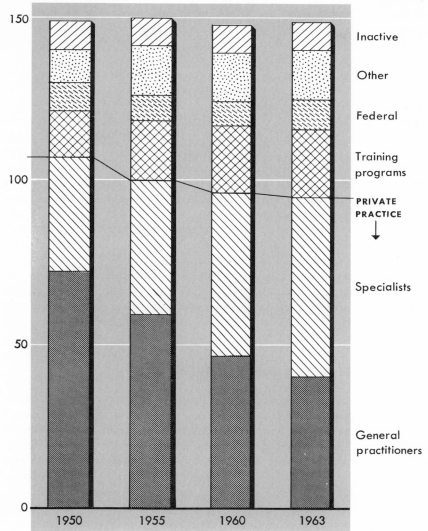

Fig. 10.1 Physicians in relation to population. (*Manpower in the 1960s,* Health Manpower Source Book No. 18, Public Health Service Publication No. 263.)

tended to reduce the important interpersonal relationship the person in distress needs with his physician. Medical practitioners today make greater use of the office, clinic, and hospital and less use of the patient's home than they did in the past. They believe that treatment can be more effective when administered at some centralized location where better therapeutic tools are available. Some of the tasks formerly handled by the physician can now be safely delegated to the hospital's highly trained staff. This has made it possible for the physician to carry a heavier case load. On the other hand, these practices have tended to give the physician less contact with home conditions and thus have deprived him of background information that would enable him to know the whole patient.

Physicians are expected to keep abreast of the mounting mass of medical data. The physician is faced with increasingly informed patients who want to know the nature of their ailments. Thus even though the physician has been professionally trained to communicate in concise technical terms, he must successfully bridge the communications gap between the forefront of research and the understanding of his patients in order to warrant their confidence.

Medical costs have risen sharply during the past two decades and will continue to rise. Although hospital costs have risen faster than other medical costs, the lay public tends to place the blame for these higher costs on the physicians. It is understandable that these higher costs are the price to be paid for improved but costlier diagnosis and therapy. However, it is important that rising costs of medical care not get out of reach of the public and prevent some people from receiving adequate medical care.

CHANGES IN THE MEDICAL PROFESSION

As a result of rapid social changes during the past two decades, there have been certain changes in traditional methods of medical practice. The medical profession has been increasingly conscious of the problem of preparing professional people who are sufficiently broad in their training to treat the whole man, yet who have adequate depth in the specialties to utilize and apply the latest information. There is increasing concern for giving emerging specialists more experience in general practice and in giving more specialized information to the general practitioner both before and after graduation. This change amounts to a de-emphasis on narrow specialties and a re-emphasis on general medicine.

There is a general feeling in the profession that health insurance must be extended. This extension is necessary if low-income families are to be sufficiently covered against mounting medical costs. Unfortunately, much energy has been lost in long arguments between the medical profession and the government on private versus public methods of providing such coverage. The federal government has felt a responsibility to provide health insurance when, in its eyes, private methods have not kept abreast of the need.

The patterns of medical practice have been changing. More group practices combining varying specialties are being established, providing a kind of unified medical service. There is increasing use of clinics and out-patient departments of general hospitals. In the past, as better medical tools became available in city or general hospitals, physicians tended to move their practices closer to urban areas. This centralization has, in some cases, left large territories in which few, if any, medical services were readily available. But now more demand is being made for physicians to return to suburban and rural areas.

CHOOSING A PHYSICIAN

The realistic healthy person realizes he may not stay healthy without consulting a doctor. Then his question is, "What kind of a physician makes the ideal medical adviser and where do I find him?" Before this question can be adequately answered, it is necessary to become acquainted with the training necessary for each type of medical practitioner.

REQUIREMENTS TO PRACTICE

Before a man is licensed to practice medicine, he must have met certain professional and ethical requirements. Although standards vary somewhat from state to state, he must take 3 to 4 years of premedical college work. He must then complete a 4-year training in a medical school approved by the Association of American Medical Colleges and the Council on Medical Education of the American Medical Association. In addition, most states require that he serve a 1-year internship to gain hospital experience. Before a physician is allowed to practice in a given state, he must be licensed by a board of medical examiners. This license is granted only after the physician has passed either a state or a national board examination, depending upon the particular state. In addition to these basic requirements, if a physician desires to take a residency in a hospital to receive advanced training or to meet the requirements for a given specialty in medicine, he must spend additional years (2 to 5) in training.

The standards for training physicians, as well as the ethics of medical practice, are set by the medical profession itself. Insofar as possible the profession attempts to regulate the ethics of its members. Much of this regulation is handled through the local and county medical societies. Most of them have adopted standards for their members on such things as prohibiting advertising, refraining from guaranteeing cures, adhering to all legalities regarding taking of a human life and the administration of drugs, cooperating with legal authorities, and giving evidence, through all public and private contacts, of their trustworthiness. Admittedly, some physicians fail to meet all of these standards. In choosing a physician, we have both the right and the obligation to be satisfied with the reputation, private and public, of the man to whom we entrust our lives.

A FAMILY PHYSICIAN

Everyone should have a physician whom he can regard as a personal or family physician. This physician should know his patients well and provide their basic medical care. In addition, he should advise the services of specialists when required. General family care can usually be provided by either the general practitioner or the general internist.

GENERAL PRACTITIONER

Traditionally, Americans looked to a single physician to diagnose and treat all family's illnesses. The physician practiced general medicine and attempted to handle the full range of health conditions. Twenty years ago general practitioners (GPs) outnumbered specialists three to one. Today less than half of the licensed physicians are in general practice (Fig. 10.1). They are more commonly found practicing in rural, semirural, and suburban areas.

A physician may practice general medicine after he has completed his basic training and has served his internship. Although not required, more of them today are taking additional, or postgraduate, training of some kind. Many of them have completed at least 2 years of residency training and are members of the American Academy of General Practice. Some of them direct this postgraduate study to a given area of medicine and confine their practice more or less to a type of specialty.

Some unique problems face the general practitioner today. First, in order to have a high-quality practice, he must keep abreast of the mass of new scientific information and developments. Second, he must face a demanding load of work. The average GP puts in an 11-hour workday, many seeing as many as 150 patients a week. Third, he is called upon to treat most of his patients' illnesses, since he is in the best position medically to minister to the whole person.

GENERAL INTERNIST

The specialist in internal medicine may or may not fill the role of family physician. He is generally better qualified to serve as a personal physician to adults than to children. To become an internist, he must have completed six years of training in an approved hospital after medical school and have successfully passed the examination given by the American Board of Internal Medicine. Since his training is primarily in diagnosis, he is particularly suited for preventive medicine as well as for coordinating the work of specialists needed to treat the specific problems the patient faces. Not all internists desire to practice general medicine; some confine their work to subspecialties such as allergy, heart disease, digestive-tract problems, or lung ailments. Generally, internists do not deliver babies, practice surgery, deal with troubles of the eye, or treat children.

THE SPECIALTIES

The more a physician concentrates his attention on a given system of the body, the less time he has for the whole person and the less proficient he is in general practice. To know one area of medicine in depth, he must confine himself to it to the exclusion of other areas. Such concentration has enabled medicine to make its great strides in heart surgery, cancer therapy, psychiatry, and other areas. Usually, a recognized specialist must have completed the hospital residency and passed the examination required of his particular specialty. He is then recognized as a *board diplomate* by that particular specialty.

Here is a brief description of several common fields of specialization:

INTERNAL MEDICINE

Although internal medicine often deals with the total person, the practice of internal medicine is recognized as one of the specialties. The characteristics of that specialty have already been described.

OBSTETRICS AND GYNECOLOGY

Obstetrics, the care of the woman in pregnancy and childbirth, is frequently combined with gynecology, the care of woman's diseases. Stressing preventive medicine, the obstetrician sees the mother early in pregnancy, supervises her health, and handles the delivery. Such attention has reduced infant mortality to a low rate in this country.

PEDIATRICS

Pediatricians specialize in the care of infants and children. They advise parents, give checkups, diagnose congenital deformities, administer immunizations, treat childhood diseases, and so on. Some pediatricians confine themselves to certain types of children's illnesses, such as cardiology or pediatric allergy.

SURGERY

The surgeon is concerned with operating upon the patient to correct an unwanted condition. Surgery may involve removing a cancer, repairing a damaged heart, stopping a brain hemorrhage, or setting a broken bone. This specialty commonly tends to be subdivided into specific areas—neurosurgery, thoracic surgery, orthopedic surgery, and so on.

PSYCHIATRY

The psychiatrist deals with emotional illnesses and disturbances. He generally treats his patients through psychotherapy, shock therapy, drugs, or combinations of these. Some psychiatrists are also neurologists. To be a psychiatrist a person must first earn an M.D. degree, then study psychiatry.

Other fields of medical specialty include:

Anesthesiology, the administering of general and local anesthetics;

Dermatology, the treatment of diseases of the skin;

Neurology, the treatment of physical diseases of the brain and nervous system;

Ophthalmology, the treatment of the eye and its diseases;

Otorhinolaryngology, the treatment of diseases of the ear, nose, and throat;

Pathology, the study of the structural changes which cause or are caused by disease;

Proctology, the treatment of diseases of the rectum and anus;

Radiology, the diagnosis and treatment of disease by means of X rays, radium, and other radioactive sources;

Urology, the treatment of diseases and abnormalities of the urinary tract in the female and urinary and genital (urogenital) tract in the male.

In all, there are 20 recognized fields of medical specialization. Each is governed by its respective American Board for purposes of examination and certification.

OSTEOPATHY

Recent development in the relationship between osteopathy and medicine in certain states requires that something be said here about this field. Originally, osteopathy was based on a theory proposed in 1870 by Dr. Andrew Still. This theory held that disease could be based on disturbed nerve functions resulting from a pinching of the nerves as they leave the spinal column. This theory considered a disease or condition in any particular organ of the body to be due to a malcondition in the nerve supplying that organ.

The medical profession has considered this theory unfounded and contradictory to our knowledge of human anatomy and pathology. Over the course of years, however, osteopathic physicians have been quietly abandoning many of the peculiar tenets originally held in osteopathy and have increasingly emphasized the practice of sound medicine. This change has progressed to the point where their training and practice is similar to that of traditional medicine. However, osteopaths are usually barred from practicing in medical hospitals. Moves have been initiated in various states by state medical societies to unite the osteopathic profession with medicine, but unification has been accomplished in only one state so far. California, recognizing the quality of osteopathic training in that state, classified most of its osteopathic physicians as Medical Doctors (M.D.s) in 1962. All former osteopathic colleges in that state now bestow the M.D. degree upon their graduates. Significantly, this move came about as the result of a joint effort between osteopathic and medical societies within that state.

Some families prefer the services of an osteopathic physician. A qualified osteopathic physician may satisfactorily serve as their family physician.

TYPES OF PRACTICE

In recent years there has been another significant change in the nature of medical practice. Physicians have increasingly favored banding together in various kinds of groups to provide better care than they could give when located in isolated, single-man offices. Although the clinic idea has been commonly used for years in larger medical centers, such as the Mayo Clinic in Rochester, Minnesota, the average local physician practiced independently prior to World War II. Since 1946 the number of medical groups and the number of physicians in the groups have tripled. Various types of group practices can now be found in any community.

The tendency is for group practices to represent something more than simple office-sharing. More commonly, it is an organization of full-time physicians with centralized bookkeeping and laboratory facilities. In the main, medical groups consist of physicians from different specialties banding together with the idea of giving complete medical care to their patients. The majority of them include fewer than six physicians. Since the physicians work to some extent as a team, this arrangement allows for more frequent consultation and for less inconvenience to the patient in making and keeping appointments.

SELECTING THE RIGHT PHYSICIAN

In seeking medical care, an individual will have to determine what his family's needs are and then settle on what is available. If he is seeking general medical care, he may prefer either a physician in general practice or several specialists in selected branches of medicine. Since some general practitioners further restrict themselves to a narrow branch of practice, the family will need to know the nature of a physician's practice. If there are young children in the family, the physician chosen should be one who enjoys working with children. Elderly people may prefer choosing one who enjoys geriatrics. If a family cannot find the single ideal physician, it may be desirable to settle for several specialists, such as a pediatrician for the children and an internist for the adults.

In choosing a physician, a family may find it useful to follow some or all of the following suggestions:

1. Select the names of a number of family physicians in the general area. A physician's office should be located close enough to make medical care readily accessible. It is a good idea to choose one whose office is located either in the patient's home town or in his part of the city. Compose a list of names from suggestions given by friends, a local hospital, or the local medical society.

2. Look into the credentials of each physician on the list by contacting the local or county medical society. Find out whether he is licensed to practice in this state. Determine if he has taken additional training beyond basic medical training, and if so, where and when. Check on how long he has been practicing. If he is a general practitioner, find out if he is a member of the American Academy of General Practice; if he is an internist, see if he has been accepted as a fellow in the American College of Physicians. Although these memberships do not necessarily guarantee a good medical man, they are some indication of a physician's interest in improving himself. Membership in the local medical society is important. Not all physicians who are licensed to practice are accepted for membership in these societies. Acceptance is based upon a physician's adherence to the ethical standards of the society.

3. Find out if a physician is a staff member of, or practices in, an accredited hospital. A phone call or visit to the hospital administrator can supply a person with this answer. Good hospitals select their members with care. Remember, if a person must go to a hospital, he will be permitted the services of his family physician only if the physician is allowed to practice there.

4. Evaluate the physicians on the list with friends and neighbors who have gone to them. Look for reasons why individuals like or dislike their physicians. If a person detects any pattern or repetition of complaint, it could well be a problem with the physician and not just the grievances of a patient. The person should likewise overlook excessive praise if he suspects it is unrealistic rather than an objective evaluation.

5. The patient should make an appointment to see a physician he would most like to have. He should find out if the physician is accepting new patients and if his office is neat and clean and well run.

The patient should discuss his family needs with the physician, determine whether or not the physician could supply most of them, discuss the specialists he consults with. He should find out whether the physician can be expected to make house calls, if he is usually available for emergencies and, if not, whether another physician fills in for him and who that other physician is. The patient should be frank in discussing with the physician his fee schedule in relation to those of other physicians in the same community.

6. When the patient has left the physician's office, he should review his visit. Is he pleased with the physician's personality? Does he seem to be the sort of physician he would want to confide in? Was he businesslike and thorough? If he can answer these questions affirmatively, he has found his family physician.

THE PATIENT-PHYSICIAN RELATIONSHIP

The patient will, in all probability, expect a satisfying relationship with his physician. However, neither the patient nor the physician should be exposed to unreasonable expectations about human relationships. As a patient one is entitled to receive careful, effective service, including use of necessary laboratory tests and consultations with appropriate specialists in order to provide himself with adequate treatment. Although it is not always within the physician's power to cure—and sometimes not even to provide relief—the patient should always be able to feel that his physician is doing his best.

The physician should administer inoculations or have them administered. He should advise the family, particularly when it includes children, as to when inoculations should be given. A careful physician will notify adults when certain kinds of periodic examinations should be made. Then his suggestions should be acted upon. In the practice of preventive medicine, it is sometimes hard for patients to grasp the full benefit of medical care and to justify the cost of it. A good physician will not suggest treatment or prescribe medicines he does not think the patient needs. Remember, a physician would much rather keep a person from getting ill than attempt to bring a patient back to health once he is ailing. Prevention of illness is not only easier, but also less painful—and cheaper.

If a patient is not completely satisfied with a physician's diagnosis and treatment, he ought to ask for further consultation with his or another physician. If the patient is convinced that he can no longer trust the medical care provided by his physician, he may seek out a new one. However, before this step is taken, the patient should be sure that a new physician will be able to offer him better treatment. There are often various ways to treat a given malady. Every physician will have his weak spots, his moments of fatigue, his failings. There is value to be gained in building up a personal health history with one physician. In the event the patient seeks a new physician, he should first be sure a basic improvement in medical care will be gained rather than mere relief from petty grievances.

If he is to expect medical care, the patient should be acquainted with a physician who will be able to provide medical care when it is needed. Some individuals moving into a new community fail to contact a new physician until they need him in an emergency or late at night. Then, if they encounter any difficulty in obtaining care, they make complaints against the medical profession. It is legitimate for a physician to question what responsibility he has toward a nonpatient who has made no attempt to acquire a family physician, but who expects care in the middle of the night.

If a patient is not satisfied with a physician's fee schedule, it is the patient's obligation to discuss it frankly with the physician. If the cost of medical care is imposing a hardship on the patient or his family, the physician wants to know about it. Often, low-cost medical care is provided where conditions warrant it. The patient should be open and fair in discussing costs with his physician, and the physician should be expected to be understanding and fair in return.

In relations with his physician, the patient should treat him the way the patient would want to be treated and expect that the physician will behave similarly. A physician can give his best service when he feels his patients appreciate his efforts. As much as he would enjoy being able to cure every physical ailment, medical research has not provided him with all the necessary answers to accomplish this aim. But a good physician will go just as far in diagnosis and treatment as his ability, training, available facilities, and patients allow him to go.

PARAMEDICAL PROFESSIONS

Complete health service requires the services of a number of professions. These workers are employed in many places—hospitals, pharmacies, nursing homes, laboratories, and private offices. Below is a limited discussion of a few significant paramedical workers.

DENTISTRY

Dentistry treats ailments or abnormalities of the gums and teeth and attempts to prevent their recurrence. The dentist does this by locating and filling cavities; extracting teeth, if such procedure is warranted; straightening crooked teeth; treating gum and mouth diseases; and replacing missing teeth with artificial dentures (prostheses) constructed to give each patient chewing comfort and efficiency. As in preventive medicine, there has been increasing emphasis on prevention of tooth diseases by routine cleaning of teeth, fluoridation of water supplies, and adequate periodic brushing. The majority of dentists are general practitioners who provide many types of dental care, although the small number of specialists is increasing. The specialties of dentistry deal with *orthodontia,* straightening teeth; *oral surgery,* extraction of teeth and surgical procedures involving the soft tissues of the oral cavity as well as the body structures of the mandible and maxilla; *periodontia,* treating the tissues that support the teeth; *prosthodontics,* making artificial teeth or dentures; *pedodontia,* dentistry for children; and *oral pathology,* treating diseases of the mouth.

Dental training consists of four years of professional training following two to four years of required college work. The dental specialties usually require two or three years of additional professional training.

NURSING

More people are engaged in the nursing services than in any other health occupation (Fig. 10.2). The nursing team is led by the professional or *registered nurse* (R.N.), but also includes the vocational nurses, nursing aides, orderlies, and attendants.

Registered nurses handle the largest share of nursing services. They administer medications and treatments prescribed by physicians; observe, evaluate, and record symptoms and the progress of patients; assist in patient education and rehabilitation; improve the surroundings of the patients; and instruct other medical personnel and students. Although the majority of them work in hospitals, they also perform in private duty, offices, public health, industrial plants, and nursing schools.

Professional nursing training requires two to three years of professional training with or without other college work. Additional training can be taken to qualify for a nursing specialty in obstetrics, pediatrics, psychiatry, or surgical nursing.

MEDICAL TECHNOLOGY

As the physician works to detect, diagnose, and treat diseases, he will frequently call for laboratory tests to confirm the presence or absence of a condition. Much of the laboratory work can be time-consuming. Therefore *medical technologists* are trained to assist the physician. Generally working directly under the supervision of a pathologist, the technologist makes blood counts, urinalyses, and skin tests; examines body fluids and tissue samples microscopically; runs cultures of microorganisms to determine their identity and reaction to drugs; types and cross-matches blood samples; measures basal metabolism; and analyzes food, water, or other materials for bacteria.

The great majority of medical technologists work in hospitals and conduct tests in connection with the examination and treatment of patients. The medical technologist is not to be confused with the medical

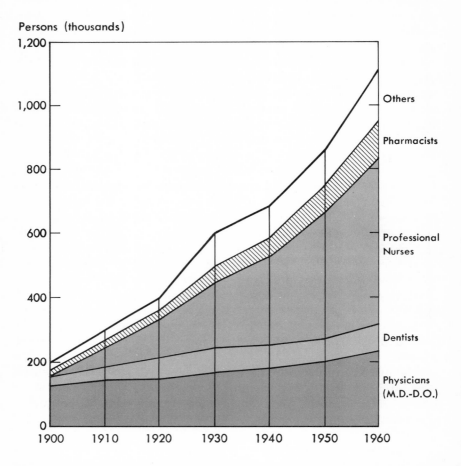

Fig. 10.2 Growth of selected health populations. (*Manpower in the 1960s,* Public Health Manpower Source Book No. 18, Public Health Service Publication No. 263.)

technician or laboratory assistant. The technologist has one or more years of professional training, based heavily on the basic biological and physical sciences; and, usually, schools of medical technology require at least three years of preprofessional college work.

PHARMACY

Pharmacists help in medical care through making drugs and medicine available and providing information on their use. They dispense prescriptions ordered by medical practitioners and sell general drugs and medical supplies. They are trained to understand the composition of drugs and to be responsible for the drug's purity and strength. Only a registered pharmacist may fill a prescription. A registered pharmacist must be a graduate of an accredited college of pharmacy and have passed a rigorous examination in the state in which he practices. The training of four years of professional study and one year of internship includes the compounding of drugs. However, many drug products today are manufactured in the form in which the patient purchases them, not requiring compounding by the retail druggist. But this fact does not diminish the importance and responsibility of the pharmacist. He is responsible for all drugs dispensed and has the prerogative to question any prescription as being dangerous in either quantity or kind. If not fully satisfied as to a drug's safety, he can validly refuse to fill a prescription.

PHYSICAL THERAPY

This branch of the healing arts serves in the rehabilitation of people with injuries or diseases affecting muscles, joints, nerves, and bones. The *physical therapist* works under the direction of a physician to administer therapy through the use of therapeutic exercise and massage, and various types of treatment with heat, water, light, and electricity. Physical therapy has been invaluable in the treating of victims of poliomyelitis, cerebral palsy, arthritis, and muscular dystrophy. Preparation for this type of work usually calls for a one- or two-year graduate program.

OPTOMETRY

The *optometrist* is especially trained and licensed to examine and refract eyes, determine the deviation from normal, and prescribe lenses and visual training that does not require drugs or surgery. He should not be confused with *ophthalmologists* or *oculists* (medical specialists dealing with the medical and surgical care of the eyes and their refractive corrections) or *opticians* (those who interpret the prescription of the ophthalmologist or optometrist and select the frames to hold the lenses). The usual training consists of two years of preoptometry education and three or four years of professional education. Most graduate optometrists are in private practice.

PODIATRY

Sometimes called a *chiropodist,* the *podiatrist* diagnoses and treats diseases and deformities of the feet or tries to prevent their occurrence in his patients. His work is important since more than half of the people in the United States have foot troubles ranging from simple corns to difficulties requiring special shoes or foot appliances, or even to problems requiring the attention of a medical specialist. The field of podiatry is far from overcrowded. Most podiatrists, when they have completed their four years of professional training after the required preprofessional training, engage in private practice.

CHIROPRACTIC

Chiropractic is a system of treatment based on the belief that the nervous system largely determines a person's state of health and that any interference with this system impairs normal functions and lowers the body's resistance to disease. Patients are treated primarily by specific adjustment of parts of the body, especially the spinal column. X ray is used extensively to aid in locating the source of the difficulty. Supplementary therapeutic measures such as diet, exercise, rest, water, light, and heat are used. Chiropractic treatment *does not* include the use of drugs or surgery. The training of chiropractors, although ranging from two to four years, consists in most states of four years of training in a chiropractic school following graduation from high school. Graduation does not qualify a chiropractor to practice in all states, since not all states license the practice of chiropractic.

The training of a chiropractor limits him to the degree that it does not stress knowledge of the diseases to which the body is subject. Since many of the body's ailments are due to infectious or degenerative diseases, any field of the healing arts that does not qualify a practitioner in the diagnosis and treatment of these kinds of maladies restricts his usefulness. Most chiropractors are better trained in therapeutics, such as body manipulation and adjustment, than they are in any adequate understanding and diagnosis of the underlying disease. Consequently, although the chiropractor may bring relief to conditions where the spinal column is maladjusted, there are many common medical conditions he is not prepared to care for. Accordingly, a chiropractor should not be sought out as a family physician.

FACILITIES FOR PATIENT CARE

As modern medicine has progressed, the providing of improved medical care has become more involved. Not too many years ago the majority of patients were seen in their homes by the traveling family physician. The diagnosis and treatment was limited to either what was on hand or what the physician could bring with him. The home served as a kind of "hospital" for the delivery of babies and the treatment of pneumonia and tuberculosis, and as a nursing home for those suffering from chronic diseases. Only patients with the most complicated conditions were admitted to the town hospital.

Today only minor illnesses are cared for at home. Improved standards of diagnosis and treatment require facilities that are available only in physicians' offices, clinics, nursing homes, and hospitals.

CLINICS AND NURSING HOMES

The services of hospitals are frequently supplemented by the services of clinics and nursing homes. Clinics are often set up in conjunction with a hospital to provide various types of specialized services for patients with venereal diseases, tuberculosis, cancer, and communicable diseases, and for patients needing maternal and child dental care. Their services are for patients whose cases are not severe enough to require hospitalization, yet who need medical care. Although dealing in diagnosis and treatment, they direct their effort toward instructing expectant mothers, providing social services, and giving advice on matters of nutrition and other public health problems. Patients who can afford the service are charged; however, many patients pay little or nothing.

Nursing homes provide services for convalescing patients or for those with chronic illnesses, but not on as large a scale as a hospital supplying qualified services. They help to free needed hospital beds for more acute illnesses. The quality of their care should be no different from that of a hospital.

HOSPITALS

Hospitals provide complete medical facilities for the acutely ill, including expensive, centralized equipment and services not available in the local physician's office. The centralized hospital enables the busy physician to see his patients as a group. It also serves to protect the public from individuals with easily communicable diseases. The greater use of hospitals today, compared to that of a few years ago, along with the natural increase in population, has substantially increased the demand for available hospital facilities.

Generally, hospitals have been constructed with funds from communities, private philanthropists, local or state tax dollars, and grants of federal monies. During the past two decades the number of available hospital beds in the United States has doubled. In addition, costly hospital facilities have been increased. Although many communities have been able to keep up with the demand in providing up-to-date hospital facilities, some parts of the country today either lack hospital facilities or have substandard ones. Yet in spite of the continuing need for more and better hospital facilities, considerable thought must precede the locating of new hospitals and the enlarging of existing ones. Preliminary questions that need to be answered include: Will the hospital be large enough to provide necessary equipment and facilities? Are there enough physicians in the vicinity to staff it adequately? Are enough nurses, trained technicians, and other qualified personnel available to man it? Can it be large enough to make the operation of the hospital plant self-supporting? Is the surrounding population large enough to warrant the cost of operating it? If there is already an existing hospital in the area, would it be cheaper to add more beds to it than to build an entirely new hospital and duplicate expensive equipment?

KINDS OF HOSPITALS

Obviously hospitals are not all alike. Hospitals are often established to provide certain kinds of medical services to certain groups of people. Generally, hospitals can be grouped according to their type of ownership and method of operation. The grouping includes (1) governmental hospitals, (2) voluntary hospitals, and (3) proprietary hospitals.

GOVERNMENTAL HOSPITALS

The federal government has established institutions for personnel in the military services and the Public Health Service and their dependents, for American Indians, for merchant seamen, for veterans, for patients of leprosy, and for narcotics addicts. Individual states have established either *specialized* hospitals for individuals such as the emotionally disturbed patients or those with tuberculosis, or *general* hospitals, which are usually associated with a state-supported medical school. City and county hospitals are commonly general hospitals providing general medical care, but frequently giving special attention to communicable disease control and the care of the indigent. In many cases, the government hospital is set up for the long-term patient.

VOLUNTARY HOSPITALS

Voluntary hospitals are public hospitals set up on a nonprofit basis. They have been established by churches, philanthropic individuals, charitable organizations, or the local community. They are run by governing boards, selected from the community, which are responsible for all phases of operation, financing, and construction. Mostly short-term institutions, these hospitals provide for more than two thirds of all hospital admissions. Although these hospitals attempt to meet their own expenses, they frequently are underwritten financially by local organizations. Since the end of World War II, the federal government has aided somewhat in the construction of voluntary hospitals by making monies available under the Hill-Burton Act.

PROPRIETARY HOSPITALS

Owned and administered by individuals or corporations, proprietary hospitals are set up as profit-seeking investments. They are often established by real estate promoters and then leased to groups of physicians at no cost to the community. Although this arrangement frequently appeals at first to the community, the operations of proprietary hospitals in many places have raised some degree of controversy and question. They are primarily short-term hospitals catering to the most profitable type of hospital business. They hesitate to admit patients who are unable to pay their way. Frequently they are small and unaccredited (only about one third of them are accredited). Although not all of them are poorly administered, they generally have gained a questionable reputation.

ACCREDITATION OF HOSPITALS

Concern over standards of hospital care resulted in the establishment in 1952 of the Joint Committee on Accreditation of Hospitals (JCAH). A voluntary, nonprofit organization, it is sponsored by the American College of Physicians, the American College of Surgeons, the American Hospital Association, and the American Medical Association. Its functions have been to set up national standards of hospital care, to accredit hospitals meeting these standards, and to see that these standards are maintained in accredited hospitals. In order to become accredited, a hospital must have 25 or more beds, have been in operation at least one year, be listed with the American Hospital Association, and have passed a rigid inspection by JCAH physicians. Upon application, a hospital is thoroughly evaluated in all respects, including cleanliness; laboratories; food handling; records; and, in particular, the practice of its staff physicians. A full accreditation is good for three years, following which the hospital must be re-examined.

Increasing value is being given to JCAH accreditation. A nonaccredited hospital may not train interns, residents, or nurses, all of whom contribute to making a better hospital. The Blue Cross insurance organizations have, in some cases, refused to make payments of insurance monies to nonaccredited hospitals. Since many of the larger hospitals in the country are accredited, hospitals representing over 85 percent of the total bed space are accredited. Over three fourths of all voluntary hospitals are accredited, compared to only one third of all proprietary ones.

HOW TO CHOOSE A HOSPITAL

Although many individuals today live in communities in which there is but a single hospital, an increasing majority of people live within easy commuting distance of two or more hospitals. Some of these individuals at some time or another have the choice of selecting a hospital. The choice of a physician may be based in part on which hospital he practices in. In our larger cities, a physician may have access to more than one hospital; in this case, the patient may select the one he prefers. Even though he may never have the choice of a hospital, any individual concerned with the quality of health care he is getting should want to be informed on his local hospital. For these reasons, one should have some basis for judging a hospital. In so doing there are three basic questions that should be asked.

1. *Is the hospital accredited?* Accreditation by the JCAH will not guarantee a first-rate hospital, but it will mean that it has met certain minimal standards, both in facilities and in staff practice.

2. *Is it a teaching hospital?* A hospital that has a program for training personnel is equipped to provide better medical service. The higher the level of this teaching, the better. The best situation is one in which a hospital is associated with a medical school. Here one can expect to find well-qualified specialists as instructors and qualified resident physicians training in the specialties. Although there are only about 200 medical school hospitals in the country, many more hospitals have some type of resident training program. If this type is not available, one should look for a hospital that at least trains interns or nurses.

3. *Who owns the hospital?* In other words, is it a voluntary, non-profit community hospital or a privately owned, proprietary hospital? Generally, a voluntary hospital is to be preferred over a proprietary one. Ultimate responsibility for the conduct in a voluntary hospital rests with its board of trustees chosen from the community, whereas in the proprietary hospital responsibility rests only with its "owners," and its quality will rise and fall with the owners' dedication, sense of ethics, or desire to make a profit.

DECISIONS BEFORE ENTERING A HOSPITAL

Even after a person is satisfied that his hospital is a good one, it is advisable, when it is suggested that he or a member of his family enter the hospital, to learn whether the hospital is the best place to obtain the needed services. For instance, could the suggested treatment be taken care of just as well in a clinic providing infant or child care or in a nursing home for older individuals? Elderly people sometimes develop serious psychological problems over entering a hospital. Cost, also, is not to be overlooked, even by those holding some form of hospitalization insurance. Even if one has such insurance, the more it is utilized, the higher will be the premium rates among its subscribers. Accordingly, hospitalization for convenience only cannot be sanctioned. Generally speaking, if a person is fortunate in having a reliable physician, he should be able to rely upon that physician's recommendation on matters of hospital admission. A good physician will always be concerned with his patient's best interests.

Upon entering a hospital, a person may have the choice of a ward or a semiprivate or private room. Although a ward location costs less, the patient will also have less privacy. The room selection should depend upon the need for privacy and other personal requirements, and financial ability.

Patients admitted to teaching hospitals and those who are not under the care of a specific physician are often assigned to intern or resident physicians. Since such students are being trained in diagnosis and treatment, patients attended by them will also be under the observation of teaching specialists. Such patients often, therefore, receive the best of professional care.

SUMMARY

I. Modern Medicine
   A. Aims
      1. Good medical care must be available to all people.
      2. Prevention of disease must be given top attention.
      3. The needs of the whole man must be ministered to, not just that bit of him that is diseased.
      4. Research into unconquered diseases and better methods of treatment must continue to be pursued.
   B. Problems
      1. Shortage of physicians.
      2. Rapidity of change in medical knowledge and technology.
      3. Rise in medical costs.
   C. Changes in the Medical Profession
      1. De-emphasis of narrow specialties and re-emphasis of general medicine.
      2. Feeling that more people must be covered by health insurance.
      3. Increased use of group practices, clinics, and out-patient departments of general hospitals.
II. Choosing a Physician—involves choosing a satisfactory medical adviser and knowing the facts regarding his training and background.
   A. Has he obtained the requirements to practice.
   B. Family physician
      1. General practitioner (GP)—practices general medicine, either by choice or because he lacks training in one of the specialties.

      2. General internist—a specialist who confines himself primarily to diagnosis, and will, if necessary, refer a patient to other specialists.

  C. The specialties

      1. Internal medicine—diagnosing internal ailments and treating them with medicine if advisable.

      2. Obstetrics and gynecology—care of women in pregnancy and childbirth, and care of women's ailments.

      3. Pediatrics—care of infants and children.

      4. Surgery—operating for unwanted conditions.

      5. Psychiatry—treating emotional illnesses and disturbances.

      6. Anesthesiology—administering general and local anesthesia.

      7. Neurology—treating brain and nervous system diseases.

      8. Ophthalmology—treating the eye and its diseases.

      9. Pathology—identifying body structural changes and diseases.

     10. Proctology—treating diseases of the rectum and anus.

     11. Urology—dealing with diseases of the urogenital tracts.

  D. Osteopathy

      1. Originally considered diseases due to nerve malconditions.

      2. Present training and practice generally based on sound medical principles.

      3. Being incorporated with medical profession some places.

      4. Serves satisfactorily as a family physician.

  E. Types of practice

      1. The past favored the independent, single-man office.

      2. Has moved toward the group or clinical practice idea.

  F. Selecting the right physician—depends upon one's personal needs and preferences.

  G. The patient-physician relationship should

      1. Be reasonable for both.

      2. Respect a physician's professional advice.

      3. Begin with a patient contact before an emergency arises.

      4. Include satisfaction with fees charged and payments made.

III. Paramedical Professions—include medical services which help the physician to provide complete medical care; they include the following professions:

  A. Dentistry

      1. Treats abnormalities of the gums and teeth and attempts to prevent their recurrence.

      2. Includes the following branches of practice:

        a. General practice—providing general dental care.

        b. Orthodontia—straightening teeth.

        c. Oral surgery—extracting of teeth and surgical procedures.

        d. Periodontia—treating tissues that support the teeth.

        e. Prosthodontics—making artificial teeth and dentures.

        f. Pedodontia—providing children's dentistry.

        g. Oral pathology—treating diseases of the mouth.

  B. Nursing—done by a team led by the professional or registered nurse (R.N.); the team includes:

      1. Vocational nurse.

      2. Nursing aide.

      3. Orderly.

      4. Attendant.

  C. Medical technology—involves performing laboratory tests under the supervision of a pathologist.

    D. Pharmacy—involves making general drugs and medical supplies available for sale, and dispensing prescriptions ordered by a medical practitioner.
    E. Physical therapy—aids the rehabilitation of people with injuries or diseases affecting muscles, joints, and bones.
    F. Optometry—involves testing the refractive ability of the eyes, determining any deviation from normal, and prescribing lenses to provide correction without use of drugs or surgery.
    G. Podiatry (chiropody)—treats diseases and deformities of the feet, and correction and prevention of foot problems.
    H. Chiropractic—a system of treatment based on the belief that the nervous system determines a person's state of health and that physical impairments are basically related to the nervous system.

IV. Facilities for Patient Care
    A. Clinics and nursing homes supplement the services of hospitals.
    B. Hospitals provide complete medical facilities for the acutely ill patient.
        1. Kinds of hospitals grouped according to their type of ownership and administration.
            a. Government hospitals—may be federal, state, city or county.
            b. Voluntary hospitals—public hospitals operating on a nonprofit basis, governed by a board of community leaders.
            c. Proprietary hospitals—owned and administrated by individuals or corporations and are set up as profit-seeking investments.
    C. Accreditation of hospitals determined by the hospital's meeting the standards of excellence set by the Joint Committee on Accreditation of Hospitals (JCAH).
    D. Choice of a hospital may be based on the consideration of various factors, including:
        1. Is the hospital accredited (by the JCAH)?
        2. Is it a teaching hospital?
        3. Who owns the hospital?
    E. Decisions before entering a hospital should include:
        1. Whether hospital admission is required.
        2. Whether the needed care could be provided just as well in a clinic or nursing home.
        3. Whether a private or semiprivate room is required or desired.
        4. How the cost of services provided is to be paid.

Glossary

If you cannot find the word you wish in this glossary, check the index for text and glossary references.

anesthesiology (an əs thē zē ol'ə jē) (G. *an*, without; *aisthesis*, sensation). The science of anesthesia (the partial or complete loss of sensation with or without loss of consciousness resulting from the administration of drugs).

chiropodist (kī rop'ə dist) (G. *cheir*, hand; *pous*, foot). A person who specializes in the minor disorders and care of the human foot.

chiropractic (kī'rə prak'tik) (G. *cheir*, hand; *pratein*, to do). A system of therapy based upon the claim that disease is caused by abnormal function of the nervous system.

dentistry (den'tis trē) (L. *dens,* tooth). That branch of medicine dealing with the care of the teeth and related structures, as practiced by the dentist.

dermatology (dur mə tol'ə jē) (G. *derma,* skin; *logos,* understanding). The branch of medicine dealing with diagnosis and treatment of diseases of the skin.

diplomate (dip'lə māt) (G. *diploos,* double; L. *atus,* to become). A holder of a certificate of the National Board of Medical Examiners or of one of the American Boards in the Specialities.

general practitioner (prak tish'ə nər) (G. *praktike,* business). One who practices the general, usually unrestricted, profession of medicine.

government hospital (hos'pi təl) (L. *hospitalis,* pertaining to a guest). A hospital which is owned and operated by some level of government, federal, state, or city.

gynecology (gī'nə kol'ə jē) (G. *gyne,* women). The study of the diseases of the female, particularly of the genital, urinary, or rectal organs.

internal medicine (in tur'nəl med'i sin) (L. *internus,* within). That department of medicine which deals with diseases that cannot be treated surgically.

internist (in'tur nist, in tur'nist) (L. *internus,* within). One who treats internal organs and diseases (not a surgeon) and who frequently confines his practice to adults.

medical technology (med'i kəl tek nol'ə jē) (L. *medicus,* physician; G. *techne,* art). The practice of medical laboratory procedures.

National Board Examination. A national examination in the medical, dental, or paramedical professions given by Board of Examiners from that particular profession, which if passed, qualifies a person to practice in that profession. Certain states require a state examination to be passed in the profession before one is entitled to practice in that state.

neurology (nyoo rol'ə jē) (G. *neuron,* nerve). That branch of medicine dealing with the nervous system and its diseases.

obstetrics (əb stet'riks) (L. *obstetrix,* midwife). That branch of medicine which deals with the care and treatment of women during pregnancy, childbirth, and the period immediately after.

oculist (ok'yə list) (L. *oculus,* eye). A physician specializing in the treatment of diseases of the eye; also called an *ophthalmologist.*

ophthalmology (of thal mol'ə jē) (G. *ophthalmos,* eye; *logos,* study). The branch of medicine dealing with the eye and its diseases.

optician (op tish' ən) (G. *optikos,* pertaining to the eye). A person who makes or sells eyeglasses and other optical instruments.

optometry (op tom'ə trē) (G. *optos,* seen; *metron,* measure). The profession of testing the refractive powers of the eye and fitting glasses to correct eye defects.

oral pathology (or'əl pa thol'ə jē) (L. *os, or,* mouth; G. *pathos,* disease). The branch of dentistry treating the nature of diseases of the teeth. Also known as *dental pathology.*

oral surgery (or'əl sur'jə rē) (ME. *surgerie* from G. *cheirourgia,* handwork). The branch of dentistry which treats conditions of the mouth and associated structures, especially the teeth and jaws, by surgical methods.

osteopathy (os tē op'ə thē) (G. *osteon,* bone; *pathos,* disease). A system of treating ailments based on the belief that they generally result from the pressure of displaced bones on nerves, and are cured by manipulation.

otorhinolaryngology (ō'tō rī'nō lar ing gol'ə jē) (G. *otos*, ear; *rhis*, nose; *larynx*, larynx). The branch of medicine dealing with the ear, nose, and larynx and their functions and diseases.

paramedical (par ə med'i kal) (G. *para*, beyond; L. *medicari*, to heal). Having a medical aspect, or secondary relation to medicine.

pathology (pa thol'ə jē) That branch of medicine dealing with the nature of disease, especially the structural and functional changes caused by disease.

pediatrics (pē dē at'riks) (G. *paidos*, child; *iatreia*, cure). The branch of medicine which treats the development and care of children and the diseases of children and their treatment.

pedodontia (pē də don'shə) (G. *paidos*, child; *odous*, tooth). The branch of dentistry which deals with the teeth and mouth conditions of children.

periodontia (per'ē ə don'shə) (G. *peri*, around; *odous*, tooth). The branch of dentistry dealing with the study and treatment of diseases occurring around the tooth.

pharmacy (fahr'mə sē) (G. *pharmakon*, medicine). The profession which prepares and dispenses drugs and medicines.

physical therapy (fiz'i kəl ther'əpē) (G. *physikos*, natural; *therapein*, treatment). The treatment of disease by physical means (nonmedical).

physician (fi zish'ən) (Fr. *physicien* from G. *physikos*, natural). A person authorized by law to practice medicine.

podiatry (pō dī'ə trē) (G. *pous*, foot; *iatreia*, cure). The diagnosis and treatment of disorders of the foot. See **chiropodist.**

proprietary hospital (prō prī'ə ta rē) (L. *proprietarius*, pertaining to property). A hospital owned and operated by private individuals or corporations as profit-seeking investments.

proctology (prok tol'ə jē) (G. *proktos*, anus). The branch of medicine dealing with the rectum and its diseases.

prosthodontics (pros tho don'tiks) (G. *prosthesis*, "a putting to"; *odous*, tooth). The branch of dentistry dealing with the mechanics of making and fitting dental appliances and substitutes.

psychiatry (sī kī'ə trē) (G. *psyche*, soul; *iatreia*, healing). That branch of medicine which deals with the diagnosis, treatment, and prevention of mental (emotional) illness.

radiology (rā dē ol'ə jē) (L. *radius*, ray). The branch of medicine which deals with roentgen rays and other radiant energy in the diagnosis and treatment of disease.

registered nurse (rej'īs tard nurs) (L. *regere*, to record; *nutrix*, a nurse). A graduate nurse who has been registered and licensed to practice by a State Board of Nurse Examiners or other state authority.

specialist (spesh'ə list) (L. *specialis*, special). A practitioner who restricts himself to a special type of disease.

State Board Examination. A state examination in the medical, dental, or paramedical professions given by a State Board of Examiners from that particular profession, which, if passed, qualifies a person to practice that profession in that particular state. See National Board Examination also.

surgery (sur′jə rē) (ME. *surgerie,* from G. *cheirourgia,* handwork).   The branch of medicine which treats diseases, partially or completely, by manual and operative procedures.

urinalysis (yoo ri nal′i sis) (L. *urina,* urine; G. *ana,* apart; *lysis,* a loosening). Chemical or microscopic analysis of the urine.

urology (yoo rol′ə jē).   That branch of medicine dealing with the urine and urinary tract. Includes the genitourinary tract.

voluntary hospital (L. *voluntas,* will; *hospitalis,* pertaining to a guest).   A public hospital owned and operated on a nonprofit basis.

CHAPTER 11

QUACKERY

WHO IS A QUACK?

WHY PEOPLE TURN TO
QUACKERY

SOME MAJOR TYPES OF
HEALTH QUACKERY TODAY

PROTECTION AGAINST
QUACKERY

THE PERSISTENCE OF
QUACKERY

SUMMARY

Although the colorful "snake oil" salesman with his medicine show is a thing of the past, his counterpart is still very much on the scene. Today's quack is much more sophisticated than his predecessor, but his goal remains the same—to separate the unsuspecting from their money. Regardless of how sincere his interest in a person's health may seem, his real interest is financial. Today over a billion dollars a year is spent in the United States for worthless or fraudulent remedies. Although much of today's quackery involves a direct "doctor"-patient relationship, a still larger field is promotion through the mail and in drug and "health food" stores of various patent medicines and remedies of questionable value.

341

WHO IS A QUACK?

A *quack* may be defined as a boastful pretender to medical skill or one who promises medical benefits which he cannot deliver. He may attempt to go beyond the limits of medical science or to exceed the limits of his own training. The quack often sells or treats patients with a *nostrum,* a cure-all drug or machine. (Any drug, machine, or treatment for which broad, sweeping claims are made may be called a nostrum.)

A common stereotype of a quack is probably that of an odd or sinister-looking individual. On the contrary, the real quack usually inspires confidence. Quacks possess varying types of educational backgrounds. A very few licensed physicians enter into quackery, sometimes authoring books which have great sales success. More common is the quack who has chiropractic or naturopathic training. There also exists today a certain amount of "corporate quackery," where proprietary compounds ("patent medicines") are sometimes overzealously promoted by advertising departments. Any individual may enter into quackery if he has attempted to diagnose and treat a serious illness by himself, for *self-treatment is quackery.*

WHY PEOPLE TURN TO QUACKERY

FEAR, IGNORANCE, AND GULLIBILITY

Much quackery preys upon fear. Sometimes the fear already exists. For example, a man who has been told by his physician that he has an incurable disease lives in fear—fear of death, fear of pain, fear of the unknown. He will grasp at any hope offered by the quack, regardless of how unscientific or expensive the remedy may be. Sometimes fear keeps a person from seeing an ethical physician in the first place. Afraid of surgery, he turns instead to the quack, who always promises a cure without surgery. Sometimes the quack must create fear where none exists. A common approach of the food quack, for example, is the use of scare tactics which will be further discussed later in the chapter.

Gullibility, especially in combination with ignorance, is the chief ally of the quack. A segment of the American public is almost unbelievably gullible. There are those who accept anything they hear as truth and anything they read in print as absolute gospel. The quack is able to make his sales talks, lectures, and literature seem entirely credible, often to well-educated people who should know better. Education does, however, provide the best protection against the claims of the quack.

TEEN-AGER TO SENIOR CITIZEN

Although no age group is immune to the quack, the teen-ager and the senior citizen contribute significantly to his support. The teen-ager is particularly receptive to mail-order quackery. He finds many deceptive advertisements in some of the magazines which appeal to his age group and may receive many direct mail advertisements, since his name is often sold for "sucker lists." Since the teen-ager is often very self-conscious about his appearance, most of the products offered promise good looks, sex appeal, and popularity. Some of the current offerings include products to add weight, take off weight, build muscles, and add to the bust line. Other popular products offer more attractive skin or hair.

The senior citizen finds appeal in products that promise to renew lost youth and vigor. He is often duped in schemes to relieve arthritis, prostate conditions, colitis, and "tired blood." The nutrition quack finds a ready market in elderly people who are eager to believe that all their aches and pains can disappear through the use of a food supplement. In addition, the elderly are attracted to so-called "clinics," "health ranches," and "hospitals" which claim cures for all types of chronic diseases through chiropractic, diet, and other limited measures. Such places offer the hope of a quick, easy, painless treatment, usually provided by practitioners who are not licensed physicians.

SOME MAJOR TYPES OF HEALTH QUACKERY TODAY

CANCER QUACKERY

Cancer quacks are estimated to make about $50 million a year for worthless treatments. Although some of their methods have repeatedly been exposed as quackery by agencies of the United States Government, these charlatans continue to prosper. Cancer quackery can be one of the most tragic of rackets when a person having an early cancer spends vital time waiting for a worthless remedy to cure his cancer. In too many such cases the cancers reach an incurable stage before the victims seek ethical treatment, although early treatment by an ethical physician using standard methods might have resulted in a complete cure.

The strongest ally of the cancer quack is many people's fear of surgery. The quack always offers treatment without surgery, but the ethical physician knows that surgery is the most positive treatment for most types of cancer.

The quack is very successful in treating cancers which never existed and thereby gains some of his most solid supporters. The patient who feels he may have cancer, not having seen an ethical physician, will almost always have his suspicions confirmed by the quack. After a series of expensive treatments, the quack will pronounce the nonexistent cancer cured. The patient is then forever grateful to the quack for having saved his life and is eager to write letters of testimonial, picket the state capitol, testify in court, or do whatever will aid the quack in his running battle with the authorities.

ARTHRITIS QUACKERY

Arthritis is a general term used to indicate an inflammation of the joints. About 12 million Americans suffer from this painful, crippling condition. The ethical physician can offer a complete cure for very few of the many types of arthritis. Thus the door is wide open for one of the most lucrative fields of quackery. An estimated 10,000 arthritis quacks sell about a quarter of a billion dollars worth of useless drugs, devices, and treatments each year. Half of all arthritis sufferers try some of these worthless remedies.

The least offensive (though often extremely high priced) of the arthritis remedies are the glorified aspirin products. At the other extreme are the dangerous drugs and the treatments which may actually be harmful. Since by their nature some types of arthritis tend to come and go, a worthless treatment is often given credit for curing arthritis when actually the symptoms would have disappeared even if nothing had been done. As with every other disease, the ethical physician can still be relied upon to offer the most effective, up-to-date treatment.

"REDUCE WITHOUT DIETING"

There is always a ready market for any treatment which promises weight loss without unpleasant diets. Since one out of every four Americans attempts to lose weight each year, any device offered is sure to find acceptance among some of these 50 million people. Some of the most common schemes are

Reducing pills sold by mail or over the counter without prescription. Such pills, if strong enough to be effective, should be used only under medical supervision.

Dietless reducing plans of every description. Many plans, although advertised as dietless, actually do involve a strict diet which must be followed if any weight is to be lost.

Vibrators. It is impossible to vibrate weight away.

Massaging devices. Neither can weight be massaged off.

Spot reducing. It is absolutely impossible to control from which part of the body fat is lost.

Reducing creams. Obviously worthless, yet their sales are brisk.

This is but a sampling of the many approaches available to the person who is looking for an "easy" way to lose weight. Some of the plans promoted are worthless but harmless; others can actually be dangerous.

FOOD FADS

Ten million Americans are today living in the shadow of confusion cast by the food faddists and "health food" quacks. These unfortunate people find themselves following expensive, complicated, and often unpleasant diets; rather than being better fed, they are actually more likely to suffer a nutritional deficiency than those who eat ordinary diets, following the simple rules of basic nutrition.

In addition to their sale in "health food" stores, "health food" products and food supplements are commonly promoted in two other ways. One method is by door-to-door selling, in which the salesman takes advantage of the privacy of the home to prescribe his expensive food supplement product as a remedy for any disease or condition the resident may mention. The other widespread approach is through "health food" or "nutrition" lectures. The lecturer, posing as a highly qualified scientist, gives an emotionally appealing presentation of a mixture of scientific fact and superstition concerning nutrition, never failing to mention repeatedly whatever product he happens to be pushing. What appears to be science is in reality *pseudo-science,* with lectures and slick-paper brochures emphasizing half-truths, quarter-truths, and false implications.

Regardless of the sales approach used, the food quack makes use of scare tactics, basing his presentation on certain modern myths used by almost all operators in his field. Although each idea contains an element of truth, the conclusions drawn are not supported by scientific evidence. Commonly used misrepresentations include the following:

1. *Myth that all diseases are due to faulty diet.*   There is absolutely no basis for such a claim.

2. *Myth of the indispensable food product.*   Promoters often represent their products as being the *only* source of a vital food substance. Every substance known to be important in nutrition is available from a variety of common grocery store foods. The promoter often counters this fact with the implication that his product contains a substance not yet known to science. Of course, there is absolutely no basis for such a claim.

3. *Myth that soil depletion causes malnutrition.*   A common story is that repeated cropping of the land has removed some substance, which is therefore lacking from the foods produced. The only substance for which a deficiency in the soil is reflected in the crop produced is iodine. Since people today obtain adequate iodine through diet and the use of iodized salt, iodine deficiency is rare. If any other mineral is lacking from the soil, this deficiency is reflected in a lowered

quantity of produce, but the nutritional *quality* is not affected.

4. *Myth of "organic" or "natural" foods.* If there is a key word in the "health food" business, it must be either "organic" or "natural." According to the biological or chemical definitions of the word organic (see a dictionary), all foods are organic. The claim is often made that foods grown with commercial fertilizers are inferior to those grown with "natural" fertilizer (manure). The fallacy of this claim lies in the fact that a plant can absorb from the soil only certain simple inorganic nutrients. If manure is used as fertilizer, the organic compounds present must be broken down by bacteria into the same simple compounds present in commercial fertilizers before any absorption into the roots of the plant can take place.

A related claim is that the synthetically produced vitamins are inferior to naturally occurring vitamins. This statement is usually made by salesmen of high-priced food supplement products to indicate the superiority of their products over lower priced products. Actually, the man-made vitamins are chemically identical to the naturally occurring vitamins, are absorbed in the same manner, and function in the body in exactly the same way.

The very word *chemical* is often used in a derogatory manner by the salesman who apparently does not know or chooses to ignore the fact that all food is nothing but a mixture of chemicals. He deplores the use of chemical food additivès such as antioxidants, coloring agents, mold inhibitors, and numerous other additives important to modern food processing. Since the 1958 amendment to the Federal Food and Drug Law, such chemicals have been thoroughly screened by their manufacturers for any possible harmful effect before the Federal Food and Drug Administration permits their use in foods. In the amounts used, today's additives are perfectly safe. The same salesman is apt to decry even the use of pasteurization, a process of indisputable value and importance for milk and certain other food products.

5. *Myth of overprocessing.* The food quack exaggerates the loss of food value through modern food-processing methods. Although some loss definitely does occur. the public today is much better fed than at any time in the past as a direct result of modern food technology. Highly nutritious processed fruits, vegetables, and meats are available throughout the year, rather than just during limited seasons. Today's processing methods are often less destructive to vitamins than were those of the past.

BEAUTY AIDS AND BALDNESS REMEDIES

Human vanity provides a steady income for numerous beauty and baldness quacks and companies preparing "miracle" cosmetics. There is always something new in the beauty cream business, often featuring such exotic ingredients as mink oil, orchid pollen, royal jelly, vitamins, and turtle oil. Excessively dry skin is definitely benefited by the use of a simple oil, lotion, or cream, but any effort to "nourish" the skin through the external application of vitamins or other substances is futile. Skin is nourished from within, and beautiful skin is usually the result of good diet, cleanliness, and general good health. Hormones *are* absorbed through the skin, but because of their possible side effects a person should consult a physician before using hormone skin creams.

Expensive baldness treatments are sold by mail through magazine and newspaper ads, and traveling baldness "clinics" often temporarily operate in hotels and motels. Although the baldness quacks sometimes include in their ads a brief statement that they can't cure hereditary baldness, the implication is always left that they can cure *your* case of baldness. The person who is losing excessive hair should see a qualified dermatologist (M.D.), who can determine whether or not the baldness is of a type that can be treated. Baldness of an irregular, blotchy nature may be the result of some disease or local infection and may be treatable by the dermatologist. Certainly, the ethical dermatologist is able to offer every method of treatment available from the quack, along with many effective types of therapy the quack cannot use. If the baldness is of an incurable type, the dermatologist will not hesitate to say so and will not administer a useless series of expensive treatments as the quack often does. As progress is made in the prevention of hereditary baldness, the dermatologist will have the latest, most effective treatments.

PATENT MEDICINES

In a typical drugstore one is confronted with literally hundreds of highly advertised remedies for the common ailments of man. Although such products are commonly called *patent medicines,* a more correct name is *proprietary* compounds, since the formulas are seldom patentable. Most patent medicines are of little value and usually do not cause any direct harm. However, some do have potential harmful effects if used to excess or by a physiologically sensitive person. Certain medicines that are normally harmless become very dangerous when used in combination with a particular physical condition. For example, usually harmless laxatives may be quite hazardous when taken by a person with appendicitis. Other products may produce drowsiness to the extent that driving a motor vehicle becomes hazardous.

A major problem with patent medicines occurs when their use replaces or delays the diagnosis and prompt treatment of a serious disease by a qualified physician. The user then may suffer from *self-diagnosis* and treatment unsupported with adequate knowledge. It is an all-too-familiar event in many drug and "health food" stores to observe customers prescribing patent medicines for each other, often with the aid of helpful, but medically untrained, clerks, when the symptoms they describe could easily indicate a very serious disease.

It is important that patent medicines be used only for minor symptoms and that their use be discontinued and a physician consulted if those symptoms do not disappear in a very few days.

Probably the most effective substance sold without a prescription is aspirin (acetylsalicylic acid), which today forms the basis for a myriad of proprietary compounds. The beneficial properties of aspirin, in addition to relief of pain, are that it reduces fever and inflammation. The "glorified aspirin" products—which usually contain aspirin, phenacetin, and caffeine, or just aspirin and caffeine—along with the buffered aspirin products have been shown to be no more effective for most individuals than plain aspirin. Several products which originally contained phenacetin no longer contain this substance, since (in large doses) it has been shown to cause permanent kidney damage. Aspirin should be purchased in small quantities (about a 3-month supply) because it breaks down in storage. The breakdown is indicated by a vinegary odor in the bottle, owing to the presence of acetic acid.

Of the more than 1 billion dollars spent in the United States each year on nonprescription remedies, about $350 million goes for aspirin and its products and another $350 million goes for cold remedies. Every year new "miracle" cold remedies are offered to the public with great fanfare from their manufacturers, only to drop quietly out of the picture a few years later when the producer releases a newer "miracle." The fact remains that, despite the many advances in other areas of medicine, there is still no way to prevent or cure the common cold. Some of the products offered do provide some symptomatic relief, such as opening a stuffed nose, drying up nasal drip, and reducing fever. But the best advice for the early cold sufferer is still that he go to bed for 24 hours. This rest helps him avoid secondary infections and complications. The actual cold will last no longer than a week, but these secondary problems may last considerably longer. Antibiotics have no effect upon the actual cold, since antibiotics are not effective against viruses. Antibiotics should be reserved only for those cases in which secondary bacterial infections occur. The cold sufferer should not pressure his physician to prescribe antibiotics.

PROTECTION AGAINST QUACKERY

PERSONAL PROTECTION

Although governmental agencies are actively and fairly successfully combating quackery, it is still everyone's responsibility to be able to recognize deception and avoid its snare. Some of the signs which may be useful for recognizing quackery are given below. The first five signs pertain to mail order quackery and patent medicines. The following ten pertain to the more direct practices of quackery—those given in offices, clinics, and such. Several of the signs listed apply equally to both types of quackery.

DIAGNOSIS BY MAIL

This is *pure* quackery. Not even the most skilled physician could accurately diagnose all disease by a mailed-in description of symptoms or sample of blood or urine. Yet such a diagnosis is the basis for much mail-order medicine.

FREE TRIAL PACKAGE

Many mail-order health or beauty aids offer a free or low-cost trial package. Others send a free book which promotes their product. The generous provider of the "free 30-day trial supply" knows that since man is a creature of habit, after 30 days the user will probably continue with the product, which he will then purchase at a high price. People often feel that a product is physically benefiting them, when the only actual effect may be imaginary. Another practice of the mail-order house is to sell names of customers for "sucker lists," often for promotion of products even more shoddy than the original.

"LIMITED SUPPLY—ACT AT ONCE"

"Don't miss this once-in-a-lifetime opportunity." This sales approach, so commonly used in all lines of business, is intended to stampede the customer into acting without taking time to think about the offer and check its validity. The salesman who successfully applies this high-pressure tactic is referred to as a "closer" because he closes a sale before the customer realizes what is happening to him. Usually, an ample supply of any product can be promoted in this way.

"RECOMMENDED BY DOCTORS AND NURSES"

The advertisement seldom states *which* doctors or nurses, or even what type of doctors they are.

"APPROVED BY INDEPENDENT RESEARCH LABORATORIES"

It is not difficult for the patent-medicine producer to find some chemist who is willing to set up an "independent research laboratory," perhaps in his garage, and for a fee approve almost any product. He may test its safety without checking its effectiveness, or, conversely, he may find it to be effective without checking its safety.

OFFER OF FREE OR LOW-COST DIAGNOSIS

The practitioner who gives a free diagnosis must make his living from the treatment he renders, so he is naturally inclined to make a diagnosis that is going to lead to some of his treatments. In ethical practice, accurate diagnosis is often much more costly than the resulting treatments, since the treatment of an accurately diagnosed condition may be very efficient.

BOASTFUL ADVERTISING

The code of ethics of most medical, dental, and similar professional societies prohibits or restricts the advertising of services by members.

LOCATION

The ethical practitioner usually chooses a professional environment for his office, rather than renting space in a department or discount store. Medical offices often are centered around a large hospital.

CLAIM TO CURE DISEASE THAT OTHERS CANNOT CURE

The quack often claims that he can cure a condition that the physician cannot cure, such as cancer, arthritis, or the common cold.

GUARANTEE OF CURE OR SATISFACTION

The ethical doctor never guarantees a cure; medical science has not progressed to the point where treatment is that certain. Even though the quack may guarantee his treatments, it is doubtful that he often refunds money.

TESTIMONIAL LETTERS

The testimonial letter is a common device of the quack. His letters are often from several sources:

1. The paid testimonial. Some people, including celebrities, will say anything if they are paid enough.
2. Person cured of a nonexistent disease. (Such cases are discussed under cancer quackery.)
3. Author of letter dead. Often during legal investigations of quacks following their arrests it is discovered that persons who wrote letters

of testimonial died a short while later of the same disease of which they claimed to have been cured.

CLAIMS OF SECRET MACHINES OR FORMULAS

Claims for wonder-working machines and magic formulas are meaningless, because the ethical physician will have knowledge of and access to any effective therapy.

USE OF SEEMINGLY IMPRESSIVE DEGREES

The quack often lists several high-sounding degrees after his name and plasters his walls with the corresponding diplomas. Such degrees can easily be obtained through nonaccredited "diploma mills" or can be made up to order in print shops.

BELITTLING THE USE OF SURGERY AND DRUGS

The quack is quite naturally against the use of valuable treatment methods such as surgery and drugs, since the M.D. can use them and the quack cannot. He therefore noisily claims the superiority of his own nonsurgical and nondrug (and worthless) methods of therapy.

CLAIMS OF PERSECUTION

The quack often takes a very defensive stance, crying that the government and the medical associations are out to get him. And for once he is right. The government agencies and ethical medical societies are determined to make life miserable for the quack and eventually to eliminate quackery from the United States.

PUBLIC PROTECTION

GOVERNMENTAL AGENCIES

At every level of government efforts are being made to control fraudulent health practices. The Federal Trade Commission is active in cases involving fraudulent or deceptive advertising. The Post Office Department may move rapidly in cases of mail-order fraud. The Food and Drug Administration regulates the purity, safety, and proper labeling of drugs and food products moved across state lines. Certain state, county, and city governments are also active in suppressing quackery. In 1967 the state of California became a leader in the fight against quackery by enacting laws making fraudulent practices a felony.

NONGOVERNMENTAL ORGANIZATIONS

Several privately financed groups actively participate in the restraint of health frauds. Among these are the Bureau of Investigation of the American Medical Association, Better Business Bureaus, and Chambers of Commerce. Although these organizations have no legal regulatory powers, they can bring cases of fraud to the attention of the public and the proper legal regulatory authorities.

When one is in doubt about the merit of a particular product or treatment, it is often worthwhile to check with a local Chamber of Commerce, Better Business Bureau, local medical society, or a licensed and registered physician.

THE PERSISTENCE OF QUACKERY

How does quackery persist in spite of intensive efforts by government and individuals to suppress it? The reason is that although the quack might not be very skilled in treating disease, he is very adept in other areas. He often operates at the very borderline of legality, perhaps obeying the letter but not the spirit of the law. When he is convicted, he usually serves a short jail sentence, pays a stiff fine (which he can well afford), then immediately changes his location and perhaps his name and is back in business again.

Often even getting a conviction proves to be very difficult. Juries may be swayed by the emotional testimonies of former patients of the quack. Large corporations engaged in sales of proprietary compounds retain excellent lawyers to fight their battles with the authorities, and the corporations often win. It took the federal government, for example, 16 years to get the word *liver* removed from the name of Carter's Little (Liver) Pills on the basis that they had nothing to do with the liver.

The private citizen can aid the campaign against quackery through reporting incidents of suspected quackery to his local district attorney's office or the local medical society. It is often only through such complaints that authorities are alerted to a fraudulent operation. It is apparent, then, that today, as always, it is the responsibility of the individual to be alert to health fraud and quackery and to avoid falling into its trap.

SUMMARY

Quackery today includes fraudulent treatments, "health" foods, patent medicines and remedies of questionable value.

I. Who Is a Quack?
  A. One who promises medical benefits he cannot deliver.
  B. One who promotes cure-all drugs, machines, and treatments.
  C. One who practices self-treatment.

II. Why People Turn to Quackery
  A. Fear of death, pain, and surgery; ignorance; gullibility.
  B. Desire by teen-agers and senior citizens to achieve attractiveness or regain youthful vigor.

III. Some Major Types of Quackery Today
  A. Cancer quackery
    1. Cure promised without surgery.
    2. Diagnosis and treatment of cancer when none exists.
  B. Arthritis quackery
    1. Ethical physician can cure only a few of the many types of arthritis.
    2. Half of all arthritis patients try quack remedies.
  C. "Reduce without dieting"
    1. One out of four Americans tries to lose weight each year.
    2. Some common "easy way" schemes are
      a. nonprescription reducing pills.
      b. dietless reducing plans of many types.
      c. vibrators.
      d. massaging devices.
      e. spot reducing.
      f. reducing creams.
  D. Food fads
    1. "Health foods" and "food supplements"—often sold by:
      a. "health food" stores.
      b. door-to-door salesmen.
      c. "health" lecturers.
    2. Commonly used misrepresentations include the following *myths:*
      a. that all diseases are due to faulty diet.
      b. that some food products are indispensable.
      c. that soil depletion causes malnutrition.
      d. of "organic" or "natural" foods.
      e. of overprocessing.
  E. Beauty aids and baldness remedies
    1. Skin creams often feature exotic ingredients.
      a. Most of these ingredients are of no value.
      b. Physician should be consulted before one uses hormone skin creams.
      c. Beautiful skin is usually the result of good diet and general good health.
    2. Expensive baldness treatments are sold through baldness "clinics" and by mail, whereas the dermatologist is the one best qualified to treat baldness.
  F. Patent medicines
    1. Most are of little or no value.
    2. Probably the most effective substance sold without a prescription is aspirin.
      a. Aspirin is the basis for many proprietary compounds.
      b. Aspirin should be purchased in small quantities, because it breaks down in storage.

3. None will prevent or cure the common cold.
   a. Bed rest remains best treatment.
   b. Antibiotics should be reserved only for those cases where secondary bacterial infections occur.

IV. Protection Against Quackery
  A. Personal protection
    1. Personal responsibility is to recognize and avoid quackery.
    2. Signs of mail-order or patent-medicine quackery are:
      a. diagnosis by mail.
      b. free trial package.
      c. "limited supply—act at once."
      d. "recommended by doctors and nurses."
      e. "approved by independent research laboratories."
    3. Signs of direct quackery are:
      a. offer of free or low-cost diagnosis.
      b. boastful advertising.
      c. location.
      d. claim to cure disease that others cannot cure.
      e. guarantee of cure or satisfaction.
      f. testimonial letters.
      g. claims of secret machines or formulas.
      h. use of seemingly impressive degrees.
      i. belittling the use of surgery and drugs.
      j. claims of persecution.
  B. Public protection
    1. Governmental.
      a. Active federal agencies:
        (1) Federal Trade Commission.
        (2) Post Office Department.
        (3) Food and Drug Administration.
      b. State, county, and city governments.
    2. Nongovernmental organizations.
      a. Bureau of Investigation of the American Medical Association.
      b. Better Business Bureaus.
      c. Chambers of commerce.

V. The Persistence of Quackery
  A. Operates at the borderline of legality.
  B. Getting conviction is very difficult.
  C. If convicted, the quack:
    1. pays a stiff fine.
    2. serves a short jail term.
    3. is soon back in business.
  D. Private citizens should be alert to health fraud and report incidents to the local district attorney's office or medical society.

Glossary

If you cannot find the word you wish in this glossary, check the index for text and glossary references.

nostrum (nos′trəm) (L. *noster,* our). A medicine recommended by its preparer; a quack remedy; a cure-all.

patent medicine. A nonprescription medicine advertised to the public; often of secret composition.

proprietary compound (prō prī′ə te rē). A preparation for the treatment of disease, protected against free competition as to name, composition, or manufacturing process by secrecy, patent, copyright, trademark, or other means.

pseudo-science (soo′dō sī′əns) (Gr. *pseudes,* false). False science.

quack (kwak). A boastful pretender to medical skill.

CHAPTER 12

FINANCING
MEDICAL
SERVICES

WHY THE HIGH COST
OF MEDICAL CARE?

PUBLIC MEDICAL CARE

PRIVATE HEALTH
INSURANCE PROGRAMS

PURCHASING HEALTH
INSURANCE

PERIODIC REVIEW OF A
PREPAYMENT PLAN

SUMMARY

Through application of the principles presented in the previous chapters, one should be able to obtain good medical care. There remains, however, the problem of paying for this care. Good medical care today can be *expensive*. In the minds of many people there arises the question of why good medical care must be as expensive as it is. Is medical care overpriced today? Is a greater share of the average wage earners' paycheck going to pay for medical and dental expenses than in past years? Have the costs of all medical services risen uniformly or are some more costly to the patient today than others? Are people today less desirous of good (yet expensive) medical care and more interested in using their dollars to possess those highly advertised home luxuries than in the past? In this chapter some of these questions will be answered.

Any comparison of the cost of medical care today with that of some past date is futile, because there is no standard of comparison. Medical care has become much more complex and the quality of treatment expected today far exceeds that expected in the past. Although we would be happy to return to the "old-fashioned" costs, we would indeed be reluctant to forego any of our current diagnostic or therapeutic methods.

WHY THE HIGH COST OF MEDICAL CARE?

Since World War II, the cost of medical care has been increasing faster than the Consumer Price Index, according to the Bureau of Labor Statistics (Fig. 12.1). Not all kinds of medical care costs have risen equally. Hospital rates have risen three times as much as the CPI. Doc-

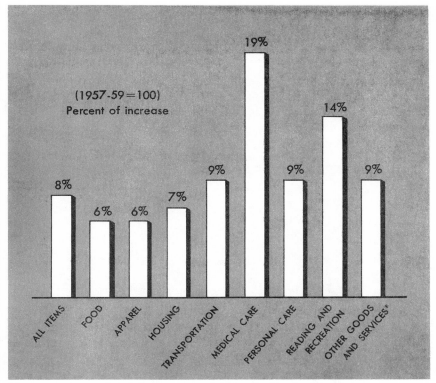

*Comprises tobacco, alcoholic beverages, legal services, banking fees, etc.

Fig. 12.1 Increases in medical care and other major groups in the Consumer Price Index in the United States, 1957–59 to 1964. (U.S. Department of Labor, Bureau of Labor Statistics.)

tors' fees, on the other hand, have risen just as much as the CPI, and the costs of drugs have not risen as much. Thus drugs have been costing the public proportionately less than they did before World War II.

There are several reasons for the great increase in hospital rates. The number of hospital admissions is twice what it was 20 years ago; physicians make greater use of hospitals today because they want their patients where the best care is available. This increasing demand has brought pressure for new hospital construction, but the cost of hospital building is today more than double what it was in 1950. Major scientific equipment used in hospitals is being improved so rapidly that a new piece of major equipment is obsolete long before it is worn out. Labor costs for hospital personnel are more than double today what they were in 1950. All of these factors have increased the cost of hospital confinement.

It is the boast of the health insurance field that over 77 percent of our population holds some form of health insurance (Fig. 12.2). However, health insurance benefits cover only about one third of the medical expenses of the average family. Consequently, the typical American

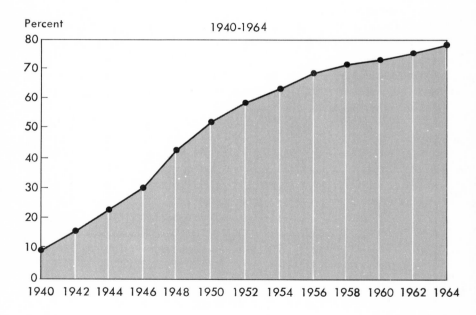

Fig. 12.2 Percentage of the U.S. population with some form of health insurance protection. (Population consists of the total civilian population.) (Health Insurance Council and U.S. Department of Commerce, Bureau of the Census.)

family looks with some suspicion on the rising costs of medical insurance. Insurance companies are facing the predicament of balancing higher benefit costs against premium rates. They have the choice of either increasing rates or reducing the benefits. Still, as far as policyholders are concerned, medical care tends to be a little cheaper in the form of a prepaid plan. They are protected somewhat against sudden large medical costs by being forced systematically to lay away funds.

The percentage of a family's income spent on medical care has actually not risen greatly since World War II. In 1950 it took about 4.5 percent of a family's disposable income, whereas in 1963 it took about 5.9 percent according to the Health Insurance Institute of America. In light of the enormous strides being made in such recent developments as open-heart surgery, where chances for recovery have risen from almost nothing to over 80 percent, such increases in cost do not seem completely out of line.

Nevertheless, it remains the job of all of us, and of the health plans in particular, to insist upon efficient administration of local hospitals. If such a watch is maintained, it will help to keep hospital costs as low as possible.

The traditional method of financing medical costs has been for each family to pay medical bills as they arise, hoping to have sufficient savings for the major episodes. This individual financing has been a "pay-as-you-go" matter for some and a matter of budgeting for others. Were medical expenses "average" and predictable from month to month, much like rent, food, or other recurring expenses, a family could budget a certain amount of money for this purpose. But because of the unpredictable nature of medical expenses, such budgeting is impossible. Medical expenses are usually erratic, with periods of heavy expense separated by periods of little or no expense. Also, some families are repeatedly hit by heavy expenses which go far beyond the average.

As a result of these problems, there has been an increasing trend toward collective financing of medical expenses. This is not a new concept, but one which dates back to ancient times. The current methods of collective financing fall into one or two basic approaches—public (tax-supported) medical services and private (voluntary) health insurance.

PUBLIC MEDICAL CARE (Tax-Supported)

Public medical care has been made available to some extent to a great number of Americans through a number of programs. These include federal, state, county, and sometimes city facilities and services. These many programs can be categorized into several main groups.

CARE OF THE INDIGENT

The oldest of the public programs for specific groups are the organized medical programs for the poor, or indigent. In 1935 the Federal Social Security Act, a milestone in the organization of health services in the United States, provided medical services for three principal categories of indigent persons: (1) the aged, (2) the blind, and (3) dependent children.

The aged includes any person 65 years of age or older. To be eligible for public medical care his income and assets must be below an amount specified by each state as being inadequate for the support of the individual or his family. The blind category includes any individual who, by state standards, is legally blind. Any child considered a minor by the state who is a member of a family unable to provide adequate support is classified as a dependent child. These people, under the 1935 Act, are entitled to medical care with the aid of federal funds administered generally through the state and local welfare departments.

In the mid-1950s a fourth category was added. It provided aid to the totally and permanently disabled (called ATPD). Essentially, it was an extension of the medical aid given to the blind. Since that time a fifth category, representing all other indigent persons, has been added. This category is conventionally spoken of by the welfare people as the "general welfare cases," as distinguished from the specific categories already described. In some communities the term "home relief" has been applied to these general welfare cases.

AID TO THE AGED

Because of their age, elderly citizens are generally in need of more health services than younger citizens (Fig. 12.3). In recent years public medical care programs have been started for elderly people not defined as indigent under earlier legislation. This elderly group, those 65 years and older, is increasing in size. Their number now stands at over 18 million (10 percent of the total population) and is expected to reach 20 million by 1970, according to the President's Council on Aging. Although more than half of them had coverage by some private health insurance program, a significant number had no coverage of any kind before Medicare. Among the uninsured were the unemployed, the very old, those in poor health, or those with low incomes—all of whom needed some form of health care protection. According to the President's Council on Aging, health insurance has not met more than one sixth of the total medical costs of the insured or one fourteenth of the total for all the aged. The plain fact has been that the income of most older Americans has been too small to allow them to afford the premiums of comprehen-

sive private health plans. According to the American Hospital Association, only one in four older people in the country held adequate
hospital insurance prior to 1965.

In response to these needs, the federal and state governments have, in
recent years, initiated programs providing some measure of medical
assistance to the great mass of older people.

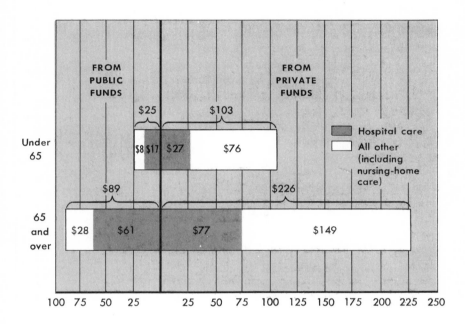

Fig. 12.3 Per capita expenditures for medical care, 1961. (U.S. Department of
Health, Education, and Welfare, Social Services Administration.)

MEDICAL ASSISTANCE TO THE AGED

In 1960 the Kerr-Mills Act was signed into law providing medical
assistance to the aged. It was a form of medical relief for individuals
considered to be "medically indigent" (those 65 years and older who
were not poor enough to qualify for welfare checks, yet who could not
afford to pay their medical bills).

Financed jointly by the United States Treasury and the states, it is
administered by state, county, or local agencies. Federal grants are made
available to those states enacting public medical programs in line with
the Federal Medical Aid to the Aged program.

Participating states have made available to these people services such
as hospital care, outpatient and clinical care, physician and dental serv-

ices, laboratory services, and drugs. Most states now participate in the program. Medicare legislation has expanded the Kerr-Mills program to include certain non-elderly individuals who are needy or near needy.

MEDICARE

By 1963 certain deficiencies in the Medical Aid to the Aged program were evident. First, only the elderly within the 25 states participating then were eligible for aid; second, persons already under Old Age Assistance and Railroad Retirement programs were not eligible for MAA; third, less than 1 percent of the elderly benefited from this program during any 1 year. Although the MAA program supplied some medical aid, a large segment of the needy elderly of the country did not have access to it. Therefore, a new federal medical aid law, commonly known as "Medicare" (also called the King-Anderson Act), was enacted in 1965.

The major provisions of Medicare are as follows.

1. *Basic benefits.* For certain persons 65 years of age and older (those under Social Security and certain others), Medicare provides some hospital care and a few medical services without cost to the patient, such as,

   a. Providing up to 90 days of hospital care for each siege of illness after the patient has paid the first $40, plus $10 for each day after the first 60 days.
   b. Providing up to 100 days of care in a nursing home for the same sickness, the patient paying $5 for each day after the first 20 days.
   c. Providing up to 100 visits a year to the patient's home, following hospitalization, by part-time nurses, physical therapists, and similar health aides.
   d. Providing for some hospital diagnostic tests and certain psychiatric hospital care.

Not covered in the basic benefits are doctors' bills, fees for private nurses, or payment for drugs prescribed outside a hospital or nursing home. Consequently, some have aptly described this program as actually providing "hospicare."

2. *Supplemental benefits.* The new law also makes it possible for persons 65 years and older to buy health insurance providing additional benefits. The premium costs of this optional insurance is shared by the individual and the federal government, each paying half. This supplemental insurance covers doctors' bills in or out of a hospital, certain dental bills, visits by part-time nurses and other health personnel to a patient's home under conditions not covered by the basic Medicare plan, some psychiatric care outside a hospital, and various other health

benefits not provided for by Medicare. Elderly individuals holding such policies pay the first $50 of the expenses and one fifth of the balance.

All individuals 65 years or older are eligible for basic Medicare, provided they (1) were born before 1903, (2) have paid into Social Security before reaching the age of 65 years, or (3) are entitled to Railroad Retirement benefits. The supplemental medical insurance is offered to anyone 65 years or older who is eligible for basic Medicare benefits, or to federal employees who would not qualify for basic benefits. Eligibility to receive these benefits is not based on "without-ability-to-pay" tests. Regardless of an individual's financial resources, he is eligible if he meets the above qualifications.

The basic Medicare provisions are financed largely through payroll deductions paid into Social Security by individuals of all ages who are covered by its provisions. Some of the cost is provided out of the annual federal budget.

Along with the above provisions of Medicare, some states have expanded the Kerr-Mills programs to include certain medically indigent individuals *under* 65 years. These include children under 21 years, the blind, and persons totally and permanently disabled.

AID TO VETERANS

A third category of tax-supported medical care is of tremendous importance in the United States. This is the system of care for veterans. The veterans' program is extremely interesting because it is an illustration of a system of socialized medicine. The veterans' program is divided into two principal parts: care of service-connected and care of non-service-connected disabilities.

Any condition that was inflicted or activated during service, if noted on the individual's medical service record, will be taken care of at government expense through the Veterans Administration. For treatment of non-service-inflicted disabilities or conditions, the individual must be able to prove inability to pay for treatment before the Veterans Administration will accept the patient for treatment.

A great network of hospitals and clinics provide this care. There is also a so-called "home town" program for veterans, which makes provision for local care of service-connected disabilities for a veteran who lives in a place distant from a Veterans Administration hospital. Some of these facilities have been consolidated in recent years, reducing the number of local centers.

AID TO MILITARY DEPENDENTS

A program of importance in recent years is that for military dependents. The wives and children of military personnel who are on active or inactive duty or who are retired from the service are the objects of this program. Children are covered until they are 18 years of age. It is interesting how this program grew during World War II. It started as a small token of appreciation to the men overseas. The government passed what was called the Emergency Maternity and Infant Care Program to see to it that service wives having babies were cared for. This program was dropped at the end of the war, but was later reintroduced as it became harder to recruit military personnel and have them stay on beyond their 6-month to 4-year tours of duty. The government said that it would see that the dependents of the military personnel received adequate medical care. This is a program extending medical care to several million people either at a military post or at a freely chosen place.

SPECIAL GROUPS (GENERAL GOVERNMENT MEDICAL CARE)

Several other groups of citizens are of interest to the government for various reasons.

1. *Military personnel.* Military persons receive all medical care while on active duty or upon retirement from the military service. Many of the young people in our country have had their best experiences with first-class medicine during the time they were in the service.

2. *American Indians.* Over half a million Americans who are Indians are entitled to medical care through a network of hospitals and clinics operated by the United States Public Health Service.

3. *United States Merchant Marine.* The Merchant Marine members' government-financed medical care goes back to 1798 and represents the first public, tax-supported medical care program.

SPECIAL DISEASES

There are tax-supported programs for special diseases. The most important is emotional disorders. For about 80 years care of the emotionally ill, especially hospital care, has predominantly been a public function. In recent years the whole approach to care of the emotionally ill has been revitalized, and the financial support of local, state, and federal agencies is in the process of revision. Hospital benefits through public or private insurance plans have not covered emotional illness. There has been a reversal of this trend in recent years, which may cause a reassessment of the role of tax-supported, centralized care of the emotionally ill.

Clinics for alcoholism and drug addiction are maintained by local, state, and federal agencies. These clinics are the major treatment centers for these conditions in the United States. This trend will continue so long as there is a strong connection between these two conditions and the law. Nearly all commitments to these institutions are legal, made by the courts.

COMMUNICABLE DISEASES

Tax-supported medical care involves all those with communicable diseases. The care of tuberculosis has been a predominantly public function in most states. Tuberculosis sanitariums have been about 85 percent government-owned and operated. Fortunately, with improved early detection, the number of sanitariums is smaller now than it once was.

Venereal disease diagnosis and treatment is of high public concern. Programs for control of venereal diseases have changed as the nature of the treatment has changed. During the early 1940s treatment of venereal disease was a long process. Most of the venereal disease therapy was given through public clinics. Then came penicillin in the mid-1940s and the picture changed. The treatment of this disease became relatively rapid and, therefore, inexpensive. The therapy shifted largely to private offices. The venereal disease programs in most health departments today are now largely concerned with public education and the epidemiological conditions of this disease. Then there are rare diseases like leprosy for which there is a public hospital in Carville, Louisiana. In some of the larger cities there are special hospitals for other infectious diseases.

CRIPPLED CHILDREN

For many years there has been special provision for medical care of crippled children, administered usually by the state health departments and to some extent by welfare departments. Crippled children receive both medical and educational care. The Crippled Children's Program is one of the best examples of a service in which the leadership has been very insistent on high standards. A child who gets medical care under the Crippled Children's Program must be treated by a specialist certified in his field. Whether it be in orthopedics, physical medicine, or surgery, the crippled child receives a higher standard of treatment than that usually received by the general population.

CRIPPLED ADULTS

There are two principal kinds of organized medical care programs for crippled adults. Oldest are the programs growing out of litigation over industrial injuries—workmen's compensation insurance. Although the cost of this program is not tax-supported, the program in each state is the result of legislation, and thus a kind of public program. Work-

men's compensation laws in the states cover both occupational disease
and injuries, but well over 90 percent of the cases are traumatic accidents. The medical care is financed under law through the insurance
carried by the employer. The workmen's compensation insurance program of the states is a form of compulsory health insurance that industry
has been living with since 1911. There are great variations among the
states, but generally speaking, the workmen's compensation insurance
program provides a good method of medical care to workers injured
in the course of their employment.

Other kinds of disabilities affecting adults, which may or may not be
related to their employment, are also covered by medical care programs.
A special program of vocational rehabilitation was initiated after World
War I and then greatly extended in World War II, so that we now have
a federal-state program of medical services. The vocational rehabilitation program is usually administered by the State Department of Education, because an important feature of it is job retraining. The chief
limitation in the selection of cases for this program is that the physical
condition for which the person is being rehabilitated must be relatively
static. Thus, a person with active pneumonia or appendicitis may not
be treated under this program because the condition is progressive; it
will lead either to prompt recovery or to death. Conditions such as amputation, blindness, or serious crippling arthritis are relatively static
and thus are the kinds of cases covered by this program.

GENERAL HOSPITAL CARE

General public hospitals are tax-supported to provide general medical
care for people with any condition. These are usually operated under
city or county governments. In most cities throughout the country the
special publicly operated hospitals are strongly oriented to the care of
persons with chronic illnesses.

LOCAL OR COUNTY HEALTH DEPARTMENTS

Finally, under the tax-supported services is the local health department, providing various special services. Although these services vary
in kind and extent from county to county, the following list includes
many of the services provided, particularly in better-organized counties:

COMMUNICABLE DISEASE CONTROL

According to the laws of most states, communicable diseases and suspected communicable diseases are reportable to the local public health
office. Public health department physicians are available to the general

public for diagnosis of communicable diseases. Immunizations against diphtheria, whooping cough, tetanus, and poliomyelitis are commonly offered to young children. Vaccination services for diseases such as smallpox and poliomyelitis are sometimes available to people of all ages.

HEALTH OFFICE

Local health centers maintain office hours for consultations on public health programs, immunizations, and diagnosis of communicable diseases. A local health center should be contacted for specific hours.

TUBERCULOSIS CONTROL

Diagnosis, which includes a chest X ray and other necessary tests, is made for suspected cases of tuberculosis. Clinical care is provided for patients when private care is not available. Supervision and correction of home conditions are arranged in cases where there is danger of contagion.

VENEREAL DISEASE CONTROL

Health centers offer examinations for diagnosis of venereal diseases, as well as necessary laboratory tests, consultation, and treatment.

PUBLIC HEALTH NURSING SERVICE

Public health nurses carry on generalized nursing programs in homes and health centers for people with acute communicable diseases, tuberculosis, venereal disease, chronic illnesses, and mental illnesses, and for maternal and child health. Nursing consultation may be provided to public and parochial schools, industrial establishments, hospitals, and nursing homes.

PUBLIC HEALTH SOCIAL WORK

Social services are provided to patients with economic, social, and emotional problems relating to illness.

PUBLIC HEALTH NUTRITION

Public health nutritionists serve as consultants to organizations in the community interested in the proper feeding of individuals or groups. They help in planning appetizing meals of high nutritive value with a minimum expenditure of time, effort, and money.

CHILD HEALTH

Conferences on child health may be arranged by parents; they may include physical examinations and consultation on food, health habits, and parent-child relationships. These conferences are usually restricted to parents with children under 2 years of age who are not under private medical supervision.

MATERNAL HEALTH

Health supervision may be provided by physicians and public health nurses for expectant mothers eligible for care. Immunizations against poliomyelitis and tuberculin tests may also be available, along with cervical cytology studies (cancer detection) for eligible expectant mothers. Some local health departments conduct classes for expectant parents on the process of birth and care of the new infant.

PUBLIC HEALTH DENTISTRY

Dental examinations and mouth health education are sometimes provided for young children. Dental hygienists and dentists are sometimes made available to public schools through local health departments. In some localities corrective care is provided for children eligible for such care. Diagnostic services and care for such diseases as Vincent's infection (trench mouth) may be available to anyone.

SANITATION

Services of inspectors are available for sanitation problems pertaining to dairies and dairy products, food and drugs, mountain and rural sanitation, rodent control, water and sewage, and other matters involving sanitation supervision.

VITAL RECORDS

Births and deaths are recorded in the health center in the district in which they occur. Certified copies of these records are obtainable at the local health centers within 60 days after a birth or death. If this service is not available, the local health department will guide a person to the correct office for obtaining these records. Help may also be given in the procurement or correction of older records.

INDUSTRIAL HEALTH

Industrial health services are designed to protect employees from health hazards while they are at work. These can include studies and consultation in industrial health matters by specially trained individuals.

PUBLIC HEALTH EDUCATION

Health department work is aided through public educational programs; through health education activities in communities, including public and parochial schools; and through spreading public health information via newspapers, radio, television, films, exhibits, and pamphlets.

AIR POLLUTION CONTROL

Air pollution control in some counties is handled either by a separate agency or by the health department. In either case there is regulation of air pollutants such as exhaust fumes from cars and trucks, industrial and residential smoke, industrial gases, and other contaminants. Included within regulation is the legal power to prohibit the burning or exhaust of certain substances at certain times.

SCHOOL HEALTH

Public and parochial schools are provided with health services such as teeth examinations and cleanings, eye examinations, tuberculin skin tests, chest X rays, vaccinations, and nursing consultations. The department may also assume responsibility for sanitation, food handling, and physical education facilities.

The fundamental duties of a health department are the control of those diseases for which there are practical means of prevention and the promotion of better health for the public. Any service that will better the general health of the public rightfully comes under the direction of a public health department.

PRIVATE HEALTH INSURANCE PROGRAMS

The several widespread forms of private health insurance presently available are based upon the idea that individuals cannot successfully budget against the potential costs of illness. The best hope for protection then lies in large numbers of persons' pooling the risks through health plans so as to spread both the chances and the costs. Insurance companies sell these health plans through employee groups, professional organizations, and individual subscriptions.

KINDS OF SUBSCRIPTIONS

The most reasonable premium rates have been gained through the formation of groups of subscribers. Group plans are available only through the employer. Typically, only one type of plan is available, with a set, group-wide premium charge for each subscriber with the same contract (with some differences, depending upon the size of the family of the subscriber). An individual, nongroup subscription will frequently cost more than a comparable group policy or will provide fewer benefits. The majority of people covered by health insurance today belong to a group of some kind, according to the Health Insurance Institute (Fig. 12.4).

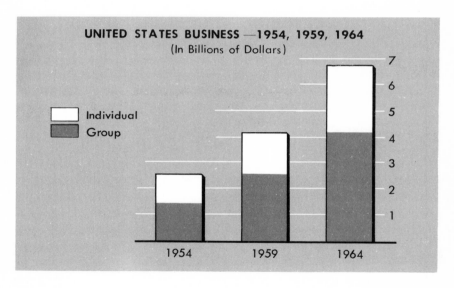

Fig. 12.4 Health insurance premiums of insurance companies by type of policy. (Health Insurance Association of America.)

TYPES OF BENEFITS

In terms of benefits, there are three general types of plans: service benefits (full payment), cash indemnity benefits, and a combination of the two. The majority of subscribers are enrolled in combination plans.

The service plans are generally in the form of contracts between the policyholder and the hospital or physician. The hospital agrees to provide certain services upon presentation by the policyholder of his policy identification card. The hospital or physician then agrees to accept fee allowances under that plan as full or near-full payment for care rendered. After the service is rendered, a claim form is filled out and sent to the insurance company by the hospital or physician. Reimbursement is then made directly to hospital or physician according to the provisions of the policy.

The cash indemnity plans pay benefits in the form of cash to the policyholder. He is reimbursed for the medical costs he has incurred or paid. The patient is usually required to present either a physician's or hospital statement showing the exact amount due or a receipt for payment already made.

TYPES OF INSURERS

There are many types of health insurance available today. Several main examples will be discussed here.

BLUE CROSS

Blue Cross is a nonprofit operation with over 50 million members. Through 77 plans it insures members against costs of hospital care, physicians' services, drugs, and laboratory tests.

Prepaid hospital plans first started in Dallas, Texas, in 1929, with a contract between the local teachers and the Baylor Hospital. Hospitals were being faced with both patients' unpaid bills and empty hospital beds. This situation was typical of the Depression years' dilemma faced by both hospitals and patients. Through the efforts of the American Hospital Association, the prepaid Blue Cross idea came into being. People discovered that through Blue Cross insurance they could have their hospital bills taken care of in return for the payment of small monthly premiums. Hospitals benefited by being able to keep their facilities in use, collect their bills, and thus balance their budgets. During the 1940s and 1950s Blue Cross grew rapidly as large employee groups came under its coverage through employer-paid or employee-shared arrangements. Today 32 percent of the United States population is enrolled under Blue Cross (according to Blue Cross).

Owing to the number of Blue Cross plans across the country, it is difficult to describe a typical plan. Each plan is a separate, regional, autonomous organization under the national name of Blue Cross. Each plan sets its own policies, rates, and benefits, and makes its own contracts with hospitals in its territory. Each Blue Cross organization reserves the right to contract only with those hospitals meeting its standards of acceptability. Consequently, not all hospitals are eligible to receive Blue Cross payments.

The majority of Blue Cross plans are combination plans providing some service benefits plus some benefits in the form of cash indemnities. Types of coverage range from several weeks to a full year of hospital service. The most widely sold policies cover the partial or complete cost of 30 days of hospital care. Other plans also cover services of physicians, anesthetists, X-ray diagnosis and therapy, drugs, and laboratory tests. Some plans are also now including *extended coverage,* benefits payable in the event of a long siege of illness. Claims under the Blue Cross plans are paid directly to the contracting hospital or physician, rather than to the subscriber as with the cash indemnity plans.

BLUE SHIELD

Set up along the same general lines as Blue Cross, these nonprofit physicians' plans today have over 50 million subscribers through 76 different plans. Started by a few local medical societies late in the 1930s, Blue Shield plans are designed to provide prepaid coverage for physicians' services and at the same time help to assure physicians the collection of their fees. Coverage is based upon annual family income. Members whose family incomes are under a set level, and whose physicians choose to accept the Blue Shield schedule of rates, are completely covered according to the payment schedule. If family income is over this set level, the plan covers only a percentage of the physicians' charges. Generally the accepted level of family income which determines the amount of coverage ranges from $4200 to $7500 a year, depending upon which plan a family belongs to.

Blue Shield is available in most states. Certain other physicians' insurance plans are available in individual states, such as the California Physicians' Service plan in California.

COMMERCIAL

Today the majority of the hospital and surgical policies are being written by commercial insurance companies (Fig. 12.5). Although their coverage is similar to that of Blue Cross and Blue Shield, the approach of the insurance companies is often different. Their plans are the cash indemnity type or combination service–cash indemnity. The commercial insurance company in no way engages in contracts with hospitals or physicians and, consequently, does not seek to control the quality of medical services rendered to their policy holders. These plans sometimes involve deductibles and coinsurance features, and often a wide variety of plans are available which can be tailor-made to the wishes of the individual applicant.

Commercial companies have led the way into other forms of health insurance.

1. *Major medical.* These plans are designed to give large amounts of coverage for major expenses. They are not designed to pay for the expenses the insured can easily pay out of his own pocket or which can be covered by the regular type of hospital, surgical, and medical contract. Consequently, major medical plans usually contain a deductible of $100 to $500. The policyholder is expected to pay this amount him-

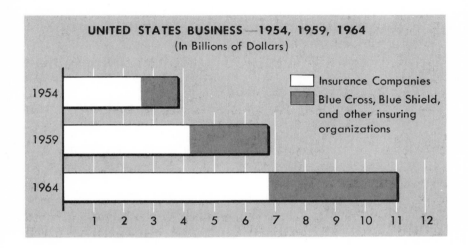

Fig. 12.5 Health insurance premiums by type of insurer. (Health Insurance Association of America, U.S. Department of Health, Education, and Welfare and *Health Insurance Review.*)

self or with a regular type of policy. In addition, a coinsurance feature provides that the insured himself must bear the cost of 20 to 25 percent of the expenses above the deductible amount, and the insurance company pays the other 75 to 80 percent. Major medical plans cover expenses resulting from both accidents and sickness.

2. *Comprehensive plans.* Comprehensive contracts are newer than major medical plans. Contracts of this type are designed to provide regular (basic) medical care plus major medical coverage. In other words, they are a basic and a major medical plan combined into a single policy. Available on either an individual or a group basis, they are designed to combine the best features of the other two types of policies.

3. *Age 65 programs.* The age 65 programs were set up by insurance companies in an attempt to prevent federal intervention in health insurance to the elderly. Going under such names as Golden 65, Fund 65 Plan, and Senior Security, these private plans sought, through mass

enrollments, to provide up to $10,000 lifetime insurance for people age 65 and over. No restrictions were placed upon a subscriber because of past or present conditions of health.

Unfortunately, during the several years these plans have been in force, the companies have met with difficulty in keeping the premium rates down. Also, with annual premium rates for an elderly couple going as high as $500 a year, many subscribers have been hard pressed to continue their policies. Some of the companies have had little or no increase in subscribers since the original enrollments. As the subscribers get older, more use is made of the policies.

In the face of these problems, along with the enactment of Medicare, some of the "65" programs are being discontinued. Medicare is providing the care it was hoped these plans would provide.

INDEPENDENTS

This label is generally applied to the 300 smaller local plans which do not fit any of the previous categories. They have been organized by labor unions, corporate managements, physicians, and laymen. Most of them have their own staffs of salaried physicians, some their own hospitals, and many their own clinics. Their main emphasis is placed on diagnostic services and on care outside the hospitals. They go under such names as Health Insurance Plan of Greater New York, Kaiser Foundation Health Plan, and the Community Health Association of Detroit. Not uncommonly, the patients must use a staff physician under these plans and may not bring a nonstaff physician in from the outside. Plans lacking their own hospitals have agreements with existing hospitals for service to their members. Although the Independents are generally local, many are large organizations. New York State and California have a number of such plans. Nevertheless, their growth has been relatively slow in relation to the growth of other health insurance plans.

DENTAL PLANS

A fairly recent development in health insurance is that of plans providing benefits for dental care. In the past, ordinary dental care has usually been excluded from health care plans except as a necessary provision in accident insurance.

Some group dental plans are now available. The Group Health Dental Insurance, Inc., in New York State has been a leader. More recently, some labor unions have participated in various groups.

Rates depend upon the type of coverage provided and the makeup of the particular group. Most coverage provides a limited amount of care, the patient's paying a portion of the cost. These plans are set up to cover necessary procedures for a sound, healthy mouth. Usually excluded are dental services not deemed necessary for normal chewing.

PURCHASING HEALTH INSURANCE

The sale of hospital, health, and accident insurance is too serious a matter to become a battle of wits between buyer and seller. Buyers can be misled as much by the omission of facts as by the deliberate distortion of facts; also, they can be presented with so many facts that truths become lost. Quite often the buyer can unwittingly put himself in a position where he has only limited legal action if his claim is disputed.

PROVISIONS TO LOOK FOR WHEN PURCHASING HEALTH INSURANCE

POLICY TERMINATION AND RENEWAL PROVISIONS

Some insurance companies make advertising claims such as

No automatic termination age, no increased costs, or reduced benefits after policy is issued.
You and your family are covered from 1 to 75 years.
This policy is absolutely NONCANCELLABLE.

Actually, most of the health insurance policies sold are renewable solely at the option of the company. Each new premium purchases insurance for a new term. The majority of these policies can be cancelled by the company at the end of any term for any reason. Cancellation is done by refusing to accept the premium payment. The right of the insurance company to refuse renewal does not exist with *noncancellable* and *guaranteed renewable* contracts. The subscriber can expect to pay more for this feature, although it is undoubtedly worth the extra cost.

EXTENT OF COVERAGE

Advertising claims which state that benefits will be paid in cases of accident or sickness generally may be open to misinterpretation. A typical claim may read, "It pays up to $15 a day for 100 hospital days—for each sickness or accident." There are in fact many cases of accident or sickness for which policies so represented do not provide payment. Most insurance companies will exclude some of the following.

1. Plastic or cosmetic surgery.
2. Elective surgery (surgery which can be done at the patient's convenience). In most policies this is covered 6 months from the date of purchase of the policy.
3. Maternity benefits. Coverage usually starts 10 months after the policy begins.
4. Venereal diseases.
5. Psychiatric care.
6. Pre-existing illnesses. These are usually not covered; there may be a waiting period before coverage commences.
7. Tuberculosis.
8. Heart disease.
9. Dental operations.

Other exclusions definitely decrease the value of the policy. A buyer will certainly have to accept some exclusions, but he should be sure he knows what the exclusions are and should take them into account when appraising each contract.

MAXIMUM DOLLAR LIMITS

Many of the companies state that claims *up to* a specified amount will be payable for certain medical, hospital, and surgical services. For example, "We pay up to $525 for each surgical operation" or, "Surgical fees, up to $400." These claims imply that if a person has a surgical operation he will receive up to that amount specified, depending on the cost of the operation. Actually, many policies provide that the full amount payable is for one or two comparatively rare operations. The maximum amount payable for the average operation is one fourth of the specified amount, or even less.

One of the main purposes of insurance is usually protection against very large medical and hospital bills. Therefore, any provision limiting the insurance companies' liabilities leave the buyer with the possibility of losing protection just when he needs it most. All policies will have limits of liability, but the buyer should make sure they are as liberal as possible.

COMMENCEMENT OF COVERAGE

Certain companies represent that their coverage is effective at the date of issuance, when actually coverage for many sicknesses is delayed until the policy has been in effect for a specified period of time. For example, many policies state that tuberculosis or heart disease will not be covered until the policy has been in effect for 6 months.

DISABILITY INCOME BENEFITS

Some companies have made representations which imply that a specified income will be paid so long as the insured is disabled, even if for life. For example, "It pays you a regular monthly income up to $200 when disabled by sickness or accident—even for life." As a matter of fact, such payments are payable for a limited period of time in cases of disability due to sickness or cases of partial disability due to accident. Only in cases of absolute total disability due solely to accidental bodily injury are the payments made as represented.

Disability insurance is only as good as the policy's definition of the term "disability." Some policies proclaim, "You are disabled when you are unable to carry out gainful employment." A person claiming fraud found that the definition of "disability" by the insurance firm limited all benefits as soon as the person was capable of selling magazines by telephone, and so on.

Another term which will vary according to the policy is "partial disability." Some such clauses refer to what the insured *can* do; others define partial disability in terms of what the insured *cannot* do.

CLARIFICATION OF TERMS USED IN POLICY

The buyer should go over the entire contract word by word whenever he purchases any form of health insurance or income protection insurance. He must rely mainly upon the reputation of the individual agent and the company issuing the policy.

If there are statements or definitions which are not completely clear to the buyer, he may ask the insurance company for a letter of clarification; the buyer may write out all terms that are not completely clear to him, mail this to the main office of the insuring company, and request them to return to him the official definitions of these terms. Upon receipt of the reply, he should study it very carefully, and if the definitions are acceptable, then—and only then—sign the contract for the insurance. When he receives his copy of the insurance policy, he should clip his letter of clarification onto the policy. Whenever presented with a claim, the insurance company is legally bound to the definitions as they have been defined.

ADVICE FROM A PHYSICIAN OR HOSPITAL

It is also advisable to ask a personal physician his reactions to a specific medical plan. It is a good idea to contact the hospital in the area to see if the amounts payable for specific hospital care are adequate to pay for at least 80 percent of their charges.

PERIODIC REVIEW OF A PREPAYMENT PLAN

At certain times a person should take time out to review his medical insurance coverage. (1) During a three-year period changes may occur in income, the relative needs of a family, and possibly even the number in a family. For this reason it is wise to review every three years. (2) Every time a person changes his employment he should review his insurance coverage, because he may lose certain types of coverage with one employer and receive new coverage with another employer. (3) Whenever there is a change in residence, he should review his insurance to bring his address up to date. Many policies are issued in a specific area and are not in force when the individual leaves this specific area. (4) Whenever a family's situation changes—as by divorce, death, or birth—the insured should review his insurance policy to be sure of exact coverage.

During these periods the insured should write down the following information as a guide to the information he is looking for: Any facts that will help determine the coverage he needs (auto coverage, life insurance, health, and so on); how large a premium he can afford with his current income (for example, can he afford coverage against catastrophic illness and events?). With this information, he must also take into account facilities and services available through the state and federal agencies. He should also determine if he would qualify for such aid if it were needed. Next, what demands income protection—car, home, school, food, clothing, and so on. Now he should write out the coverage that he has through sick leave, disability benefits, workmen's compensation, and any insurance provided through his employer. He should note any discrepancies that can be eliminated, and take action.

Regardless of *how* a family provides for its medical care, there can be no question that such care must be available. The human life has a clear value which, to some extent, can be guaranteed through a reliable insurance program. Since the great majority of people depend upon their ability to work and thereby to earn money, the protection of their lives from physical disability will be one of their most important assets. A family *must* be protected in its ability to earn money, as well as against unnecessary loss of money owing to medical and hospital costs.

SUMMARY

I. Why the High Cost of Medical Care?
   A. People expect far better medical care today than in the past.
   B. More complex medical care has boosted medical costs.

C. Hospital costs have risen the most.
D. Medical care is cheaper in prepaid insurance plans.
E. Individual financing is pay-as-you-go or budgeted.
F. Collective financing is provided by:
    1. Public (tax-supported) medical services.
    2. Private (voluntary) health insurance.

II. Public Medical Care
  A. Care of the poor (indigent).
  B. Aid to the aged.
    1. Medical Assistance to the Aged (MAA).
    2. Medicare
      a. Basic benefits—covering primarily hospital care.
      b. Supplemental benefits—covering primarily the physician's care.
  C. Aid to veterans.
  D. Aid to military dependents.
  E. Special groups (general government medical care).
  F. Special diseases.
  G. Communicable diseases.
  H. Crippled children.
   I. Crippled adults.
  J. General hospital care.
  K. Local or county health departments.
    1. Communicable disease control.
    2. Health office.
    3. Tuberculosis control.
    4. Venereal disease control.
    5. Public health nursing service.
    6. Public health social work.
    7. Public health nutrition.
    8. Child health.
    9. Maternal health.
    10. Public health dentistry.
    11. Sanitation.
    12. Vital records.
    13. Industrial health.
    14. Public health education.
    15. Air pollution control.
    16. School health.

III. Private Health Insurance Programs
  A. Kinds of subscriptions:
    1. Group plans—set up by employer in a given firm.
    2. Individual (nongroup) plans—set up for each person or family.
  B. Types of benefits:
    1. Service (full payments)—contract between policyholder and hospital or physician.
    2. Cash indemnity—pay cash benefits to the policyholder.
    3. Combinations of service and cash indemnity policies.
  C. Types of insurers:
    1. *Blue Cross*
      a. Nonprofit policy for hospitalization.
      b. Plan provides mostly service benefits, with some cash indemnity provisions.
    2. *Blue Shield*—nonprofit policy for physician's services.

3. *Commercial*
    a. Usually provides cash indemnity benefits.
    b. Engage in no service contracts with hospitals or physicians.
    c. Include many forms of coverage.
       (1) Major medical.
       (2) Comprehensive plans.
       (3) Age 65 programs.
4. *Independents*—set up by special groups to provide for prepaid medical service from hospitals, clinics, nurses, and physicians.
5. *Dental*—provide a limited amount of care, with patients paying portion of the costs.

IV. Purchasing Health Insurance
  A. Provisions to look for:
    1. Policy termination and renewal provisions.
    2. Extent of coverage.
    3. Maximum dollar limits.
    4. Commencement of coverage.
    5. Disability income benefits.
  B. Clarification of terms used in policy—should be obtained in writing from the insuring company *before* the contract is signed.
  C. Advice from a physician or hospital should be sought before the contract is signed.

V. Periodic Review of a Prepayment Plan
  A. Changing needs of a family insurance program should be reviewed:
    1. Every three years.
    2. With every change in employment.
    3. With every change in residence.
    4. With every change in family situation.
  B. Guideline for future purchases should include:
    1. What facilities and services are already provided through public facilities and workmen's compensation.
    2. Amount of coverage needed.
    3. Extent of a person's present commitments for essential items.
    4. How large a periodic premium can be afforded.

Glossary

If you cannot find the word you wish in this glossary, check the index for text and glossary references.

cash indemnity benefit. A cash benefit paid by a health insurance policy to the policyholder for an insured loss.

coinsurance. A policy provision, often found in major medical insurance, by which the insured person and the insurance company in a specific ratio share the hospital and medical expenses resulting from an illness or injury.

collective financing. The financing of medical expenses through the prepayment of fees, either through public taxes or through a private insurance plan.

deductible. That portion of covered hospital and medical charges which an insured person must pay before his policy's benefits begin.

disability. A physical condition which makes an insured person incapable of doing one or more duties of his occupation.

exclusion. A specific hazard for which a policy will not provide benefit payments.

extended coverage. Coverage providing benefits for extended medical care due to severe injury or prolonged sickness, usually in addition to basic coverage for short-term medical care.

guaranteed renewable. A policy which the insured has a right to continue in force by the timely payment of premiums to a specified age, during which period the insured has no right to, on his own, make any change in any provision of the policy while it is in force.

indigent (in'di jənt) (L. *indu,* in; *egere,* to need). Poor or needy.

individual financing. The financing of medical expenses without the benefit of any prepayment or insurance plan, either on a pay-as-you-go basis or by budgeting for expected expenses.

pre-existing condition. A physical condition of an insured person which existed prior to the issuance of his policy.

service benefits. A contract benefit which is paid directly to the provider of hospital or medical care for services rendered.

CHAPTER 13

THE
HEART
AND
CIRCULATION

CIRCULATION

TYPES AND CAUSES
OF CIRCULATORY DISEASES

ENVIRONMENTAL EFFECTS
ON THE CIRCULATORY
SYSTEM

HEART DISEASE AS A
CAUSE OF DEATH

PREVENTION OF HEART
DISEASES

SYMPTOMS AND TREATMENT

SUMMARY

During the past 60 years a change has occurred in United States public health in that the noninfectious chronic diseases have replaced the acute infectious ones as the most pressing health problem. Dr. Paul Dudley White, the famous heart specialist, recalls that when he was a young physician hospital staffs had difficulty making hospital beds available fast enough to take care of the many cases of typhoid fever. Today typhoid fever is no longer a major health problem in the United States.

Adults in this country can expect to live much longer today than they could in 1900. Medicine and public health have successfully overcome the two great killers—acute infection and malnutrition—which have devastated mankind for centuries. The average life expectancy of 45 years in 1900 has risen to over 70 today. Dimming this bright picture, however, is the fact that the chronic diseases continue largely unreduced in incidence. Among the chronic diseases, the *cardiovascular* ailments are by far the chief producers of illness, disability, and death among both middle-aged and elderly people. One of them, arteriosclerotic heart disease, accounts for almost one third of all deaths. Researchers, public and private, have mounted a massive campaign against this number one villain—not only in terms of treating those already afflicted, but also of identifying the factors causing cardiovascular diseases and preventing their complications. Although there are encouraging omens, the task is far from complete. This chapter attempts to describe the structure and functions of the circulatory organs and their disorders, and to survey the present state of heart research.

CIRCULATION

The billions of cells of the human body must have not only a sure source of food and oxygen, but also protection against the waste materials that are produced as food is turned into energy. Various organs of the body have specific assignments in seeing that the all-important cell is maintained in peak condition.

CIRCULATORY SYSTEM

The *circulatory system* is responsible for the continuous and rapid movement of materials to and from the cells. It carries its materials in a fluid medium called *blood*. It directs blood to the lungs, where oxygen is obtained, then carries it to the cells and tissues (groups of cells). Wastes are picked up from the cells and carried by the blood to the kidneys and other excretory organs, from which they are excreted; digested foods are picked up from the digestive tract and carried to tissues for storage or use; and hormones are carried around the body to regulate and coordinate activities. The blood also regulates body temperature and protects the body against disease. The blood is kept circulating by two muscular pumps contained in a single organ, the *heart* (Fig. 13.1).

Vessels called *arteries* carry the blood away from the heart; other vessels called *veins* return it to the heart. The arteries are large as they leave the heart, but divide into smaller and smaller vessels (*arterioles*) the farther they go from it. These arterioles lead into microscopic vessels called *capillaries*. The capillaries are profuse and form extensive networks through the various body tissues. Through their very thin walls the exchange of materials between the blood and the tissues occurs. Thus each cell is bathed in *tissue fluid* from the blood. The tissue fluid coming from the blood to the cell is rich in food and oxygen and is rich in waste products as it returns from the cell to the blood. As the tissue

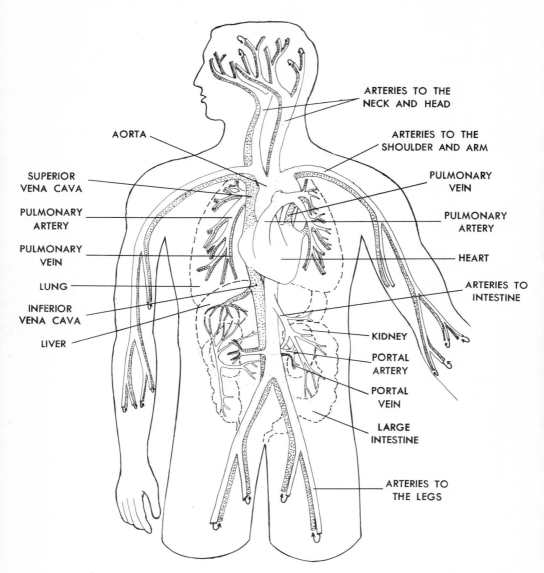

Fig. 13.1 Human circulatory system showing principal arteries and veins.

fluid from the cells collects in the capillaries, it passes to small veins, called *venules,* which combine into larger veins, the largest of which open into the heart.

THE HEART

STRUCTURE OF THE HEART

Approximately the size of a person's fist, the heart is an amazing bundle of muscle fibers richly interwoven with blood vessels. Nerves connecting the brain to the heart transmit information, telling the heart the amount of work required of it. For its size (about three fourths of a pound) this little pump turns out an astonishing amount of work. It is centrally located between the lungs, a bit to the left of the midline of the body. The heart is shaped like a cone; its tip *(apex)* is directed downward and to the left. It is divided into four chambers, two on each side (Fig. 13.2). The two upper chambers are called the *atria;* the two lower ones, the *ventricles.* The ventricles, or pumping chambers, are

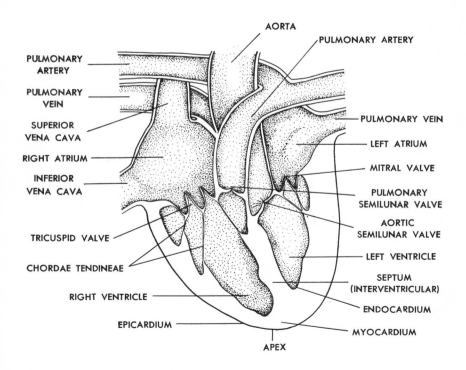

Fig. 13.2 Heart showing chambers and major vessels.

386 HEALTH SCIENCE

larger and have thicker muscular walls than the atria, or receiving chambers. The two halves of the heart are separated by a partition called the *septum*. The upper portion separating the atria is called the *interatrial septum;* the lower portion separating the ventricles, the *interventricular septum*.

The walls of the heart are composed of three different layers. The interior is lined by a thin, smooth, shiny membrane called the *endocardium* (Fig. 13.2). This lining is continuous with the lining of the blood vessels and of the *valves* inside the heart. Inflammation of this lining is referred to as *endocarditis*. The middle and thickest layer is composed of muscular tissue; it is called the *myocardium*. The muscular tissue of the myocardium is somewhat layered, with thicker layers in the ventricles than in the atria. Externally, the heart is covered by a membrane, the *epicardium*. The wall of the heart is supplied with blood from the *coronary arteries,* which lie on its surface (Fig. 13.3).

The right atrium receives deoxygenated blood from the heart muscle and from all other body areas by way of a network of veins. These veins terminate as the *superior vena cava,* which collects blood from the upper

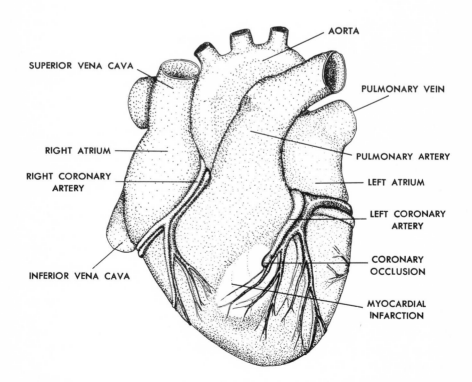

Fig. 13.3 Heart showing coronary vessels and a myocardial infarction.

portions of the body, and the *inferior vena cava,* which collects blood
from the lower portions of the body. It transmits this blood into the
right ventricle through the *tricuspid valve,* which allows blood to pass
from the atrium into the ventricle but prevents its movement in a backward direction. Blood passes through this valve when the right atrium
contracts, after which the right ventricle contracts. When the ventricle
contracts, blood cannot pass backward through the now closed tricuspid
valve, but instead must pass on through the *pulmonary valve* into the
pulmonary artery and on to the lungs for oxygenation. The pulmonary
valve is also called a *semilunar valve,* because it is made up of three
halfmoon-shaped leaflets that prevent blood from passing back from the
pulmonary artery into the right ventricle. Following oxygenation, the
blood returns to the left side of the heart by way of the *pulmonary veins,*
which empty into the left atrium. Upon contraction of the two atria,
the blood on the left side passes into the left ventricle via the *mitral
(bicuspid) valve.* Upon contraction of the ventricles, the blood passes
through the *aortic valve* into the *aorta,* the largest artery of the body.
The aortic valve, also called a semilunar valve, prevents blood from
flowing back into the left ventricle from the aorta.

The two atria contract simultaneously and drive the blood through
the tricuspid and mitral valves at the same moment. These valves both
close when the ventricles contract. Then both the right and the left
ventricles contract at the same moment and drive the blood through
these two semilunar valves into the respective arteries, after which these
valves close. To prevent the tricuspid and bicuspid valves from collapsing when the ventricles contract, strong cords—the *chordae tendineae,*
which are attached to the valves at one end and to the papillary muscles
in the ventricle wall on the other end—contract and shorten.

PHYSIOLOGY OF THE HEART

When the body is at rest, more than 10 pints of blood are passed
through each of the heart's chambers each minute. During strenuous
activity, the capacity of the heart increases 5 to 10 times. This organ
begins its activities months before birth and never ceases until the
moment of death. To give the muscle some measure of rest, there is a
rhythmic alternation of the contraction phase *(systole)* with a resting
phase *(diastole).* The time needed for contraction and relaxation varies.
At the usual rate of 70 beats per minute, the diastole is twice as long as
the systole. As activity becomes more strenuous, the rest period becomes
shorter. The systole phase begins in the atria, then passes into the ventricles. The systole phase results in the familiar "lubb-dupp" sounds of
the heart. The "lubb" sounds are caused mostly by the closure of the
atrioventricular valves (tricuspid and mitral); and the "dupp" sound,
by the closure of the semilunar valves. If a valve fails to close properly,

blood moves back through the valve, causing a "swishing" sound, called a *murmur*. (Other abnormalities of the heart will be discussed later.)

The heart muscle operates in a manner completely different from that of any other muscle of the body. Although the heart is under the control of the central nervous system, its beat originates independently inside the heart. The beat starts in the right atrium at a spot called the *sino-atrial node (SA node)*, also called the "pacemaker." From the right atrium the impulse travels over the entire atrial muscle, causing the atria to contract. The wave action is passed to a second specialized area, the *atrioventricular node (AV node)*, located in the septum between the right atrium and the ventricle. From this spot the wave action is transmitted to the *bundle of His,* a band of specialized cells which pass down the interventricular septum and divide into two main branches, called the *Purkinje fibers.* These fibers spread throughout the ventricular walls. As a result the muscles of the ventricle contract almost all at once.

BLOOD VESSELS

The *pulmonary circulation* carries the blood from the right ventricle toward the lungs; the *systemic circulation,* from the left ventricle to all parts of the body. Blood traveling to the heart muscle leaves the aorta through the *coronary circulation* (Fig. 13.3).

The blood vessels, together with the four chambers of the heart, form a closed system of circulation. The blood cannot escape unless there is a break in some wall. Blood vessels may be divided into three groups: *arteries, capillaries,* and *veins.*

ARTERIES

Arteries carry blood away from the pumping chambers of the heart to other parts of the body. The arterial system begins with the main artery of the body, the aorta, from which lesser arteries branch off until the entire body is supplied with blood (Fig. 13.1).

Arterial walls are relatively thick, since they must sustain the pressure created on the blood by the heartbeat. The walls are composed of three layers: the inner, or *tunica intima;* the middle, or *tunica media;* and the outer, or *tunica externa.* The elastic quality of the arteries allows them to stretch, but prevents them from collapsing upon themselves. The walls contain muscle tissue that contract when the nerves supplying them are stimulated. Such contraction narrows, or constricts, the internal diameter of the arteries. When the nerves are not stimulated, the muscles relax, or dilate, giving a larger internal diameter. These actions are called *vasoconstrictions* and *vasodilations,* respectively. (The prefix *vaso-* refers to a vessel.) Through branching, the arteries eventually become very small. The smallest subdivisions, the arterioles, lead into the capillaries.

CAPILLARIES

The capillaries are minute, thin-walled tubes connecting the arterioles with the *venules* (smallest veins). Because the capillaries have thin walls, materials carried by the blood move through them very slowly, allowing for an interchange of materials. The capillaries are exceedingly numerous. No living cell of the body is more than a few cells away from a capillary.

VEINS

Veins drain the tissues and the organs and return the blood to the heart. Their walls are much thinner than those of arteries, have much less muscle and elastic tissues, and are easily collapsed. Consequently, they are less extensible and elastic. Since the blood pressure is reduced as it moved through the capillaries, the veins cannot depend solely upon heart pressure to move the blood through them. They are thus provided with one-way *valves* that prevent the blood from flowing back into the capillaries. Many veins are located in the skeletal muscles. As one exercises and stretches, he assists the movement of the blood through the veins.

LYMPHATICS

The food and oxygen leave the blood in the capillaries and enter the tissue fluid. This tissue fluid, which bathes all cells of the body and which acts as a connecting link between the blood and the cells, is known as *lymph*. It is made up of certain fluid portions of the blood. Lymph accumulates faster than it is able to move back into the blood capillaries. It is continually drained from the tissue spaces through a system of tubules called the *lymphatic system* (see Fig. 14.2). Completely separate and apart from the blood capillaries, these lymph, or collecting, capillaries begin as microscopic, blind (closed) ducts. Becoming larger, they finally converge into the *thoracic duct,* which enters the right subclavian vein near the right side of the neck (from the upper parts of the body). In the intestinal wall the lymphatic capillaries are called *lacteals* (see Chapter 6).

The lymphatic vessels are thin walled and are provided with valves, like the valves of the veins, to prevent backflow. Exercise and changes in body position help to maintain the flow of lymph. The lymphatic system has no pump, or heart, to push the lymph along.

As the lymph is returned to the veins, it passes through a series of filters called *lymph nodes* (lymph glands). Here certain undesirable particles are taken out of circulation. Made of specialized tissues, called *lymphoid tissue,* the nodes remove and to some extent destroy impurities such as carbon particles, cancer cells, dead blood cells, and pathogenic organisms. These foreign proteins and bacteria are ingested and partly destroyed by certain white blood cells normally present. The nodes manufacture *lymphocytes,* which make up about one-fifth of all white blood cells, and produce antibodies (see Chapter 15). *Gamma globulin* (see Chapter 15) is formed in the lymph nodes as the result of the formation and destruction of lymphocytes; through the lymph it is made available to the body for protective tasks.

Lymph nodes are quite variable in size and tend to occur in groups. They are located in chains of from several nodes up to several hundred, the greatest masses being found along the side of the head and neck, in the nose-throat area, under the armpits, and in the groin. Lymph nodes close to cancer sites tend to collect wandering cancer cells; thus nodes near known cancer sites are commonly surgically removed along with the cancerous tissue. An example would be the removal of lymph nodes in the armpit of a woman at the same time that her cancerous breast is removed.

Lymphatic tissue is also found in the tonsils, thymus gland, and spleen (see Chapter 6). Although the functions of the tonsils and thymus gland have long been debated, it is thought that they function in a manner similar to that of other lymphatic tissue. Abnormalities in tonsil size as a result of the development of diseased tissue can be a detriment to health; consequently, the tonsil and adenoid lymphatic tissue are sometimes removed surgically. The spleen undoubtedly performs the same task as other lymphatic tissue, in addition to serving as a reservoir for red blood cells and a filter for disintegrated blood cells. Hodgkin's disease and lymphosarcoma, cancerous disorders of the lymphatics, will be discussed in Chapter 14.

FETAL CIRCULATION

During fetal life the blood of the unborn child travels through the umbilical artery (in the umbilical cord) to the mother to be oxygenated. It returns to the child from the mother by way of the umbilical vein, is passed to the liver, and thence into the right atrium (see Fig. 13.4). Accordingly, the blood in the right atrium is rather well oxygenated. Since the child's lungs are not yet functioning, and since much of the blood entering the right side of the heart is already oxygenated, the child is normally provided with two short circuits that allow much of the blood to bypass the lungs. An opening in the interatrial septum, the *foramen ovale,* provides for some of this short-circuiting; and a connection between the pulmonary artery and the aorta, the *ductus arteriosus,* provides for the rest. The main volume of blood passes through the foramen ovale.

At birth the child's lungs become functional and the placental circulation is broken. Normally, during the first year a septum closes over

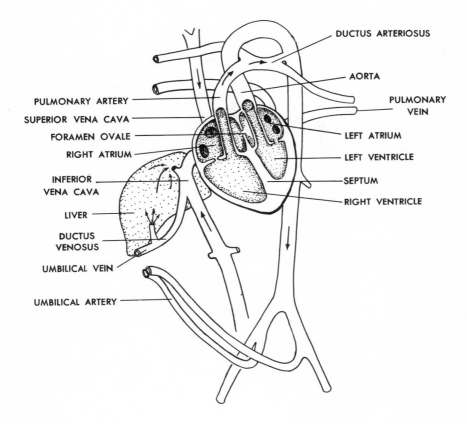

Fig. 13.4 Fetal circulation.

the foramen ovale. This closure is incomplete in about 20 percent of all individuals. The ductus arteriosus normally closes during the first month of life.

BLOOD

Blood is the fluid that circulates through the closed circulatory system to all tissues of the body. Under normal conditions it consists of a straw-colored fluid, or *plasma,* in which are suspended the *corpuscles*—the red blood cells, or *erythrocytes;* the white blood cells, or *leucocytes;* and the *platelets* (see Fig. 13.5). The fluid portion makes up about 55 percent of the whole blood; the cells, or solid portion, about 45 percent. Since blood is continuously exchanging materials with tissues it services, its composition is constantly changing.

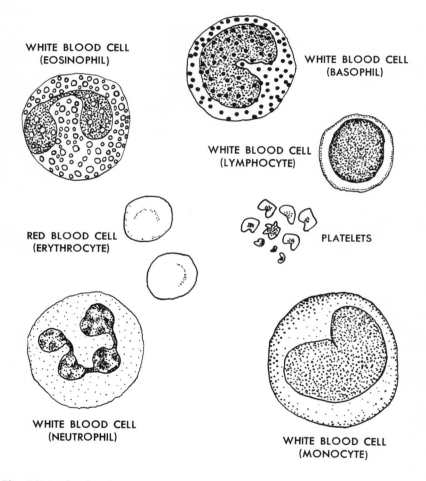

WHITE BLOOD CELL
(EOSINOPHIL)

WHITE BLOOD CELL
(BASOPHIL)

WHITE BLOOD CELL
(LYMPHOCYTE)

RED BLOOD CELL
(ERYTHROCYTE)

PLATELETS

WHITE BLOOD CELL
(NEUTROPHIL)

WHITE BLOOD CELL
(MONOCYTE)

Fig. 13.5 Blood cells.

PLASMA

The liquid portion of the blood consists of about 90 percent water. The remaining 10 percent of the plasma contains many different substances, including proteins, carbohydrates (principally in the form of glucose), lipids (fats), mineral salts (including compounds of calcium and sodium, carbonates and phosphates, and potassium and magnesium salts), waste products, hormones, and gases.

RED BLOOD CELLS

The red blood cells are tiny disc-shaped bodies. Normally formed in the bone marrow, they usually live no longer than 120 days. Their main purpose is to carry oxygen from the lungs to the tissues. This function is made possible by the ingredient *hemoglobin,* which is also responsible for the red color of these cells. The more oxygen present, the brighter red their color; the less, the darker red their color. They are by far the most numerous of any corpuscle in the blood, averaging from 4.5 to 5.5 million per cubic millimeter of blood.

WHITE BLOOD CELLS

The white blood cells consist of various types of colorless cells. They are outnumbered by red cells by about 700 or 800 to 1. Although generally in the shape of a ball, they have the ability to change shape. Their ability to change shape allows some of them to leave the capillaries, which the red blood cells cannot do. Attracted to any area of tissue in which *pathogens* are present, such as at the site of a wound or infection, they engulf (or ingest) the pathogens and thus destroy them. Often they are affected by the poisons given off by the pathogens and die. They then become a part of the accumulation of material we know as an *abscess* or *pus.* The white blood cells that return to the blood stream generally do so by way of the lymph.

PLATELETS

Fragments of larger cells, *platelets (thrombocytes)* are essential to blood clotting, or *coagulation.* When a blood vessel is damaged, platelets release *thromboplastin* (also released by damaged tissues). This reacts in stages with two plasma proteins *(prothrombin* and *fibrinogen)* to form a meshwork of *fibrin* threads which entrap blood cells, thus forming a *clot.* Fibrin threads are sticky and adhere easily to any blood vessel opening.

BLOOD GROUPS

If, for any of a number of reasons, the amount of blood in the body is too severely reduced, a person may need additional blood in the form of a *transfusion*. Before the twentieth century transfusions often had disastrous results. Later, it was discovered that red blood cells contained protein antigens, substances which, when present in the body, cause the production of antibodies. Four main antigen types have been identified. Type A persons have A antigen, type B persons have B antigen, type AB persons have both, and type O persons have neither. The percentage of each type varies with different races. Among Caucasians about 43 percent are type O, about 40 percent type A, about 13 percent type B, and 4 percent type AB. The plasma may also contain antibodies *a* or *b* which react with the corresponding antigen and cause red blood cells to clump. The plasma of a type B person contains *a* antibodies, the plasma of a type A person *b* antibodies, the plasma of a type AB person neither antibodies and the plasma of an O type person both *a* and *b* antibodies. If we mix type A blood with plasma containing *a* antibodies, the cells will gather together in clumps. If these cells clump in the blood vessels, the capillaries will be clogged and death is likely to follow. In transfusions it is always best to give blood of the recipient's own type. It is possible, however, to give another type blood. A type O person can give blood to a recipient of type O, A, B, or AB, and for this reason can be called a *universal donor*. A type AB person can receive blood from donors of type O, A, B, and AB, and for this reason can be called a *universal recipient*. Prior to transfusion small volumes of both the donor's and the recipient's blood should be *cross-matched* to determine compatibility. This is done by both placing red blood cells of the donor in *serum* of the recipient and red blood cells of the recipient in serum of the donor. Absence of agglutination indicates that the two blood specimens are compatible.

The main blood types are inherited characteristics. As a consequence, they may be of some value in determining the disputed paternity of a child.

Another blood protein, the Rh factor, is now recognized to be of significance not only in transfusions, but also in childbirth. About 85 percent of the white population in this country possesses this factor. (A more detailed discussion of the Rh factor can be found in Chapter 9.)

BLOOD COUNT

The normal white blood cell count is about 6000 to 8000 per cubic millimeter of blood, compared with 4.5 to 5.5 million red cells per cubic millimeter. An apparatus for counting the number of blood cells, called a *hemocytometer*, is generally used to make blood counts. Since the number of red and white blood cells varies rather quickly in response to certain physical conditions, a count can be used for certain diagnostic purposes.

BLOOD DISORDERS

There are several abnormalities involving the blood. They can be conveniently divided into four groups.

THE ANEMIAS

Reduction in the number of red blood cells or the amount of hemoglobin in red blood cells is called *anemia*. A reduction in the number of red blood cells may be due to hemorrhage (loss of blood); destruction of red blood cells by organisms such as malarial parasites or by coal tar products; abnormalities in the red blood cell–forming mechanism as a result of overexposure to X rays, radioactive substances, or organic poisoning; or defects in the formation of the red cell. Since hemoglobin contains iron, an iron deficiency may reduce the hemoglobin concentration and cause an iron-deficiency type of anemia, the only type of anemia that responds well to treatment.

NEOPLASTIC BLOOD DISEASES

Neoplastic blood diseases, characterized by an enormous increase in the number of white blood cells of one or more kinds, are the *leukemias;* they represent forms of cancer. Since Chapter 14 deals with forms of cancer, discussion of these diseases will be found there.

LEUKOPENIAS

Leukopenias are diseases or conditions which reduce the number of white blood cells below a satisfactory level. They occur in many infections, such as typhoid fever, measles, influenza, and malaria. They also develop from chronic hemorrhage; malnutrition; lead, mercury, and arsenic poisoning; and from alcohol and morphine poisoning.

HEMORRHAGIC DISORDERS

In hemorrhagic disorders the normal coagulation process is disrupted, leading to abnormal bleeding. *Hemophilia,* one of these disorders, is a hereditary disease in which the platelets fail to dissolve in the proper manner. A hemophiliac is in danger of bleeding to death with even the smallest cut. *Purpura* is a disease in which hemorrhages occur in the skin and the mucous membranes. This malady is due to a reduced number of platelets caused by one of several factors.

PULSE AND BLOOD PRESSURE

With each beat of the heart, which average 70 per minute in man, blood is forced out of each ventricle. It flows into the aorta from the left ventricle with great force, and from the right ventricle into the pulmonary artery with moderate force. The rapid contraction of the heart makes this discharge of blood rapid, spurtlike, and intermittent. During the interval of each beat the heart collects as much blood from the body as it discharges. With each beat of the left ventricle (Fig. 13.2), a wave of pressure starts at the heart and travels along the arteries. This wave is called the *pulse*. The pulse can be felt on any arteries that are close to the surface of the body, such as on the wrist, the sides of the throat, or the temple. The pulse is the result of the pressure of the blood on the walls of the arteries—the *blood pressure*. This pressure is highest in the aorta; it gradually decreases as it travels through the arteries, capillaries, veins, and into the right atrium. Although the blood pressure is greater after the left ventricle contracts, there is always some pressure in the arteries. The blood pressure at the moment of contraction is the *systolic pressure;* it should normally be sufficient to displace about 120 mm of mercury in a glass tube. The blood pressure at the moment of relaxation of the heart is the *diastolic pressure;* it should normally displace about 80 mm of mercury. Thus the reading of blood pressure in a normal young person should be about 120/80 ("one-twenty over eighty").

The usual instrument for determining arterial blood pressure is called a *sphygmomanometer*. It consists of a rubber cuff wrapped around the arm and connected by a tube to a scaled mercury column. The cuff is inflated so that it collapses an artery in the arm. By listening to the flow of blood through the artery with a *stethoscope* as the air in the cuff is let out, a physician can determine systolic and diastolic blood pressure.

FACTORS INFLUENCING PULSE RATE

A number of things can influence pulse rate. It tends to be faster in smaller people and in women. It tends to be faster in a newborn infant than in an adult. It increases proportionately with increases in bodily activity and it decreases during sleep. It increases under emotional excitement, even where no muscular activity is involved. Many infections will increase the pulse rate as the temperature increases.

FACTORS INFLUENCING ABNORMAL BLOOD PRESSURE

The nature of the blood pressure may indicate any number of factors of importance in a person's circulation. It can indicate the strength of the heart action. It can reflect the volume of blood in circulation. A decrease in volume, as through shock or hemorrhage, will cause a drop in blood pressure. An increase in volume will cause a corresponding increase in pressure. Blood pressure can indicate whether the elastic quality of the artery walls is normal. In the event an artery becomes "hardened" (sclerotic) and loses this elasticity, the blood pressure will increase, since the same volume of blood is being forced through a smaller opening. Any impediment along the circulatory route will hinder the flow of blood and increase its pressure. Consequently, increased blood pressure may indicate kidney disease, uremia, or cancerous growths. *Hypertension*, or high blood pressure, will be discussed more fully later in the chapter.

ELIMINATION OF BLOOD WASTE

After the food brought by the blood to the cell has been metabolized, certain waste products remain. These include urea, carbon dioxide, water, and salts. These are eliminated from the body by one of three main routes: the skin, the lungs, or the kidneys. Although the skin and lungs are important, the kidneys are the most important in blood purification.

THE KIDNEYS

The kidneys serve to eliminate most of the urea and salts and much of the water from the body. As the body uses proteins, it produces nitrogenous wastes, which are excreted as urea. In addition, certain salts from the blood plasma are also excreted. Excretion is only one of the functions of the kidneys. They also aid in maintaining water balance and aid in regulating the acid-base balance of the body.

The amount of blood that is filtered through the kidneys depends upon the blood pressure. This amount of blood flow is reflected in the amount of urine produced. If the blood pressure falls too low (below 40 mm of mercury), urine ceases to flow. In the filtering of blood plasma, the kidneys extract water from the blood along with dissolved substances. Blood cells, droplets of fat, and other very large molecules are held back.

A large volume of blood is filtered by the kidneys. The rate is about one quart per minute. A volume of blood equal to the entire amount in the body flows through the kidneys every four to five minutes. Since only the larger components of the blood are held back in filtration, certain useful substances are filtered out along with waste products. These the kidneys reclaim before the wastes are passed out as urine. Although not all useful substances are reclaimed, most of them are returned to the blood. On occasion these useful substances may appear in the urine in more than normal amounts if they appear in the blood in higher than normal concentrations, such as excess glucose in diabetics.

The general body blood pressure tends to increase if the *renal* (kidney) arteries are obstructed or narrowed. Occasionally such rise may be due to tumors of the kidneys. Either of these can be a persistent cause of hypertension.

THE ROLE OF EXERCISE

During muscular activity much of the oxygen in the blood is used up by the contracting muscles and the amount of carbon dioxide is increased. There is increased respiration in the lungs, which is enhanced by an increased heart rate and an increase in the flow of blood through the pulmonary and systemic circulation. Inversely, the amount of activity a person can perform is influenced by the action of his heart, the size of the blood vessels, and the characteristics of his blood.

The body can maintain sufficient oxygen supply and elimination of carbon dioxide during light or moderate exercise. During severe exercise, however, the carbon dioxide concentration begins to increase faster than the supply of oxygen and it takes the body some time after the exertion has ceased to catch up on the necessary elimination of the oversupply of carbon dioxide.

TYPES AND CAUSES OF CIRCULATORY DISEASES

Like any other tissues of the body, those of the heart and circulatory system are subject to disease and infection. Diseases in tissues in an arm or leg may cripple a person, but diseases of the heart muscle frequently lead to early death. For that reason the heart and possible structural or functional disorders of that vital organ will be of major concern in the following discussion, although the entire circulatory system and its disorders is the subject under consideration in this chapter. Some of the conditions to be discussed occur during fetal development and therefore are *congenital* disorders; others occur later in childhood or adulthood and therefore are *degenerative*.

CONGENITAL DISORDERS

Abnormalities in the development of the heart may occur during the first three months of fetal life. Although the specific causes of congenital malformations of the heart are generally unknown, known causes include certain maternal illnesses or metabolic upsets during the first three months of pregnancy, such as German measles, mumps, or influenza. Ionizing radiations (such as X rays) and certain drugs may have similar effects. According to the President's Commission on Heart

Disease, Cancer and Stroke (Volume II), more than 20,000 babies with heart deformities are born each year in this country. These malformations are common to all parts of the world and all races, and most of them present a severe handicap to the child. Such inborn heart defects are not thought to be inherited. A mother with a congenital heart defect has about a 2 percent chance of passing such a malformation on to her children.

KINDS OF CONGENITAL HEART DEFECTS

Heart malformations may take many forms. They may affect any part of the heart. The extent of the malformation may be slight or extensive. Because some of them cause reduction in the normal supply of oxygenated blood, the skin takes on a bluish hue; thus they are generally called "blue baby" conditions.

1. *Septal defects.* An abnormal opening in the septum may occur between the two atria (upper chambers) or the two ventricles (lower chambers). The most common is the persistence of the foramen ovale, the fetal opening between the two atria (Fig. 13.4). Incomplete closure, called a *patent foramen ovale*, occurs in about one out of every four individuals. This ovale allows the deoxygenated blood from the right side to move to the left atrium, which should be transmitting oxygenated blood. In a small number of cases the presence of sufficient impure blood passing into the aorta may give a bluish hue to the skin, hence the term "blue baby."

A ventricular septal defect has a different effect. Since the blood in the left ventricle is under more pressure than that in the right ventricle, such a defect allows some of the blood to move from the left ventricle into the right ventricle rather than into the aorta. Thus less blood is available for the aortic flow. To compensate, the heart usually works harder, thus placing an extra load on it and causing it to fail at an earlier age.

2. *Patent ductus arteriosus.* Earlier it was noted that in the fetal circulatory system a duct exists between the pulmonary artery and the aorta and that this duct normally closes during the first month of life (see Fig. 13.4). If it fails to close, it is called a *patent ductus arteriosus*. Since aortic blood is under greater pressure than pulmonary blood, some of the pure aortic blood passes into the pulmonary artery. The systemic (body) circulation is thus deprived of some blood. To compensate, the heart works harder. This condition allows the person less reserve for strenuous activities and high altitudes and also reduces the life span of his heart. If this condition is uncorrected by surgery, the patient usually dies between the ages of 20 and 40. Since this defect is in the arteries just above the heart, corrective surgery does not involve the heart itself; it has been quite effective.

3. *Coarctation of the aorta.*   An abnormal constriction, or "pinching in," of an artery is called a *coarctation.* It is most severe when it occurs within the aorta. Since such a "pinching shut" impedes the flow of blood through the aorta, it increases the work load required of the heart. Formerly, individuals with this disorder often failed to reach middle age. Today surgery brings about a complete cure in most cases.

4. *Stenosis.*   A stenosis is a fusing of the leaflets of either of the semilunar valves, pulmonary or aortic. Such fusion (narrowing) hampers the flow of blood and increases the work the heart must do. Surgery can be performed on selected patients. A severe, uncorrected case can place such a work load on the heart that the heart is likely to fail earlier than normal.

5. *Tetralogy of Fallot.*   This condition, caused by a combination of defects, results in poor oxygenation of the blood. It involves abnormal aortic location, pulmonary stenosis, a defective ventricular septum, and an enlarged right ventricle. Formerly a condition causing a very early death, it can today be treated relatively successfully by surgery, which can increase the life expectancy of the victim by 30 to 50 years.

FUTURE FOR CONGENITAL DEFORMITIES

Until 25 years ago about one out of every three congenital heart patients survived to the age of 10. Today the development of the *heart-lung machine,* a device which takes over the functions of the heart and lungs while they are bypassed for surgical repair, has made *open-heart surgery* possible. Such surgery involves operating on the heart directly. The heart-lung machine is also used where repair is called for in a major artery or vein. Although new improvements are being made in congenital heart surgery, the ultimate goal of cardiology is to discover what causes congenital heart defects and to find ways of preventing them.

DEGENERATIVE HEART DISORDERS

Although the heart is very resistant to disorders, many things can impair its efficiency. Heart disease may result from infections, toxins, injuries, insufficient nutrition, or other disturbances that weaken that organ. Unfortunately, diseases of the heart and blood vessels, called cardiovascular diseases, are the leading causes of death among adults all over the world. The following kinds of degenerative heart disorders are common.

RHEUMATIC HEART DISEASE

As explained in Chapter 16, about 3 percent of persons suffering from certain streptococcal infections develop, two or three weeks later, the

symptoms of *rheumatic fever*; these symptoms are swelling and pain in
the joints, accompanied by fever. The original infection may be in
any part of the body, but it is commonly a "strep throat" or tonsilitis.
Rheumatic fever is an allergic response to such streptococcal infection.
In about 60 percent of cases the heart is inflamed and may be permanently damaged.

Although other layers of the heart may be affected, the most common
damage is to the endocardium, the inner lining of the heart. This
endocarditis (inflammation of the endocardium) causes the heart valves,
particularly the mitral valve, to become scarred, since the valves consist mostly of endocardium. Material from the blood deposits on the
scarred valves; they thicken and tend to stick together, and thus are
prevented from opening properly. This obstruction of the flow of
blood is called stenosis. In addition, the scarring may prevent the valve
from closing tightly, so that blood leaks back through the valve,
forcing the heart to pump harder in order to circulate an adequate
supply of blood. Open-heart surgery has been increasingly effective in
relieving such damage. The scar tissue may be removed, or the damaged
valves may even be replaced with effective artificial valves.

Antibiotic therapy has lowered the incidence of and death rate from
rheumatic fever. As a preventive measure, all streptococcal infections
should be promptly treated. The person with a history of rheumatic
fever must be particularly prompt in seeking treatment for infections,
as one attack of rheumatic fever leaves a person highly susceptible to
repeated attacks for the rest of his life.

ARTERIOSCLEROSIS

"Hardening of the arteries" involves the middle of the three layers of
the artery wall, the *tunica media*. When the fibrous tissue accumulates
calcium deposits, such arteries become "hard," or sclerotic. Their
rigidity can be felt in such spots as the wrists, and X rays depict them
clearly because of the calcium. Although such arteries are hard, they
commonly retain adequate space inside, and circulation remains adequate. But hardened arteries have lost much of their elasticity and are
easily ruptured or hemorrhaged.

ATHEROSCLEROSIS

Atherosclerosis is a disease principally of the large arteries. Platelike
lipid (fat) deposits, called *plaques*, appear at one or more points in the
inner walls (*tunica intima*) of the arteries. As these plaques enlarge, they
commonly protrude into the channel (*lumen*) of the artery. The roughness of this inner surface may cause blood clots (*thrombi*) to develop
at these sites. A thrombus may cause the partial or complete obstruction

(*occlusion*) of the vessel at this spot and shut off blood flow. On occasion, a thrombus may break loose into the blood stream. Such a moving clot, or *embolus,* may be carried to a point where it completely blocks the flow of blood. Although other substances, such as air, fat plaques, or tumerous material may also cause emboli, clots are the most common cause. Owing to the absence of calcium in atherosclerotic arteries, X rays do not show a clear picture of them unless some dye is injected into the artery before the X ray.

Although atherosclerotic damage may occur in any vessel, it is most severe in certain places. If it occurs in the heart muscle, the patient has a heart attack; if in the brain, a stroke; if in the foot, gangrene; if in the kidney, high blood pressure. The patient may be fortunate and be able to develop *collateral circulation* (enlargement of other vessels in the same area to make up for the lost circulation). Although the consequences of atherosclerosis usually appear during old age, there is evidence of atherosclerosis in some young adults. The full-blown disease in older people is likely the result of a lifetime of lipid deposition within the arteries.

Although some medical scientists believe that cholesterol in the diet is the chief contributor to atherosclerosis, it appears that there are other contributing factors. In certain parts of the world where people consume considerable amounts of saturated animal fats with a high rate of cholesterol, blood cholesterol levels are low. Our present understanding of the causes of atherosclerosis is incomplete.

HYPERTENSION

Hypertension simply means high arterial blood pressure. Sometimes it can be traced to a known disease, and that disease can be cured. Most commonly, however, it is a hereditary factor, called *essential hypertension,* that tends to run in families. Whatever the cause, the increase in blood pressure puts added strain on the left ventricle, sometimes causing it to enlarge and thus reducing its ability to respond to the demands made on it.

The causes for essential hypertension are known in a minority of cases. These include chronic inflammation of the kidneys and certain diseases of the endocrine glands. Fortunately, a number of effective drugs are available, including sedatives which can satisfactorily reduce the blood pressure if prescribed in time. Some sufferers from hypertension have been successfully treated by a drastic reduction of the quantity of sodium in their diets, but the resulting reduction in blood pressure brought about by this treatment involves an incompletely understood mechanism which probably has something to do with the kidneys.

CORONARY DISEASE

The blood vessels surrounding the heart derive their name from the fact that they encircle the heart like a crown, or *corona* (see Fig. 13.3). They transport almost one-half pint of blood every minute over the heart muscle. Any sudden obstruction of one of the coronary arteries will deprive that respective part of the heart of its blood supply and will cause the muscle to cease to function. This deadening of an area of heart muscle is called a *myocardial infarction;* it is manifested by a typical pain in the chest and sometimes by an arrest of the heart. If a coronary artery is completely obstructed, whatever the cause, the condition is called a *coronary occlusion* or *heart attack.* Sudden death usually occurs if the occlusion occurs in a main coronary artery. If the obstruction is only partial or is in a smaller coronary tributary, sufficient nutrition and rest may lead to the patient's recovery. The agonizing pain caused when such an area of dead tissue is formed may be felt in the region of the heart and in the left arm and shoulder. Such pain is called *angina pectoris.* Angina pectoris may be accompanied by a feeling of suffocation and of doom.

Fortunately, the great majority of coronary disease patients recover and are able to lead active, useful lives, provided they get proper treatment under good medical supervision. Approximately one third of all deaths in the United States, however, result from coronary artery disease. Almost all elderly persons have at least some impairment of coronary artery circulation.

In all cases the best medical care is essential. Great care is necessary, particularly during the critical time of the second and third days after the attack, when the rhythm of the heart may be disturbed. Following the infarction, the dead portion of the heart is replaced in a few weeks by fibrous tissue. At the same time new blood vessels begin taking the place of the occluded artery. Eventually, if full recovery is made, all that will remain on the heart will be a scar.

It is important to distinguish between a coronary attack and a coronary failure. An attack may be mild or severe and may or may not lead to death. A coronary failure is the stoppage of the heart and, in most cases, will lead to the death of the patient unless emergency treatment is successful in reviving the victim.

CEREBROVASCULAR ACCIDENTS

The brain demands more than one fifth of all the blood pumped by the heart. As with the heart, any interruption in the normal flow of blood to the brain can have serious consequences. Such interruptions, commonly called *strokes* or *apoplexy,* may come about in several ways: (1) blockage of an artery by the formation of a clot (thrombus); (2) blockage due to an embolus carried from some other place in the body; (3) rupture of a blood vessel in the brain as a result of high blood pressure, arteriosclerosis, or an *aneurysm* (ballooning of a vessel at a weakened spot), or (4) cutting of the flow of blood by a tumor that places pressure on a blood vessel.

Depending upon its size and location, the stroke may be severe enough to cause rapid death or be too slight to be noticed. The common symptoms of moderately severe strokes include speech impediments, loss of memory or mental activity, and often partial paralysis. Since nerve cells on one side of the brain control the muscles on the opposite side of the body, a cerebrovascular accident in one side of the brain usually causes paralysis on only one side of the body, a condition called *hemiplegia.*

Considerable progress has been made both in the treatment of stroke patients and in their rehabilitation. Most patients who survive the acute phase are able to lead a life which, although restricted to some extent, is nevertheless satisfying.

SYPHILITIC HEART

Reference is made in Chapter 17 to the cardiovascular complications of certain venereal diseases and to syphilis in particular. In the late stage of this disease there is destruction of cardiovascular tissue. The organism infiltrates blood vessel walls, and the lesions formed are scarred over with fibrous tissue. These late lesions are destructive and chronic, in some cases occurring for many years. Such lesions, even though they are scarred over, represent weak spots; they lead to the development of aneurysms, which may give way under pressure or form clots.

HEART BLOCK

As a result of degeneration or disease in the nerve cells of the heart, the rhythmic transmission of nerve impulses regulating the heart beat may be disturbed. The exact type of heart block produced will depend upon the location of the destruction, although in all cases some degree of impulse interference, or blockage, occurs. A *sinoatrial block* affects the nerve transmission through the atria. The ventricles pick up a new rhythm and perform normally. An *atrioventricular block* prevents the transmission of the impulse from the AV node to the ventricles. Although a complete stoppage of the ventricular beat would mean death, this type of blockage often only reduces the number of ventricular contractions in relation to the atrial contractions. For every two atrial beats the ventricles may beat only once, creating a 2:1 rhythm, or perhaps a 3:2 or a 3:1 rhythm.

VASCULAR DISORDERS

In addition to the abnormal conditions of the blood vessels already discussed, there are several others.

1. *Aneurysms.* As previously defined, an aneurysm is a sac-like or ballooned section of the wall of an artery or vein resulting from a localized weakness in that part of the vessel. Most commonly, the aorta is the vessel affected. Such damage may result from lesions caused by syphilis or from the effects of arteriosclerosis. Regardless of the cause, aneurysms tend to enlarge, thus weakening the walls affected. Under excess pressure, the aneurysm may suddenly burst; if it bursts in a critical location, such as the aorta, immediate death results. In some cases modern surgery can replace weakened aortic sections with synthetic materials.

2. *Hemorrhage.* Hemorrhage is the profuse escape of blood from the vessels. It may occur from any vessels, external or internal, regardless of size or location. If only a small vessel is involved, normal clotting mechanisms will usually stop the flow. Loss of blood from a larger vessel, particularly an artery, may often be rapid and fatal. Immediate first aid through the use of direct pressure on the wound or the manual compression of the artery at a critical pressure point where the artery crosses a bone may successfully halt the loss of blood.

3. *Shock.* Shock is a general, highly dangerous condition in which circulation is suddenly reduced. A state of shock may be brought on by a number of conditions—severe hemorrhage, a sudden nervous disturbance, burns, prolonged surgery, certain drugs, cold or exhaustion, or anything causing a lack of oxygen in the blood. One or more of these factors may cause the small vessels to expand, with the result that blood drains from the large vessels into the small vessels of the tissues and stops circulating. Thus the blood volume is markedly reduced and essential organs needing constant circulation are deprived of the contents of the blood and soon begin to die. The victim will die quickly unless steps are taken to restore adequate circulation. A transfusion of whole blood is the best therapy, although plasma and plasma substitutes (such as glucose solutions) have been used. These increase blood volume and help restore the circulation to normal.

A person in shock will usually have cold, clammy skin, lowered body temperature, very low blood pressure, and shallow breathing. Temporary relief, such as keeping the patient warm and tilting his body so that it is either horizontal or in a tilted position with the feet up, is desirable until better measures can be taken.

4. *Varicose veins.* Since blood in the veins is under less pressure

than that in the arteries, the veins are equipped with internal valves arranged so that the movement of the blood through them can only be toward the heart. These valves, along with any muscular movement, "squeeze" the nearby veins, helping to "pump" the blood back to the heart. Unfortunately, the valves are frequently destroyed. This destruction occurs when the veins have been overstretched (undue pressure placed on them) for an extended period of time, as for example from pregnancy or prolonged standing; it is more frequent in women than in men. The veins stretch so that the valves can no longer block the backflow of blood, and eventually the valves are destroyed. As a result the person develops *varicose veins,* large swollen veins either beneath the skin or deep in the tissues. Although these disfiguring veins may occur in various places on the body, they commonly are found along the lower leg. The resulting accumulation of venous blood in these damaged vessels creates pain and weakness in the affected muscles. (Varicose veins in the rectum are commonly referred to as hemorrhoids.)

Treatment includes elevation of the patient's legs, wearing of elastic stockings or bandages, and injection of sclerosing (hardening) solutions to restrict the swelling. Surgery may be resorted to in cases where the vein lies just under the skin. Called *stripping* the veins, the process involves ligating (tying-off) the affected section of vein and then pulling it out. The flow of blood is then rerouted through other connecting veins.

5. *Phlebitis.* Phlebitis is an inflammation of a vein, resulting in distinct pain and considerable swelling at the point involved. The general inflammation and irritation may lead to the formation of a blood clot, a condition called *thrombophlebitis.* The same danger exists with this clot as with any other clot in the body. An embolism might break loose, enter the right side of the heart, and then be circulated to the lungs (*pulmonary embolism*), where it could form an obstruction and cause sudden death. Phlebitis has been reduced in recent years through greater use of anticoagulants, earlier exercise after surgery to insure proper circulation, and prevention of infections.

ENVIRONMENTAL EFFECTS ON THE CIRCULATORY SYSTEM

According to the World Health Organization, cardiovascular disease is common to all races. It is not, as is sometimes claimed, a disease confined mainly to people of Europe and North America. Any differences in frequency and distribution of the major cardiovascular diseases can be explained by differences in environment, in nutrition, and in the general way of life. These diseases are particularly prevalent among middle-aged men.

Heart research has been unable either to place these factors in order of importance or to show that any one of them might be decisive. Nevertheless, evidence is accumulating that some factors tend to increase the risk of cardiovascular disease. These studies have made it possible to pick out individuals who are high risks for the development of arteriosclerotic heart disease. Some of the risk factors that are clearly important will be discussed here.

SERUM CHOLESTEROL LEVELS

Coronary heart victims show a higher level of serum (blood) cholesterol than does the population as a whole. A man with a serum cholesterol of over 240 mg has more than three times the possibility of acquiring arteriosclerotic heart disease (ASHD) than does a man with a serum cholesterol of less than 200 mg.

BLOOD PRESSURE LEVELS

Blood pressure was discussed earlier under Hypertension. Individuals with a systolic blood pressure greater than 160 have four times the risk of acquiring ASHD as do individuals with a systolic blood pressure of less than 120. This risk has been shown to be particularly true when the higher blood pressure of the patient has caused his left ventricle to enlarge.

SMOKING

Various studies have been conducted on the relationship of cigarette smoking and coronary disease. Present research has shown the cigarette smoker to be nearly twice the risk for developing heart disease as the nonsmoker, his chances varying somewhat according to the number of cigarettes smoked. Those who have stopped smoking cigarettes have lower rates than those who have continued. Pipe and cigar smoking does not appear to be associated with an excessive risk for developing coronary heart disease.

OBESITY

Heart researchers have not completely agreed with the insurance companies in finding obesity a cause of heart disease. Insurance companies have maintained for years that all overweight persons show a higher mortality. Other recent research, however, has shown that there is increased likelihood of development of coronary heart disease only among the grossly obese.[1]

[1] *A National Program to Conquer Heart Disease, Cancer and Stroke,* Vol. II, Washington, D.C., The President's Commission on Heart Disease, Cancer and Stroke, 1965, p. 77.

SOCIAL FACTORS

Men from rural areas appear to have a lower incidence of coronary heart disease than men from urban areas, and as rural areas become urbanized, men living in these areas show an increasing rate of heart disease. Men of European backgrounds tend to show a lower incidence than American-born men. Men with frequent changes of residence or occupation seem to have a higher frequency than other men.

OTHER FACTORS

Patients with diabetes mellitus and hypothyroidism show higher risk factors for cardiovascular disease. The Framingham study[2] has demonstrated that the incidence of coronary heart disease rises progressively as risk factors are combined. The absence of risk factors accompanies a distinctly lower incidence of coronary heart disease. Although some factors not mentioned appear to be involved, further study is needed to confirm their relevance.

HEART DISEASE AS A CAUSE OF DEATH

Diseases of the cardiovascular system account for more than 50 percent of deaths from all causes in this country today. In 1900 only one fifth of all deaths were charged to these diseases. This apparent increase must, however, be properly interpreted. During the past half century there has been a distinct increase in the percentage of older people in the population. (When a correction is made for the age changes in the population since 1930, there has actually been a decline in the death rate from cardiovascular diseases.) However, owing to recent advances in medical science, deaths attributable to rheumatic, congenital, and syphilitic heart disease have been on the decline since the end of World War II.

The preponderance of deaths from cardiovascular diseases today is attributed to degenerative and arteriosclerotic causes. Among these, coronary heart disease is responsible for the greatest number of deaths (over 50 percent of all cardiovascular diseases). Causes for other cardiovascular disease deaths, in order of decreasing importance, are stroke and hypertension. These three diseases are responsible for over 80 percent of all cardiovascular disease deaths. Since the methods of accumulating statistical information have changed in recent years, it is so far impossible to project the long-term trends of these diseases.

[2] *The Framingham Heart Study, Detection of Factors Increasing Risk of Coronary Disease,* Washington, D.C., National Heart Institute, 1964.

Incidence of death from the major cardiovascular diseases increases markedly with age (for both sexes and among all races in this country). The only pronounced decline in deaths during the past three or four decades has been among those under 35 years of age. The greatest decline has been for those under 25 years of age. For those between 25 and 34 the mortality decline has been less for males than for females. Beyond age 35 the death rate from cardiovascular diseases has been either leveling off or increasing since 1930. The most evident increase in death rates is among those over 65 years of age. Cardiovascular death rates in terms of geography show a higher mortality in the East and Far West and a lower rate in the Central and Mountain areas. The rates are higher in metropolitan than in nonmetropolitan areas. It must be noted once more that this general decline in cardiovascular deaths, although encouraging, has not been substantial and for the most part reflects a reduction in death rates from rheumatic and syphilitic heart disease. Furthermore, deaths from coronary arteriosclerotic heart disease have increased during the past decade.

Aside from the deaths they cause, cardiovascular diseases have also been responsible for more illness and disability than any other group of diseases. According to the Report by the President's Commission on Heart Disease, Cancer and Stroke,[3] among persons aged 18 to 79, almost 25 percent had definite or suspected cases of heart disease.

PREVENTION OF HEART DISEASE

Whether or not heart disorders are preventable depends upon their nature. Heart diseases due to infection or malnutrition are largely preventable. Congenital malformations of the heart and vessels can in most cases be corrected by surgery, although little is known about their prevention. The incidence of rheumatic fever can be considerably reduced by proper and prompt use of antibiotics in treating streptococcal infections. Circulatory problems of the lungs can be reduced through prevention or early treatment of respiratory infections and through reduction of air pollution and cigarette smoking.

The reduction of coronary sclerosis appears to depend upon a reduction in cholesterol and other lipids in the blood, control of excessive blood pressure, and the receiving of sufficient regular physical exercise. But more study needs to be done before we can answer some questions. What is an ideal diet? How are health and disease influenced by physical activity and rest? What part is played by nervous tension and chronic anxiety? What are the positive or negative effect of our environment upon us? Some additional points in reducing heart disease might include

[3] Op. cit., p. 20.

1. Getting proper nutrition, including all the basic food elements in reasonable amounts.
2. Avoiding or adequately treating infections of all kinds, including those of the teeth.
3. Avoiding excessively emotional upsets and smoking of any tobacco products (particularly where such smoke is inhaled).
4. Living a balanced life; getting balanced activity. Adequate and regular rest is important, as is regular moderate physical exercise.
5. Getting regular periodic physical examinations.

SYMPTOMS AND TREATMENT OF HEART ATTACKS

SYMPTOMS

The presence of cardiovascular disease may become apparent in several ways. It may be revealed by a routine physical examination, electrocardiogram, or chest X ray in a patient who may have had asymptomatic (without symptoms) heart disease for many years. It may manifest itself by affecting other organs, so that the true diagnosis becomes apparent only after detailed diagnostic studies. The physician must be alert to the identification of the cardiac basis for symptoms which appear to be those of other diseases, such as allergy, pulmonary disease, or disease of the gastrointestinal tract.

Most patients of heart disease, however, come to the physician complaining of common indications of heart disease. The following are some important symptoms that should be looked for.

PAIN

Cardiac pain is due to oxygen deficiency. The pain is often in the center of the chest, is very pressing, and occurs for a brief time after a period of exertion. It may radiate to the shoulders, down both arms, into the neck or jaws, and through to the back. It is described as heavy, squeezing, bursting, or burning. Occurring especially after exertion, it forces the patient to stop or slow down, then disappears shortly. In more severe cases it may continue for hours or days.

BREATHLESSNESS

Breathlessness is both the most common and most important of all symptoms. It signals a marked oxygen shortage at some place in the body. The intensity of it will vary considerably from person to person, depending upon his physical size, his lung capacity, and the severity of the attack. It tends to be more intense where there is pulmonary congestion along with heart disorder.

EDEMA

Edema is a swelling due to abnormally large amounts of fluid in the tissues of the body. It is attributed to the body's retention of sodium. In some cases it may be the result of heart disease. Other causes of edema should not be confused with cardiac edema.

FATIGUE

Heart patients are apt to complain of a heaviness of the limbs during exertion, weakness, lack of vigor, and general tiredness. Fatigue can be from both cardiac and noncardiac causes. Cardiac fatigue is usually related to or follows effort and exertion. Fatigue from anxiety and mental conflict is not related to exertion.

CYANOSIS

Cyanosis is the blueness of skin caused by insufficient oxygen in the blood. When hemoglobin is not carrying oxygen, it becomes somewhat purplish; this color shows on the surface of the body. There may be various causes for a reduction in oxygen supply, most of which can be associated with some type of circulatory abnormality.

LOSS OF CONSCIOUSNESS

Loss of consciousness may occur because of epilepsy, coma, concussion, or asphyxia. However, it can also be caused by an inadequate flow of blood to the brain due to vascular constriction, vascular obstruction, cardiac failure, or other malfunctions.

PALPITATIONS

Palpitations, fluttering of the heart or an abnormal rate or rhythm, may or may not be due to cardiovascular abnormalities. Since palpitations of any kind draw attention to the heart, a person having them may feel unnecessary anxiety over the condition of his heart. When palpitations are noticed or suspected, a physician should be consulted.

RECURRENT BRONCHITIS

Chronic cough and bronchitis may or may not be related to heart attacks. In some cases they may result from congenital abnormalities or

from pulmonary circulatory congestion. These represent the most prom-
inently recognized danger signs of cardiovascular disease. In cases of
either chronic cough or bronchitis, a physician should be consulted.

TREATMENT

The kinds of treatment selected for the heart patient will depend
upon the nature of the disease and how critical the case is. A chronic
illness slowly affecting the patient should allow for planned diagnosis
and treatment. Surgery for the repair of congenital conditions may
often be planned well in advance. In critical, sudden cardiovascular
illness, however, the story is far different. Of most common concern is
the kind of treatment used for heart seizures.

EMERGENCY CARE

The heart-attack patient is in need of emergency care; his life is at
stake. In most cases, he should be taken to a hospital immediately. The
first medical care will depend upon his general condition. It may include
the use of oxygen, drugs to dilate obstructed blood vessels, electric or
drug stimulators to revive his faltering heart, measurements for pulse
and blood pressure, electrocardiograms to record the electric impulses
of his heart, or X-ray and fluoroscopic examinations to measure the size
and outline of his heart. All efforts must be made to reduce the load
placed on his heart. He should be physically and mentally relaxed and
given absolute rest to preserve his strength. The extent of heart tissue
death will depend upon the severity of the coronary obstruction and the
care he receives after the attack. Dead cells cannot be revived. However,
heart cells alive but starving for adequate oxygen-food supply may be
saved if the load on the heart can be reduced.

The first week is the most critical. Most deaths occur during the first
48 hours after the attack. The danger lessens from the second week on.
Gradually new blood vessels form around the obstructed vessels, setting up a new circulation and adequate oxygen-food supply to the deprived cells. Fibrous scar tissue forms over the affected area. Blood
cells work to remove the dead cells. Slowly, as the heart returns to
normal, the patient can resume normal activities.

LONG-TERM CARE

The cardinal rule of all treatment for heart patients is to prevent
anginal discomfort (pain brought on by inadequate oxygen supply).
Drug routines are often established—digitalis to cause a fuller heartbeat; nitrates, such as nitroglycerine, to dilate coronary blood vessels;
anticoagulants to reduce the possibility of clotting; sedative drugs to

quiet the patient; and drugs to cause specific actions to take place in the kidneys. A selective diet must be set up, including dos and don'ts. The patient must learn the need for rest and for limitation of activity. Schedules of moderate exercise must be established.

Through careful control the patient may be enabled to resume much or all of his previous routine. As a rule, the patient lives a good many years after the first attack of angina pectoris. This longevity will depend, however, upon his properly understanding his condition, faithfully using all medicine prescribed, and preventing situations that tend to precipitate other attacks.

SUMMARY

I. Circulation
  A. Circulatory system—provides the cells of the body with food and oxygen and eliminates wastes.
  B. Heart
    1. Structure of the heart
      a. Three layers:
        (1) endocardium.
        (2) myocardium.
        (3) epicardium.
      b. Supplied with its own vessels.
      c. Two separate pumps, with an intervening septum:
        (1) receives deoxygenated blood from the body and pumps to the lungs.
        (2) receives oxygenated blood from the lungs and pumps to the body.
      d. Four chambers:
        (1) left and right atria.
        (2) left and right ventricles.
      e. Four valves: tricuspid, pulmonary (semilunar), mitral (bicuspid), aortic.
    2. Physiology of the heart
      a. Cardiac cycle:
        (1) contraction phase (systolic phase), creating "lubb-dupp" heart sounds.
        (2) relaxation phase (diastolic phase).
      b. Action regulated by a nervelike conduction system in the heart: sinoatrial node (pacemaker), atrioventricular node, and bundle of His.
  C. Blood vessels carry blood to all parts of the body.
    1. Arteries—carry blood, under considerable pressure, away from the ventricles.
    2. Capillaries—small, thin-walled tubes which lie between the arterioles (at the supply end) and the venules (at the delivery end).
    3. Veins—carry blood from all parts of the body into the venae cavae.
  D. Lymphatics
    1. A system of tubules carrying lymph, made up of certain fluid portions of blood that bathe all cells of the body.

2. Begin as blind ducts and converge into larger ducts which enter veins of the neck.

3. Are lined with series of filters called lymph nodes.

E. Fetal circulation

1. Fetal oxygen supply obtained from the mother's blood through the placenta.

2. Fetal blood largely bypasses the lungs by means of the foramen ovale and ductus arteriosus (both of which normally close shortly after birth).

F. Blood—composed of:

1. Plasma.

2. Red blood cells.

3. White blood cells.

4. Platelets.

G. Blood groups

1. Based on various types of protein antigens in the blood

a. A group.

b. B group.

c. AB group.

d. O group.

2. Plasma may contain antibodies, which in some cases will agglutinate with a given type antigen.

3. Rh factor another significant blood protein.

H. Blood count—determines the ratio of white to red blood cells (normally about 1:700–800).

I. Blood disorders

1. Anemias—reduction either in number of red blood cells or the amount of hemoglobin in these cells.

2. Neoplastic blood diseases—great increase in the number of white blood cells (also called leukemias).

3. Leukopenias—reduction of white blood cells below the normal level.

4. Hemorrhagic disorders—disruption of normal coagulation.

J. Pulse and blood pressure

1. Pulse is expansion and contraction of an artery wall due to the passage of blood following each heart beat.

2. Blood pressure is the pressure of the blood in the arteries.

3. Factors influencing the pulse rate.

4. Factors influencing abnormal blood pressure.

K. Elimination of blood wastes

1. By means of the kidneys.

2. In relation to the role of exercise.

II. Types and Causes of Circulatory Diseases

A. Congenital disorders—those occurring before birth

1. Kinds most commonly include:

a. septal defects.

b. patent ductus arteriosus.

c. coarctation of the aorta.

d. stenosis.

e. tetralogy of Fallot.

2. Future for congenital deformities is to strive for medical prevention.

B. Degenerative heart disorders affecting adults are classified according to kind:

1. Rheumatic heart disease.

    2. Arteriosclerosis.
    3. Atherosclerosis.
    4. Hypertension.
    5. Coronary disease.
    6. Cerebrovascular accidents.
    7. Syphilitic heart.
    8. Heart block.
    9. Vascular disorders:
       a. aneurysms.
       b. hemorrhage.
       c. shock.
       d. varicose veins.
       e. phlebitis.

III. Environmental Complications—considered the main causes for the major cardiovascular diseases, although no one factor can yet be considered the *most* important.
    A. Serum cholesterol levels.
    B. Blood pressure levels.
    C. Smoking.
    D. Obesity.
    E. Social factors.
    F. Other factors include chronic diseases or combinations of the preceding factors.

IV. Heart Diseases as a Cause of Death
    A. Cardiovascular diseases account for more than 50 percent of all deaths from all causes in the United States.
    B. Majority due to degenerative and arteriosclerotic causes.
       1. Coronary heart disease causes death in over 50 percent of all cardiovascular diseases.
       2. Stroke and hypertension cause death in over 30 percent of all cardiovascular diseases.
    C. Mortality incidence in the past several decades shows:
       1. Pronounced decline for those under 25 years of age.
       2. No significant change for those between the ages of 25 to 65.
       3. Evident increase in those over 65 years of age.
       4. Higher rate in the East and in metropolitan areas in general.

V. Prevention of Heart Disease
    A. Largely preventable if caused by infection or malnutrition.
    B. Little known about prevention of congenital malformations.
    C. Rheumatic heart disease prevented by treating streptococcal infections in time.
    D. Heart diseases relating to the lungs may be prevented by early treatment of respiratory infections and reduction of:
       1. Cigarette smoking.
       2. Air pollution.
    E. Coronary sclerosis reduction *may* depend upon:
       1. Reduction in cholesterol intake.
       2. Control of excessive blood pressure.
       3. Sufficient physical exercise.
    F. Heart diseases in general may be reduced by:
       1. Proper nutrition.
       2. Avoiding or adequately treating infections.
       3. Avoiding emotional turmoils.

4. Balanced living—sufficient rest and moderate physical exercise.
5. Regular periodic physical examinations.

VI. Symptoms and Treatment of Heart Attacks
    A. Symptoms—vary according to the nature of the illness, may be common to other conditions, should be called to immediate attention of a physician.
        1. Pain in the chest, shoulder, arm, and neck areas, especially after exertion.
        2. Breathlessness.
        3. Edema—swelling due to abnormally large amounts of fluid in the body tissues.
        4. Fatigue.
        5. Cyanosis—blueness of skin caused by insufficient blood in the body tissues.
        6. Loss of consciousness.
        7. Palpitations—fluttering of the heart or an abnormal heart rate or rhythm.
        8. Recurrent bronchitis.
    B. Treatment
        1. Emergency care.
        2. Long-term care.

Glossary

If you cannot find the word you wish in this glossary, check the index for text and glossary references.

abscess (ab'ses) (L. *ab-*, from; *cedere*, to go).   Swollen, inflamed area of body tissues, in which pus gathers.

anemia (ə nĕ'mē ə) (G. *an-*, not; *haima*, blood).   A condition in which there is a decrease in the number of red blood cells or in the amount of hemoglobin or in both.

aneurysm (an'yə rizm) (G. *aneurysma*, a widening).   A sac-like bulging of the wall of an artery or vein, resulting from weakening of the wall by disease or abnormal development.

angina pectoris (an jī'nə pek'tə ris) (G. *anchein*, to squeeze; L. *pectus*, breast).   Pains in the chest, and often in the left arm and shoulder, arising from insufficient blood supply to the heart muscle.

antigen (an'ti jen) (G. *anti-*, against; *gennan*, to produce).   A substance that induces the production of antibodies.

aorta (ā or'tə) (G. *aorte*).   The main artery of the body, carrying blood from the left ventricle of the heart to all parts of the body except the lungs.

aortic valve (ā or'tik).   The valve at the junction of the aorta and the left lower chamber of the heart. Formed by three cup-shaped membranes and also called a semilunar valve.

apex (ā'peks) (L. *apex*, summit).   The blunt rounded end of the heart, directed downward, forward, and to the left.

apoplexy (ap'ə plek sē) (G. *apo-*, down; *plessein*, to strike).   Sudden paralysis with partial or total loss of consciousness and sensation, due to breaking or obstruction of a blood vessel in the brain. Also called a stroke.

arteriole (ahr tē′rē ōl) (L. *arteriola,* small artery). The smallest arterial vessels resulting from repeated branching of the arteries.

arteriosclerosis (ahr tē′rē ō sklə rō′sis) (*artery;* G. *skleros,* hard). Commonly called "hardening of the arteries." Includes any conditions causing artery walls to become thick and hard and lose elasticity.

artery (ahr′tə rē). Any one of a system of tubes or vessels carrying blood from the heart to all parts of the body.

atherosclerosis (ath′ə rō sklə rō′sis) (G. *athere,* gruel; *skleros,* hard). A disease of the arteries in which the inner layer of the wall becomes thick and irregular by deposits of fat. These deposits decrease the inside diameter of the vessel.

atrioventricular block (ā′trē ō ven trik′yə lər) (L. *atrium,* hall; *venter,* belly). Also called "heart block." Interference with conduction of electrical impulses from upper to lower chambers of the heart and throughout the lower chambers.

atrioventricular node Small mass of special muscular fibers in septum between right atrium and ventricle which forms beginning of bundle of His. It receives electrical impulse from sinoatrial node. Abbreviated AV node.

atrium (ā′trē əm). One of the two upper chambers of the heart.

bicuspid valve (bī kus′ pid) (L. *bi-,* twice; *cuspis,* pointed end). Usually called mitral valve. A valve of two cusps located between the upper and lower chambers in the left side of the heart.

blood pressure. The pressure of the blood in the arteries.

bronchitis (brong kī′tis) (G. *bronchos,* windpipe; *-itis,* inflammation). Inflammation of the mucous lining of the bronchial tubes.

bundle of His (his) (Wilhelm His, Jr., German physician, 1863–1934). A bundle of specialized muscular fibers running from the AV node along the septum down to the lower heart chambers. It serves to conduct electrical impulses to the ventricles.

capillary (kap′i ler ē) (L. *capillus,* hair). One of the very small tubes or vessels forming a network between the arterioles and the venules. Through its walls materials leave and enter the blood.

cardiovascular (kahr′dē ō vas′kyə lər) (G. *kardia,* heart; L. *vasculum,* a vessel). Pertaining to the heart and blood vessels.

cholesterol (kə les′tə rol) (G. *chole,* bile; *stereos,* solid). A fat-like substance found in animal tissue. An excess amount in the blood is often associated with high risk of coronary atherosclerosis.

chordae tendineae (kor′dē ten din′ē ē) (G. *chorde,* string; *tendene,* to stretch). Fibrous chords which serve to hold the valves between the upper and lower chambers of the heart secure when they are forced closed by pressure of blood in the lower chambers.

circulatory (sur′kyə lə tor ē) (L. *circulari,* to form a circle). Pertaining to the heart, blood vessels, and the circulation of the blood.

coagulation (kō ag yə lā′shən) (L. *co-,* together; *agere,* to move). Process of changing from a liquid to a thickened or solid state. The formation of a clot.

coarctation (kō ahrk tā′shən) (L. *co-,* together; *arctare,* to make tight). A pressing together or a narrowing of a blood vessel, usually the aorta.

collateral circulation (kə lat′ə rəl) (L. *co-,* together; *lateralis,* lateral, side).

Circulation of the blood through nearby smaller vessels when a main vessel has been blocked.

congenital (kən jen′i tal) (L. *con,* together; *genere,* to beget). Pertaining to presence at birth, resulting from heredity or prenatal environment.

coronary artery (kor′ə ner ē) (G. *korone,* wreath). One of two arteries, arising from the aorta, arching over the top of the heart, and conducting blood to the heart muscle.

coronary disease. A destructive process involving the blood vessels conducting blood to the heart muscle.

coronary occlusion (ə kloo′zhən) (L. *ob-,* toward; *clausere,* to shut). An obstruction (generally a blood clot) in a branch of a coronary artery which hinders the flow of blood to some part of the heart muscle.

corpuscle (kor′pus əl) (L. *corpusculum,* little body). A blood cell.

cross-match. A determination of the compatibility of the blood of a donor with that of the recipient before transfusion by placing red blood cells of donor in serum of recipient and red blood cells of recipient in serum of donor. Absence of agglutination indicates that two blood specimens are compatible.

cyanosis (sī ə nō′sis) (G. *kyanos,* blue). Blueness of the skin caused by insufficient oxygen in the blood.

deoxygenated blood (dē ok′si jə nā ted). Blood that has lost or been deprived of oxygen.

diastole (dī as′tə lē) (G. *diastole,* dilation). In each heart beat, the period of dilation of the heart.

ductus arteriosus (duk′təs ahr tē′rē ō sis) (L. *ducere,* to lead). A small duct in the heart of the fetus between the artery leaving the left side of the heart (aorta) and the artery leaving the right side of the heart (pulmonary artery). This duct normally closes soon after birth.

edema (i dē′mə) (G. *oidein,* to swell). Swelling due to abnormally large amounts of fluid in the tissues of the body.

electrocardiogram (i lek′trō kahr′dē ə gram) (G. *elektron,* amber; *kardia,* heart; *gramma,* mark). Often referred to as EKG or ECG. A graphic record of the electric currents produced by the heart.

embolus (em′bə ləs) (G. *embolos,* plug). A blood clot (or other substance such as air, fat, tumor) inside a blood vessel which is carried in the blood stream to a smaller vessel where it becomes an obstruction to circulation.

endocarditis (en′dō kahr dī′tis) (G. *endon,* within; *kardia,* heart; *-itis,* inflammation). Inflammation of the inner layer of the heart (endocardium) usually associated with acute rheumatic fever or some infectious agent.

endocardium (en′dō kahr′dē əm). A thin, smooth membrane forming the inner surface of the heart.

epicardium (ep′i kahr′dē əm) (G. *epi,* upon; *kardia,* heart). The outer layer of the heart wall. Also called the visceral pericardium.

erythrocyte (e rith′ro sīt) (G. *erythros,* red; *kytos,* cell). A red blood corpuscle.

fibrin (fī′brin) (L. *fibra,* fiber). An elastic protein which forms the essential portion of a blood clot.

fibrinogen (fī brin′o jən) (L. *fibra,* fiber; G. *gennan,* to produce). A soluble protein in the blood which, by the action of certain enzymes, is converted into the insoluble protein of a blood clot.

foramen ovale (fo rā'mən ō vā'lē) (L. *forare*, to bore; *ovum*, an egg). An oval hole between the left and right upper chambers of the heart of the fetus which normally closes shortly after birth.

gamma globulin (gam'ə glob'yə lin) (G. *gamma*, greek letter g; L. *globulus*, globule). That portion of serum with which most of the immune antibodies are associated.

heart block. Interference with the conduction of the electrical impulses of the heart; blockage can be either partial or complete.

hemiplegia (hem'i plē'jē ə) (G. *hemi*, half; *plege*, a stroke). Paralysis of one half of the body caused by damage to the opposite side of the brain. It is sometimes caused by a blood clot or hemorrhage in a blood vessel in the brain.

hemocytometer (hē'mō sī tom'ə tər) (G. *haima*, blood; *kytos*, hollow vessel; *metron*, measure). An instrument used in counting the blood corpuscles.

hemoglobin (hē'mə glō'bin). The oxygen-carrying red pigment of the red blood corpuscles.

hemophilia (hē'mə fil'ē ə) (G. *philein*, to love). A hereditary condition in which the blood fails to clot quickly enough, causing prolonged, uncontrolled bleeding from even the smallest cut.

hypertension (hī'pər ten'shən) (G. *hyper*, over; L. *tendere*, to stretch). Commonly called "high blood pressure." An unstable or persistent elevation of blood pressure above the normal range.

inferior vena cava (in fēr'ē ər vē'nə kā'və) (L. *inferus*, low; *vena*, vein; *cava*, hollow). The venous trunk for the lower extremities, pelvis, and abdominal viscera which empties into the right atrium.

interatrial septum (in'tər ā'trē əl sep'təm) (L. *inter*, between; *atrium*, heart; *septum*, partition). The muscular wall dividing the left and right upper chambers, or atria, of the heart.

interventricular septum (in'tər ven trik'yə lər sep'təm). The muscular wall, thinner at the top, dividing the left and right lower chambers, or ventricles, of the heart.

lacteal (lak'tē əl) (L. *lacteus*, milky). Any one of the intestinal lymphatics that take up digested fats.

leukemia (loo kē'mē ə) (G. *leukos*, white; *haima*, blood). A fatal disease of the blood-forming organs, characterized by a marked increase in the number of leukocytes in the blood.

leukopenia (loo'kə pē'nē ə) (G. *leukos*, white; *penia*, poverty). Reduction in the number of leukocytes in the blood.

lipid (lip'id) (G. *lipos*, fat). Fat.

lymph (limf) (L. *lympha*, water). A tissue fluid confined to vessels and nodes of the lymphatic system.

lymphatic (lim fat'ik). Pertaining to or containing lymph.

lymph node (limf nōd) (L. *lympha*, water; *nodus*, knob). Small oval collection of lymphatic tissue interposed in the course of lymphatic vessels.

lymphocyte (lim'fə sīt) (G. *kytos*, hollow). A variety of small colorless corpuscles found in lymph.

lymphoid tissue (lim'foid) (L. *eidos*, form). Connective tissue infiltrated with lymphocytes.

mitral valve (mī'trəl) (G. *mitra*, headband). Sometimes called bicuspid valve.

A valve of two cusps located between the upper and lower chambers in the left side of the heart.

murmur (L. *murmurare,* murmur). An abnormal heart sound, sounding like fluid passing an obstruction, heard between the normal "lubb-dubb" heart sounds.

myocardial infarction (mī ō kahr'dē əl in fahrk'shən) (G. *mys,* muscle; *kardial,* heart; L. *infarcire,* to stuff in). The damaging or death of an area of the heart muscle (myocardium) resulting from a reduction in the blood supply reaching that area.

myocardium (mī ō kahr'dē əm). The muscular wall of the heart. The heart muscle. The thickest of the three layers, lying between the endocardium (inner) and epicardium (outer).

neoplasm (nē'ō plazm) (G. *neos,* new; *plasma,* formation). Any new or abnormal growth, such as a tumor.

neoplastic (nē'ō plas'tik) (G. *neos,* new; *plasma,* formation). Pertaining to or like a neoplasm.

occlusion (ə kloo'zhən) (L. *occlusus,* to shut). The closing or blocking of a passage, such as a blood vessel.

palpitation (pal pi tā'shən) (L. *palpitare,* to feel). A fluttering of the heart of abnormal rate or rhythm, experienced by the person himself.

patent ductus arteriosus (pā'tənt duk'təs ahr tē'rē ō'sis) (L. *patens,* open). A congenital defect in which the ductus arteriosus fails to close. See *ductus arteriosus.*

patent foramen ovale (pā'tənt fo rā'mən ō vā'lē). A congenital defect in which the foramen ovale fails to close. See *foramen ovale.*

pathogen (path'ə jən) (G. *pathos,* disease; *gennan,* to produce). A microorganism or substance capable of producing a disease.

phlebitis (flə bī'tis) (G. *phlebos,* vein; *-itis,* inflammation). Inflammation of a vein, often in the leg. A blood clot may be formed in the inflamed vein.

plaque (plak) (Fr. *plak,* a disc). A flat or patchlike deposit of lipid (fat) in the inner walls (tunica media) of the arteries.

plasma (plaz'mə) (G. *plasma,* form). The cell-free fluid portion of uncoagulated blood.

platelet (plāt'lit). Roundish discs, smaller than red blood cells, found in the blood, and associated with clotting.

pulmonary artery (pul'mə ner ē ahr'tə rē) (L. *pulmo,* lung). The large artery which conveys unoxygenated (venous) blood from the lower right chamber of the heart to the lungs.

pulmonary circulation. The circulation of the blood through the lungs, flowing from the lower right chamber of the heart through the lungs, back to the left upper chamber of the heart.

pulmonary valve. The valve formed by three cup-shaped membranes at the junction of the pulmonary artery and the right lower chamber of the heart; also called a semilunar valve.

pulmonary vein. One of four veins (two from each lung) which conduct oxygenated blood from the lungs into the left upper chamber of the heart.

pulse (puls) (L. *pulsus,* stroke). The expansion and contraction of an artery which may be felt with the finger.

Purkinje's fibers (pər kin'jēz) (Johannes Purkinje, Bohemian physiologist,

1787–1869). Atypical muscle fibers lying beneath the endocardium of the heart which constitute the impulse-conducting system of the heart.

purpura (pur′pyoo rə) (G. *porphyra,* shellfish yielding purple dye). A condition characterized by hemorrhages in the skin and the mucous membranes.

rheumatic fever (roo mat′ik) (G. *rheuma,* a flow). A disease, usually occurring in childhood, which may follow a few weeks after a streptococcal infection.

rheumatic heart disease. The damage done to the heart, particularly the heart valves, by one or more attacks of rheumatic fever.

SA node. See *sinoatrial node.*

sclerosis (sklə rō′sis) (G. *skleros,* hard). A hardening of body tissues, usually as the result of an accumulation of fibrous tissue.

semilunar valves (sem ē loo′nər) (L. *semis,* half; *luna,* the moon). Cup-shaped valves. The aortic valve at the entrance to the aorta, and the pulmonary valve at the entrance to the pulmonary artery are semilunar valves. They consist of three cup-shaped flaps which prevent the backflow of blood.

septum (sep′təm) (L. *septum,* partition). A dividing wall. The atrial or interatrial septum is a muscular wall dividing the left and right upper chambers of the heart. The ventricular or interventricular septum is a muscular wall dividing the left and right lower chambers of the heart.

serum (sēr′əm) (L. "whey"). The fluid portion of the blood which remains after the cellular elements have been removed by coagulation. It is different from plasma which is the cell-free liquid portion of uncoagulated blood.

sinoatrial block (sī′nō ā′trē əl). Also called a heart block. Interference with conduction of electrical impulses throughout the upper chambers of the heart and to the atrioventricular node.

sinoatrial node. A small mass of specialized cells in the right upper chamber of the heart which give rise to the electrical impulses that initiate contractions of the heart. Also called the SA node or "pacemaker."

sphygmomanometer (sfig′mō mə nom′ə tər) (G. *sphygmos,* pulse; *manos,* thin; *metron,* measure). An instrument for measuring blood pressure in the arteries.

stenosis (sti nō′sis) (G. *stenosis,* narrowing). A narrowing or stricture of an opening. Mitral stenosis or aortic stenosis indicate narrowing of those valves.

stethoscope (steth′ə skōp) (G. *stethos,* chest; *skopein,* to examine). An instrument for listening to sounds within the body.

stroke (strōk). Also called apoplectic stroke, cerebrovascular accident, or cerebral vascular accident. An impeded blood supply to some part of the brain caused by a clot, hemorrhage, embolus, or tumor.

superior vena cava (sə pēr′ē ər vē′nə kā′və). The venous trunk for the upper extremities, thorax, head, and neck which empties into the right atrium.

systemic circulation (sis tem′ik) (G. *systema,* to set together). The circulation of the blood through all parts of the body except the lungs, the flow being from the left lower chamber of the heart, through the body, back to the right upper chamber of the heart.

systole (sis′tə lē) (G. *systole,* to draw together). In each heartbeat, the period of contraction of the heart. Atrial systole is the period of contraction of the atria. Ventricular systole is the period of contraction of the ventricles.

tetralogy of Fallot (te tral′ə jē uv fa lō′) (G. *tera-,* four; *logos,* word; E.-L. A. Fallot, French Physician, 1850–1911). A congenital malformation of the heart involving four defects. See discussion of Congenital Heart Defects in Chapter 13.

thoracic duct (tho ras'ik dukt) (G. *thorax,* chest; L. *ducere,* to lead). The largest lymphatic vessel of the body. Originates in the abdomen, passes upward through the thorax, and empties into the left subclavian vein.

thrombocyte (throm'bə sīt) (G. *thrombos,* clot; *kytos,* a hollow). A blood platelet.

thrombus (throm'bəs) (G. *thrombos,* clot). A blood clot which forms inside a blood vessel or cavity of the heart. See *embolus.*

transfusion (tranz fyoo'zhən) (L. *trans,* across; *fundere,* to pour). The introduction of whole blood, plasma substitutes, or other solutions directly into the blood stream.

tricuspid valve (trī kus'pid) (L. *tri-,* three; *cuspis,* a point). A valve consisting of three cusps located between the upper and lower chamber in the right side of the heart.

tunica externa (tyoo'ni kə ek'stər nə) (L. *tunica,* coating; *externus,* on the outside). The outer layer of wall of artery or vein.

tunica intima (tyoo'ni kə in'ti mə) (L. *intimus,* within). The inner layer of wall of artery or vein.

tunica media (tyoo'ni kə mē'dē ə) (L. *medius,* middle). The middle (intermediate) layer of wall of artery or vein.

valve (L. *valva,* leaf of a folding door). A structure in a canal or passage which prevents the backflow of the contents, such as the valves of the heart.

varicose veins (var'i kōs) (L. *varix,* enlarged vein). An abnormally or irregularly swollen vein.

vasoconstriction (vas'ō kən strik'shən) (L. *vas,* vessel; *con,* together; *stringere,* to draw). The narrowing of blood vessels, especially constriction of arterioles, leading to decreased blood flow. Such narrowing may be caused by nervous or chemical stimulation.

vasodilation (vas'ō dī lā'shən) (L. *dilatare,* to bring apart). The enlarging of blood vessels, especially dilation of arterioles, leading to increased supply of blood to the part. Such enlarging may be caused by nervous or chemical stimulation.

vein (vān) (L. *vena,* vein). Any of a series of vessels of the vascular system which carries blood from the various parts of the body back to the heart.

vena cava (vē'nə kā'və). See *inferior* and *superior vena cava.*

ventricle (ven'tri kl) (L. *ventriculus,* little belly). One of the two lower chambers of the heart.

venule (ven'yool) (L. *venula,* vein). A very small vein.

vessel (ves'əl) (L. *vas,* a vessel). A tube circulating a body fluid, as a blood vessel or a lymph vessel.

CHAPTER 14

CANCER AS A HEALTH PROBLEM

One of the great generalizations of science is the *cell theory,* that all living plants and animals consist of cells and cell products. This theory implies that the basic unit of living organisms is the cell. Cells, however, are not all alike. They vary in size, shape, and structure, according to the functions they perform. In spite of these differences, new living cells can arise *only* when pre-existing cells reproduce them. Thus, life is a continuous process.

WHAT IS CANCER?

The human begins life as a single cell which is the product of fertilization between an ovum and a spermatozoon (see Chapter 9). This cell

423

then grows by adding new cells through *mitosis*. This addition of cells is very rapid and random at first, and, up to a point, all of the cells appear the same. Upon reaching this point, the cells undergo a process of differentiation wherein they begin to take on identity. Some become bone, others skin, and others nervous tissue; thus the complex structure of the human takes shape. After a time, limiting processes come into play and growth begins to taper off, slightly, throughout infancy, becomes more slow in childhood, and finally stops in old age, except for the replacement of worn-out, injured, or shed cells.

From birth to death each living thing is constantly changing. It is growing, degenerating, being injured, repairing damage, reproducing, and adjusting. All of this activity normally involves the death and orderly replacement of millions of cells every day. If for any reason a disorderly replacement of these worn-out cells continues as an abnormal growth, the individual has cancer. Such uncontrolled, cancerous growth may appear in man or in any animal or plant.

Cancer, the *uncontrolled* growth of cells, does not heed the signals that govern normal cell and tissue behavior within the body. Normally, when a finger is cut, growth and cell division occur to a point, and then stop as soon as healing is complete. But cancer cells grow abnormally and have a tendency to invade adjacent structures and spread to distant parts of the body. Such growth often leads to death.

CELLULAR STRUCTURE

Cancer cells, like normal cells, consist of a nucleus, cytoplasm, and a cellular membrane which separates the cell from other cells and from its surroundings. (These subcellular structures which make up the cell are discussed in Chapter 9.) Cancer cells are structurally similar to normal cells; yet they show clear differences. Cancer cells do not necessarily resemble each other; there are important differences depending on the organ and tissue in which the cancer originates.

The nucleus in cancer cells, as in normal cells, is the site of the genetic material DNA, the center of cellular reproduction, which directs the cell's over-all functions. Cancer cells are, however, distinguished from normal cells principally by the nucleus. Their nuclei are usually larger than those of comparable normal cells and may vary significantly in size and shape within a group of cancer cells. These large nuclei deviate from the normal in the number and appearance of chromosomes, as well as in the number of nucleoli present. Cell division is abnormal, resulting in the above deviations in chromosomes.

The cytoplasm is similar in cancer and normal cells. No single cytoplasmic difference (structural or chemical) that would specifically characterize a cancer cell has been identified.

The normal cell membrane has the ability to allow the inward passage of nutrients and the outward passage of products of cell metabolism and secretion. The cancer cell membrane appears to differ from that of healthy cells in this ability. Cancer cell membranes adhere to each other less firmly than comparable normal cells and tend to shed very readily.

At the cellular level the cancerous changes are slight. In time the amount of cytoplasm increases, altering the size and shape of the cell; these changes may take months or even years. While the cancerous growth remains confined to the epithelium (Fig. 14.1), the cancer cells show fewer abnormalities than those in advanced tumors. The earliest detectable sign of cancer is an increase in the number of chromosomes produced. Often *tetraploid* cells, those having twice the normal number of chromosomes, are found in cancerous organisms. Advanced invading cancers show odd and irregular numbers of chromosomes as well as abnormally shaped chromosomes.

CELLULAR PROCESSES AND BEHAVIOR

The processes of cell growth and behavior have been studied through tissue cultures. In this study, living cells are put into glass vessels containing sterile (germ-free) nutrient solutions. From time to time they are given new nutrients. Periodically the excess cells are removed and discarded. Such a tissue culture of cells from the embryonic heart of a chicken was started in 1912 under the direction of Alexis Carrel (early cellular physiologist at the Rockefeller Institute) and flourished for 27 years.

Cells of any kind grown in a tissue culture outside of the body are described as being grown *in vitro* (within glass). Cells growing within the body are *in vivo* (within the living body).

The in vitro growth of cells is of great value to research. Cells grown in this manner may be observed growing and undergoing mitosis. The effects of substances added to the medium which would normally kill or harm an individual may also be observed. When cells growing in vitro touch each other, the normal active movement of the cell membrane is inhibited. There is at the same time a pronounced decrease in the synthesis of protein, RNA, and DNA within the cell, resulting in slower growth. Under certain conditions cell growth can be speeded up. For example, in skin the normal rate of cell division can be *increased* up to 90 times by removing successive layers of epidermal cells, simply with the aid of cellulose tape. But how does the cell know when new cells are needed and how does it know when to stop growing?

In a normal human, every cell is compressed against other cells and each has a fluid medium that brings nutrients to the cell from the blood

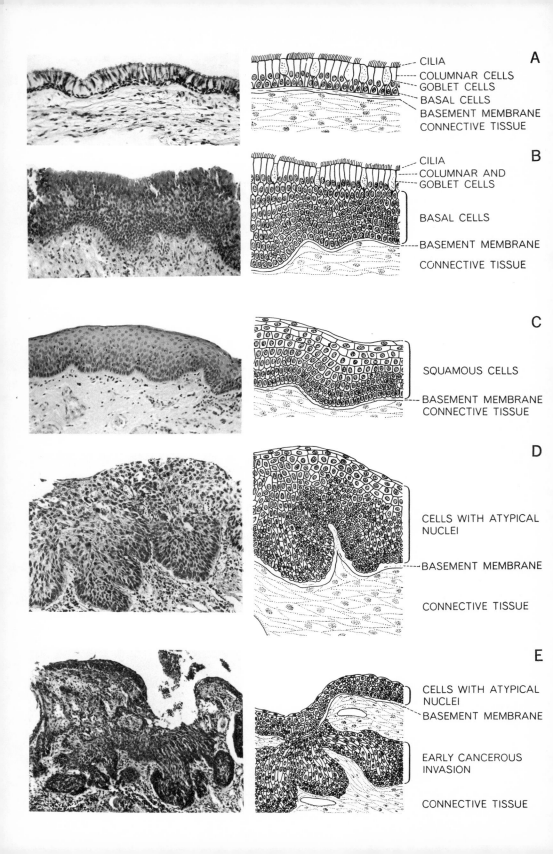

CILIA
COLUMNAR CELLS
GOBLET CELLS
BASAL CELLS
BASEMENT MEMBRANE
CONNECTIVE TISSUE

A

CILIA
COLUMNAR AND
GOBLET CELLS

BASAL CELLS

BASEMENT MEMBRANE

CONNECTIVE TISSUE

B

SQUAMOUS CELLS

BASEMENT MEMBRANE
CONNECTIVE TISSUE

C

CELLS WITH ATYPICAL
NUCLEI

BASEMENT MEMBRANE

CONNECTIVE TISSUE

D

CELLS WITH ATYPICAL
NUCLEI
BASEMENT MEMBRANE

EARLY CANCEROUS
INVASION

CONNECTIVE TISSUE

E

and carries away waste materials. This body fluid is also a chemical communication system. Special chemicals, when released into this fluid, may turn on or off specific chemical activities in the cells they enter. One group of chemicals, called *hormones*, has been found to control the whole body by such activity. But it is also believed that there exists a *general chemical feedback mechanism* among all cells which may be used to control either a cell's own functions, the functions of other cells, or both. Although these mechanisms of feedback are not now readily understood, the outstanding feature of cancer cells appears to be their failure to obey signals of the normal cells in the body and their lack of such a feedback, self-controlling mechanism. They start to grow, produce large amounts of DNA, RNA, and protein, but never find out when to stop.[1]

TUMORS

A growth which persists, grows, and serves no useful purpose is called a *tumor* or *neoplasm*. Tumors are divided into two classes: *benign* (harmless) *tumors* and *malignant tumors* or *cancers*.

BENIGN TUMORS

Benign tumors are growths that may increase slowly in size, are usually surrounded by a fibrous membrane, and remain localized. Such a growth does not invade other tissues or produce secondary growths in other parts of the body. Benign tumors may, however, cause discomfort by pressure on adjacent structures.

Common benign tumors may occur on the skin as *warts, wens,* and *birthmarks;* in the uterus as *fibroid tumors;* on the skeleton as growths of bone tissue; and in the breast or ovary as *cysts.* Some benign tumors,

[1] *A National Program to Conquer Heart Disease, Cancer and Stroke,* Vol. II, Washington, D.C., The President's Commission on Heart Disease, Cancer and Stroke, 1965, pp. 218–220.

Fig. 14.1 Progression of cancer through epithelium. Bronchial epithelium is the original site of almost all lung cancer, which often develops as shown on the photomicrographs. (A) Shows one of the first effects of smoking on normal epithelium—hyperplasia. (B) In this section there is an increase in the number of basal cells. (C) The epithelium is lost and the cells become squamous, or flattened, and show atypical nuclei. (D) This stage is termed carcinoma *in situ.* (E) Finally, when these cells break through the basement membrane, the *cancer* may spread through lungs and to the rest of the body. (From "The Effects of Smoking" by E. Cuyler Hammond. Copyright © 1962 by *Scientific American, Inc.* All rights reserved. Photomicrographs by Dr. Oscar Auerbach of the Veterans Administration Hospital, East Orange, N.J.)

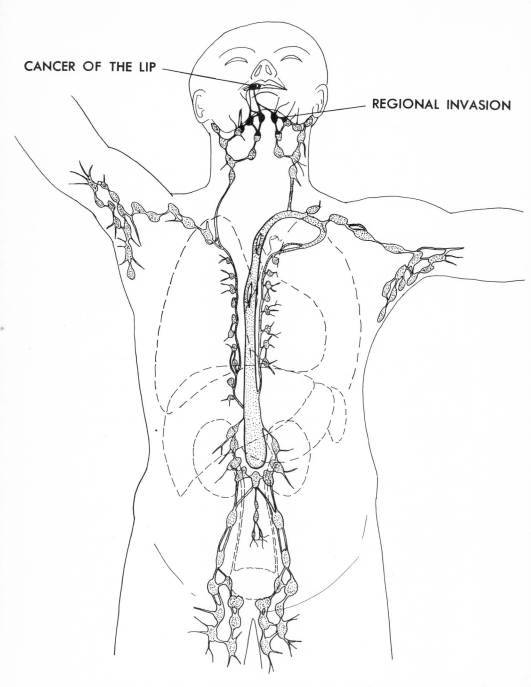

CANCER OF THE LIP

REGIONAL INVASION

Fig. 14.2 Lymphatic system of the body showing regional invasion (metastases) of cancer of the lip.

if subjected to certain harmful effects (explained later), may change into malignant tumors.

MALIGNANT TUMORS

Cancer is the term commonly used to designate all malignant tumors or neoplasms regardless of their origin. Cancers are divided into two main classes: malignant tumors arising from epithelial tissue are called *carcinomas,* and those arising from connective or supportive tissue are called *sarcomas.* Table 14.1 lists the more common cancers, their sites of origin, names, and possible complications.

HOW CANCER SPREADS

The most serious complication in curing cancer is the tendency of cancer cells to spread. This spreading may occur in one of three ways:

1. *Invasion.* Malignant tumors having no surrounding capsule or limiting membrane possess an unlimited ability to enlarge, extend, and invade the spaces between the normal cells of the tissues in which they are located. Such growths (primary cancer growths) may remain unnoticed until, because of enlargement, they interfere with the functions of important structures and organs of the body. This interference occurs as the result of pressure, or size, or by the destruction of normal tissues because their nourishment and blood supply has been cut off.

2. *Metastasis.* Metastasis is the process of transferring disease from

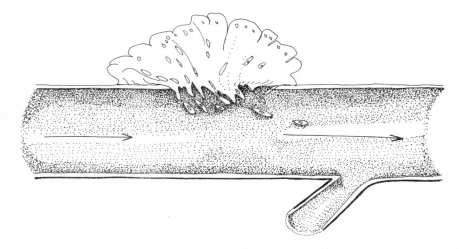

Fig. 14.3 Invasion (metastases) by cancer of a blood vessel.

TABLE 14.1 **COMMON SITES**

Common Sites	Common Types	Signs and Symptoms
Cartilage	Chondrosarcoma	Pain resembling rheumatism, arthritis, or sprain; fever; slowly growing tumor
Bone	Osteogenic sarcoma; Ewing's tumor	Same as above
	Multiple myeloma	Pain on pressure; fractures of non-weight-bearing bones
Brain and central nervous system	Neuroblastoma; medulla blastoma; astrocytoma; and craniopharyngioma	Enlargement of the head; loss of neurologic function; headache; blurred vision
Spinal cord	Neuroblastoma	Local twitching pain; motor and sensory impairment; tenderness of the spine
Breast	Carcinoma	Lump; abnormal discharge from the nipple; "dimpling" or "pigskin" appearance of the skin; elevation of the affected breast; retraction of the nipple
Esophagus	Squamous cell carcinoma; adenocarcinoma	Difficulty in swallowing, hoarseness
Stomach	Adenocarcinoma	Persistent chronic indigestion; aversion to rich food and meat; decreasing appetite; dark, tarry stools

AND TYPES OF CANCER

Common Sites of Metastases	Complications	Additional Information
Lungs	Weight loss; fractures	Contrary to usual cancer pattern, pain is an early symptom
Lungs	Weight loss	Occurs frequently in young males
To other bones, lymph nodes, spleen, and liver	Anemia; fractures; renal failures	Occurs predominantly in males, 40 years of age and over
	Vomiting, drowsiness, convulsions	May occur in all ages and both sexes; rapid growth in a young child
Axillary lymph nodes; lungs; pleura, liver, and bones; opposite breast	Hemorrhage, anemia	Develops more frequently in women who have not lactated
Local lymph nodes; mediastinum; liver, bones, and kidney	Weight loss; paralysis of larynx; excessive salivation; starvation	First difficulty in swallowing solids, then soft foods and finally, after 6 to 9 months, inability to swallow even liquids
Regional lymph nodes; liver, lungs, and bones	Hemorrhage; starvation	Most patients wait too long for treatment; the earliest symptoms are those of persistent chronic indigestion

TABLE 14.1 **COMMON SITES**

Common Sites	Common Types	Signs and Symptoms
Small intestine	Adenocarcinoma, myosarcoma	Intermittent pain; nausea; constipation and/or diarrhea; blood in stools and hemorrhage
Colon	Adenocarcinoma	Bleeding from rectum; foul flatus; change in size, color, or odor of stools; blood in stools; difficulty in swallowing; loss of appetite; nausea, vomiting, and loss of weight
Rectum	Adenocarcinoma	Same as above
Anus	Squamous cell carcinoma	Itching; an urgent feeling of the necessity to defecate
Liver	Malignant hepatoma	Feeling of fullness; abdominal pressure; jaundice, constipation, and pain
Gallbladder	Adenocarcinoma	Strong nausea at onset; belching, loss of appetite, jaundice, weakness, and diarrhea

AND TYPES OF CANCER (Continued)

Common Sites of Metastases	Complications	Additional Information
Regional lymph nodes, liver, lungs and bones; general metastases	Obstruction, starvation, hemorrhage, secondary anemia	Rare; slightly higher in females than in males
Regional lymph nodes; pancreas, gallbladder, liver, spleen, lungs; bone and bladder in males; uterus in females	Obstruction, uremia, hemorrhage, bronchopneumonia, anemia, pain, starvation	The average experience has shown that 9 months usually elapse between the onset of symptoms and treatment. Signs and symptoms tend to occur early but they are neither intense nor dramatic and simulate those of other fairly common gastrointestinal disorders
Same as above	Obstruction, hemorrhage, anemia	Hemorrhoids may coexist and are frequently erroneously considered to be source of bleeding
Regional lymph nodes	Hemorrhage, bladder invasion	Tends to occur more frequently in females
Heart, lungs, brain, skeletal system, and regional lymph nodes	Circulatory changes; hemorrhage, edema of the extremities	Primary cancer of liver is rare; however, the liver is a common site of metastasis
Regional lymph nodes, lungs, bones, suprarenal glands, spleen, and other organs	Liver abscess	About 70 percent of the patients have a long history of repeated gallbladder attacks

TABLE 14.1 **COMMON SITES**

Common Sites	Common Types	Signs and Symptoms
Ovary	Adenocarcinoma	Abdominal discomfort and pain; pressure, constipation, swelling of abdomen
Uterus	Adenocarcinoma, adenocanthoma	Intermenstrual bleeding; post-menopausal bleeding; foul, watery discharge; hemorrhage
Cervix	Squamous cell carcinoma, adenocarcinoma	Elongation of menstrual period; post-coital bleeding; foul, yellow, watery discharge
Vagina	Squamous cell carcinoma	Bloody vaginal discharge, pain, painful urination
Prostate	Adenocarcinoma	Frequent, painful, or difficult urination
Malignant lymphomas and leukemias	Hodgkin's disease	Painless enlargement of lymph nodes; pain in the abdomen and back, or in the legs; fatigue; persistent sore throat; trouble in swallowing
	Lymphosarcoma	Same as for Hodgkin's disease

AND TYPES OF CANCER (Continued)

Common Sites of Metastases	Complications	Additional Information
Regional lymph nodes, lungs, and liver	An urgent feeling of the necessity to urinate when there is no need	The growth may become quite large before producing abdominal discomfort
Regional lymph nodes, iliac nodes, inguinal nodes, vagina, vulva, liver, lungs, brain, and bone	Anemia, hemorrhage	Most cancers develop after menopause and in women who have not borne children
Regional metastases, lung, liver, bone, and brain	Hemorrhage, constipation, anemia, vomiting, weight loss	Occurs more frequently in women who have borne children; the most common form of cancer found in the female reproductive organs
Regional lymph nodes	Anemia, ulceration	
Bones, lung, and liver	Bladder obstruction; renal insufficiency	Very common in males past the age of 50
General throughout body	Debility, marked anemia, pneumonia	The leukemias and malignant lymphomas occur predominantly in males. The cervical lymph nodes are often affected
General throughout body		Found frequently in children

TABLE 14.1 **COMMON SITES**

Common Sites	Common Types	Signs and Symptoms
	Chronic leukemia	Sudden onset; weakness, loss of weight, fatigue, bleeding from mucous membranes, enlarged liver and spleen
	Acute leukemia	Sudden onset; fever, ulceration and death of the oral tissues, hemorrhage from the skin and mucous membrane
Mouth	Squamous cell carcinoma	Swelling or thickening of mucous membrane, wartlike growth, inability to chew
Upper lip	Basal cell carcinoma	Pearly-white nodular growth, superficial ulceration; scab may fall off and reform
Lower lip	Squamous cell carcinoma	Thickening of lip; smooth, flat, ulcerated surface with an indurated base
Tongue	Squamous cell carcinoma	Thickening of speech, slight pain, ulceration, hypersalivation, earache, trouble in swallowing, limited movement of the tongue, persistent desire to clear the throat

AND TYPES OF CANCER (Continued)

Common Sites of Metastases	Complications	Additional Information
General throughout body	Debility, pneumonia, cerebral hemorrhage, gastrointestinal hemorrhage	
General throughout body	Pneumonia, circulatory collapse, hemorrhage, debility, pallor	Found frequently in children
Submaxillary region lymph nodes; rarely distant spread	Destruction of oral structures, bleeding, pain, ulceration	Cancer of the oral cavity is often associated with pipe smoking or poor oral hygiene and is usually found in older males; may arise from leukoplakia
Regional lymph nodes	Destruction of adjacent structures	Basal cell cancer is sometimes called "rodent ulcer"
Regional lymph nodes	Destruction of adjacent structures	The majority of lip cancers are on the lower lip
Regional lymph nodes	Hemorrhage, pneumonia, starvation	Muscular action of the tongue may force cancer cells into the adjacent tissues, lymphatics, and blood vessels

TABLE 14.1 **COMMON SITES**

Common Sites	Common Types	Signs and Symptoms
Pharynx	Squamous cell carcinoma	Foul breath, hoarseness, cough, earache, painful and progressive inability to swallow
Lung	Squamous cell carcinoma, adenocarcinoma	Irritating cough; wheezing, chest pain; emphysema
Retina	Retinal gliosarcoma or retinoblastoma	Distorted pupil; frequent stumbling; gray, white, bluish green, or red glassy streak across the pupil of the eye ("cat's eye"); disturbed vision; pain
Skin	Squamous cell carcinoma	Small crusty lesion, bleeding easily; ulceration
	Basal cell carcinoma	Crusty lesion or small node, pearly-white raised edge; ulceration
	Malignant melanoma	Change in size or color of any mole, especially the blue-black or slate blue ones

AND TYPES OF CANCER (Continued)

Common Sites of Metastases	Complications	Additional Information
Internal jugular chain of lymph nodes	Pneumonia	In some instances, metastatic nodes may be the first signs
Regional lymph nodes; systemic movement to brain, bone, and liver	Empyema, pulmonary problems	The majority of lung cancers occur in men over 45 years of age, heavy smokers
Liver, spleen, and lungs	Loss of vision	Occurs in children of both sexes; average age is about 14 months
Regional lymph nodes	Deformities	Skin cancer is the commonest form of cancer and the easiest to cure; most develop on the face; common to individuals who spend many hours in the sun, such as farmers, sailors, and others exposed to the sun
Does not seem to metastasize	Local destruction and deformities	
Regional lymph nodes; liver, lungs, brain, spine	Widespread metastases, ulceration, bleeding	Rare before puberty

TABLE 14.1 **COMMON SITES**

Common Sites	Common Types	Signs and Symptoms
Kidney	Adenocarcinoma	Dull or burning painful sensation in the lower back; painless and intermittent blood in urine
	Wilms' tumor	Pain; loss of appetite; weight loss, fever
	Squamous cell carcinoma	Painless but profuse bleeding; costovertebral pain; fever
Bladder	Squamous cell carcinoma, adenocarcinoma	Abrupt, painless blood in urine; frequent painful urination

one organ or part of the body to another. This results in the formation of new (secondary) sites of disease. Rapidly growing and invading cancer cells shed very easily and may be filtered into the lymphatic system and thereby transported into the regional lymph nodes, as shown in Fig. 14.2. Or they may actually invade an adjacent blood vessel, as shown in Fig. 14.3, be carried to remote parts or organs, lodge there, become established, and produce a new site of cancer. Such a process occurs when secondary cancer of the liver is produced by metastasis of breast cancer.

3. *Implantation.* Because cancer cells are so easily shed, they may become dislodged easily and implant themselves in some adjacent organs, where they will continue to grow and produce their destructive effects. This type of spreading occurs quite frequently in cancers of the abdominal and thoracic cavities.

Malignant tumors, at the beginning, are always localized and often remain so for a time. Early diagnosis, while the growth is still localized,

AND TYPES OF CANCER (Continued)

Common Sites of Metastases	Complications	Additional Information
Lungs and bones	Fever, pyelonephritis, uremia	
Lung, brain, and liver; regional lymph nodes	Uremia, pyelonephritis	The majority of cases are found in children under 5 years of age
Regional lymph nodes; ureters, and bladder	Uremia, pyelonephritis	
Regional lymph nodes; liver, lungs, and bones	Uremia, pyelonephritis	One urination may be bloody while the next is entirely clear, or the bloody urine may change slowly to a normal color over a period of days; blood may not reappear for several months

and complete removal offer the greatest chance of cure, but may be impossible after widespread metastasis or implantation has taken place.

HOW CANCER KILLS

In cancer patients the inability or failure of cancer cells to obey the normal feedback of body signals results in a number of deficiencies which seriously interfere with bodily functioning. At least three deficiencies are important in the resulting death of an individual—*anemia, infection,* and *debility.*

Anemia and infection are closely related to bone marrow deficiencies. Complete bone marrow failure is not common; the deficiency usually occurs from the victim's inability to produce specific cells of the usual number or quality needed by the body. In anemia, the primary effect of cancer is its causing either insufficient production of red blood cells or defective red cells that do not survive long in circulation. In chronic lymphocytic leukemia and Hodgkin's disease (see Table 14.1), the red cell life span is shortened by some factor which produces premature red cell destruction.

Intestinal bleeding that causes anemia may result directly from the tumor, or indirectly, as shown by cancers associated with deficiencies of the bone marrow in reducing the production of platelets. Platelets control clotting; when they are markedly reduced, as in the leukemias and other diseases, hemorrhage results. When growth of the cancer involves the blood supply of a specific tissue or organ, bleeding may result, as in lung cancer.

Because of the above conditions which cause a depression of the host's defenses against infection, serious infections frequently occur in cancer patients. In patients with acute leukemia, infection is the most common direct cause of death. Bacterial, fungal, and viral diseases are common in people who have had massive damage to their lymphocyte-producing tissues, as is caused by Hodgkin's disease and the leukemias.

The other example of physical damage is debility, the wasting away of the body. This is quite common in cancer patients. It may result from simple undernutrition, as might occur in a specific damage of the mouth or stomach; or debility might be the result of treatment by drugs, surgery, or radiation. Loss of appetite associated with continuous pain or emotional depression arising from neglect or loss of hope is common.

DIAGNOSIS IS NOT DEATH

Many cancers can be cured if they are diagnosed and treated in the early stages. One of the most serious deterrents to cancer control is that many patients do not seek medical advice during the time the disease can be cured.

The greatest need in the cancer program is to minimize the time between the appearance of early symptoms, their diagnosis, and the taking of corrective action. *The most important single weapon in detecting cancer before any symptoms appear is the painstaking periodic health examination of the presumably well individual.* Since no age group is totally without cancer, regular cancer examinations are essential for everyone.

Age is an important factor in the over-all diagnosis of cancer. Studies have revealed that the death rate from cancer for females under 10 years of age is less than 10 per 100,000 population. At age 40 it is 100, and over 75 years it is 1000 per 100,000.[2] On this basis, a lump in the breast of a girl under 10 is almost certainly *not* cancer, in a woman

[2] Charles S. Cameron, *A Cancer Source Book for Nurses*, New York, American Cancer Society, 1962, pp. 16–17.

aged 40 there is a chance it *is* cancer, and in a woman aged 75 it is almost *certainly* cancer. Also, different types of cancer appearing at selected body locations tend to have a maximum incidence within definite age groups. The most frequent sites of cancer according to the age of the individual infected is shown in Table 14.2. Everyone should keep these facts in mind and have a regular, at least yearly, physical examination that investigates the common sites of cancer for his age group.

PREVENTION OF CANCER

Many kinds of cancer may be prevented by avoiding or correcting long-continued irritations or inflammations. This prevention includes avoiding both unnecessary exposure to X-ray radiation as used in medicine and excessive exposure to ultraviolet radiation as found in strong sunlight; using safeguards in occupations involving exposure to known cancer-producing chemicals and dusts; and avoiding exposure to tobacco, particularly cigarette smoke, which has been proven to play an important part in causing cancer of the lip, mouth, larynx, and lung.

TABLE 14.2 **MOST FREQUENT TYPES OF CANCER BY AGE**

Age	Most Frequent Types of Cancer (except skin cancer)[a]
0–10	Leukemia; cancer of the brain, kidney, eye, and bone
10–20	Leukemia, Hodgkin's disease, cancer of the brain and bone
20–30	Leukemia; Hodgkin's disease; cancer of the testis, uterus, and ovary
30–40	Males—Hodgkin's disease, cancer of the genitals Females—cancer of the uterus, breast, and ovary
40–50	Males—cancer of the lung, colon, rectum, and stomach Females—cancer of the breast, uterus, and ovary
50–60	Males—cancer of the lung, stomach, colon, and rectum Females—cancer of the breast, uterus, and colon
60–70	Males—cancer of the lung, stomach, colon, and rectum Females—cancer of the breast, uterus, colon, and stomach
Over 70	Males—cancer of the prostate, stomach, colon, lung, and rectum Females—cancer of the breast, colon, stomach, and uterus

[a] Cancer of the skin is omitted from this table since there is seldom adequate reason for failure to diagnose it correctly and early.

SOURCE: Adapted from Charles S. Cameron, *A Cancer Source Book for Nurses,* New York, American Cancer Society, Inc., 1962.

EARLY SYMPTOMS

The identification of the earliest detectable signs of cancer is important. A knowledge of the seven danger signals of cancer cannot be overemphasized. No one symptom or group of symptoms is invariably characteristic of the onset of cancer. However, certain symptoms, which can be easily recognized, frequently tend to show themselves as the *first* expressions of the commonest forms of cancer. These "Seven Danger Signals of Cancer" include:

1. Any sore that does not heal, particularly those about the mouth, tongue, or lips
2. A lump or thickening in the breast or elsewhere, such as on the lip or tongue
3. Unusual bleeding or discharge from the nipple of the breast or irregular bleeding from any of the natural body openings
4. Any change in a wart or mole, such as a progressive change in color or size
5. Persistent indigestion or difficulty in swallowing, which may be followed by a sudden, unexplained loss of weight
6. Persistent hoarseness or cough
7. Any change in normal bowel habits

Recognition of one or more of the seven danger signals may or may not indicate the beginning of cancer—but it is not worth the time to wait and find out. The person who manifests any of these danger signals should consult a physician as soon as possible. Table 14.1 may give some insight into the formation, characteristics, and complications of the early symptoms of cancer.

The absence of pain in early cancer has been overemphasized. This is a generalization which should not be completely overlooked. A pain, or sensation of discomfort, which lasts more than a few weeks, always in the same place, and which can be localized with the tip of the finger, may be regarded with suspicion and calls for a medical examination. As shown in Table 14.1, one type of cancer of the bone first expresses itself through the symptom of pain.

Every woman should inspect her breasts monthly, immediately following the end of her menstrual period. Examination during the menstrual period is unsatisfactory because of the temporary changes and tenderness which normally may occur in the breasts at that time. As shown in Fig. 14.4, breast self-examination is performed in two stages. The *first stage* is performed while the woman is sitting before a mirror. With her arms at the side and posture erect, she examines her breasts for symmetry in size and shape, noting any changes in *dimpling of the skin* or *depression of the nipple*. Then with the arms overhead, she repeats the above procedure. The second stage is performed while she is reclining on a bed. During this portion of the examination she places a flat pillow or folded towel under her shoulder on the same side as the breast to be examined. This prop raises the side of the body and distributes the weight evenly over her chest wall. Now she systematically examines the flat, sensitive portions of the breast, extending her examination well into the armpit area. If any abnormal lump or thickening is found, she consults a physician immediately.

Fluids from bronchial, uterine, cervical, urethral, and rectal areas may contain cancer cells if these regions are either producing or being bathed by secretions containing tumors. Such fluids may be sampled a number of ways for microscopic study. The sample is usually smeared upon a glass microscope slide, stained by a method first suggested by Dr. George N. Papanicolaou in 1942, and studied for the presence of exfoliative cancer cells. Such a smear is called a Papanicolaou or "pap" smear.

The pap smear technique may be used for any of the above areas but is used most commonly for diagnosis of cervical cancers. A smear of the fluid and any exfoliative cells of the cervix may be harmlessly and painlessly obtained by the introduction into the uterus, by way of the vagina, of either a cotton-tipped applicator (cotton swab), a wooden tongue depressor, or a spatula, and a speculum (an instrument for dilation or opening for viewing of a passage or cavity of the body). The dry speculum is inserted into the vagina before a general pelvic examination is made, and the cervix is exposed. With a spatula, swab, or tongue depressor, the opening of the cervix (Fig. 9.5) is thoroughly scraped and the material placed on a glass slide. Another spatula is then placed in the vagina's interior (Fig. 9.5), and any discharge obtained is removed and placed on another glass slide.[3] Such a uterine-vaginal smear can be obtained with ease and without any discomfort to the patient during a physician's routine physical examination. If the smear is obtained carefully and the material adequately spread on the slides, sufficient diagnostic evidence is usually obtained for staining by the Papanicolaou method to produce either a negative or positive diagnosis of cervical cancer.

Sufficient evidence has accumulated at this time to indicate that *invasive epidermoid* or *squamous cervix cancer* (Fig. 14.1) develops from a diseased, cancerous surface epithelium known as *in situ carcinoma* (international stage O; see Fig. 14.7, p. 458). If all carcinomas of the cervix could be discovered and treated while still in this readily curable in situ (pre-invasion) stage, the possibility of eradicating cervical cancer as a cause of death would be very good indeed.[4]

[3] C. E. Lyght, ed., *The Merck Manual*, 11th ed., Rahway, N.J., Merck & Co., 1966, p. 663.

[4] L. G. Koss, *Diagnostic Cytology*, Philadelphia, Lippincott, 1961, p. 81.

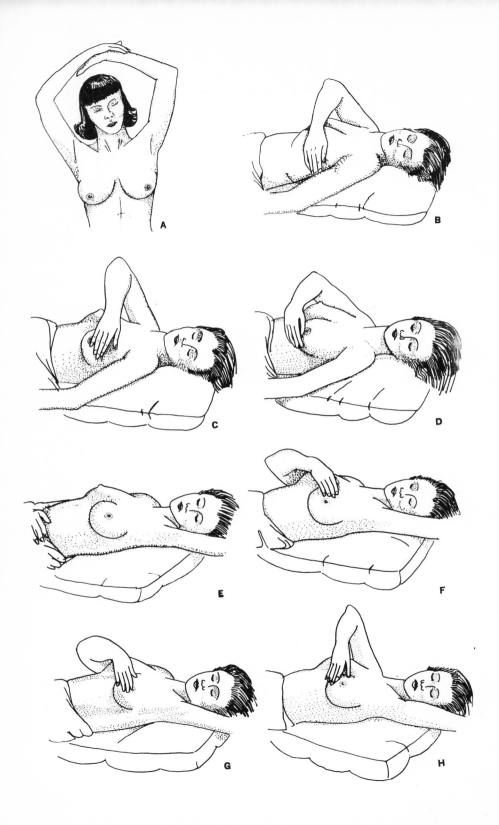

Unfortunately, in situ carcinoma may not produce alterations of the cervix visible to the naked eye, and their discovery cannot be left to a chance biopsy. The diagnosis of in situ carcinoma can be established only by a microscopic examination of tissues or cells derived from the cervix. A cytologic examination of Papanicolaou smears from the cervix is a reliable and accurate means of diagnosis of cancer of the cervix in its early stages.

It is generally assumed that the average age at the time of discovery of in situ carcinoma is from 5 to 10 years younger than the average age of the time of discovery of the invasive carcinoma.[5] This fact is of considerable importance, inasmuch as it indicates a very good chance of discovery of cancer of the cervix in the in situ stage if a systematic

[5] *Ibid.*, p. 86.

Fig. 14.4 Steps for the systematic self-examination of the breast. (A) Sitting before a mirror, arms at the sides and posture erect, the breasts are examined for symmetry in size and shape, noting any dimpling of the skin or retraction of the nipple. With arms over head repeat observations. (B) With padding in place under the shoulder, and arm at the side, the woman begins the self-examination of her breast by careful feeling of the tissues which extend well into the armpit area. Any lump or thickening is noted. (C) The woman now proceeds to inspect the upper, outer portion of the breast. She makes use of the sensitive flats of her fingers instead of their tips, and she gives this portion special attention. Again, any lump or thickening is noted. (D) Having covered the armpit region and the upper, outer portion, the woman now goes over the remainder of the outer half of the breast, feeling in successive stages from the outer margin to the nipple. Lumps or thickenings are noted. (E) When the entire outer half of the breast has been examined, with the arm at her side, the woman now raises the arm over her head. This spreads and thins the tissue for the remaining steps. (F) Beginning at the breast bone, she gently presses the tissue of the inner half of the breast against the chest wall, moving in a series of steps from the breast bone to the middle of the breast. (G) At this point, the woman carefully palpates the nipple area and the tissues lying beneath it. Using the flats of her fingers still, she notes the normal structures of her breast, and any new lumps. (H) She now completes her examination of this breast by feeling the rest of the inner half systematically. Along the lower margin she will find a ridge of firm tissue which is normal, and should not alarm her. Any new lumps or thickenings which she had not noted in the past should be reported to her physician. (National Cancer Institute, Public Health Service, Department of Health, Education, and Welfare.)

search for the disease is conducted along with an annual physical examination from the teens on through middle age.

CANCER THERAPY

Treatment of cancer does not result in a "cure" in the usual sense of the word. When a physician speaks of "curing cancer," he means that the patient has not had a sign of the disease for five years after diagnosis and treatment. The three major types of cancer therapy are *surgery, radiation,* and *chemotherapy.*

SURGERY

Surgery in the treatment of cancer is an attempt to remove completely all of the cancerous tissue in the involved organ. Because of the spreading nature of cancer, large amounts of normal tissue are always removed along wtih the malignant growth. Surgery is used to remove certain endocrine glands (ovaries, pituitary or adrenal glands) in an effort to check the growth of cancer in organs which depend on the hormones produced by those glands for growth. It is also used to relieve pain in cases of incurable cancer by severing nerves serving the site of pain.

Numerous recent improvements in cancer surgery permit modern operations to be performed with far more safety than in the past. Even as early as 1953, the operative mortality rate had decreased considerably; today, the five-year-surgical-cure rate for some types of cancer has been greatly improved. However, it must be remembered at all times that the chance of a cure is still dependent on the stage of the disease at the time surgery is attempted. *The earlier the diagnosis the better the chance of survival.*

Surgery, radiation, and chemotherapy are being combined in an effort to find the most effective cancer cures possible. Chemicals are now being fed directly into the surgical wound to prevent the spread (metastasis) of any remaining cancer cells into the blood or lymph. Preoperative radiation to prevent implantation and growth of tumors in areas adjacent to the surgical area is being used. It is hoped that such preoperative radiation may materially reduce the degree of spread of cancer following surgery.

RADIATION

Radiation has been used as a cancer treatment for about 50 years. Amounts of radiation which seem to have no effect on normal tissue cause considerable damage to cancerous tissue, sometimes even destroying the cancer completely. Radiation now is used to treat about six out of every ten cancer patients. Some types of cancer, however, are not affected by doses of radiation that are safe for normal tissue. Three sources of radiation are used in cancer therapy—high-voltage X-ray machines, radioisotopes (elements which release energy and nuclear particles as they change to other elements at a predictable rate), and laser radiation.

X rays are controlled beams of electrons at variable high-energy levels. X rays of extremely high energy levels readily penetrate tissue and can be used to arrest the growth or kill cancerous cells in deep internal organs. Relatively low-energy X rays are used for superficial cancers, such as skin growths.

Radioisotopes give energy in the form of alpha and beta particles and gamma rays (see Chapter 18). The advantage of radioisotopes is that they are picked up by the body through the digestive system like other chemicals. A physician may select the radioactive isotope according to the area or organ he wishes to reach. Certain glands and organs tend to collect specific chemicals. Small harmless doses of a radioisotope introduced into the body will then accumulate at such sites. The thyroid gland, for instance, tends to collect and accumulate iodine. Consequently, in treatment of cancer of the thyroid, a radioisotope of iodine (I^{131}) is introduced into the body and is accumulated by the thyroid. Its destructive energy is thus in a strategic spot to attack the tumor with a controlled dose.

Radioactive cobalt is also used, but the procedure is similar to that used in X-ray therapy. Cobalt therapy involves a carefully calculated placement of the patient in such a position that he or the cobalt can be rotated during exposure to the radiation beam so that the tumor is at the center of rotation in line with the radiation beam. This placement and rotation permits a maximum amount of radiation to be given to the tumor and a much smaller dosage to any one area of intervening tissue. An example of a cobalt machine is shown in Fig. 14.5.

Chemical compounds are now being used in conjunction with radiation. These drugs markedly increase the radiosensitivity of cancer cells. In some conditions doses of radiation in combination with drugs are much smaller than those required when radiation was used alone.

Laser radiation is a relatively new type of light energy which was first made available for biomedical research in the late 1950s and early 1960s. In cancer therapy the beams are focused on an accessible tumor or focused internally through special glass rods. This radiation has to some degree produced death in cancerous cells. The extent of such tumor control is dependent upon the amount of pigmentation of the tumor. The more highly pigmented the tumor, the greater the damage by lasers. Lesions that have been readily affected are basal cell carcinoma, squamous cell carcinoma, adenocarcinoma of the breast, and superficial and deep melanomas (see Table 14.3). Reduction in such tumors, followed by their surgical removal, has been successful. To increase pigmentation

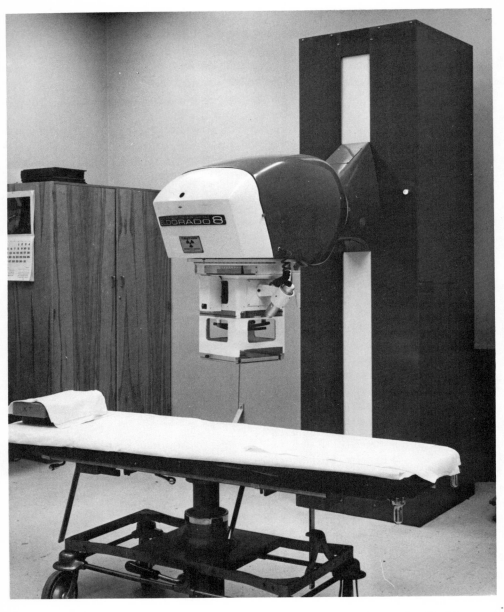

Fig. 14.5 Cobalt machine for radiation therapy. (UCLA, Center for Health Sciences.)

in tumors, vital dyes such as Janus green and Evans blue are painted on or injected into the arterial supply of the tumor to saturate the area.

After laser radiation the cells have shown chromosomal changes, which emphasize that cellular changes induced by lasers are more than just heat reactions. But the greatest limitations to date have been the

TABLE 14.3 **LASER RADIATION TREATMENT AREAS**

Type of Tumor	General Characteristics	Areas of the Body Affected	Additional Information
Basal cell carcinoma (rodent ulcer)	Begins as a small nodular growth in the skin, slowly enlarges, and ulcerates on to the surface; ulcer may crust over, fall off, and reform; contains pigmented chromatic cells	Characteristically a tumor of the face, nose, upper lip, and ears	Because of the pigmentation and surface characteristics of this tumor, treatment by laser radiation has been effective
Squamous cell carcinoma (epidermoid carcinoma)	First recognizable lesion is either an elevated papillary growth or a hardened, raised growth beneath the surface, in which a central ulcer develops	May originate in any organ or tissue with epithelium, but is most common in those containing squamous (cell) epithelium; such as the skin, oral cavity, lips, tongue, larynx, lung, pharynx, esophagus, anus, vulva, vagina, cervix, penis	A well-developed tumor shows small, round, paper-white islands, embedded in a gray stroma; the high coloration of the gray stroma and the affinity of the other cells for vital dyes gives the laser light beam a better target for treating; surface tumors are more accessible to laser treatment
Adenocarcinoma of the breast	Has the same microscopic appearance in the breast as in other parts of the body; this will be a firm, grayish-white node with fibers extending into the surrounding breast	The breast has greater recovery rate because of fast rate of discovery and treatment	The pigmentation (gray-white) of the tumor helps in the use of laser radiation
Superficial and deep melanomas	These tumors are composed of pigment-producing cells; they are black (or darkly pigmented) masses of soft, pliable cells	The most frequent site is the skin. The usual sites of origin are the face, leg, foot, back, neck, and arm	The extremely large amounts of pigment in these tumors make the use of laser radiation very effective

low-energy densities available; the small, inadequate impact areas produced by such small beams; and the lack of prolonged follow-up studies on patients who have been treated with laser radiation.

CHEMOTHERAPY

Although surgery or radiation can often remove or arrest localized cancers, rarely can they cure cancers that have spread beyond their point of origin. They cannot be used to cure cancers of the blood or blood-forming tissues which are widespread from the beginning. For many years scientists felt that the only way to treat such cancers would be with drugs or chemicals that would destroy cancer cells and yet not harm normal tissues, but before the 1940s there was no evidence that drugs could be useful in treating cancer.

The first success in chemotherapy came as a by-product of wartime research. Accidental exposure to nitrogen mustard gas was found to lead to a fall in the white cell count in the blood. Since leukemia results in overproduction of malignant white cells, nitrogen mustard gas was tested as a means of controlling this overproduction. The chemical proved more successful than anything previously tried.

Today some twenty drugs are being used in the treatment of cancer. These drugs are of three main types—*hormones, cell poisons (alkylating agents)*, and *metabolic antagonists*. None of them are cures, but they temporarily stop the growth of certain cancers, relieve pain, and allow the patient to live longer. Five or six of these drugs have been found to be particularly promising in the treatment of leukemia.[6]

Hormones, as explained earlier, are chemicals which are produced and secreted by the endocrine glands of the body. They influence or control many of the body's activities, such as growth and reproduction. Many cancers occur in hormone-controlled tissues, such as the breasts, prostate gland, and uterus. Cancer tends to appear in these organs at a time in life when the body hormones are changing. These changes seem to produce an environment very suitable to cancerous growth. Hormone therapy acts by changing the hormone environment upon which cancers are dependent for growth.

The cell poisons interfere with the cell division of cancer cells and stop their growth. However, they also damage normal cells in the same manner and have had limited use until recently. Nitrogen mustard gas and urothane are examples of such cell poisons.

Metabolic antagonists are drugs very similar to the materials cancer cells use in synthesizing DNA. Flooding the cancer site with these drugs keeps the cells from building the chemicals needed to form DNA, thus blocking cell division and slowing or stopping the growth. They are

[6] M. J. Rodman, "New Drugs in the Fight Against Cancer," *RN*, Nov. 1964, pp. 79–89.

often effective in treating acute leukemia in children, producing remissions that last several months.

CANCER INCIDENCE

It is not known how many people actually have cancer. Some cancers, for example, skin cancer, are observable shortly after the malignant growth begins. But many forms remain undetected until late in the course of the disease. In addition, some individuals fail to seek medical care even after the disease is noticeable. These conditions make the total number of persons who actually have cancer much larger than the number with diagnosed cancer. All published statistics are based on the number of persons who have been diagnosed as having cancer.

The magnitude of any disease problem is measured by (1) incidence, the number of new cases per year; (2) mortality, the number of deaths per year; and (3) prevalence, the number of cases under treatment or care at any one time during a given year. With information such as the incidence and mortality from all diseases, it is possible to estimate what proportion of the population may be expected to develop cancer (or any other disease) during life or at any specified age. A projection of the increase in death from lung cancer is shown in Fig. 14.6.

A cancer morbidity reporting system has been in operation in New York State since 1940. These reports indicate that during 1941–1943, the total cancer incidence rate was higher in females than in males. In 1958–1960, this situation was reversed, the male rate (261.3 per 100,000 population) exceeding the female rate (244.7 per 100,000 population). This change was due almost wholly to the marked rise in lung cancer, which has increased more rapidly in males. If lung cancer incidences are excluded from the 1958–1960 figures the female rate (239.9) continues to exceed the male rate (232.7). Although lung cancer has increased in both sexes, the increase among males has been more than twice that among females.

It is estimated that approximately 830,000 persons are under treatment for cancer during any year; the annual hospitalization cost for such a large group is over $666 million per year. More than 40 percent of cancer deaths occur during the productive years from 25 to 64.

CANCER IN CHILDREN

Cancer as a cause of death in children in the United States has increased since 1930. At that time only 0.7 percent of all deaths under age 15 were attributed to cancer; in 1962, cancer accounted for 4468 deaths (2.4 percent) of all deaths under 15.

Since 1955, recorded cancer deaths in this country among children under 15 have been distributed according to specific body sites, such as

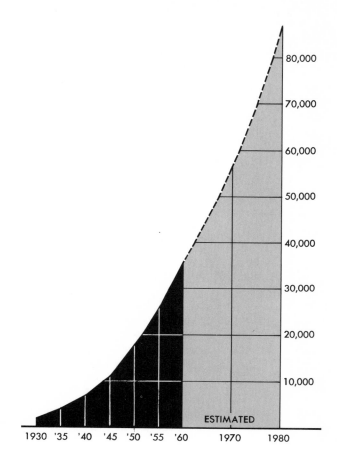

Fig. 14.6 Projection of the increase in lung cancer deaths to 1980, assuming present trends continue. Based on lung cancer deaths for the period 1930–1960. (Reprinted from the June 1963 issue of *Consumer Reports* with permission. Copyright 1963 by Consumers Union of U.S., Inc., a nonprofit organization.)

brain and nervous system (21 percent), lymphomas (8 percent), and Wilms' tumor of the kidney (about 7 percent).

CANCER IN MALES

The ten most common causes of death by cancer in males are shown in Table 14.4. Cancer of the lung is now the leading cause of cancer death in men. Over the last 50 years cancer of the lung has shown a

TABLE 14.4 CANCER DEATHS BY SEX AND TEN MAJOR SITES

Site	MALE Number of Cancer Deaths by Site	Percent of All Cancer Deaths
Lung	35,312	23
Prostate	15,173	10
Colon[a]	13,561	9
Stomach	11,947	8
Pancreas	8,725	6
Lymphomas[d]	7,896	5
Leukemia	7,493	5
Rectum	6,131	4
Bladder and urethra	5,575	4
Buccal cavity (mouth) and pharynx	4,920	3
Total of 10 major sites	116,733	78
Total of all sites	150,009	100

Site	FEMALE Number of Cancer Deaths by Site	Percent of All Cancer Deaths
Breast	24,733	19
Colon[a]	16,276	13
Uterus[b]	14,290	11
Ovary[c]	8,340	6
Stomach	7,431	6
Pancreas	6,294	5
Lung	6,064	5
Lymphomas[d]	5,859	5
Leukemia	5,504	4
Liver and biliary passages	3,601	3
Total of 10 major sites	98,392	77
Total of all sites	128,553	100

[a] Excluding rectum.

[b] Corpus uteri and cervix.

[c] Including fallopian tube and broad ligament.

[d] Including lymphosarcoma, Hodgkin's disease, multiple myeloma.

SOURCE: "Vital Statistics of the United States, 1962," "Mortality," Vol. 2, pp. 1–22. Taken from *A National Program to Conquer Heart Disease, Cancer and Stroke*, Vol. II, Washington, D.C., The President's Commission on Heart Disease, Cancer and Stroke, 1965, p. 119.

much greater rise in frequency than any other type of cancer. Cigarette smoking is associated with this sharp increase. The effects of cigarette smoking and other diseases will be discussed in a separate section later in this chapter.

The majority of lung carcinomas arise in the main bronchi or their immediate divisions. These primary cancers consist of either squamous cell carcinoma, adenocarcinoma, or the rather rare undifferentiated carcinomas (Table 14.1). Further extension of these cancers gives rise to lymphatic metastases early in their course by involving the regional lymph nodes very early. Cancer cells move upward to the nodes of the neck and downward to nodes around the abdominal aorta and on to the liver and adrenal glands. Metastasis by way of the blood stream is frequent, so that brain cancer often occurs.

Carcinoma of the prostate accounts for 5 percent of the total cancer death rate, and 10 percent of male deaths from cancer. It is the second commonest cancer in men, the first being cancer of the lung. Over 90 percent of cases of prostate cancer occur after the age of 60, but only one in five cases of enlarged prostate is malignant. The chief symptoms of the disease are the same as those for benign enlargements—frequency, urgency, and difficulty in urination. Later there is pain, especially during urination. The primary carcinoma is slow growing, but it gains early access to the surrounding venous and lymphatic channels, giving rise to metastases in the spine, pelvis, or regional lymph nodes.

Cancers of the buccal cavity and pharynx are the tenth commonest types of cancer in men, yet they account for 3 percent of the male deaths from cancer (Table 14.4). *There is a strong link between these cancers and smoking.*

A few simple observations and safeguards practiced by all individuals could help in the prevention of mouth cancer. A heavy smoker in whose mouth white patches develop and persist should give up smoking. Any dental condition such as pyorrhea, gingivitis, decaying teeth, or ill-fitting dental prostheses should be corrected before they cause irritation, sores, or other damage to appear upon the gums, tongue, or lip. If, after removal of the cause, an irritated area should fail to heal promptly, the persistent sore may be an early cancer; thus medical advice should be sought. A crack in the skin of the lip which fails to heal, or any growth or patches on the tongue or in the mouth, which enlarge, thicken, or bleed, should be regarded as danger signals and medical advice should be sought immediately.

People with head and neck cancer are often undernourished by the time they seek treatment. They have neither taste nor desire for food, and for them eating may be difficult, uncomfortable, or even painful. This group of cancers produces constant discomfort from excessive salivation, sensations of obstruction, difficult swallowing, soreness, and pain.

Tumors of the bladder occur about twice as frequently in men as in women, and most are papillary carcinomas (Table 14.1). Many of these growths seem to be benign when they first appear, but have a pronounced tendency toward malignant change and recurrence. The natural course of bladder cancer is very prolonged, but treatment is quite successful. The average age of patients diagnosed to have bladder cancer is about 57 years, and it accounts for 3 percent of the total cancer death rate.

Metastasis to the pelvic lymph nodes is not uncommon, but distant metastasis is rare. The symptoms and complications are explained in Table 14.1.

CANCER IN FEMALES

Cancer of the breast accounts for one in every five female deaths from cancer. It is more common in women who have not had children; the average age of patients is 51, which approximates the menopausal phase of life.

Most carcinomas of the breast arise in the small ducts leading from the glands. Skin nodules may occur at any time and usually develop over the breast in the untreated individual, or around the scar in those operated upon. Cancer of both breasts is not uncommon, although it is difficult to say whether one is a metastasis from the other breast or a new primary growth. Some tumors metastasize so early and spread so widely that they often prove fatal within one year of onset.

The factors causing cancer of the breast seem to be as diverse as the various forms the disease may take. Endocrine factors often seem important and, occasionally, inherited susceptibility appears significant. There is, however, no known way in which cancer of the breast can be prevented, making it very important that a tumor be detected at the earliest possible stage. Detection is accomplished by Breast Self-Examination (BSE), shown in Fig. 14.4 and explained elsewhere in this chapter.

Cancer of the uterus may be divided into cancer found in two areas: the cervix and the body of the uterus (*corpus uteri*). Cancer of the cervix is the second most common cancer in women; deaths are distributed by age in a manner similar to that for breast cancer. This cancer is more common in women who have borne children than in women who have not.

The growth usually begins as a node near the opening of the uterus, with an ulceration soon appearing. In the early stages of the disease the only outward symptom may be a slight watery discharge or an occasional spotting of blood during a nonmenstrual period. Lengthening of menstrual period may be an early symptom and, of course, any bleeding after the menopause is suspicious and demands immediate examination.

The degree of growth at the time of diagnosis and treatment is of

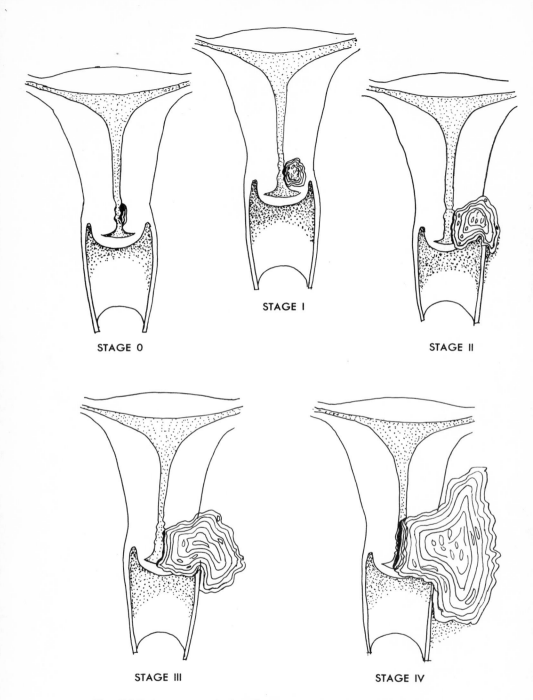

STAGE 0

STAGE I

STAGE II

STAGE III

STAGE IV

Fig. 14.7 International classification of carcinoma of the cervix.

great significance in the outcome of cancer of the cervix. The Cancer Committee of the League of Nations in 1929 initiated an international classification of carcinoma of the cervix, dividing the degree of involvement of the disease into four stages. The clarification of these stages is shown in Fig. 14.7 and is as follows:

In stage I carcinoma of the cervix is established when a growth is found which is strictly confined to the cervix. Only about 10 percent of the patients first seen are at this stage.

In stage II the growth has spread into the upper part of the vagina or into the second layer of tissue of the cervix, but at no point has it reached the pelvic wall. About 30 percent of the patients are in this stage when treated.

In stage III the growth has reached the pelvic wall at one point, so that no operation can remove such a growth. About 40 percent of the patients are in this stage when first seen.

In stage IV the growth has invaded the bladder or rectovaginal area and may have filled the pelvis or given rise to distant metastases. Twenty percent of the patients are in this very advanced stage on their first examination.

When this criterion for the four stages of uterine cancer was established, it made no provisions for a flat noninvading type of cancer cell that seemed to exist for years before spreading began. Since that time this noninvading cancer has been called *in situ epidermoid carcinoma* and is now designated Stage O in the international classification of carcinoma of the cervix. Such early cases of cancer are now discovered very frequently in women, as a result of finding cast off (exfoliate) cells in Papanicolaou smears. When found in this preinvasion stage (in situ carcinoma), the disease is always curable. For this reason *every* woman should be examined once a year.

Cancer of the body of the uterus is uncommon and usually occurs in older age groups (early 60s). Such cancers arise from the endometrial lining, where frequently a pre-existing growth has been present.

Ovarian tumors are benign in about 80 percent of cases. There are no distinctive signs of a malignancy until metastases take place. Consequently, a suspected ovarian tumor always requires an exploratory operation.

CANCERS COMMON IN BOTH SEXES

Cancer of the skin is the commonest of all cancers, but its frequency does not show in mortality statistics because it seldom involves vital organs, is recognizable in an early stage, and is easily cured.

The most common type of skin cancer is basal cell carcinoma (Table 14.1). It occurs mainly on the face and, in some patients, seems to be associated with prolonged exposure to the sun. Its highest incidence is among outdoor workers. It grows very slowly and usually begins as a small pearly plaque in the skin. After a year or two it ulcerates in the center and covers over with a scab or crust. In the late stages it may extend to the underlying cartilage or bone and ultimately will destroy the nose, eye, or any other involved part. Unlike other cancers, it practically never metastasizes, not even to the lymph nodes in the immediate area.

Squamous cell carcinoma (Table 14.1) is physically similar to basal cell carcinoma, less frequent, and shows a greater tendency to metastasize to regional lymph nodes after a year or two. It may also appear on other than the exposed areas of the body.

Malignant melanoma (Table 14.1) is rare, but is highly malignant. It generally arises in a mole that has been subjected to constant irritation by a shoe, belt, brassiere strap, and so on. The melanoma metastisizes quite readily by spreading through the blood stream to all organs of the body.

Cancers of the cecum, colon, and rectum (Table 14.1) taken together make up about 15 percent of the total cancer death rate. Although these diseases are seen mostly in older age groups, 4 percent of the cases occur in young people under 30 years of age.

The most common symptom of cancer in the large intestine is blood in the fecal material. The patient has usually ignored the early minor symptoms (such as repeated attacks of constipation, increased mucus in the stools, mild colicky pain before and after defecation, or a sensation of incomplete bowel movements), but he regards the bleeding as more serious and sees his doctor.

Cancer of the stomach (Table 14.1) accounts for about one tenth of the total cancer mortality. Its early symptoms are very indefinite—slight indigestion and, perhaps, a distaste for meat. The persistence of these two symptoms in an individual over 40 demands an X-ray examination. The later symptoms are mainly pain, anemia, and loss of weight. By this time there are usually metastases in the regional lymph nodes, soon followed by a spread of the cancer to the liver and abdominal walls.

Malignant lymphomas and leukemias (Table 14.1) are primary malignant diseases of the lymph nodes, spleen, liver, and bone marrow. There are three recognized conditions: leukemia, Hodgkin's disease, and lymphosarcoma.

The leukemias generally run a chronic course in adults, the average length of life from onset being from 2 to 5 years. In older men it may be 5 to 10 years or longer. Some cases of lymphoid leukemia may have very long periods of remissions, when all symptoms may disappear. There is an acute form of leukemia which affects young children, especially those about 2 to 5 years old; it causes a rapid wasting away. Death may ensue in a few months.

Hodgkin's disease has several forms. The term is usually used to designate malignant growths of the lymph nodes and the spleen, those not affecting the bone marrow, liver, and other organs. Hodgkin's disease, along with some forms of leukemia, mainly affects young adults in the 20–30 age group. Since 1949, the International List of Diseases, Injuries, and Causes of Death[7] has included the leukemias and Hodgkin's disease as forms of cancer; leukemia has accounted for about 4 percent of the cancer mortality and Hodgkin's disease for 1 percent.

Lymphosarcoma is a rare disease. In most cases it affects either the lymph nodes of the chest or the tonsils and lymph nodes of the neck. It spreads very slowly and may be entirely curable if treated before it becomes generalized.

Cancer of the urinary system accounts for 3–4 percent of the total cancer death rate. The most frequent type is a carcinoma of the kidney called *hypernephroma* (Table 14.1), which may occur at middle age; it is more often encountered in males than in females.

Wilms' tumor of the kidney is one of the forms of cancer which affects young children. Over half of the cases are found in the age group under 3 years, and nearly all cases are in children under 5.

Tumors of the bladder seem to be benign when they first appear but have a tendency toward malignant changes and recurrence. The average age of patients at diagnosis is about 57 years. Bladder cancer accounts for 3 percent of the total cancer mortality.

RESEARCH TRENDS

For many years researchers have probed the nature of cancer; now they share an attitude of optimism concerning the eventual understanding of that complex disease.

CHEMICAL CARCINOGENS

Knowledge of the role of the chemical compounds in cancer comes primarily from clinical observation of the occurrence of certain types of cancer in men associated with particular occupations. A limited number of human cancers are unquestionably caused by exposure to particular *chemical carcinogens*. Examples of such occupational carcinogens are (1) soot, tar, and creosote; (2) petroleum-based oils; (3) aniline dyes; (4) metals and ores (notably chromates and nickel); and (5) asbestos.

Chemical studies have led to the identification of at least one powerful carcinogen in coal tar (3, 4-benzpyrene); the other carcinogenic compounds of coal tar as yet have not been identified. Substances in the aniline dyes are among the best known of human carcinogens. The mining and processing of chromates is associated with a high incidence of

[7] World Health Organization, Geneva, Switzerland.

carcinoma of the lung, and nickel refining is associated with carcinoma of the sinuses.

In cancers related to occupational exposure, the carcinogenic hazard is pinpointed by studies of the occurrence of specific tumors and then proved by studies of animals in which similar types of cancer are induced by exposure to the suspected carcinogenic compounds whose carcinogenic activity is measurable only in laboratory animals. These compounds are being introduced into the environment in steadily increasing numbers as a result of industrialization, urbanization, and the other changes of modern living. This situation has created an urgent need to identify, characterize, and assess the ability of chemical agents to induce human cancer. In the meantime, agents that are proven to be carcinogenic should be regarded as hazardous. Such was the procedure in establishing the hazardous role of cigarette smoking in lung cancer.

RADIATION

Cancer induced by exposure to radiation was first reported more than 60 years ago. Since then, the ability of radiation to induce tumors has been well documented in laboratory animals and human beings. Studies of irradiated animals and men indicate that radiation of almost any part of the body increases the incidence of malignancy roughly in proportion to dosage. But it is impossible to say how much human cancer is induced by radiation, X ray, or radionuclides lodged in the tissues.

VIRUSES

More than 50 years ago the relation of viruses to cancer in fowl was first demonstrated. Research since then has yielded numerous viruses that induce tumors in various animals, including mammals. But, to date, no human cancer-causing virus has been identified.

The task of solving the puzzle of tumor-producing viruses assumes a degree of urgency because of the role of these viruses in the leukemias of birds and rodents, and possibly in man. The infecting virus, upon entering the cell, takes over the cell's protein-synthesizing machinery. Then the cell synthesizes viral DNA and protein, instead of normal cell DNA and protein, just long enough to produce a crop of new complete viruses, after which the cell dies. These cell-destroying viruses are called *cytolytic* viruses. In non-cell-destroying viruses the cell does not turn off the synthetic processes, but produces a slightly different DNA, which transforms the cell into a new cell type, differing in some respects from the original infected cell. This infected cell is very likely malignant. The viruses which have been shown to perform this transformation are termed *oncogenic* viruses (tumor-producing).

The precise role of the invading virus in the transformation of normal host cells into cancerous cells remains to be established, but the stage has now been set for such investigations.

ENDOCRINE FACTORS

The suspicion that endocrine factors may participate in cancer in man has long interested researchers. Observations have shown that hormones profoundly influence the rates of biochemical and physiological processes within the body. However, no evidence is available that cancer in man may arise as a primary result of the production in the body of one or more hormones. Tumors, in both experimental animals and man, may regress to some degree following endocrinologic therapy.

Human malignancies such as cancer of the prostate, breast, uterus, and the lymphomas and leukemias can be inhibited by hormone changes. Although life has been prolonged, cures have never been obtained through the use of hormones.

GENETIC FACTORS

A few uncommon types of human cancer are considered to be hereditary. These include *Xeroderma pigmentosium,* a recessive condition in which the skin is quite sensitive to sunlight, so that exposure may result in skin cancers. Retinoblastoma, a type of cancer of the eye (Table 14.1), follows a dominant pattern of inheritance. Children with mongolism, a commonly inherited condition, have 20 times more leukemia than nonmongoloid children.

Information from studies of the more common types of cancer is difficult to analyze genetically because of the general make up of the population. A family's tendency toward cancer in a particular site is suggested when statistical studies show a frequency greater in one family than would be expected in the general population. Family tendencies have been reported for cancer of the breast, uterus, prostate, stomach, colon-rectum, and lung. However, these hereditary factors are not considered to be strong.

IMMUNITY TO CANCER

No certain evidence exists that human tumors possess specific *antigens.* Most of the difficulties in translating observations from animals to man stem from the genetic variables which cannot be controlled in man as they are in experimental animals. Studies concerning the general immunities of the cancer patient are being made, as are intensive efforts to find specific antigens in human tumors. A patient does have some body defenses against his own cancer, but he also has certain immunity problems. Cancer patients are highly susceptible to infection. In the leu-

kemias and similar diseases, infection may be related to the advance of
the disease, tumor invasion, and replacement of the tissues that produce
white blood cells which normally ingest foreign material.

Research in the future may attempt to stimulate body defenses by
utilizing cancer vaccines made from a patient's own tumor or other
patients' tumors.

SMOKING AND HEALTH

The relationship of smoking to health has received a great deal of
attention. Research brought to light by the 1965 President's report on
smoking and disease has shown a definite link between smoking and the
occurrence of a variety of diseases (Table 14.5). In particular, the association of cigarette smoking with increased likelihood of developing
lung cancer has been well demonstrated. Table 14.6 contains the associations that have been shown between different types of cancer and
various kinds of uses of tobacco. On the whole, these relationships seem
to be *definitely* or *probably* established.

TABLE 14.5 **EXPECTED AND OBSERVED DEATHS FOR SMOKERS OF
CIGARETTES ONLY AND MORTALITY RATIOS IN SEVEN PROSPECTIVE
STUDIES**

Underlying Cause of Death	Expected Deaths	Observed Deaths	Mortality Ratio
Cancer of lung (162-3)[a]	170.3	1,833	10.8
Bronchitis and emphysema (502, 521.1)	89.5	546	6.1
Cancer of larynx (161)	14.0	75	5.4
Oral cancer (140-8)	37.0	152	4.1
Cancer of esophagus (150)	33.7	113	3.4
Stomach and duodenal ulcers (540, 541)	105.1	294	2.8
Other circulatory diseases (451-68)	254.0	649	2.6
Cirrhosis of liver (581)	169.2	379	2.2
Cancer of bladder (181)	111.6	216	1.9
Coronary artery disease (420)	6,430.7	11,177	1.7
Other heart diseases (421-2, 430-4)	526.0	868	1.7
Hypertensive heart (440-3)	409.2	631	1.5
General arteriosclerosis (450)	210.7	310	1.5
Cancer of kidney (180)	79.0	120	1.5
All causes[b]	15,653.9	23,223	1.68

[a] International Statistical Classification numbers in parentheses.
[b] Includes all other causes of death as well as those listed above.
SOURCE: *Smoking and Health*, Washington, D.C., U.S. Department of Health, Education, and Welfare, February 1964.

Association of smoking with cancers of the upper digestive and respiratory tracts seems reasonable, because there may be a direct exposure of these organs to carcinogenic agents in tobacco. But such reasoning does not explain the cigarette smoking–bladder cancer association, although this relationship has been observed. Therefore, this association is indicated as being *suggestive*.

LUNG CANCER AND SMOKING

The upward trend of lung cancer was first noted by a University of Minnesota pathologist, Dr. Moses Barron. He reported his findings to the Minnesota State Medical Society in August 1921. His report revealed that from 1899 to 1918 only four cases of lung cancer had been identified at autopsy by University of Minnesota pathologists. In 1919 there was only one case, but in 1920 this trend was reversed. From July 1, 1920, to June 30, 1921, eight lung cancer patients (0.9 percent of autopsies performed) died at that medical center.

Another series of autopsy records was studied and reported on by Dr. David M. Spain of the Presbyterian Hospital in New York City. Since the diagnosis of lung cancer depends primarily on the microscopic examination of cells taken from the lungs, this hospital had maintained microphotographs of cancer cells from its earlier autopsies and had actually preserved stained slides of the cells of later autopsies. Dr. Spain was able to review, confirm, or correct all of the diagnoses of cancer of the lungs which had been seen in that hospital from 1912 to 1956, a 45-year period. His findings are contained in the following figures:

1912–1921	0.6%	(6 deaths in 992 autopsies)
1922–1931	1.3%	(21 deaths in 1649 autopsies)
1932–1941	2.8%	(83 deaths in 2950 autopsies)
1942–1946	3.4%	(49 deaths in 1449 autopsies)
1947–1956	3.7%	(120 deaths in 3250 autopsies)

Many other studies have shown similar results and upward trends such as these. Information compiled from studies of the causes of deaths recorded on death certificates fully confirm the above data from autopsies.

In the United States in 1914 only 371 deaths were attributed to lung cancer. This number has since climbed to 36,420 in 1960. The rate is still on the rise, and if present trends continue, the American Public Health Association has stated, "Lung cancer will claim the lives of more than 1,000,000 present school children in this country before they reach the age of 70 years." (A projection of this trend was shown in Fig. 14.6.)

TABLE 14.6 **ASSOCIATION OF TOBACCO CONSUMPTION WITH
HUMAN CANCER OF VARIOUS SITES**

Type of Tobacco	Cancer Site	Assessment
Cigarettes	Lung	Definite
	Larynx (intrinsic and extrinsic)	Probable
	Bladder	Suggestive
	Oral cavity[a]	Suggestive
Pipe	Oral cavity[a]	Probable
	Extrinsic larynx	Probable
Cigars	Oral cavity[a]	Probable
Chewing tobacco	Oral cavity[a]	Probable

[a] Includes lip, tongue, tonsil, mouth, and pharynx.

SOURCE: P. E. Sartwell, *Preventive Medicine and Public Health,* New York, Appleton-Century-Crofts, 1965, p. 545.

Cigarettes contain over 100 distinguishable chemical compounds. One of the most prominent components is the narcotic *nicotine.* This compound seems to play an important part in the paralyzing of cilia, causing the loss of ciliary action, but it plays an even more important role in the cardiovascular diseases (see Chapter 13). The smoke which results from the burning of tobacco contains more than 270 chemicals, of which *15 are known carcinogens* whose abilities to induce cancer either in animal experiments or in humans themselves has been thoroughly demonstrated. In addition, there are many substances whose carcinogenic qualities have not been tested.

This carcinogen-saturated smoke, when inhaled, actually reaches the cells which are the major sites of primary growth for the most prevalent types of lung cancer (squamous cell carcinoma, adenocarcinoma, or undifferentiated carcinomas). By referring to Fig. 14.8, a drawing of the respiratory system, the reader will note that smoke entering the body first enters the mouth and throat. If an individual does not inhale, as when smoking a pipe or cigar, the smoke is exhaled. This individual runs little chance of lung cancer but does run quite a risk of cancer of the oral cavity and pharynx. After being inhaled (most cigarette smokers who do contract lung cancer inhale), the smoke passes down the throat and through the trachea and bronchi to the lungs. The bronchi branch extensively into smaller and smaller subdivisions, which then end in an expanded, sac-like alveolus. The alveolus is the actual structure where the oxygen is supplied to the blood and the waste carbon dioxide is removed from the blood. The reader should note that each tube in the respiratory system is much wider where it forks than in the tube itself. This widening, mainly at the branching of the bronchi, causes the air or smoke to slow down, stagnate slightly, and deposit any particles that are being carried. The carcinogenic particles that may cause damage or induce cancer are deposited in this area. Normally, and early in the career of a smoker, all tubes leading to the alveoli are lined with minute cilia (Fig. 14.1, drawing and photomicrograph A), small whiplike fingers which beat rhythmically. Present on the surface is mucus, secreted by the lining membrane. Any foreign material which is able to enter the lungs is trapped by this mucus and expelled up and out of the trachea into the esophagus and the digestive system by the action of the cilia.

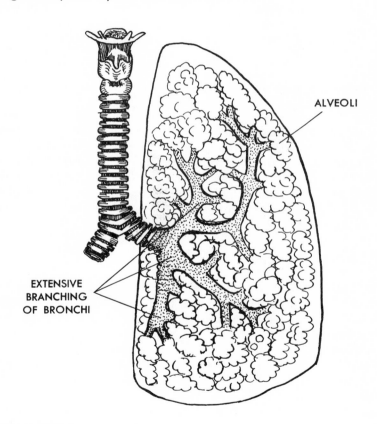

ALVEOLI

EXTENSIVE
BRANCHING
OF BRONCHI

Fig. 14.8 Respiratory system.

Cigarette smoke, in time, will paralyze the action of the cilia, causing the cilia to die and disappear altogether. When the cilia die, foreign material trapped by the mucus builds up in the lungs and either closes the alveoli, reducing their efficiency and adding strain to the heart, or is expelled very poorly by a reflex "smoker's cough" which develops for this purpose. Autopsies upon hundreds of human lungs show the dead or missing cilia, the accumulation of mucus, and the precancerous or cancerous changes taking place in the widened areas (bifurcations) where the smoke has deposited its carcinogens. This is the progression which is induced in the lungs by smoking, but what are the results?

In 1964 the U.S. Department of Health, Education, and Welfare published a booklet, "Smoking and Health, Summary of the Report of the Advisory Committee to the Surgeon General." This booklet states that the risk of developing lung cancer increases with duration of smoking and the number of cigarettes smoked per day, and is diminished by discontinuing smoking. In comparison with nonsmokers, average male smokers of cigarettes have approximately a nine- to ten-fold risk of developing lung cancer and heavy smokers at least a twenty-fold risk.

SMOKING AND ALL DISEASES

It is further stated in the HEW pamphlet that, in general, the greater the number of cigarettes smoked daily, the higher the over-all death rate at premature ages. For men who smoke fewer than 10 cigarettes a day, the death rate from all causes is about 49 percent higher than that for nonsmokers; for those who smoke from 10 to 19 cigarettes a day, it is about 70 percent higher than for nonsmokers; for those who smoke 20 to 39 a day, 90 percent higher; and for those who smoke 40 or more, it is 120 percent higher from all causes.

CHRONIC BRONCHITIS

Bronchitis is an inflammation of the lining of the bronchial tubes. When the bronchi become inflamed, they are easily infected. Such inflamed and infected bronchi impede air flow to and from the lungs, causing labored breathing and heavy mucus or "phlegm" to be coughed up. A brief attack of acute bronchitis with fever, coughing, and spitting occurs in severe colds. *Chronic bronchitis* is the term applied to coughing and spitting that continues for months and returns periodically.

Cigarette smoking and air pollution are the most important causes of chronic bronchitis in the United States. Smoking also increases the chances of dying from chronic bronchitis. This disease seems, at first, just to hang on after a cold; the cough is usually dismissed as only "smoker's cough." But the colds become more frequent, the coughing and spitting last longer. After a while, without the individual's realizing it, the condition is lasting the year around. At this stage, without medical attention, the individual is open for a wide range of very serious respiratory diseases.

PULMONARY EMPHYSEMA

Pulmonary emphysema is a condition characterized by chronic short-ness of breath and evidence of obstruction to the flow of air into and, particularly, out of the lung. Very advanced conditions show destruc-tion of the alveoli.

The two main complications are *ventilatory failure* and *congestive heart failure*. These constantly threaten an individual who has emphy-sema. Ventilatory failure occurs when the obstruction to breathing becomes so severe that air is not moved in and out of the lungs in amounts adequate to maintain a normal composition of gases (oxygen and carbon dioxide) in the arterial blood. Congestive heart failure is most commonly encountered in patients who have had ventilatory failure, which has made it impossible for the heart to maintain its increased activity.

The individual developing pulmonary emphysema is usually a male between 50 and 70 who has smoked for years; has had colds, accompa-nied by a heavy cough (sometimes amounting to chronic bronchitis); and begins to feel short of breath in the morning and/or evening. He may seek medical advice at this time or he may wait until the coughing produces blood or the obstruction and shortness of breath interfere with his normal daily activity. Unless the condition is promptly treated, the lungs may be permanently damaged, resulting in a day in, day out struggle to keep the lungs working. Every breath is labored and may be a major effort.

Doctors do not know how to prevent emphysema, but the best avail-able advice is (1) don't smoke, and (2) clear up any infection of the respiratory system (mouth, nose, throat, sinuses, or lungs) as quickly as possible, because such infections set up a possible starting place for pulmonary emphysema.

CARDIOVASCULAR DISEASES

Male cigarette smokers have a higher death rate from coronary artery diseases than nonsmoking males. This association is not completely clear, but it was discussed at some length in Chapter 13.

PEPTIC ULCER

Studies indicate an association between cigarette smoking and peptic ulcer. Smoking's irritation of ulcers greatly interferes with the healing process.

TOBACCO AMBLYOPIA

This is a condition of dimness of vision without any organic lesions in the eyes or nervous system. Studies have substantiated an implication of this disease with pipe and cigar smoking as well as cigarette smoking.

CIRRHOSIS OF THE LIVER

The increased mortality of smokers from cirrhosis of the liver has been shown, but there is not sufficient evidence to support more than a suggestive association.

MATERNAL SMOKING AND INFANT BIRTH WEIGHT

Women who smoke cigarettes during pregnancy tend to have babies of lower birth weights. It is not known whether this decrease in birth weight has any further implications.

There have been many studies showing the direct and indirect relationships between smoking and health. These are documented by scientists in countries throughout the world. Reports, beginning with the report on lung cancer by Dr. Barron and continuing through the release of the "Smoking and Health" report of the Advisory Committee to the Surgeon General, have made it quite clear that the habit of smoking is very injurious to health. But how does the general public feel about smoking? The sales of tobacco have not diminished to any great extent, and people are still dying at an increasing rate from lung cancer, emphysema, heart disease, and other diseases directly associated with smoking.

Starting on p. 471 is an open letter from a physician, a specialist in internal medicine with a particular interest in cardiology. The four children it is addressed to were in their teens.

SUMMARY

I. What Is Cancer?
   A. An uncontrolled, disorderly replacement of worn-out cells which continues as an abnormal growth.
   B. Cancer cells are distinguished by the nuclei which:
      1. Are usually larger than those of comparable normal cells.
      2. Vary significantly in size and shape within a group of cancer cells.
      3. Deviate in number and appearance of chromosomes.
   C. Cellular processes and behavior
      1. Cancer cells fail in obeying feedback and self-controlling mechanisms.
      2. They produce large amounts of DNA, RNA, and protein.

This letter was written by Dr. Robert R. Montgomery, a 40-year-old Washington physician with six children. Four are in their teens, and it is to them that the letter is addressed. For some years, Dr. Montgomery has been an unofficial consultant to Changing Times on medical matters, and that is how the editors chanced to see his manuscript. They felt that it should be read by teen-agers and parents everywhere and asked Dr. Montgomery to share this message to his own children with yours. Professionally, Dr. Montgomery is a specialist in internal medicine with a particular interest in cardiology.

What a Doctor Tells His Own Kids About Smoking [7]

Dear Susie, Kathy, Tom and Chris:

Each of you is a very important person, especially to me. You may feel that I can't understand what it's like to be a teen-ager today. Maybe you're right. But I am interested in you, and I'm vitally concerned when anything threatens your life or your health. This is why I'm writing you about smoking.

Besides being your father, I am a doctor. Though doctors don't know everything, they do know more about health than almost anyone else. I was a teen-ager, too. It was a while ago, but I do remember what it was like.

When I was your age, I did smoke. A girl taught me how when I was only 16.

I met her one summer. I met her father, too. He was very stern, and classed smoking along with such vices as drinking, dancing and playing cards. He forbade them all for reasons we thought were poor. We didn't listen.

My girl smoked. She let me understand that she would feel uncomfortable dating a boy who didn't. So I learned.

I went through a few horrible days when I couldn't smoke without coughing or making a fool of myself some way. It took a month or so before I could hold the cigaret right.

Soon I was hooked. But I didn't mind. All my friends were smoking, too. And SHE liked it.

I couldn't smoke at home, though. My father did, but he wouldn't let me. I couldn't smoke at school, either. There wasn't any such thing as a smoking area for students. But we found ways, as kids always can.

[7] Reprinted by permission from *Changing Times*, the Kiplinger Magazine, September 1964 issue. Copyright 1964 by the Kiplinger Washington Editors, Inc., 1729 H. Street, N.W., Washington, D.C.20006.

Later, smoking was such a fixed habit that I couldn't stop. I remember feeling quite smug in college because the soccer coach never caught me at it. But the laugh was really on me because smoking kept me from building up good wind.

And movies! They were horrible as long as I was a smoker. I found myself waiting for the end, not to find out how the picture came out, but to get a smoke. I remember *Gone With the Wind* partly because it had an intermission, a chance for a smoke.

In medical school there were many long hours of studying and boning for exams. My ashtrays always were full of butts.

In the war, I was on an aircraft carrier where we all learned the danger of a lighted cigaret around aviation gasoline. We obeyed the rules and didn't smoke in restricted areas or when the "smoking lamp" was out. I wanted to smoke, though. And I didn't stop even though it often was pure torture to wait till someone called, "Smoking lamp is lit."

Later, in my hospital training and in medical practice, I learned more about the effects of smoking. Still I did not stop. I smoked for a total of 16 years, averaging two packs a day in the last few of them.

One day—I remember the date, hour and place—another doctor and I were reviewing methods of testing blood flow in certain arteries. His was normal; mine was not. When the test was repeated after two hours with no cigarets, mine was normal, too. Smoking was affecting my own arteries! I stopped smoking on the spot, permanently.

In the next few weeks, I began to notice some changes. My resting pulse rate dropped 20 beats per minute. The cold, wet feeling my hands always got when I was tense gradually disappeared. The little cough I had been disregarding went away. My senses of taste and smell became very sharp again.

I suppose this all seems so long ago to you. But it shows that I do understand about smoking, both as a teen-ager sees it and as a doctor sees it.

The medical reasons for not smoking are far better known now than they were then. They are all contained in the Surgeon General's report on *Smoking and Health*. This extensive, thorough, unbiased review of all the available evidence makes two big points.

1. The general death rate for smokers is higher than for nonsmokers.

2. Death rates from lung cancer and coronary heart attacks are much higher for smokers.

These are facts. Oh, I know the arguments smokers use to laugh off these facts. "Not all the evidence is in. Other factors may play a part." Which is true enough. They also say: "What's the difference? You've got to die of something." Which is true enough, too.

But neither comment gets around another big fact, which is this: While the search for the exact cause of lung cancer continues, it is the smokers who will most likely have to have their lungs removed because of that cancer.

If your generation smokes the way mine has, at least half of you will be ordered to stop by your doctor at some time in your lives. Believe me, it is much easier to stop when you are young and healthy than when you're in bed just trying to live through your heart attack or your operation.

So both as a parent and a doctor, my most earnest advice to you on smoking is NEVER START. As far as I know, you don't smoke. But if you have started already, I urge you to stop now, before years of the habit make stopping seem impossible.

All habits are hard to break, but this is one of the hardest. It is almost an addiction. It just cannot be stopped unless you have a very strong desire or need to do so.

Stopping a true addiction is usually impossible without medical help, often including time in a hospital. Fortunately, the smoking habit is not that hard to kick. Many of my patients, though, say they can't stop and want some medicine to "cure" the habit. I do not advise any medicine. I have not yet found a safe one that truly works. Nor do I recommend a substitute, like chewing gum. I find that the smoker who uses a substitute habit usually returns to smoking.

I think it often takes a real and almost immediate threat to your own life to make you stop the habit once it is firmly established. Anyone can stop for a while on a bet, for Lent, or for most of the football season. These are only pauses in the habit, though; smoking starts again at the end of the test period.

How could you, a teen-ager, stop smoking?

First, you must decide that you never want another smoke *in your entire life.*

Then don't carry cigarets, don't bum any, and try to avoid groups where there is a lot of smoking going on. In a month or so, you won't miss it much. In a few months, you'll be glad you stopped.

One of the hardest things to stand will be taunts of "goodie-goodie," "fink" and "show-off" from those who haven't yet stopped. Endure the name-calling. It will die out soon.

You see now the dangers of smoking. You see how hard it is to stop. Why, then, do teen-agers start to smoke? What can you do about it?

Often you hear that teen-agers start smoking "because you want to look big and important." Usually old fogies say this, and it is a galling thing to hear. I don't believe it.

I think the smoking habit starts as a social act. Usually it begins with a group of friends. Later it becomes such a personal need that you have to smoke even when you are alone. But at first, it's a group thing. You smoke because "everyone does."

So that suggests the constructive thing you can do. If you don't smoke and if most of your friends don't smoke, there will be no compulsion for someone else coming into your group to start smoking.

You are the ones, the only ones, who can control teen-age smoking. We parents can offer our advice and assure you of our support as you try to curb this habit. But you alone can stop it. I sincerely hope you will.

DAD

D. Tumors—growths which persist, grow, and serve no useful purpose.
   1. Benign tumors are growths that increase in size slowly, are surrounded by a fibrous membrane, and remain localized.
   2. Malignant tumors are growths that increase in size rapidly, are not surrounded by a membrane or capsule, and tend to spread and invade other tissues.
     a. cancer—usually used to designate all malignant growths.
     b. carcinomas—malignant tumors arising from epithelial tissues.
     c. sarcomas—malignant tumors arising from connective tissues.
E. Cancer spreads by:
   1. Invasion—extension into spaces between normal cells.
   2. Metastasis—process of transferring cancer from an organ or part of the body to another, forming secondary cancer sites.
   3. Implantation—dislodged or shed cancer cells that implant themselves in adjacent organs grow, and produce their destructive effects.
F. How cancer kills.
   1. Anemia:
     a. insufficient production of red blood cells.
     b. production of defective cells that do not survive long in circulation.
     c. intestinal bleeding either directly from a tumor or indirectly (example: bone marrow deficiencies).
   2. Infection—frequently occurs because of the reduction of white blood cells, which causes a depression of the body's defenses against infection (Chapter 15).
   3. Debility (wasting away of the body) which might result from:
     a. damage to mouth or stomach.
     b. treatment by drugs, surgery, or radiation.
     c. loss of appetite from pain or emotional depression.

II. Diagnosis Is Not Death
  A. Cancer can be cured if diagnosed and treated in early stages.
  B. Prevention of cancer:
    1. Periodic health examination of the presumably well individual.
    2. Avoidance of long-continued irritations or inflammations.
    3. Knowledge of first symptoms of the commonest forms of cancer, the "Seven Danger Signals of Cancer."
  C. Cancer therapy.
    1. Surgery—used to remove completely all of the cancerous tissue in an involved organ.
    2. Radiation—used to damage or destroy cancerous tissues.
    3. Chemotherapy—use of drugs or chemicals to destroy cancer cells without harming normal tissues.

III. Cancer Incidence
  A. Actual number of cases is not known; all statistics based on number of persons diagnosed as having cancer.
  B. Cancer in children has increased since 1930.
  C. In males, the most common sites for cancer are the lungs, prostate, colon, and stomach.
  D. Cancer in females occurs most often in the breast, uterus, and colon.

IV. Research Trends
  A. Chemical carcinogens are chemical compounds unquestionably causing cancer.
  B. Radiation has cancer-producing qualities.

C. Viruses can invade and transform normal cells into cancerous areas.

D. Genetic factors have produced only a few uncommon types of human cancers.

V. Smoking and Health

A. Research shows a definite link between smoking and the occurrence of a variety of diseases.

B. Lung cancer and smoking.

1. Upward trend linked with increased consumption of cigarettes.

2. Carcinogens in cigarettes are known to have definite cancer-producing properties.

C. Smoking and all deaths—the greater the consumption, the higher the over-all death rate at premature ages.

D. Respiratory diseases due to smoking:

1. Chronic bronchitis.

2. Pulmonary emphysema.

E. Other conditions linked to smoking include:

1. Cardiovascular disease.

2. Peptic ulcer.

3. Tobacco amblyopia.

4. Cirrhosis of the liver.

5. Reduced infant birth weight in those whose mothers smoked during pregnancy.

Glossary

If you cannot find the word you wish in this glossary, check the index for text and glossary references.

anemia (ə nē'mē ə) (*an*, negative; G. *haima*, blood). A condition in which the blood is deficient either in quantity or quality.

benign tumor (bi nīn') (L. *benignus*). An abnormal swelling or growth that is not malignant or cancerous.

birthmark (burth'mark). Some peculiar mark or blemish found on the body at birth and retained throughout life.

cancer (kan'sər) (L. "crab"). A cellular tumor showing uncontrolled growth. The natural course is fatal and usually associated with formation of secondary growths.

carcinogenic (kahr si nō jen'ik). Causing or producing cancer.

carcinoma (kahr si nō'mə) (G. *kardinōma* from *karkinos* crab, cancer). A new tumorous growth made up of epithelial cells invading the surrounding tissues and giving rise to secondary growths throughout the body.

cell poison (sel poi'zn) (L. *cella*, compartment; L. *potio*, to drink; G. *toxicum*, toxin). Any substance which by its chemical action may cause damage to the structure or function of the cell.

cervix (sur'viks) (L. *cervix*, neck). The lower and narrow end of the uterus.

chemotherapy (kem'ō ther'ə pē) (G. *chemeia*, chemistry; *therapeia*, treatment). The treatment of disease by administering of chemicals which affect the causative factor unfavorably but do not injure the patient.

chromosome (krō'mə sōm) (G. *chromo*, color; G. *soma*, body). A small dark-staining and more or less rod-shaped body which appears in the nucleus of a cell at the time of cell division. They contain the genes, or hereditary factors, and are constant in number in each species.

cobalt (kō'bawlt). A metal with atomic number 27; a radioactive isotope of the element cobalt is used in the treatment of cancer.

cyst (sist) (G. *kystis,* sac, bladder). Any vesicle or sac of membranous tissue.

debility (de bil'i tē) (L. *debilis,* weak). Lack or loss of strength.

emphysema (em fi sē'mə) (G. *emphysema,* inflation). Presence of air in the tissues of the lungs as a result of distention and rupture of the pulmonary alveoli.

empyema (em pē ē'mə) (G. *en,* in; *pyon,* pus). Accumulation of pus in a cavity of the body, especially the chest.

endocrine glands (en'də krin) (G. *endo,* within; *krinein,* to separate; L. *glans,* acorn-like). Glands or organs whose function is to secrete into the blood or lymph a substance (hormone) that has a specific effect on another organ or part.

endocrinologic therapy (en'dō krin'ə loj'ik ther'ə pē). Treatment of disease by the administration of endocrine preparations (hormones).

endometrial lining (en'dō mē'trē əl) (G. *endo,* within; *metra,* womb). The mucous membrane that lines the cavity of the uterus.

epithelium (ep i thē'lē əm) (G. *epi,* on, upon; G. *thele,* nipple). The covering of internal and external surfaces of the body, including the lining of vessels and other small cavities.

fibroid tumor (fī'broid), **fibroma** (fī brō'mə). A tumor composed mainly of fibrous or fully developed connective tissue.

hormone (hor'mōn) (G. *hormon,* excite). A chemical substance secreted into the body fluids by an *endocrine gland,* which has a specific effect on the activities of other organs.

incidence (in'si dəns) (L. *incidens,* falling upon). The range of occurrence of a disease.

infection (in fek'shən) (L. *infectio,* to dip in). Invasion of the body by pathogenic microorganisms and the reaction of the tissues to their presence and to the toxins generated by them.

in situ (in sī'too). (Latin term meaning "in the natural place.") In situ epidermoid carcinoma is a changing of the surface epithelium of the cervix which histologically resembles cancer but shows no evidence of invasion of the underlying fibromuscular stroma.

in vitro (in vē'trō) (L.). Within a glass; observable in a test tube.

in vivo (in vē'vō) (L.). Within the living body.

laser (lā'zər) (Light, Amplification, by Stimulated Emission of Radiation). An instrument for producing an enormously intense and sharply directed beam of light.

lymphoma (lim fō'mə) (L. *lympha,* water; G. *oma,* from *onkoma,* a swelling). Any tumor made up of lymphoid tissue.

lymphomatosis (lim'fō mə tō'sis). The development of multiple lymphomas in various parts of the body.

malignant (mə lig'nənt) (L. *malignans,* acting maliciously). Ability to invade the tissues of an individual; tending to go from bad to worse.

metabolic antagonist (met ə bol'ik an tag'ə nist) (G. *metabolos,* changeable; G. *antagonistes,* to struggle against). A substance which reverses or inhibits the physical or chemical processes by which living organisms produce and maintain life.

metastasis (mə tas′tə sis) (G. *meta,* after, beyond; *stasis,* stand). The transfer of disease from one organ or part to another not directly connected with it. It may be due either to the transfer of pathogenic organisms or to transfer of cells, as in malignant tumors.

mortality (mor tal′i tē) (L. *mortalis,* mortal, living). The death rate; the ratio of total number of deaths to the total population.

mucous membranes (myoo′kəs) (L. *mucosus,* slimy). The lining membranes of the body.

nucleus (nyoo′klē əs) (L. *nucleus,* a little nut). A spheroid body within a cell which controls the cell's activities.

platelet (plāt′lit) (G. *plate,* flat). Discs found in the blood of all mammals, which are concerned in coagulation of the blood and formation of clots.

prostate gland (pros′tāt) (G. *prostates,* one who stands before). A gland which in the male surrounds the neck of the bladder and the urethra.

radiation (rā dē ā′shən) (L. *radiatio,* to emit rays). The giving off of electromagnetic waves such as light, or particulate rays such as the alpha, beta, and gamma rays (see Chapter 18).

radioisotopes (rā′dē ō ī′sə tōp) (L. *radius,* ray; G. *isos,* equal; *topos,* place). An element, with radioactive properties, of chemical character identical with that of another element occupying the same place in the periodic table, but differing from it in its atomic characteristics. Radioisotopes are used as tracers or indicators by being added to the stable compound under observation, so that the course of the compound in the body can be detected and followed by the radioactivity thus added to it. The stable element so treated is said to be "labeled" or "tagged."

radiosensitivity (rā′dē ō sen si tiv′i tē) (L. *radius,* ray; *-sensus,* to perceive). Being sensitive to, or destroyable by, radiant energy, as radium, X-ray, or electric radiations.

remission (ri mish′ən) (L. *remittere,* to send back). A decrease or abatement of the symptoms of a disease.

sarcoma (sahr kō′mə) (G. *sarkos,* flesh; *onkōma,* a swelling). A form of cancer arising from cells of nonepithelial tissue, such as connective tissues, lymphoid tissue, cartilage, or bone.

tetraploid (tet′rə ploid) (G. *tetraple,* fourfold). Having four full sets of homologous chromosomes; they are found in cancerous organisms.

tumor (tyoo′mər) (L. from *tumere,* to swell). A mass of new tissue which persists and grows independently of its surrounding structures, and which has no physiologic use (neoplasm).

ultraviolet (ul′trə vī′ə lit). Radiation beyond the violet end of the light spectrum. Ultraviolet rays have powerful electrochemical properties.

wart (wort) (L. *verruca,* elevation). A small tumor on the skin.

wen (wen) (AS. wenn, *ultimate*). A lump on the body; a sebaceous cyst.

X ray (*X,* unknown; L. *radius,* ray). Penetrating electromagnetic radiation discovered by German physicist Wilhelm Conrad Roentgen in 1895, and also called roentgen ray.

CHAPTER 15

DISEASE

Disease has been with man since he first arrived on earth and will always be present in some form. When the body is unable to maintain a healthy state, it is because destructive forces from within or without are interfering with the body's proper functioning. Such a state is called *disease*. Disease, the result of many factors, is *any* abnormality of the body, its parts, or its functions.

CAUSES OF DISEASE

NUTRITIONAL DEFICIENCIES

Many distinctive diseases result from lack of essential vitamins, minerals, or organic foods in the diet. Examples of such diseases were discussed in Chapter 6.

PHYSICAL AGENTS

Damage from such agents as excessive heat or cold or electricity, and some kinds of mechanical damage to tissues may be classified as *accidental* disease. Mechanical damage such as cuts, fractures, or crushing of tissues is called *trauma*.

CHEMICAL AGENTS

Many substances, when present or introduced into the body in excessive amounts, result in *poisoning*, another type of disease.

TUMORS

A tumor is an abnormal growth of cells arising in any organ or tissue of the body. Tumors are called *neoplasms*, meaning "new growths" (see Chapter 14).

ALLERGY

An allergy is a reaction by the tissues of an individual to some substance which is harmless to other people. This substance is called an *allergen*, and the victim is said to be hypersensitive to that substance.

HEREDITY

Many diseases are the result of specific defects in the genetic material (DNA) received by the individual from his parents. Often a person inherits a tendency toward a particular disease; the actual appearance of the disease may be caused by diet, stress, or other environmental factors.

SENESCENCE

Senescence refers to the degenerative conditions which appear with advancing age. Common examples of such conditions include hardening of the arteries (arteriosclerosis) or degenerative changes in the bones, joints, or other parts of the body.

EMOTIONS

As discussed in Chapter 2, the emotions may in many ways interefere with the normal functions of the body. Diseases of emotional origin are referred to as psychosomatic or psychogenic diseases.

CONGENITAL ABNORMALITIES

Congenital abnormalities are abnormalities of structure or function which are present at the time of birth. They may be hereditary in origin or the result of infectious disease or nutritional deficiency in the unborn infant. Some congenital abnormalities may be the result of isolated "accidents" in the development of the embryo.

INFECTIOUS DISEASES

The term *infection* is applied to disease produced when the body is invaded by living organisms. Any disease which is *communicable* or *contagious* (a disease that can be "caught") is an *infectious disease*. The disease is "caught" when the living parasite invades the human body. Most of the remainder of this chapter will deal with the infectious diseases.

PATHOGENS

Every communicable or infectious disease that inflicts misery upon man is the result of the parasitism of man by some living organism. These disease-producing organisms are called *pathogens*. Pathogenic organisms are commonly called "germs." Most, but not all, pathogens are microscopic in size and are, therefore, sometimes referred to as *microbes* or *microorganisms*. Only a small percentage of known microorganisms are human pathogens. Many others are highly beneficial to man, and still others produce diseases in plants and animals other than man.

A disease is usually due not to the mere presence of the pathogen, but to some aspect of its life processes. A healthy man harbors many microorganisms; some are beneficial, such as the intestinal bacteria which may produce vitamins. Others are potential pathogens, capable of producing disease under the proper conditions. Still others have been shown to be neither beneficial nor harmful. Perhaps this last category includes the best-adapted parasites, those able to derive their sustenance from man without producing any detectable harm.

For ease of study, organisms have been classified into several groups according to their basic characteristics. All known pathogens may be included in one of the following categories of living things (arranged in order from smallest to largest):

1. Viruses: subcellular, semiliving particles
2. Rickettsia: single-celled, plantlike organisms
3. Bacteria: single-celled, plantlike organisms
4. Fungi: unicellular and multicellular, plantlike organisms

5. Protozoa: single-celled animals
6. Parasitic worms: multicellular animals

VIRUSES

The viruses (Fig. 15.1), although the smallest of all pathogens, are responsible for much human misery. Viruses are the causative agents for such common diseases as colds and influenza, as well as for less common diseases such as poliomyelitis, rabies, and yellow fever. Viruses are not visible with even the most powerful light microscope but can be seen with electron microscopes. As many as a million virus particles could be placed within a bacterial cell.

Fig. 15.1 Typical virus. Viruses occur in a wide range of sizes and shapes.

Virus particles lack the more complex cellular structure that is characteristic of most plants and animals. A characteristic virus particle consists merely of a central core of genetic material, either ribonucleic acid (RNA) or deoxyribonucleic acid (DNA), enclosed within a protein coating.

Viruses lie at the borderline between living and nonliving matter and lack some of the refinements of more typical living organisms. They are incapable of unassisted self-reproduction, growth, production of energy, and other vital processes of life. Viruses must live and reproduce *within* the living cell of some host organism; thus they are all intracellular parasites. A host for a virus may be a plant, an animal, or even a bacterium. When a virus particle invades a suitable host cell, only the core of genetic material enters the cell; the protein shell of the virus remains outside. Once inside the host cell, the genetic material of the virus is believed to act as a "gene" which takes over the control of the cell and "tricks" the cell into manufacturing more virus material. The normal functioning of the cell is thereby disrupted, often with serious consequences. The cells may be only temporarily affected, producing such minor diseases as a common cold; or they may be permanently damaged, producing such serious diseases as polio.

RICKETTSIAE

The rickettsiae are in many respects intermediate between viruses and bacteria. In appearance and structure they resemble very small bacteria. However, like the viruses, the rickettsiae reproduce only within living host cells (although not in the same manner as the viruses).

One characteristic of all rickettsiae is their transmission by insects and related animals (arthropods) such as fleas, lice, mites, and ticks. Some examples of rickettsial diseases include typhus fever, Rocky Mountain spotted fever, rickettsialpox, and Q fever.

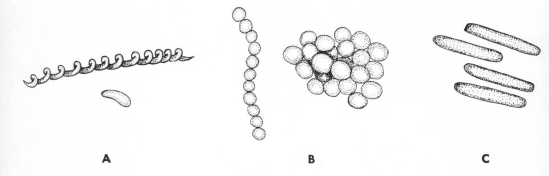

Fig. 15.2 Typical bacteria. (A) Spirilli. (B) Cocci. (C) Bacilli.

BACTERIA

Bacteria are microscopic single-celled plants (Fig. 15.2). Although much larger than viruses, they are still small enough that a million or more might be carried on the head of a pin. Unlike the viruses, however, most bacteria are neither parasitic nor pathogenic; in fact, many bacteria are very beneficial to man. That most bacteria are not pathogenic is illustrated by the fact that in most states pasteurized milk may legally contain up to 113,550,000 bacteria per gallon. The water we drink and the air we breathe also contain numerous harmless bacteria.

Unlike the viruses, pathogenic bacteria rarely enter the individual cells of man. Instead, they usually live on, around, and between the human cells. The harmful effect of pathogenic bacteria upon man is the result of their production of poisonous substances called *toxins*. Some of these bacterial toxins are among the most powerful poisons known to man—sometimes millions of times as toxic as cyanide. These toxins fall into two groups: (1) the *exotoxins*, which diffuse out of the living bacterial cells into the surrounding human tissues; and (2) the *endotoxins*, which are held within the bacterial cells and released only after the death of the cell. The significant difference in these two is that the exotoxins of different pathogens are of many different specific types and stimulate the animal body to produce specific *antibodies* (discussed later in this chapter), which act upon the toxins to neutralize them. This action makes possible the production of immunizing substances against exotoxin-caused diseases, such as tetanus and diphtheria. The endotoxins, however, are not specific and do not stimulate the production of specific antibodies by man or other animals, so it has not yet been possible to produce highly effective immunizing substances against the endotoxins. Unfortunately, there are more endotoxin-producing bacteria than exotoxin-producing ones.

The toxins of some bacteria have a localized effect, killing and dissolving the human cells near the site of the infection. The contents of the damaged cells are then available as food for the bacteria. As further cells are killed, the infection spreads deeper into the surrounding tissue. Such is the condition in the development of an abscessed tooth, where bone and supportive tissues, at the apical end of the tooth, are lost as the abscess increases in size. Other toxins are produced at one point in the body, are carried by the blood, and act upon the body at some other point. Often some specific system is then affected, as for example the nervous system in a tetanus infection.

TYPES OF BACTERIA

There are three basic groups of bacteria, the classification being based upon their shapes (Fig. 15.2).

1. *Cocci.* The cocci (an individual one would be a coccus) are the spherical bacteria. They may occur singly, in pairs (*diplococcus*), in chains (*streptococcus*), or in irregular clusters like bunches of grapes (*staphylococcus*).
2. *Bacilli.* Bacilli (the singular form is *bacillus*) are rod-shaped bacteria.
3. *Spirilli.* Spirilli (the singular form is *spirillum*) are the spiral or corkscrew-shaped bacteria.

FUNGI

The fungi are primitive plants. Some of the more common fungi include mushrooms, toadstools, and bread and cheese molds. Only a few fungi cause human diseases. Such diseases range from bothersome skin infections, such as *ringworm* and *athlete's foot,* to the sometimes fatal *histoplasmosis,* a lung infection. Fungus infections of man are most commonly associated with the skin and lungs; they are frequently very difficult to treat or cure. Treatment forces adverse conditions upon the fungi; and in response they form "spores," a dormant stage which is extremely resistant to heat (will survive boiling water for several hours as well as *dry* heat of 212°F.), drying, disinfectants, and powders or salves commonly used in treatment.

PROTOZOA

Protozoa (Fig. 15.3) are primitive single-celled animals. Although much larger than bacteria, most protozoa are still microscopic. Most protozoan diseases are associated with tropical areas, some examples

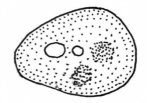

Fig. 15.3 Typical protozoan.

being malaria, African sleeping sickness, and amebic dysentery. Many protozoan diseases tend to be recurrent; that is, the patient suffers periodic relapses and the pathogen remains inactive in the body between attacks.

PARASITIC WORMS

The parasitic worms (Fig. 15.4) are multicellular animals ranging in size from about the size of the head of a pin (such as the worm causing trichinosis) up to many feet long (the tapeworms). Many parasitic worms include other animals as well as man in their life cycles. Such worms can be acquired by man through contact with these animals or through eating their incompletely cooked meat. Typical animal hosts include pigs, cows, fish, and snails.

COURSE OF A COMMUNICABLE DISEASE

Communicable disease in general follows a characteristic pattern of development. Such a course is shown in Fig. 15.5 and explained in the following sections.

TRANSMISSION AND INFECTION

In order for a person to become infected, that is, to "catch" a communicable disease, the pathogen must be carried in some manner from the source or reservoir of the disease in sufficient number to overcome

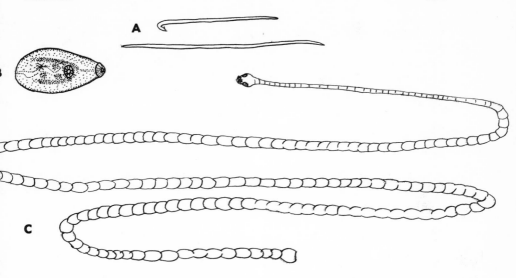

Fig. 15.4 Parasitic worms. (A) Roundworm. (B) Fluke. (C) Tapeworm.

body resistance and successfully enter the body through one of its portals of entry. This movement of disease agents from the reservoir to the victim is called *transmission*. There are various methods of transmission of communicable diseases.

PERSON TO PERSON

An infection may be caused by transmission from one person to another. This may be by *direct contact*—actual touching of an infected person through kissing, sexual intercourse, or other close personal contact—or by *indirect contact*—touching of objects contaminated by an infected person, such as toys, drinking glasses, handkerchiefs, soiled clothing or bedding. Indirect transmission may also be made by airborne droplets through the coughing, sneezing, talking, or singing of an infected person.

CONTAMINATED WATER

Diseases of the digestive tract are often transmitted by contaminated water when sewage accidentally contaminates drinking water.

CONTAMINATED FOOD OR MILK

Contaminated food or milk might result from infection in the animal food source (such as in meat or milk) or from the subsequent handling of food by an infected person.

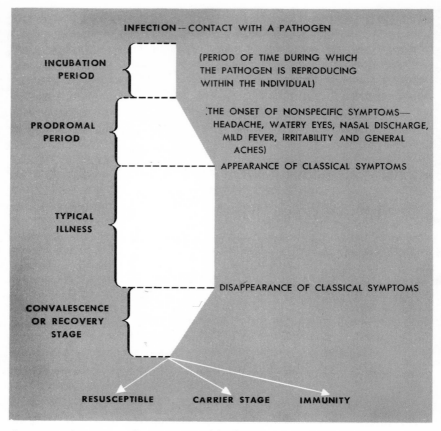

Fig. 15.5 The course of a communicable disease.

ANIMAL TO PERSON

Although most diseases that affect animals do not affect humans there are many diseases of animals to which humans are also susceptible. Transmission from animals to humans can be described as either direct or indirect. *Direct transmission* can result from the handling or the bite of an infected animal. *Indirect transmission* can result from contact with fecal material or other residue from an infected animal.

VECTORS

Some diseases are transmitted exclusively through the bites of arthropods or by contact with their feces. Such insects and related animals which are capable of transmitting a disease are called *arthropod vectors*.

The diseases they carry usually cannot be transmitted directly from one person to another, except perhaps through blood transfusion, since the pathogen often completes parts of its life cycle within the vector.

PORTALS OF EXIT AND ENTRY

A pathogen generally leaves the patient by the same route (portal) as that by which it entered. The common portals of entry and exit include the *body orifices* (mouth, nose, eyes, anus, and urogenital canals) and the *skin* and *mucous membranes*. A few pathogens may pass through the unbroken skin or mucous membrane, but most require a cut or wound for passage.

INCUBATION PERIOD

After an infectious organism has entered the body, there is a period of time during which the pathogen is reproducing within the body, but no symptoms appear. This time of reproduction is called the *incubation period*.

Most diseases are not communicable during the incubation period, although some, such as measles and chickenpox, are contagious during the latter parts of their incubation periods.

Each disease has its characteristic incubation period, which depends upon the rate of reproduction of that particular pathogen and the area of the body in which the pathogen multiplies. Incubation near the surface of the body, as with gonorrhea and diphtheria is usually rapid; incubation at remote sites, as with typhus fever and infectious hepatitis, requires a longer period of time.

During the incubation period, a person's body may build up a defense against the invading pathogens. The speed with which such defenses are mobilized plays a role not only in the incubation period, but also in the severity of the disease. The person who has previously come into contact with an organism will react faster and may be able to overcome the organism before it can become established. This fast reaction is indicative of *immunity,* to be discussed later in this chapter.

COMMUNICABLE PERIOD

The time during which an infectious pathogen may be transmitted from an infected person to another person or from an infected animal to man is called its *communicable period*.

In diseases such as tuberculosis, syphilis, and gonorrhea, the communicable state may extend over a long period of time, intermittently recurring when unhealed *lesions* of the disease permit the discharge of infectious pathogens from the surface of the skin or through any body openings. Other diseases, such as measles and chickenpox, are communicable for only a short time during the late incubation period and early stages of the diseases. In diseases transmitted by arthropod vectors, communicability extends for the time during which the pathogen occurs in the blood of the infected person.

PRODROMAL PERIOD

The onset of nonspecific symptoms occurs during the *prodromal period*. During this time the patient suffers from such discomforts as headache, watery eyes, nasal discharge, mild fever, irritability, and general aches. Many times an individual suffering from the prodromal period of a serious disease may believe that he has only a common cold. He may stay out in public and unknowingly expose a considerable number of people to the specific disease he has contracted. *During the prodromal period the individual is highly contagious.*

This is the time when the disease is becoming established. Now the agent is organizing into a recognizable clinical case. The prodromal period is very important, since the virulence of the organism is extremely high and most transmissions from infected people are made during this period. Thus, isolation of the infected person during the prodromal period is important in controlling epidemics.

TYPICAL ILLNESS STAGE

A short time later the first set of symptoms of a specific disease will appear. Now we have the typical illness—measles, whooping cough, chickenpox, and so on. The diagnosis of the specific infectious disease is made principally by the physician's recognition of characteristic symptoms or groups of symptoms. Such a group of symptoms is termed a *syndrome*. Among the factors which help the physician make a diagnosis are:

1. *The manner of onset*—whether abrupt or gradual. When did the first symptoms appear?
2. *The type of fever*—whether continuous, remittent, or intermittent. How and when did the fever terminate?
3. *The course of the disease*—its duration, the presence of symptoms on certain days.
4. *The incubation period*—the time between exposure to the disease and the first appearance of symptoms.
5. *The leukocyte count*—the number and kinds of white blood cells that are present in the body.

6. *The agglutination reaction*—whether the patient's blood causes the organisms of the suspected disease to clump together.
7. *Isolation of the organism*—whether the organism suspected of causing the disease can be found in the blood, urine, feces, spinal fluid, pleural fluid, etc.

The disease has now been recognized and treatment can begin. The illness, now at its height, is still communicable; but since the patient is ill enough to be in bed, the danger of his spreading the disease at this stage is reduced. During this time the body's defenses either begin to defeat the invading pathogens or succumb to them.

CONVALESCENCE OR RECOVERY STATE

At termination of the typical illness the patient has either succumbed or he passes into the next period, the *convalescence* or *recovery state*. During this time the patient begins to regain his health. However, if he overexerts himself at this time, he may weaken the body's defenses and give the invading organisms a fresh start, producing a rapid return of the symptoms. The body still contains large numbers of virulent organisms which, if multiplication recurs, soon reach symptomatic proportions. Such a return of disease is called a *relapse*.

During recovery a period of recuperation is needed for the patient to regain normal strength and vitality.

TERMINATION OF A DISEASE

The convalescent period is followed by one of three possible terminal states:

1. *Resusceptibility.* In one terminal state the person is resusceptible and immediately may become infected again if he comes into contact with the pathogen. This is the case in diseases such as gonorrhea.

2. *Carrier state.* A person or animal who harbors a disease, but does not show the clinical symptoms of the disease and is able to pass such a disease on to another person, is called a carrier. Several different types of carriers exist.

The person who is transmitting a disease during the communicable period of the disease is termed an *incubatory carrier*.

With some diseases the person is able to pass the disease on while he is overcoming the disease (convalescence stage) or after all symptoms have disappeared and he is considered completely normal (post-convalescence period). These persons are *convalescent carriers*.

The carrier state may occur with an infection which has not been apparent (a subclinical condition) to the individual. Such people are said to be *healthy carriers*.

Carriers are common after an occurrence of typhoid fever, diphtheria, cholera, influenza, and cerebrospinal meningitis. The carrier is probably the main reservoir of infections.

3. *Immunity.* The ability of a body to resist disease is called *immunity*. The persistence of immunity following infection varies within wide limits. After a number of viral infections, such as measles and yellow fever, it is lifelong and does not depend on reinfection in order to be maintained. After staphylococcal infection, gonorrhea, or treated syphilis, any immunity that may develop is very short-lived. Where many different organisms can produce a clinically recognized disease, such as pneumonia, it is difficult to determine the duration of immunity. Immunity conferred by influenza appears to persist less than a year.

The immunity which a vaccine gives against diseases such as smallpox is known to weaken with the passage of years; but if the disease is acquired even several years after vaccination, it is generally mild. This weakening of immunity is the general reason for "booster" doses.

SUBCLINICAL ILLNESS

The term *gradient of infection* refers to the variety of responses to an infection. At one extreme is the infection that produces a fatal illness; in the middle lie the illnesses, severe or mild, from which the person may recover; and, at the other extreme, is the unapparent infection, an infection so mild that it does not produce a "typical illness." The term "subclinical illness" has essentially the same meaning as "unapparent infection." This illness is only detectable by laboratory means, such as the discovery of the organism in the person's body, the demonstration of antibodies in the person's blood stream, or hypersensitivity to tests of the skin. This type of infection will still run the typical course of a communicable disease (Fig. 15.5), but nearly all of its periods are unrecognizable.

TYPES OF DISEASE OUTBREAKS

When a communicable disease occurs in an individual or in scattered cases throughout an area, it is termed a *sporadic outbreak*. On the other hand, when a disease is present more or less continuously in an area, it is said to be *endemic* to that specific area. An outbreak of a disease which is clearly in excess of the normal incidence for that size of a community, population, or area is an *epidemic*. Such an outbreak is frequently propagated from a single common source. A disease that sweeps over a large region (an entire country or continent) is termed *pandemic*. Influenza has been pandemic at times in the United States and throughout the world.

THE BODY'S DEFENSES AGAINST DISEASE

SKIN AND MUCOUS MEMBRANES

Commonly referred to as the "first line of defense" are the *skin* and *mucous membranes*. Although the unbroken skin and membranes form an effective barrier against most pathogens, some organisms have the ability to penetrate the unbroken skin or membranes of the body.

The trachea and bronchioles are lined with countless microscopic hairlike projections, *cilia* which clear bacteria from the lungs. These cilia, which constantly wave rhythmically, carry dust and bacteria, on a layer of mucus, from the lungs to the throat, where it is swallowed without conscious effort. These cilia are lost by the heavy smoker, who depends on his "smoker's cough" to rid his lungs of mucus and foreign matter.

The gastric juice of the stomach is highly acid. This acidity kills some, but not all, bacteria.

The eyes obtain some measure of protection against infection from the constant flow of tears, which wash away many bacteria.

INFLAMMATION

In cases where infection does become established, the body still has several means of defense. The second line of defense is called *inflammation,* a local dilation of the capillaries in response to the infection. The area surrounding the infection becomes hot, red, and swollen as a result of increased blood supply. The increased blood supply brings an abundance of white blood cells, which engulf and destroy the bacteria.

IMMUNITY

The third and most important body defense against disease is *immunity,* of which there are many types.

NATURAL IMMUNITY

Natural immunity (also called "resistance") is merely an inherited lack of susceptibility. This immunity may be characteristic of the entire human species, of certain races of man, or of certain individuals, depending upon the disease in question.

ACQUIRED IMMUNITY

Acquired immunity is always the result of *antibodies*. Antibodies are protective chemical substances produced by the body in response to the presence of an *antigen* in the body. The function of the antibody is to destroy or inactivate the antigen. (You will recall that an antigen is a foreign substance, usually a protein, which has been introduced into the body.) Antibodies are *specific;* that is, they will destroy only the antigen which caused the production of the antibody. Acquired immunity may be of two types: *active* or *passive.*

1. *Active immunity* results when a person produces his own antibodies in response to the presence of an antigen. Such antigen would usually be a microorganism or its toxic product. Natural active immunity is obtained while the person is recovering from an actual case of the infectious disease. This type of immunity is often of very long duration. Artificial active immunity is the result of *vaccines* containing antigens which when introduced into the body cause the production of immunizing antibodies. Fortunately, for many diseases there are today vaccines or *toxoids.* A vaccine or toxoid consists of an antigen which has in some way been attenuated (weakened) so that it no longer causes disease, but still stimulates the production of antibodies. A vaccine consists of a killed or weakened pathogen; a toxoid consists of a modified toxin.

2. *Passive immunity* results when antibodies are introduced into the body from some outside source. But since no antigen is introduced, there is no stimulus for the production of any new antibodies. As a result, passive immunity is of short duration, lasting only as long as the introduced antibodies remain active in the body. Like active immunity, passive immunity may be either natural or artificial.

Natural passive immunity is the *congenital* immunity conferred by the mother upon her unborn child. Antibodies are small enough to allow their diffusion across the membranes of the placenta from the mother's blood to that of the fetus. The newborn infant is thereby immune to most diseases to which the mother is immune. Since congenital immunity is passive, it lasts only as long as the original antibodies remain active, usually several months.

Sometimes a person is exposed to a communicable disease for which no vaccine or toxoid is available, or perhaps the person has neglected to take advantage of an existing vaccine. In these cases, it is possible to confer upon that person artificial passive immunity through an injection of antibodies. These antibodies are usually concentrated from the blood of an animal that has been injected with the proper antigen. It must be emphasized that this type of immunity is temporary and results in no long-lasting protection. Passive immunity for several virus diseases may be obtained through the injection of *gamma globulin.* Gamma globulin is a derivative of human blood in which a high concentration of antibodies exists. Some of these are specific antibodies, for specific diseases; others are more generalized and serve to protect the body from several diseases.

ALLERGY

Although *allergy*, also called *hypersensitivity*, is not an infectious disease, it seems appropriate to discuss allergies at this point, since an allergy is the result of an antigen-antibody reaction. When a person has an allergy, he has developed antibodies against some normal component of the diet or environment. Allergies are commonly developed against such varied substances as pollens, feathers, furs, dusts, cosmetics, and foods of all types. In fact, it is difficult to mention a substance to which no person would be allergic. (An accurate description of an allergy might be "a reaction to a substance which may be harmless to other people.")

The discomfort felt during allergic reactions is the result of a substance called *histamine*, which is released from the tissues in response to antigen-antibody reactions. Some of the effects of histamine include dilation of the small blood vessels (inflammation), sneezing, running nose, constriction of the bronchioles (*asthma*), and local swelling.

A severe allergic reaction, releasing much histamine, can lead to an often fatal condition called *anaphylaxis*, or *anaphylactic shock*, in which the blood pressure drops dangerously, owing to the dilated blood vessels. Nausea and convulsions often accompany this shock.

The cause of an allergy can often be determined through a series of skin-patch tests, in which small amounts of various antigens, such as foods and pollens, are scratched into the skin on the back. In these tests allergic reactions are indicated by local inflammation. Then the patient can often be desensitized by a series of injections of minute amounts of the offending antigen.

TREATMENT OF DISEASE

The treatment, or *therapy*, for a disease may be defined as any effort to cure the disease, arrest its course, lessen its severity, or alleviate the pain and inconvenience the disease causes. It includes:

1. *Dietary therapy*, the treatment of disease by regulation of the food the patient eats. In the treatment of all diseases it is important that a patient have proper food and a proper amount of fluid.

2. *Operative therapy*, the surgical treatment, in which disease is removed with the scalpel and other instruments of the surgeon. It is a mechanical treatment of disease. The diseased organ or area is removed, repaired, opened, drained, or manipulated.

3. *Physical therapy*, the use of physical agents in the treatment of

disease—heat, cold, light, other rays (X rays, infrared and ultraviolet rays, and radiation), electricity, and massage.

4. *Psychotherapy,* the treatment of emotional disorders. Its purpose is to remove or reduce the emotional factors in disease—to dispel the worries, doubts, and fears that are so often the cause of illness and which nearly always affect organic diseases (see Chapter 2).

5. *Chemotherapy,* the introduction into the body of substances which are designed to cure a disease, affect its course, lessen its severity, or alleviate its pain and inconvenience. Any substance or mixture administered to a sick person is medicine. Medicines are derived from various natural sources or are manufactured.

CHEMOTHERAPY

The majority of drugs exert actions which enable them to be divided into two major groups: (1) the *organotropic* drugs and the *replacement* drugs, which exert an action mainly on the body; and (2) the chemotherapeutic drugs, which exert an action against invaders of the body.

ORGANOTROPIC DRUGS

Organotropic drugs produce an action directly upon tissues or organs of the body. These drugs act specifically by causing *stimulation* or *depression* of the functions of the tissues or organs acted upon. They may cause stimulation of the central nervous system, as does caffeine, or depression of the nerve trunks and nerve endings, as is the case with cocaine and other local anesthetics. The action may be upon the heart, as with the cardiac stimulant digitalis, or upon the respiration, which may be seriously depressed by a toxic dosage of *opium* or *morphine.*

REPLACEMENT DRUGS

Replacement drugs' chief function is indicated by the name. They include the various extracts from the endocrine glands; also included are the essential vitamins, which the highly specialized human body is unable to synthesize for itself, and the sera and vaccines, which promote and intensify the body's natural resistance to infection.

CHEMOTHERAPEUTIC DRUGS

The chemotherapeutic drugs, which act mainly against the infectious invaders of the body, are usually highly selective, extending to only a single organism or group of organisms. The two most widely recognized drugs of this group are the *antibiotics* and the *sulfa drugs.*

Antibiotics are produced during the normal growth of many types of soil-inhabiting microorganisms. Antibiotics inhibit the growth of bacteria that compete with the soil microorganisms for the available food. Antibiotics were first recognized by Sir Alexander Fleming, a Scottish bacteriologist, in 1929. Since that time several hundred antibiotics have been isolated and purified for use in controlling disease-producing bacteria.

The exact response of antibiotics to bacteria is still not completely known, but evidence indicates that the antibiotics interfere with various steps in cellular metabolism vital to bacterial growth. The antibacterial activity of antibiotics is highest during the period of greatest bacterial multiplication. Thus there is a good reason for early diagnosis of a disease, followed by immediate treatment. When antibiotics are present in adequate concentrations, they kill bacteria; lower concentrations may only inhibit the growing organisms. Old cultures of bacteria beyond the stage of rapid growth show less response to antibiotics than do new cultures.

The administration of antibiotics is ordinarily by intramuscular or, occasionally, intravenous injection. Most antibiotics are readily absorbed following their injection into the tissues. The simple antibiotics are absorbed at different speeds to produce a maximum blood concentration. Penicillin is absorbed within 30 minutes; other antibiotics, such as streptomycin and the tetracyclines, are absorbed in about 60 minutes. Slowly absorbed preparations of some antibiotics are available, so that the period of effective treatment following injection can be prolonged—that is, one dose of penicillin compound can be absorbed continuously for three days, whereas another is absorbed for nearly three weeks in smaller daily amounts.

When given orally, penicillin must be protected against the destructive secretions of the stomach. It is usually prescribed for use before meals when there are less secretions in the stomach. However, even when it is protected, five times the intramuscular dose of penicillin must be administered orally to the patient to obtain equivalent blood levels. Erythromycin, which may be substituted for penicillin, need not be given in such large dosages, because it is absorbed adequately following oral administration. Tetracycline antibiotics and others are absorbed very readily from the digestive tract, but only about 10 percent of an oral dose of streptomycin is absorbed into the bloodstream; the rest of the dose remains in the digestive tract, where it inhibits many kinds of bacteria and may upset the digestive processes and cause slight discomfort to the patient.

Most antibiotics can be distributed readily through the body, but not into the central nervous system in concentrations adequate for treatment of either systemic or local infections. Although they diffuse into the central nervous system with difficulty, excessively high concentrations of antibiotics in the bloodstream will promote diffusion even into the nervous tissues.

Antibiotics must be used cautiously or their value will be lost. On the other hand, no patient should be deprived of the benefit of antibiotic therapy solely because of fear of inducing resistance in the disease germ.

The sulfonamides (sulfa drugs) were discovered in 1935. They have been very important in controlling bacterial diseases in man. Despite the subsequent introduction of the more effective and less toxic antibiotics, the sulfonamides continue to be widely used in the treatment of certain diseases.

The sulfonamides are produced by chemical synthesis; they are stable white powders administered by mouth. Since they have limited solubility in water and in the fluids of the body, there is sometimes difficulty in eliminating the drugs in the urine.

The sulfonamides inhibit bacterial multiplication during the growth phase. A bacterial cell has a complicated enzyme system functioning for the purpose of satisfying its nutritional requirements. This enzymatic activity involves a series of chemical reactions requiring vitamin-like compounds for its completion. The sulfonamide drugs interfere with the function of the enzymes, and this reduced function of the enzymes in turn damages the cell, resulting in its inability to produce energy and grow. If there is enough sulfa compound in the vicinity of a growing bacterial cell, this cell will incorporate this material in place of the vitamin-like material needed for normal growth. Consequently, the sulfonamides may be likened to "antivitamins" in their mode of action in controlling bacteria.

Because of the need for flooding a diseased area with sulfa, these drugs must be administered at regular intervals throughout a 24-hour period for general effectiveness. The goal in sulfonamide therapy is to maintain an antibacterial concentration of sulfonamide continuously in all tissues of the body where the disease germs might multiply.

If there is no impairment of kidney function that handicaps excretion, sulfonamides may be prescribed for any general bacterial disease. At all times water must be available to a patient receiving sulfonamides. If necessary, extra water is given a patient to insure nearly normal consumption. Water is the vehicle for excreting sulfonamides, which will precipitate and block the kidney if there is too little fluid.

Virus infections are not susceptible to sulfonamides, although secondary bacterial invaders may be.

SUMMARY

I. Causes of Disease (inability of the body to maintain a healthy state)
    A. Nutritional deficiencies, which are the lack in the diet of essential vitamins, minerals, and organic foods.
    B. Physical agents such as heat or cold, electricity, trauma.

C. Chemical agents—substances which, when present or introduced into the body in excessive amounts, result in poisoning.

D. Tumors or abnormal growths in any tissue or organ.

E. Allergy—reaction by the tissues of an individual who is hypersensitive to a discrete substance (allergen).

F. Heredity—abnormal conditions produced by specific genetic defects received by an individual from his parents.

G. Senescence—the appearance of degenerative conditions brought on by advancing age.

H. Emotional disorders—emotional interference with the normal functioning of the body.

I. Congenital abnormalities—abnormalities of structure or function which are present at the time of birth.

J. Infectious diseases—produced when the body is invaded by living organisms (pathogens).

II. Pathogens—disease-producing organisms.

A. Viruses—subcellular, semiliving particles.

B. Rickettsia—single-celled, plantlike organisms, intermediates between viruses and bacteria.

C. Bacteria—single-celled, plantlike organisms.

   1. Harmful effect is the result of their production of poisonous substances:

      a. exotoxins—substances which diffuse out of living bacterial cells into the surrounding tissues.

      b. endotoxins—substances released only after the death of the bacteria.

   2. Types of bacteria based on their shape:

      a. cocci—spherical bacteria.

      b. bacilli—rod-shaped bacteria.

      c. spirilla—spiral or corkscrew-shaped bacteria.

D. Fungi—primitive multicellular and unicellular plants.

E. Protozoa—primitive single-celled animals.

F. Parasitic worms—multicellular animals. The more commonly known examples are roundworms, flukes, and tapeworms.

III. Course of a Communicable Disease.

A. Transmission and infection—the passing of pathogenic organisms from one source or reservoir (transmission) into the body of a victim (infection).

   1. Methods of transmission

      a. Person to person—which may be by direct or indirect contact.

      b. Contaminated water—when sewage has accidentally been mixed with drinking water.

      c. Contaminated food or milk—infection in the animal source or handling by infected individuals.

      d. Animal to person, which may be by:

        (1) direct transmission through handling or the bite of an infected animal.

        (2) indirect transmission through contact with fecal material or other residue from an infected animal.

      e. Vectors—transmission exclusively through bites or fecal material of arthropods.

   2. Portals of exit and entry—pathogens usually leave and enter by the same route.

B. Incubation period—that period of time, after infection and prior to the appearance of symptoms, when the pathogen is reproducing within the individual.

C. Communicable period—time during which an infectious pathogen may be transmitted.

D. Prodromal period—the period of nonspecific symptoms.

E. Typical illness stage—the appearance and period of signs and symptoms of a specific disease.

F. Convalescence or recovery stage—time following a typical illness when a patient begins to regain his health.

G. Termination of a disease—three possible terminal stages follow convalescence:

   1. Resusceptibility—person is resusceptible immediately after termination of the disease if he comes into contact with the pathogen.

   2. Carrier state—harboring and ability to transmit a disease to another person without showing the clinical symptoms.

   3. Immunity—ability of the body to resist disease.

H. Subclinical illness—an infection so mild that it does not produce a "typical illness stage."

I. Types of disease outbreaks—terms used in reference to the number of cases of a particular disease in an area.

   1. Sporadic outbreak—a single or scattered occurrence of a communicable disease.

   2. Endemic—more or less continuous presence of a disease.

   3. Epidemic—outbreaks clearly in excess of the normal.

   4. Pandemic—the sweeping of a disease over large regions.

IV. The Body's Defenses Against Disease.

A. Skin and mucous membranes—the first line of defense. The unbroken skin and mucous membranes form an effective barrier against most pathogens.

B. Inflammation—the second line of defense. A local dilation of the capillaries in response to an infection.

C. Immunity—the third line of defense.

   1. Natural immunity (resistance)—inherited lack of susceptibility.

   2. Acquired immunity—the result of antibodies, produced in response to an antigen. May be of two types:

      a. active immunity results when a person produces his own antibodies in response to the presence in his body of an antigen.

         (1) natural active immunity—obtained while a person is recovering from an actual case of an infectious disease.

         (2) artificial active immunity—results from the use of vaccines or toxoids.

      b. passive immunity results when antibodies are introduced into the body from an outside source.

         (1) natural passive immunity (congenital immunity)—conferred by the mother upon her unborn child through the diffusion of antibodies across the placental membranes into the bloodstream of the fetus.

         (2) artificial passive immunity results from the use of serums.

V. Allergy—an antigen-antibody reaction which takes place within an individual who is hypersensitive to some normal component of the diet or environment.

VI. Treatment of Disease.
    A. Kinds of therapy:
        1. Dietary therapy—regulation of the food the patient eats.
        2. Operative therapy—surgical treatment, removal of diseased tissue or organ by the surgeon.
        3. Physical therapy—use of physical agents.
        4. Psychotherapy—treatment of emotional disorders by meaningful discussion between the patient and the therapist.
        5. Chemotherapy—introduction into the body of substances designed to:
           a. cure a disease.
           b. affect its course.
           c. lessen its severity.
           d. alleviate its pain or inconvenience.
    B. Chemotherapy—the use of drugs which exert actions on the body or against invaders of the body.
        1. Organotropic drugs—drugs which produce an action directly upon one or more tissues or organs of the body.
        2. Replacement drugs—drugs used to replace substances vital to the desired functioning of the body.
        3. Chemotherapeutic drugs—drugs which act mainly against the infectious invaders of the body.

Glossary

If you cannot find the word you wish in this glossary, check the index for text and glossary references.

allergen (al′ər jen) (G. *allos,* other; *gennan,* to produce). A substance capable of producing an allergy.

allergy (al′ər jē) (G. *allos,* other; *ergon,* work). A hypersensitive reaction to a particular substance.

anaphylaxis (an ə fə lak′sis) (G. *ana,* up; *phylaxis,* protection). An exaggerated reaction to a foreign substance; an antigen-antibody reaction.

antibiotic (an′ti bī ot′ik) (G. *anti,* against; *bios,* life). A chemical produced by microorganisms which has the ability to inhibit the growth of bacteria or other microorganisms.

antibody (an′ti bod′ē). Chemical agents formed by the body to help destroy antigens.

antigen (an′ti jen). A foreign substance, usually a protein, which stimulates the production of antibodies.

attenuation (ə ten′yoo ā′shən) (L. *ad,* to; *tenuis,* thin). The act of weakening, such as the weakening of a pathogen or toxin.

bacillus (bə sil′əs) (L. *bacillus,* rod). A rod-shaped bacterium.

bacteria (bak tēr′ē ə) (G. *bakterion,* little rod). Microscopic, single-celled, plant-like organisms.

carrier (kar′ē ər). An individual who harbors disease organisms in his body without suffering from the disease.

chemotherapy (kem′ō ther′ə pē) (G. *chemeia,* chemical; *therapeia,* treatment). The treatment of disease with chemicals or drugs.

coccus (kok′əs) (G. *kokkos,* berry). A spherical bacterium.

500 HEALTH SCIENCE

communicable (kə myoo'ni kə bl). Capable of being transmitted from one person to another.

contagious (kən tā'jəs). Capable of being transmitted directly from one person to another.

disease (di zēz'). Any abnormality of the body, its parts, or its functions.

endemic (en dem'ik) (G. *endemos,* dwelling in a place). Present in an area at a low level at all times.

endotoxin (en dō tok'sin) (G. *endon,* within; *toxikon,* poison). A bacterial toxin released only after the death of the cell.

epidemic (ep i dem'ik) (G. *epidemios,* prevalent). A disease attacking many people at the same time.

exotoxin (ek'sō tok'sin) (G. *exo,* outside; *toxikon,* poison). A bacterial toxin released while the cell is still alive.

fungus (fung'gəs) (L. *fungus,* mushroom). A filamentous plant which lacks chlorophyll.

histamine (his'tə mēn). A chemical occurring in all tissues which, upon release, causes dilatation of the capillaries and other affects.

hypersensitivity (hī'pər sen si tiv'i tē). An allergy or abnormal sensitivity to a stimulus of any kind.

immunity (i myoo'ni tē) (L. *immunitas,* exemption). The power which an individual may acquire to resist an infection to which most members of the species are susceptible.

incubation (ing kyoo bā'shən) (L. *incubare,* to lie on). The interval between exposure to a disease and the appearance of the first symptom.

infection (in fek'shən) (L. *inficere,* to taint). Invasion of the body by pathogens.

infectious (in fek'shəs). Capable of being communicated by infection; capable of being transmitted.

inflammation (in flə mā'shən) (L. *inflammare,* to set on fire). A tissue reaction to injury.

lesion (lē'zhən) (L. *laesio,* to hurt). An injury, wound, or infected area.

pandemic (pan dem'ik) (G. *pan,* all; *demos,* people). A widespread epidemic disease.

parasite (par'ə sīt) (G. *para,* alongside; *sitos,* food). A plant or animal that lives on or in another (host) organism at the expense of the host.

pathogen (path'ə jen) (G. *pathos,* disease; *gennan,* producing). A disease-producing organism or substance.

prodromal (prō drō'məl) (G. *prodromos,* forerunning). Indicating the approach of a disease.

protozoa (prō tə zō'ə) (G. *protos,* first; *zoon,* animal). Single-celled animals.

relapse (ri laps') (L. *relapsus,* slipping back). The return of a disease after the beginning of convalescence.

reservoir (rez'ər vwahr) (L. *reservare,* to keep back). A stockpile or pool. A reservoir of infection may be a symptomless carrier.

rickettsia (ri ket'sē ə) (Howard T. Ricketts, American pathologist, 1871–1910). Microscopic bacteria-like organisms transmitted by arthropods.

spirillum (spī ril'əm) (L. *spirillum,* coil). A corkscrew- or spiral-shaped bacterium.

sporadic (spo rad'ik) (G. *sporadikos,* scattered). Occurring only occasionally.

syndrome (sin'drōm) (G. *syndrome,* concurrence).   A group of symptoms.

therapy (ther'ə pē) (G. *therapeia,* treatment).   The treatment of disease.

toxin (tok'sin).   A poison.

toxoid (tok'soid) (G. *toxikon,* poison; *eidos,* form).   An attenuated (weakened) toxin which has lost its toxic properties while retaining its ability to cause production of antitoxins; used in immunization.

transmission (tranz mish'ən) (L. *trans,* through; *missio,* sending).   Transfer of anything, as of a disease.

trauma (traw'mə, trou'mə) (G. *trauma,* wound).   An injury or wound.

vaccine (vak sēn') (L. *vaccinus,* of cows).   A preparation of killed or attenuated microorganisms for use in immunization.

vector (vek'tər) (L. *vehere,* to carry).   An animal, usually an arthropod, which transmits pathogens from one host to another.

virus (vī'rəs) (L. *virus,* poison).   A minute infectious particle, consisting of a core of DNA or RNA contained within a protein coat. All are intracellular parasites.

CHAPTER 16

VENEREAL DISEASE

GENERAL CHARACTERISTICS

PREVENTION AND CONTROL

SYPHILIS

GONORRHEA

CHANCROID

GRANULOMA INGUINALE

LYMPHOGRANULOMA
VENEREUM

SUMMARY

Five venereal diseases are recognized in the United States—syphilis, gonorrhea, chancroid, granuloma inguinale, and lymphogranuloma venereum. All may result in serious disability or death. Although each disease varies as to the organism causing it and its particular symptoms, all have one thing in common—they are spread chiefly by sexual or close physical contact.

Modern sanitation practices in the United States, along with modern medicine, have reduced the incidence of chancroid, granuloma inguinale, and lymphogranuloma venereum. Today fewer than 2000 cases of all three are reported annually in the United States. Yet every effort should be made to detect these infections as long as they exist. Also, it is important to distinguish between these and syphilis or gonorrhea for purposes of diagnosis and treatment. An individual may have more than one venereal disease at one time. Also, reinfection may occur at any time.

Syphilis and gonorrhea are more significant because of their wide distribution. Syphilis is especially important because of its chronic nature and the serious lesions, disabilities, and deaths resulting from it. A review of reports on the trend of venereal diseases around the world indicates that both syphilis and gonorrhea are on the rise. Of 106 nations reporting to the World Health Organization, 76 report a rising rate of incidence. In comparison with the United States the rise is less marked in England, Wales, and Canada, but more pronounced in Denmark and Italy.[1]

GENERAL CHARACTERISTICS

All venereal diseases are infectious communicable diseases (see Chapter 15). The organisms which induce the diseases are very well known, and their diagnosis, treatment, and cure are equally well known. The only common factor connecting venereal diseases is the manner in which they are contracted—mainly by sexual intercourse. If eradication of these diseases is ever to be accomplished, there must be proper enlightenment of people as to discriminate sexual relations. These diseases must be regarded in the same light as any other communicable disease, without undue reference to the moral implication. Shame or guilt must not discourage victims from seeking treatment, as it often has in the past.

In recent years over 125,000 cases of syphilis, in all stages, have been reported annually in this country. Of these, over 21,000 are in the primary and secondary—the infectious—stages. What would happen if 21,000 persons living in the United States contracted smallpox or plague? The answer is obvious—there would be panic! Yet syphilis can cause more organic damage to the individual who survives the disease than smallpox can.

The actual incidence of syphilis in this country is believed to be between 75,000 and 100,000 new cases a year, all of which remain infectious for a time.[2] Because many of these are not found and treated, there exists a large reservoir of people needing treatment—probably close to 1,200,000 in the United States at any one time. Of these *untreated* syphilitics, 1 in 200 may be expected to become blind, 1 in 48 will develop *paresis* (paralysis caused by brain tissue degeneration), 1 in 25 will become crippled to some extent, and 1 in 13 will be expected to develop syphilitic heart (Chapter 13), and 1 in 400 (3000 per year) will die.[3]

---

[1] T. Guthe and R. R. Wilcox, "Treponematoses a World Problem," Geneva, *Chron. World Health Organ.*, 1954.

[2] *V.D. Fact Sheet*, Washington, D.C., U.S. Department of Health, Education, and Welfare, Public Health Service (Communicable Disease Center), annual.

[3] P. E. Sartwell, *Preventive Medicine and Public Health*, 9th ed., New York, Appleton-Century-Crofts, 1965, pp. 274–278.

The picture of gonorrhea is less dramatic but more extensive. Although it is present in all parts of the world, its actual incidence is unknown, because of self-treatment, undiagnosed cases (mainly in females), and very inadequate reporting of known cases.

In the United States *gonorrhea is the leading reported communicable disease.* Although it is estimated that there are more than 1,500,000 new cases per year, only one sixth of these are reported to public health authorities. No reliable estimate can be made of the amount of economic loss and the degree of mental and physical suffering produced by gonorrhea. For example, under the *best* conditions only 25 percent of the cases of gonorrhea in women are ever diagnosed, and the total extent of complications of such infections in females cannot be determined at all.

Why have syphilis and gonorrhea emerged as the leading communicable diseases in young people? The following are a few of the major conditions which help to spread venereal diseases.

1. Millions of young people between the ages of 15 and 24 know little or nothing about these diseases; others are saturated with misinformation passed on from one person to the other. A striking example of such misinformation was shown in a survey taken by the Los Angeles County Health Department at a "Teen-age Fair" during a recent year. Approximately 1750 true-false questionnaires were used to test the knowledge of these young people. The questionnaire and the many misconceptions about venereal disease are shown in Table 16.1.

2. Parents and society may overemphasize the moral and social implications of venereal disease to such an extent that young adults will neither present themselves for treatment, nor voluntarily submit to public health interviews, which are the only means of eventually eradicating venereal disease.

3. To avoid embarrassment, many individuals seek treatment through "quacks" or through self-medication.

4. The absolute curative powers of the antibiotics and sulfa drugs have been so far overrated that widespread apathy among young people, physicians, and society in general has resulted. Consequently the reporting of cases and the resulting contact studies are not nearly as routine as they should be. Apathy and ignorance on the part of physicians lead to misdiagnosis, inadequate follow-up studies of treated patients, and a weak response to public health pleas for reporting of venereal disease patients to be screened for investigation and interviewing. With the advent of penicillin, with its ease of administration and low cost, much venereal disease treatment is being given in the local doctor's office.

5. Uninformed homosexuals may not recognize that venereal infection can be transmitted by or contracted from homosexual or close physical contacts.

6. Greater sexual freedom for young adults has been caused by our mobile society and the relaxed restrictions of parents.

TABLE 16.1   **TEEN-AGE FAIR QUESTIONNAIRE***

Correct Answer	Percentage of Wrong Answers		Statements
false	42	1.[a]	Since syphilis germs can live a long time outside of the body, it is possible to acquire the disease in a variety of ways.
false	21	2.	Sores and rashes can always be found on people who have syphilis, therefore people usually know when they are infected.
true	64	3.[b]	The symptoms of syphilis will go away even if a person does not have proper medical treatment for the disease.
true	14	4.	If a pregnant woman has syphilis, she can transmit the disease to her unborn child, if she does not receive treatment soon enough.
false	41	5.[c]	Syphilis can be inherited and passed on for generations.
false	8	6.	Once a person has syphilis and the disease is cured in the early stage he can never get the disease again.
true	16	7.	Some people have syphilis, yet may never have any outward signs of the disease.
true	9	8.	If syphilis is not found and treated, it may cause blindness, insanity, crippling, or even cause death.
false	16	9.	Gonorrhea is often caused by lifting a heavy object (strain).
true	18	10.	If gonorrhea in the female is not found and treated, it may cause sterility (prevent the woman from ever having a baby).
true	62	11.[b]	The symptoms of gonorrhea will go away even though the person is not cured of the disease.
false	15	12.	If a person has gonorrhea once and is cured, he will never get it again because he has become immune.
true	19	13.	It is possible for a female to have gonorrhea and not know it.
false	25	14.	If gonorrhea is not treated, it will turn into syphilis.

TABLE 16.1   **TEEN-AGE FAIR QUESTIONNAIRE (Continued)**

Correct Answer	Percentage of Wrong Answers	Statements
true	14	15. Syphilis and gonorrhea are almost always acquired by sexual contact with an infected person.
true	36	16. It is possible for a person to have both syphilis and gonorrhea at the same time.
false	74	17.[d] A blood test can be used to diagnose both gonorrhea and syphilis.
false	42	18.[a] Both syphilis and gonorrhea are frequently acquired by contact with any object an infected person has used, such as toilet seats, lipsticks, and towels.
false	11	19. People with syphilis or gonorrhea have a distinctive appearance so that it is possible to tell an infected person just by looking at him.
true	5	20. Both syphilis and gonorrhea can be cured by proper medical treatment.

* Questionnaire given to 1750 individuals attending "Teen-age Fair," Easter week, 1964, in Los Angeles, Calif.

[a] 42% of the participants missed both of these questions (#1 and #18).

[b] 63% of the participants missed both of these questions (#3 and #11).

[c] 41% missed this question (#5). This result may have been caused by a confusion between *congenital* and *hereditary*.

[d] 74% missed this question (#17). Blood tests might give these teen-agers a false sense of security.

7. The increased use of alcohol and "pills" (barbiturates and amphetamines; see Chapter 4) have contributed to the increase of venereal disease infections in young adults.

PREVENTION AND CONTROL

The successful control of any communicable disease depends upon the recognition and elimination of sources of infection, a process which is especially necessary in the control of venereal disease. Venereal disease control officers agree that in order to reduce the incidence of venereal disease, a much higher percentage of cases must be interviewed, so that *all* contacts may be found, examined, and treated if infected. If cases are not reported, it is not possible for the health department to provide a trained interviewer to obtain the names of all the infected individual's close contacts. If cases are not reported, the infected individual will continue to spread the disease.

One infected individual, untreated, will usually have infected two, three, or more people, who if not found and treated will in turn infect others. Every patient interviewed yields at least one other case of infectious syphilis, the one who infected him.

THE SOCIETY'S METHODS FOR CONTROLLING VENEREAL DISEASE

INTERVIEWING PROCEDURE

The interviewing procedure will vary from area to area, but the following is the usual process.

As patients are diagnosed, they are interviewed and asked to name those people to whom they have been exposed sexually (from the beginning of the incubation period up to the time when treatment renders them noninfectious) as well as the names and addresses, if possible, of any sexual partner during the six months before the symptoms began. All of these *contacts* are then located, examined, and, if necessary, treated.

The interviewer makes these contacts by telephone or by visiting the individuals. He explains to them that they have been "exposed to a dangerous communicable disease" and asks if they would please see either their own physician or the local public health clinic as soon as possible. This contacting is done without mentioning the reporting patient's name or identifying him in any manner. If the individual elects to see his own physician, the doctor's name is asked for, and the physician is informed of the suspected venereal disease and asked to conduct the tests and inform the public health interviewer of the outcome. If the contact does not report to the public health clinic or to his physician within a reasonable period of time, the local police are asked to "pick up" the individual and bring him to the public health clinic for an examination. Under no condition is the reporting patient's name ever disclosed to anyone, including the police, the private physician, or the suspected contact.

REPORTING BY PRIVATE PHYSICIANS

Unless more private physicians are brought into the control effort, venereal disease will remain a serious hazard to the health of the public. More patients are treated in doctors' offices than in public clinics, yet the number of reports given by private physicians to the public health department for interviewing and follow-up studies are pitifully low. Private physicians hold the key to the eradication of venereal disease, but they must give more support to locating and examining all known contacts as well as to posttreatment follow-up examinations.

It is estimated that physicians are now reporting slightly more than half of the cases they diagnose and treat as compared to about one fourth in the period 1955–1958. Figure 16.1 shows the relationship between the diagnosis, treatment, and management of syphilis by public clinics and private physicians in 1961.

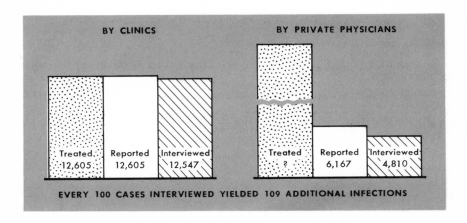

Fig. 16.1 Infectious syphilis diagnosed in 1961. (U.S. Department of Health, Education and Welfare, Public Health Service, *The Eradication of Syphilis,* 1963.)

Such apathy by physicians prompted the American Social Health Association, in cooperation with the American Medical Association, the National Medical Association, and the American Osteopathic Association to send out a questionnaire to every private physician in the United States. Over 131,000 (71 percent of the total queried) responded to the survey. They indicated that they had treated an estimated 55,720 cases of infectious syphilis during 1962. These 55,720 cases added to the 13,769 infectious cases treated in 1962 in public clinics give a total of 69,489 newly acquired cases of syphilis treated that year. Yet only 20,084 cases of infectious syphilis were officially reported to the United States Public Health Service by both private physicians and public clinics in 1962.[4]

4 *V.D. Fact Sheet—1965,* Washington, D.C., U.S. Department of Health, Education, and Welfare, Public Health Service (Communicable Disease Center), annual, p. 2.

Since 1962 such information has prompted physicians to increase their reporting of venereal disease by 11 percent annually. This interest by private physicians is helping greatly to establish a more accurate picture of the venereal disease conditions within the United States.

CLUSTER TESTING

In addition to increasing the interviewing of contacts, a new method has been introduced to control venereal disease. Patients with infectious venereal disease are, as usual, interviewed for sexual contacts but are also asked to name other persons, of either sex, who move in the same sociosexual environment, and who the patient thinks might benefit by an examination for syphilis, gonorrhea, or other venereal diseases. These other people include friends, acquaintances, neighbors, fellow employees, or anyone with sexual behavior approximating that of the patient. This type of interviewing is called *cluster testing*. Between July 1960 and March 1961 cluster testing in large metropolitan areas consisted of interviews with 5452 persons with primary and secondary syphilis[5] (Table 16.2).

PERSONAL RESPONSIBILITY IN CONTROLLING VENEREAL DISEASE

The contracting of venereal disease depends wholly upon how an individual conducts his life. If one is never exposed to a disease, he will not contract it. The best preventive measure against venereal disease is *abstinence from promiscuous sexual contact*. These sexual contacts may be either heterosexual (individuals of different sexes) or homosexual (individuals of the same sex); both contacts can transmit venereal

TABLE 16.2 RESULTS OF EXTENDING EPIDEMIOLOGIC PROCESS TO INCLUDE CLUSTER TESTING

July 1960—March 1961			
	Additional Primary and Secondary Cases Found by:		
Primary and Secondary Cases Interviewed	Contact Tracing Alone	Contact Tracing with Cluster Testing	Percent Increase in Infections Found
5452	2047	2534	23.8

SOURCE: *The Eradication of Syphilis*, Washington, D.C., U.S. Department of Health, Education, and Welfare, Public Health Service, 1963.

[5] *The Eradication of Syphilis*, Washington, D.C., U.S. Department of Health, Education, and Welfare, 1963, p. 13.

disease equally well. Married individuals having extramarital sexual relationships run the risk of exposing not only themselves, but also their spouses, to venereal disease.

If a person does place himself in a situation where there is a possibility of contracting venereal disease, he can use a few precautions during and immediately after exposure. The man may reduce his chances of infection by using a condom or other prophylactic covering during the sexual act. He may choose to use prophylactic salves or chemicals shortly after exposure. However, none of these are highly effective. Mechanical covering devices tend to spread the disease to other parts of the body when they are being removed and disposed of. For the woman, because of the generalized internal and external nature of the female sexual contact, there are no safe chemicals or devices available which will guard against possible infection. Both males and females can reduce the infective ability of gonorrhea, chancroid, granuloma inguinale, and lymphogranuloma venereum by a liberal use of soap and water to thoroughly cleanse the genitalia and surrounding areas. In the case of syphilis, however, such cleansing, no matter how quickly accomplished after exposure, may still not be in time to prevent possible infection.

The next best measure for the prevention of venereal disease is for all individuals to be aware of the venereal disease problem and the necessity for prompt and proper medical treatment if and when signs or symptoms of infection do appear.

Also, individuals must recognize and dispel misconceptions concerning venereal disease. Mistakenly, some feel that a genital sore which heals requires no further medical care, that venereal disease cannot be spread by homosexual contact, that venereal disease cannot be cured, or that some people are naturally immune. Many people mistakenly believe that a prophylactic device will absolutely prevent venereal disease or that both pregnancy and venereal diseases can be prevented by douching with water or other liquids, such as a carbonated drink, after intercourse. Then there are those with no opinions—and, often, no knowledge whatsoever. Mistaken ideas in the home, the school, the church, and between individuals must be replaced with up-to-date information.

SYPHILIS

Syphilis is a body-wide disease produced by infection with the spirochete *Treponema pallidum* (Fig. 16.2). There are two distinct forms of syphilis, *venereal* and *nonvenereal*.

NONVENEREAL SYPHILIS

Nonvenereal syphilis is referred to as *endemic syphilis* or *Bejel*. It is spread by means other than sexual contact and is confined to parts of the world where economic, social, and climatic conditions favor its development; it is not found in the United States. Bejel is found mostly in Syria and surrounding countries. It is characterized by lesions of the skin and mucous membranes, usually without an initial primary lesion; these lesions may be indistinguishable from secondary lesions of venereal syphilis.

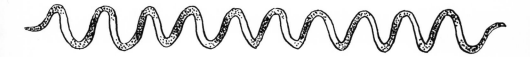

Fig. 16.2 *Treponema pallidum,* the organism that causes syphilis.

VENEREAL SYPHILIS

Throughout this discussion the word syphilis will mean *venereal syphilis.*

Venereal syphilis is of worldwide occurrence. The spirochete causing syphilis (*Treponema pallidum*) is a corkscrew-shaped organism (shown in Fig. 16.2). This organism is extremely fragile and unable to resist drying. It is destroyed by many common antiseptics and can survive only *momentarily* on exposure to air. Its normal and preferred habitat is deep in the body tissues, but when deposited from an open lesion onto moist, warm skin, it can survive long enough to establish a colony, burrow through the surface, and eventually spread throughout the body. Because of these required conditions of intimate contact, it is easy to recognize why syphilis is spread almost exclusively by sexual contact during intercourse, through a lip or oral cavity when kissing, or by close bodily contact with a secondary syphilitic rash. In few other circumstances is there the necessary combination of body surfaces and intimate contact necessary to transfer *Treponema pallidum* alive from one person to another.

Because of the great variety of potential signs and symptoms which occur in all stages of syphilis it has been called "the great imitator." There are at least 40 skin diseases that secondary syphilis may resemble, 23 diseases that the mouth lesions may resemble, and at least 16 diseases that resemble primary genital lesions.[6]

The course of the disease is divided into four distinct stages, each with its own signs and symptoms. This course is outlined in Tables 16.4 and 16.5 and explained in more detail in the following sections.

[6] Sartwell, *op. cit.*, p. 277.

TABLE 16.3 **NATURAL HISTORY OF ACQUIRED**

SYPHILIS

Reservoir for Agent	Causative Agent	Incubation Period	Mode of Transmission	Immunity
Man	*Treponema pallidum* (spirochete)	10–90 days, usually 21 days following exposure	Direct physical contact, usually during sexual relations	There is no immunizing agent (vaccine) against syphilis. Acquired immunity will eventually develop in the absence of treatment. Though early treatment halts the immunological process and readily permits reinfection, it also protects the body against the systemic advance of the disease process.

Extent of Disease Process

Syphilis: The first sign of *Primary Syphilis* is a single, painless lesion or sore called a chancre. It most often appears at the place where the germs enter the body, usually in the genital area. Sometimes this chancre does not appear or is overlooked, especialy in women. If it does appear, it goes away without treatment. In a short time, which may vary from a few weeks to six months, *Secondary Syphilis* signs appear. Although different patients have different symptoms, the most common are lesions, which may be few or many, large or small, and which may appear on various body areas. Whitish patches in the mouth or throat, "moth eaten" or "patchy" falling hair, low fever, painless swelling of lymph glands, and pain in bones and joints may all be signs of secondary syphilis. While the *Primary* and *Secondary* manifestations persist, the disease is highly contagious. With the disappearance of secondary symptoms, the disease enters a period of early latency. The degree of infectiousness associated with *Early Latent* syphilis is governed by the recurrence of secondary lesions. In any event, because of such a possibility, the disease is considered communicable for approximately four years following initial infection. The final category, noninfectious *Late Latent Syphilis,* can become destructive and may eventually cause heart disease, insanity, paralysis, blindness, or death. These end results of untreated syphilis may not take place until 10 to 30 years after the primary infection.

SYPHILIS AND GONORRHEA

GONORRHEA

Reservoir for Agent	Causative Agent	Incubation Period	Mode of Transmission	Immunity
Man	*Neisseria gonorrheae* (bacterial)	Within 5 days for 85% of males following exposure; 2–8 days for females.	Sexual contact, usually sexual intercourse.	There is no immunizing agent (vaccine) against gonorrhea. An attack of the disease does not afford protection against reinfection.

Extent of Disease Process

Gonorrhea, or GC as it is more commonly called, is a local disease of the body parts affected and is not a body-wide or systemic disease as is syphilis. In the *male,* the disease manifests itself as a burning on urination and a discharge of pus. The disease is quite painful and generally forces the patient to seek medical attention. Although not too common, chronic GC in the male may lead to involvement of other portions of the urinary or generative system and may, if not treated early, produce sterility. In the *female* the early symptoms of GC are less pronounced. The slight discomfort associated with urinary symptoms rarely motivates the infected person to seek early treatment. Progression of the disease often leads to infection of the fallopian tubes, ovaries, and lower abdomen, causing severe pain. This process often results in sterility, owing to scarring and closure of the tubes, or to emergency surgery.

SOURCE: Los Angeles County Health Department.

PRIMARY SYPHILIS

During sexual contact, *Treponema pallidum* gains entry by burrowing into the body of the partner. After entry, it reproduces at the site of entrance and within a few hours produces millions of spirochetes, which begin to spread by way of the blood and lymph throughout the body.

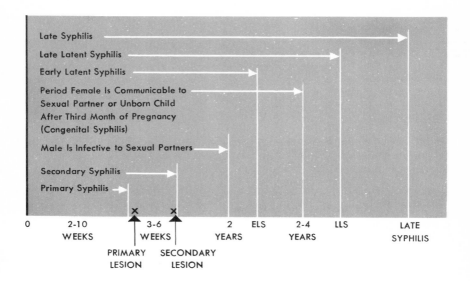

Fig. 16.3 Stages of syphilis, showing relative infectious periods. (Adapted from K. H. Sutherland, *VD Teaching Manual,* Los Angeles County Health Department.)

This stage is the incubation period (Table 16.3), which ranges from ten to ninety days (the average is three weeks).

The first indication or symptom of the disease is the *primary lesion,* called a *chancre,* which appears at the site of entry of the spirochete within three to four weeks after exposure. This highly infectious primary lesion may be a typical chancre (a painless lesion the size of a dime, pink, raised, ulcerated, and firm, with enlarged neighboring lymph nodes), or it may be so slight as to go unnoticed. Since primary syphilis may resemble many diseases, any lesion of the genital area of a male or female who has had prior sexual contact should be regarded as possible primary syphilis until it is proven, by medical consultation, to be something else. Any lesion anywhere on the body—particularly on the lips, tonsils, or fingers—which fails to heal in a reasonable length of time may be a primary syphilis lesion.

This primary lesion will disappear spontaneously without treatment before the appearance or disappearance of the secondary stage. It usually leaves no scar, but the disease agents are still present in the body. Blood tests of victims are negative when the primary lesion appears but become positive one to two weeks after the chancre is first noted (see Fig. 16.4).

SECONDARY SYPHILIS

The spread of *Treponema pallidum* throughout the body before the primary lesion appears produces the secondary syphilis symptoms in the skin, mucous membranes, eyes, and nervous system. The organism multiplies in these areas of the body, and in about four weeks to six months (Table 16.3) after the appearance of the primary chancre, the secondary signs and symptoms appear. These include a rash, which does not itch, which may be all over the body or just on the palms of the hands or the soles of the feet, and which often is diffcult to see. The victim may also have a sore throat, mild fever, or headache. Other more or less common symptoms are falling patches of hair; external or internal inflammation of the eyes; pain in the joints, from bone involvement; jaundice, from liver involvement; and, in very severe conditions, syphilitic meningitis with severe headache, convulsions, deafness, partial paralysis, and sometimes coma.

It is important for a person who is seeking a physician for an examination of the symptoms described here to divulge if he has been exposed or thinks he may have been exposed to syphilis in the past six months. These symptoms of secondary syphilis persist for a variable period of time, ranging from a few days to several months, and then disappear spontaneously. Secondary syphilis, which lasts three to six months, can always be diagnosed by blood tests (Fig. 16.4).

LATENT SYPHILIS

Latency begins with the healing of untreated secondary lesions; it may extend from a few months to a lifetime. If we consider the first two years of an untreated infection as the over-all period of potential infectiousness, latency may be divided into two stages—the potentially infectious stage, *early latent syphilis,* and a noninfectious later stage, *late latent syphilis.*

These phases, commonly called "hidden syphilis," are not recognizable by visible signs or symptoms. They are uncovered only by blood tests (Fig. 16.4). Latent syphilis is usually discovered during routine blood examinations.

Early latent syphilis. If the disease goes untreated during the secondary eruptions, there may be a series of recurring infectious lesions of the skin or mucous membranes of the mouth for the first two to four years; this is the period of early latent syphilis. Because of these possible early lesions the disease is considered communicable throughout its early latency. During this long latent period the disease loses some of its infectiousness, and after the first two years, the person can rarely transmit

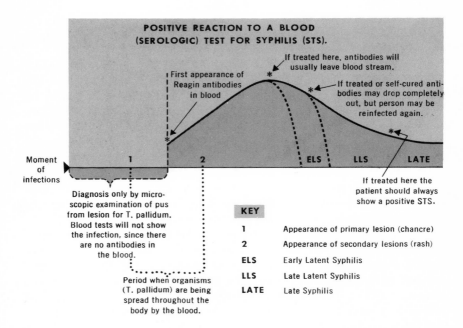

Fig. 16.4 Course of syphilis, showing effectiveness of blood serologic tests. (Adapted from K. H. Sutherland, *VD Teaching Manual,* Los Angeles County Health Department.)

syphilis through sexual intercourse, although a syphilitic pregnant woman can still transmit it to her unborn child (*congenital syphilis*) for about two more years. Such a prenatally infected child is presumptive proof of the mother's latent infection.[7]

Late latent syphilis. After the individual has lost all powers of infection, the disease has entered the period of late latent syphilis. This period may last for a few months or for a lifetime. During this time there are no apparent signs of illness. If routinely examined, the individual will show a positive blood test but will have no further symptoms.

[7] J. H. Stokes, *Modern Clinical Syphilology: Diagnosis, Treatment and Case Study,* Philadelphia, Saunders, 1944, p. 142.

In this latent stage, progressive degeneration of the brain, spinal cord, hearing, sight, or bones may be going on unnoticed. If and when the symptoms of this degeneration appear, the individual then slips into the last stage—late syphilis.

LATE SYPHILIS

Of all persons acquiring syphilis, many may be expected to develop, if untreated, a late manifestation that will incapacitate or kill them. Although almost any part of the body may be affected, only the most common manifestations are discussed below.

Cardiovascular syphilis. The lesions in most cases of cardiovascular syphilis are located in the thoracic aorta (see Fig. 13.1, Chapter 13). The elastic tissue is destroyed and the aorta dilates, producing an aneurysm; or the infection may involve the aortic valve, causing an insufficient flow of blood. The symptoms of cardiovascular syphilis differ in no unique way from other heart and vascular disorders (explained in Chapter 13).

Neurosyphilis. The process of neurosyphilis (syphilis affecting nervous tissue) may be detected by routine spinal fluid examination years before the appearance of obvious changes in the behavior of the individual. *Paresis* (general paralysis), the most dread late manifestation of syphilis, will be the eventual fate awaiting this victim.

The symptoms of neurosyphilis arise from a widespread destruction of the brain tissue by large numbers of *Treponema pallidum*. The mental changes vary, the most common being gradual changes in personality, decreased ability to work, and impairment of concentration and judgment. These changes produce abnormal behavior, including delusions, loss of memory, lack of insight, apathy or violent rages, convulsions, and disorientation. Neurosyphilis is responsible for many deaths, as well as for much of the invalidism seen in mental institutions.

Tabes dorsalis. This is a failure of muscular coordination within the body; it is the most common outcome of the destruction of the spinal cord by large numbers of spirochetes. Similar degeneration of the optic and other cranial nerves is common. The usual diagnostic signs of *tabes dorsalis* is a weakening or loss of ankle and knee reflexes. Occasionally all reflexes may be lost, including the ability to change pupil size, sense of position, or any irregularity of muscular coordination.

In treated cases life can be prolonged, but permanent care may be necessary because of the extreme degeneration that may have taken place prior to treatment.

Primary optic atrophy. This is a degeneration of the optic nerve; it is usually first noticed by a loss of peripheral vision. Central vision may be lost in advanced cases, leaving the individual completely blind. Primary optic atrophy also results from glaucoma (Chapter 3) and other conditions affecting the eyes.

SYPHILIS IN PREGNANCY

If a woman is infected with syphilis at the time of conception or shortly thereafter, the primary chancre appearing on her may be very mild or completely suppressed. Secondary symptoms in her skin are likely to be absent, and if she has not had blood tests during her pregnancy, she may have no indication that she has syphilis before the birth of her child. Infection of a fetus takes place by the spirochetes of syphilis crossing the placental membranes from the blood of the mother to the bloodstream of the child. Such infection of the fetus apparently does not occur before the fifth month of fetal life. Consequently, adequate treatment of a pregnant woman who was previously syphilitic before the fifth fetal month will insure the child's safety. Treatment given a mother after the fifth month will also reach and cure the syphilitic fetus. Because of the aforementioned conditions and because syphilis can also be acquired during pregnancy, blood tests during the first half of pregnancy and during the seventh month are considered to be adequate for detecting this disease.

In a majority of instances the infection of the fetus takes place quite late in the pregnancy; and the more recent the mother's syphilitic infection, the greater the chance that the child may be born with syphilis. A severe infection is very likely to lead to the death of the fetus before birth. Thus, syphilis is a rather common cause of stillbirths. Of the infants born alive to untreated syphilitic mothers, approximately 50 percent will have syphilis at birth. Syphilis obtained in this manner is termed *congenital syphilis*.

CONGENITAL SYPHILIS

An infant born with syphilis may show secondary lesions at birth; may appear normal at birth and develop lesions within a few months; or may remain without symptoms until adolescence, when the symptoms of late syphilis may appear. As a rule, the earlier the symptoms appear, the more severe the infection. Syphilis is capable of producing many different types of lesions, but never do all of them occur in one infant.

Of the various secondary lesions appearing at birth, *rhinitis*—an inflammation of the nose with a discharge of *Treponema pallidum* spirochetes—is the most frequent. This discharge may interfere with breathing, is extremely infectious, and accounts for many infections of individuals who handle infected children. If it is severe and continues over a long period, the growth of the nasal bones is disturbed, resulting in the deformity known as "saddle nose" (Fig. 16.5). Skin lesions at birth are frequent and are often similar to the rash seen in secondary stages of venereal syphilis. In a high proportion of children, the palms

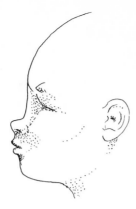

Fig. 16.5 Saddle nose. Destruction of the septum in congenital syphilis.

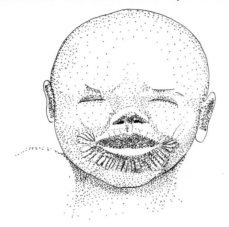

Fig. 16.6 Congenital syphilis, showing rhagades (perioral excoriations).

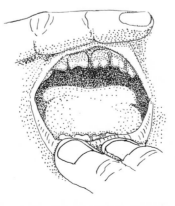

Fig. 16.7 Congenital syphilis, showing Hutchinson's teeth.

and soles or the skin about the mouth may be reddened, inflamed, and
thickened at birth or shortly after birth. When this occurs around the
mouth, fissures may radiate in all directions. After healing, these lesions
and radiating scars about the mouth are known as *rhagades* (Fig. 16.6)
and are considered as signs of congenital syphilis.

After the secondary lesions, the course of untreated congenital syphilis
is similar to that of venereal syphilis. These late symptoms may appear
in a few months, at six or seven years, or late in the teens. Some of the
more common are Hutchinson's teeth (Fig. 16.7), which are "notched" or
screwdriver-like permanent central incisors; *keratitis,* a condition of the
eyes which is uncommon in young children but very common in older
children and may cause permanent blindness (neurosyphilis); bone and
joint involvement; or a lung condition which usually leads to death
during the first few days or weeks of life.

DIAGNOSIS OF AND THERAPY FOR SYPHILIS

Early diagnosis followed by prompt and adequate treatment will
completely cure syphilis.

MICROSCOPIC EXAMINATION

The lesions of early syphilis which may begin to appear at the points
of physical contact within three to five weeks from contact are rich in
Treponema pallidum, which provides the best means for the conclusive
diagnosis of this disease. *Treponema pallidum* taken from such a
chancre of primary syphilis or from skin lesions of secondary syphilis
can readily be seen under a microscope by what is termed "darkfield
illumination." The more recent the lesion, the more readily can the
organism be discovered and the disease cured.

BLOOD (SEROLOGIC) TESTS FOR SYPHILIS (STS)

The blood tests become positive only after a general invasion of the
body by the spirochetes. The underlying principle of a blood test is the
appea.ance in the blood, after syphilis infection (and occasionally after
some other conditions), of an *antibody-like* substance called *reagin.* All
of the blood tests for syphilis, based on reagin in the blood, are mod-
ification's of the original Wasserman test (a test for determining reagin
in the blood which was much less sensitive than presently used tests).[8]

Besides the reagin tests there are other blood tests for syphilis. These
are for *Treponema pallidum* spirochetes and specific antibodies pro-

[8] *Syphilis, Modern Diagnosis and Management,* Washington, D.C., U.S. Department
of Health, Education, and Welfare, Public Health Service (Communicable Disease
Center), 1960.

duced by the body in response to the syphilis infection. They are posi- tive for syphilis only, are quite expensive, and involve complicated pro- cedures which could not be used as easily as the reagin tests for screening numbers of individuals.

SYPHILIS THERAPY

The purposes of treatment are to destroy all treponemes, to initiate the healing of existing lesions, and to prevent further damage to the body. Treatment of syphilis also serves to prevent the spread of the disease to others. The earlier this treatment is started, the more effective it is in accomplishing these purposes.

In the mid-1940s penicillin began to replace the long, expensive, and difficult treatment of syphilis with arsenical products and bismuth preparations. Since that time the use of penicillin alone in the treatment of syphilis has been standard all over the world.

The primary consideration in treatment is maintenance of a high penicillin level in the blood and tissues for a sufficient period of time to destroy all of the organisms present in the body. Consequently, the treatment varies with the stage of the disease. Unfortunately, the wide- spread use of penicillin for treatment of a variety of other disorders has frequently added some difficulties to the diagnosis of syphilis. Syphilitic infection may be masked completely or its course altered by smaller doses of penicillin than are necessary to treat syphilis adequately. When a patient's sensitivity to penicillin restricts the use of this preferable drug, erythromycin and tetracycline are good alternatives. No matter what drug is used, inadequate therapy may lead to a relapse.

GONORRHEA

Gonorrhea is an acute venereal disease which frequently progresses into a chronic state. It is initiated by a microorganism that prefers to live in the mucous membranes lining the genitourinary tract, the rectum, the mouth, and the eye. This organism is the gonococcus, *Neisseria gonorrheae* (Fig. 16.8).

All gonococcal infections, except eye infections in newborn infants and occasional accidental eye infections in adults, are the result of direct physical contact. Although the gonococcus is rarely spread by circulation of the blood, it can cause serious infection of the heart or joints (arth- ritis) when it does enter the blood.

The gonococcus is quite sensitive to conditions outside the human body. Infection requires the direct depositing of *Neisseria gonorrheae* organisms near the susceptible tissues of the genital organs. Occasionally the organism is accidentally deposited from the hand to an eye or into the eyes of the newborn as a result of its passage through an infected birth canal (*ophthalmia neonatorum*).

The incubation period of gonorrhea is usually three to five days, but occasionally varies from two to ten days. The signs, symptoms, and outcome differ between males and females. The course of the disease is

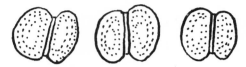

Fig. 16.8 *Neisseria gonorrheae,* the organism that causes gonorrhea.

explained in Table 16.3, and the significant differences are explained in the following discussion.

MALE GONORRHEA

The first symptoms of gonorrhea are a sensation of burning during urination and a discharge of pus from the penis, which may be severe or so mild as to go unnoticed. In the absence of treatment the organisms gradually work their way along the urethra and vas deferens into the internal organs of the male reproductive tract. The disease may damage the delicate structures of the testes and tubules through which the sperm must travel, thus causing sterility.

FEMALE GONORRHEA

The initial symptom of gonorrhea in the female, a slight vaginal discharge of pus, in most instances is so mild as to go unnoticed. Only when the infection has progressed into the fallopian tubes, generally months after infection, is a woman likely to be aware of gonorrhea. Then pain may occur in the lower abdomen and often is mistaken for appendicitis.

When exposure of a woman to gonorrhea is suspected or when there is a vaginal discharge that may be caused by gonorrhea, the physician will usually take samples of such secretions from her uterus, cervix, and vagina for both smears and cultures. Many different organisms can cause vaginal discharge, and the job of establishing which are involved may take considerable time and effort. Prolonged exposure to such infections may cause sterility from a stricture forming within the fallopian tubes. Since different drugs are effective against different organisms, a correct diagnosis is important.

OPHTHALMIA NEONATORUM

This is a condition causing blindness in the newborn children of mothers who are infected with gonorrhea at the time of birth. The source of infection is the mother's birth canal, which is infected with *Neisseria gonorrheae* organisms. These organisms rub off onto the child while it is being born, incubate in 36 to 48 hours, and start destroying the tissue of the eyes.

This condition can be prevented by the use of preparations for the protection of the eyes of babies at birth. An established effective treatment is drops of silver nitrate solution put into the eyes of children shortly after birth. Such treatment has been a law in all states for many years. Many antibiotic solutions are as effective as silver nitrate and are now being used in some areas.

DIAGNOSIS AND THERAPY

In both men and women gonorrhea remains infectious until cured, and the disease may take months or years to cure in a female.

Despite considerable talk about penicillin-resistant strains of gonococcus, penicillin is still the best treatment for gonorrhea. The resistance developed so far can be overcome by using larger doses, although the standard dosages are used first. Other antibiotics and sulfa drugs are effective in the treatment of penicillin-sensitive patients.

Both men and women who are to be treated for gonorrhea should have a blood test for syphilis before treatment begins, because the two diseases frequently occur together. The dosage of penicillin used for gonorrhea is not large enough to cure syphilis, but it can mask the symptoms of syphilis. The tracing of sex contacts is just as important for gonorrhea as for syphilis. In fact, in women the disease is often not suspected by either patient or physician until complications occur or a sexual partner is infected and contacted through the public health department.

CHANCROID

Chancroid, also known as *soft chancre,* is an acute, localized infectious communicable disease acquired through sexual contact (Table 16.4). It is induced by an organism known as the Ducrey bacillus (*Hemophilus ducreyi*). Soft chancre was distinguished from the primary lesion of syphilis in 1850 and later named *chancroid*. In 1889 Augosto Ducrey, an Italian dermatologist, identified the microorganism that caused the disease. The genital ulcerations produced by the disease are variable in

TABLE 16.4 **CHANCROID, LYMPHOGRANULOMA VENEREUM, AN**

Disease	Reservoir for Agent	Causative Agent
Chancroid	Man	*Haemophil ducreyi* (bacillus)
Granuloma inguinale (GI)	Man	*Donovania granulomat* (bacillus)
Lymphogranuloma venereum (LGV)	Man	Filterable virus

Extent of Disease Process

Chancroid: An acute localized genito-infectious disease characterized by a single, sometimes multiple, ulcerative lesion. The ulceration is usually accompanied by painful swelling of lymph nodes in the groin. The disease is usually self-limited but may persist for a long time.

Granuloma inguinale: A chronic progres disease, which begins as a small pap vesicle, or nodule, ulcerates and gradu spreads to form a smooth, velvety surf The lesion may occur in any genital area quite often involves the lymph nodes in groin. Extragenital lesions occur in 6 per

appearance and even now are occasionally confused with the chancre of syphilis.

Usually the disease is self-limiting, but when a lesion is in an area that is hard to keep clean or hidden, where it cannot be properly exposed and treated, prolonged infection will cause severe tissue destruction. Spreading of the organisms to adjacent areas of the body may cause reinfection and multiple lesions.

Chancroid occurs throughout the world and is especially common in tropical and subtropical countries. In many countries it is not a reportable disease and exact data as to its occurrence, distribution, and trends are not available.

About three to five days after exposure to the bacillus *Hemophilus ducreyi*, a small red area appears at the site of infection; this enlarges into a pimple-like growth, which soon breaks down, forming an ulcer with ragged edges and oozing pus. The ulcers are very painful and bleed easily. In about half of the cases a swelling develops in the local lymph glands within two weeks. It becomes inflamed, accumulates large amounts of pus, and may rupture spontaneously.

GRANULOMA INGUINALE (THE "MINOR" VENEREAL DISEASES)[a]

Incubation Period	Mode of Transmission	Immunity
average of to 5 days	Sexual contact, usually sexual intercourse	None
to 12 weeks	Considered to be of sexual contact, never completely proven	Acquired immunity depends on duration of untreated infection
to 21 days	Sexual contact, usually sexual intercourse	Acquired immunity depends on duration of untreated infection

Extent of Disease Process

all reported untreated cases.

lymphogranuloma venereum: The first sign is usually a small, transient lesion followed by regional swelling of lymph nodes. Constitutional symptoms are often present, including chills, headache, fever and generalized aches. The disease may disappear spontaneously or progress to more consequences. Malignancy may occur in long-standing lesions.

a National and local morbidity rates for these diseases are not significant.
   Source: Los Angeles County Health Department.

PREVENTION

The key to prevention of chancroid is cleanliness. The use of soap and water immediately after exposure is a preventive measure. But better education, better living standards, and improved personal hygiene will eliminate the infection.

GRANULOMA INGUINALE

Granuloma inguinale is a chronic venereal disease that usually affects the genital and inguinal regions of the body (Table 16.4). It is initiated by a microorganism known as the Donovan body (*Donovania granulomatis*), probably a bacterium. Among the other names given this disease are the following: ulcerating granuloma, granuloma pudendi tropicum, granuloma contagiosa, chronic venereal sore, and granuloma venereum.

The first report of a case was in India in 1882. The first case reported in the United States was in 1913. Exact data on its incidence and prevalence are not available, but it seems to be the least common of the venereal diseases. It is most frequent in the tropics but has been reported in all countries of the world. In the United States it is found quite often in the South, particularly among the lower socioeconomic groups, and is more frequent among males than females.

The incubation period has been stated to be from 8 to 12 weeks, but has run more than 100 days. The initial lesions are on the genital organs and slowly spread to involve the inguinal regions. The lesion takes the form of a deep red ulceration, which rarely heals and continues to enlarge. If secondary infections occur, pain and fever may appear. Ultimately, in most untreated cases, severe debility develops, ending in death.

LYMPHOGRANULOMA VENEREUM

Lymphogranuloma venereum (Table 16.4) is a sexually acquired *virus* infection of the lymph channels and lymph glands near the genital organs. It is also known as lymphogranuloma inguinale, climatic bubo, proadenitis, lymphopathia venereum, and Nicolas-Favre disease.

The disease was well described in.1922 and was proved to be of viral origin in 1930. It is a relatively common disease, occurring throughout the world, especially in the tropical and subtropical areas. It is found in the southern part of the United States, particularly among lower socioeconomic groups.

The primary lesion, an open ulceration, appears on the genital organs from 5 to 21 days after infection has taken place. This lesion is often of such short duration that it escapes notice; and the first symptoms of the disease may be swollen, hot, tender groups of lymph glands in the inguinal region, appearing from 10 to 30 days after exposure. Fever, chills, headache, and joint pains may also be present. The inflamed lymph nodes frequently fill with pus and drain continuously. In females, the initial lesion is frequently internal or absent, and the first symptoms are enlarged lymph glands which appear near the rectum.

SUMMARY

    I. Five Venereal Diseases—spread by sexual or close physical contact:
       A. Syphilis.
       B. Gonorrhea.
       C. Chancroid.
       D. Granuloma inguinale.
       E. Lymphogranuloma venereum.

   II. General Characteristics—all venereal diseases are infectious communicable diseases (see Chapter 15).

    A. Gonorrhea, leading reported communicable disease in the United States.

    B. Syphilis is important because of:
1. Chronic nature.
2. Serious lesions produced.
3. Disabilities.
4. Deaths.

III. Prevention and Control
    A. Depends upon recognition and elimination of sources of infection by:
1. Interviewing of patients.
2. Reporting of infected individuals by physicians.
3. Cluster testing.

    B. Personal responsibility, abstinence from promiscuous behavior.

IV. Syphilis
    A. Nonvenereal syphilis: *endemic syphilis* or *Bejel.*

    B. Venereal syphilis
1. Body-wide disease produced by *Treponema pallidum.*
2. Spread almost exclusively by:
    a. heterosexual or homosexual contact.
    b. a lip or oral cavity chancre when kissing.
    c. any close bodily contact with a "primary chancre" or "secondary rash."
3. Course divided into four stages:
    a. Primary syphilis—appearance of primary lesion or chancre.
    b. Secondary syphilis—appearance of a rash which does not itch.
    c. Latent syphilis—begins with healing of untreated secondary lesions. Divided into two stages:
      (1) Early latent syphilis (ELS)—infectious stage which may last for the first two to four years.
      (2) Late latent syphilis (LLS)—period after all powers of infection have been lost.
    d. Late syphilis—appearance of manifestations which incapacitate or kill.

    C. Syphilis in pregnancy
1. Primary chancre may be mild or absent.
2. Secondary symptoms (rash) likely absent.
3. Spirochetes of syphilis cross the placental membranes into blood of the child and produce "congenital syphilis."

    D. Diagnosis of syphilis
1. Microscopic examination of spirochetes from primary chancre or secondary lesions.
2. Blood (serologic) tests—become positive only after a general invasion of the body.

    E. Syphilis therapy should:
1. Destroy all treponemes.
2. Initiate healing of lesions.
3. Prevent further damage to body.
4. Prevent spread of disease to others.

V. Gonorrhea
    A. Acute venereal disease initiated by the microorganism *Neisseria gonorrheae.*

   B. Male gonorrhea—sensation of burning during urination and a discharge of pus from the penis.
   C. Female gonorrhea
      1. Initial symptom—a slight vaginal discharge of pus which may go unnoticed or be mistaken as part of the menstrual flow.
      2. Women likely to become aware of disease only after months of infection.
   D. Ophthalmia neonatorum—condition causing blindness in newborn children.
   E. Diagnosis
      1. In male by a microscopic study of discharge of pus from penis.
      2. In women only after complications or as the result of an infected male sexual partner being interviewed by the public health department.

   VI. Chancroid (soft chancre)
      A. Localized, raised ulcer with ragged edges and oozing pus.
      B. Self-limiting venereal disease induced by the Ducrey bacillus (*Hemophilus ducreyi*).

   VII. Granuloma inguinale
      A. Chronic venereal disease usually affecting the genital and inguinal lymph nodes of the body.
      B. Initiated by a microorganism known as the Donovan body (*Donovanian granulomatis*).

   VIII. Lymphogranuloma venereum
      A. Infection of the lymph glands and channels near the genital organs.
      B. Produced by a venereally acquired virus.

Glossary

   If you cannot find the word you wish in this glossary, check the index for text and glossary references.

arsenical (ahr sen'i kəl) (G. *arsen,* strong).   A drug containing arsenic.

bismuth (biz'məth) (L. *bismuthum*).   A silver-white metal, atomic number 83. Its salts have been used in inflammatory diseases of the stomach and intestine, and in the treatment of syphilis.

chancre (shang'kər) (L. *cancer,* crablike).   The primary lesion of syphilis developing at the site of entrance of the syphilitic organism.

chancroid (shang'kroid).   A nonsyphilitic venereal ulcer; also called soft chancre.

coma (kō'mə) (G. *koma,* a deep sleep).   An abnormal deep stuporlike sleep occurring in illness.

congenital (kən jen'i təl) (L. *congenitus,* born together).   Existing at, and usually before, birth.

contact (kon'takt) (L. *contactus,* a touching together).   In control of venereal diseases, an individual who is known to have been sufficiently near to an infected individual to have been exposed to a disease.

erythromycin (e rith'rō mī'sin) (G. *erythros,* red; *mykes,* fungus).   An antibacterial substance produced by the growth of *Streptomyces erythreus.*

genital (jen′i təl) (L. *genitalis,* genital). Pertaining to the organs of reproduction.

gonorrhea (gon ə rē′ə) (G. *gone,* seed; *rhein,* to flow). A contagious inflammatory disease of the genitourinary tract, affecting either sex.

granuloma inguinale (gran yə lō′mə ing gwi nal′ē) (L. *granulum,* a little grain; *inguinalis,* in the groin). A venereal disease characterized by deep pus-containing ulcerations of the skin of the genital organs and groin areas.

heterosexual (het′ər ō sek′shoo əl) (G. *hetero,* other; L. *sexus,* sex). One having normal attraction for the opposite sex.

homosexual (hō′mō sek′shoo əl) (G. *homo,* like, same; L. *sexus,* sex). One sexually attracted to another of the same sex.

infectious (in fek′shəs) (L. *inficere,* to stain). Capable of being spread. Infectious disease—any disease caused by the entrance, growth, and multiplication of a disease-causing organism.

jaundice (jawn′dis) (G. *ikteros,* yellow). Condition characterized by yellowness of skin due to deposition of bile pigments.

lymphogranuloma venereum (lim′fō gran′yə lō′mə ve nēr′ē əm) (L. *lympha,* water; *granulum,* a little grain; G. *oma,* a tumor; *venereus,* from Venus, the goddess of love). Specific venereal disease affecting chiefly the lymphatic tissues of the iliac and inguinal regions of the body.

paresis (pə rē′sis) (G. *paresis,* weakening). Partial or incomplete paralysis which can result from syphilis.

promiscuous (prə mis′kyoo əs) (L. *pro,* before; *miscere,* to mix). Engaging in indiscriminate, irregular, or casual sexual intercourse.

reagin (rē ā′jin) (L. *re,* back, again; *agere,* to act). An antibody associated with many diseases such as syphilis, hay fever, and asthma.

reservoir (rez′ər vwahr) (L. *reservare,* to keep). The nonclinical source of an infection.

self-limiting. A disease that runs a definite limited course.

syphilis (sif′i lis) (from an 18th century poem about a shepherd boy named *Syphilis*). An infectious, chronic, venereal disease characterized by lesions which may involve any organ or tissue of the body.

syphilitic meningitis (sif i lit′ik men in jī′tis). Inflammation of the meninges due to a syphilitic infection.

tetracycline (tet′rə sī′klēn) (G. *tetra-,* four; *kyklos,* a circle). A yellow, odorless, crystalline powder, with antibiotic activity against a wide range of organisms.

venereal (və nēr′ē əl). Due to or propagated by sexual intercourse.

Wassermann test (Wahs′ər mən) (after A. von Wassermann, 1866–1925, German bacteriologist). A test based on the *reagin* antibody in the serum of syphilitic patients. Used as a test for syphilis.

CHAPTER 17

OTHER
DISEASES
OF MAN

Medicine is concerned both with the prevention and cure of diseases as well as the prevention of accidents. Such prevention finds its most important role in the field of pediatrics (treatment of children). A program of preventive medicine for children is reflected in a healthier adult population. To understand the problems of prevention, it is necessary to know the chief causes of sickness and death among infants and children and measures that may be taken to prevent them.

CHILDHOOD DISEASES AND HAZARDS

Infant deaths are defined as deaths occurring within the first year of life. These are concentrated among the very young; one third occur during the first day of life; one third occur among infants who live only from 1 to 28 days; and the remaining one third of the deaths is among those surviving from 1 to 12 months. Because of the nature of their causes, deaths of the very young up through the first month have been more difficult to reduce than those of older infants and children. Seventy percent of these young infant deaths are caused by prematurity, birth injury, congenital malformations, and anoxia. These conditions and their lack of decline were discussed in Chapter 9. An outstanding cause of death after the first month of life is infection by communicable diseases.

Older children, 1 through 15 years old, have shown a decreasing death rate due to infectious diseases; death from accidents is now in first place as cause of death in this age group.

PREVENTION POINTERS

The prevention of childhood diseases and accidents is the responsibility of parents and all persons and agencies in contact with children. Points to be stressed include the following:

1. *Periodic physical examinations.* In Appendix C (p. 655) is a suggested Life Preventive Medicine Program. The examination schedule of this program or a similar schedule which has been modified by a physician should be followed closely.

2. *Nutrition.* Proper nutrition is essential to good health. Chapters 6 and 7 may be used as a guideline for an organized nutritional program.

3. *Physical fitness.* Proper exercise and adequate rest should be emphasized to produce good health. Educational programs conducted by the schools, Ys, Scouts, and similar organizations will provide opportunity for physical exercise in youth.

4. *Immunization program.* Appendix C includes a general immunization schedule. The immunizations available today and new ones as they are developed should be used to ensure a child's maximum protection from disease.

5. *Accident prevention.* Education and the use of protective devices will reduce accidents. Children who know dangers and respect them will have fewer accidents throughout life.

6. *Parent guidance.* One of the most important aspects of preventive pediatrics is education of the parents. The conditions that kill, injure, and maim cannot be overcome until those who have immediate responsibility for children are informed and convinced of the need for protective measures.

Preventive measures will reduce medical and dental expenses, maintain a healthier population, and stop the needless suffering to which some children are subjected.

ACCIDENTS

Accidents rank first as the cause of death in children after the age of infancy. The lower relative rank of accidents in infancy exists because the other types of deaths are more frequent, not because accidents are less frequent. The magnitude of the accident problem is further emphasized by the fact that 100 persons have *serious nonfatal injuries* for every one killed by accident. The prevention of accidents is everybody's responsibility and the chief tools for such prevention are educational.

The following topics are the leading causes of accidental death for successive age groups in children.

SUFFOCATION

About 50 percent of all accidental deaths in infancy are classified as suffocation in bed; other deaths are due to such things as an infant's choking on food or solid objects. Suffocation in bed is unlikely as a cause of death among healthy infants but may occur with an infant weakened by an illness, especially an illness which obstructs breathing. Suffocation in older infants and children is usually traced to a few common causes—such as thin plastic bags given to an infant as a toy, which adhere to his nose and mouth, obstructing breathing, or children accidentally locked into empty refrigerators or freezers.

POISONINGS

Poison control centers have been established in hospitals and health centers across the country. Every adult should know how to contact the one nearest the family home in case of an emergency.

Nearly three quarters of all poisonings take place in children between 1 and 3 years of age. An infant is likely to swallow poisons which are accessible under the sink or on the floor of a closet or cabinet. Products such as detergents, bleaches, polishes, lye, paint, and petroleum products are especially dangerous when they have been transferred from the original container to something else, such as a soft drink bottle. The 1- or 2-year-old child is able to reach drugs or cosmetics on a table or in his mother's handbag, and the 2- and 3-year-old can climb and search shelves and medicine cabinets for sweetened and flavored drugs such as aspirin, which is often the greatest hazard in the medicine cabinet.

The kitchen is the room of greatest risk, followed by the bathroom and bedroom. Normally the poison found by a child is not in its usual place, but rather has been left on a table, dresser, or desk top.

Over 90 percent of poisonings are preventable. Most poisonings are the result of parental ignorance of the poison potential of such things as furniture polish, hair solutions, insect sprays, or detergents. Parents do not realize that a child can drink enough kerosene or eat enough aspirin to be harmed.

FALLS AND BURNS

Most serious falls are preventable in infancy and the early preschool years. During the school years prevention is very difficult, because the child is learning to climb and is testing his skill and courage.

Deaths from burns are primarily concentrated in children under 4 years of age and are usually preventable. Most of these deaths are due to small children's being trapped in homes which are set on fire by faulty heating fixtures.

DROWNING

Drowning has become an important cause of accidental death. Most drownings occur while the child is swimming or playing in the water. A considerable proportion are boating accidents, related to the tremendous increase in boating as a sport.

Drowning prevention in the preschool years is largely a matter of parents' and other adults' remembering that a baby can drown if left alone in a bathtub, or that a toddler can fall into an open well or swimming pool. For older children, the best means of prevention is teaching everyone the elements of water safety and how to swim. This is done at life-saving and swimming classes in public schools, at beaches, Ys, camps, and similar places. The prevention of boating accidents is promoted by courses in boating organized by the U.S. Power Squadrons, the Coast Guard Auxiliary, Outboard Clubs, and the Red Cross, Scouts, and Ys.

MOTOR VEHICLE ACCIDENTS

Motor vehicle accidents are the leading causes of accidental death for people from 1 through 64 years of age. The highest death rate is in the 15- to 24-year age group, and most often with an unmarried driver.

Studies of the various contributing factors point to some suggestive means of prevention. One factor in accident prevention is strict enforcement of traffic laws. The raising of the minimum age for a driver's license from 16 to 18 years in all states would also contribute to a reduction in mortality. High school driver education classes have been shown to be effective and are now given to over 1,500,000 students a year. The use of policemen, housewives, and student traffic aides at street crossings near schools reduces accidents in children walking to and from school. The use of seat belts and other safety factors also reduce deaths from motor vehicle accidents (Chapter 18).

DISEASE

After the first year of life the child faces a completely new set of hazards from his expanding environment. His increased range of locomotion within and outside the home and his natural tendency to climb and investigate sets the stage for accidents. As he progresses, his expansion out of the home and into the neighborhood and school increases his exposure to communicable and other diseases.

The major killer-diseases of children are heart disease (discussed in Chapter 13) and cancer (discussed in Chapter 14). This section will deal with the common childhood diseases which predominantly affect the age group 1 through 15.

POLIOMYELITIS

Poliomyelitis is a communicable disease caused by one of three types of poliomyelitis viruses. The polio viruses, if they gain entrance into the central nervous system, produce malfunction or death of nerve cells. More commonly, however, they do not enter the central nervous system but produce an infection centering around the digestive tract, where they produce no recognizable signs of destruction. Only in about 1 out of 100 infections do the viruses progress into the central nervous system. Polio infections may occur in several degrees. For convenience these are usually grouped into the carrier state, where the individual excretes the viruses in his feces and urine with no evidence of a disease; abortive infection, with symptoms of initial poliomyelitis (brief fever, headache, sore throat, mild diarrhea, abdominal pain, nausea, and vomiting) but with no involvement of the nervous system; nonparalytic, similar to the foregoing, except that symptoms may be prolonged over several days, and there is evidence of some nervous system involvement but no paralysis; and paralytic poliomyelitis, the most severe outcome of the disease, which produces some degree of permanent crippling or involvement of the respiratory mechanisms, leading to respiratory failure, the usual cause of death in this disease.

Through the intensive administration of polio vaccines, a marked reduction in the incidence of polio in the United States has occurred. However, immunization of every child against polio remains extremely important as the viruses of polio are still present in the United States. Two vaccines are available. One is an *inactivated poliovirus vaccine* (IPV) developed by Jonas Salk, and the other, an *attenuated live oral poliovirus vaccine* (OPV) developed by Albert Sabin.

Inactivated poliovaccine is made from live Types I, II, and III poliomyelitis viruses which have been killed, placed into a single vaccine, and injected into the individual to be immunized. This was the first material successfully developed to immunize against poliomyelitis.

After much debate, the Sabin idea of using unkilled poliomyelitis viruses for purposes of immunization was accepted. Since this was an oral dosage, taken with a cube of sugar, it had great appeal to the public.

This attenuated poliovirus vaccine is fed by mouth, usually in three separate feedings, one for each type. When all three types are fed simultaneously, the more dominant type may completely suppress one or both other types so that antibodies are formed to only one or two types. This suppression is avoided if the three viruses are fed separately at intervals of about six weeks. It is considered desirable to feed the least dominant type first; the preferred order is Type I followed by Type III and last by Type II. In booster doses, however, all three types are fed at once.

Both IPV and OPV are effective and acceptable, but the oral live attenuated poliovirus vaccine has certain advantages which include ease of administration and longer-lasting immunity.

DIPHTHERIA

Diphtheria is induced by the growth of the bacillus *Corynebacterium diphtheriae* on skin or mucous membrane surfaces. This growth produces a drainage of pus cells and fibrin, an insoluble protein formed in a clotting process. This fibrin coagulates into a pseudomembrane, which seems to grow across the infected body surface. This membrane is at first grayish-white but later becomes a dirty gray, and forcible removal of the membrane results in its spreading in all directions. The most frequent locations of the infection and the membrane are in the throat (particularly on the tonsils), nose, larynx, trachea, and sometimes on the skin.

Diphtheria also produces a toxin which has severe destructive effects locally and systemically. This toxin causes degeneration and death to tissue. Such degeneration of the heart muscle (myocarditis) is one of the most serious effects. Also diphtheria toxin causes degeneration of nerves, producing paralysis, malfunctions of organs, and respiratory involvement, which may result in death.

Transfer from an infected to a noninfected individual may occur by many means since the organism survives for hours or even days outside the body. The diphtheria bacillus will grow in milk very well without appreciably changing its flavor or appearance. Unpasteurized milk has been the occasional source of diphtheria outbreaks.

The toxoid which prevents diphtheria has been available for nearly 40 years, yet diphtheria is still found in all large communities because of the apathy of parents about having their children immunized. Although it occurs to some extent in all seasons, it increases in winter, sometimes to the extent of an epidemic, and declines in late spring. Diphtheria occurs at all ages, but has the greatest frequency in children between 1 and 14 years of age. All children should be protected prior to their first birthday.

Although a single injection of toxoid may give satisfactory immunity, three or four smaller injections a month apart give more reliable protection and fewer unpleasant reactions. The time required to produce immunity varies from two weeks to six months. The majority are immune within two months. Even among those vaccinated it is desirable to verify the presence of immunity by means of a Schick test, which consists of injecting into the skin a small amount of toxin. A *positive* or *nonimmune* reaction consists of redness, swelling, and tenderness around the area of the injection, the reaction reaching its maximum usually within a few days after the injection. If there is no reaction, the individual has obtained immunity from diphtheria. Booster injections of toxoid are usually necessary to maintain immunity into adulthood.

Diphtheria toxoid is sometimes efficiently used in combination with other disease antigens. Commonly today the combination of diphtheria toxoid, tetanus toxoid, and whooping cough (pertussis) vaccine, called DPT, is used for young children. In recent years the IPV Salk vaccine has been combined with these three to produce a quadruple vaccine, which reduces the number of injections the child must receive.

WHOOPING COUGH (PERTUSSIS)

Whooping cough is caused by the bacillus *Bordetella pertussis*. It commonly occurs in children under 6 years of age, and rarely in those over 10. Very young infants are susceptible, for immunity is not transmitted across the placenta. One attack may be expected to confer lifelong immunity, although it does not do so in all instances, since second attacks of the disease occasionally occur.

The typical stage of severe cough, called a *paroxysm,* consists of a series of explosive coughs rapidly repeated on a single expiration with no time for a breath between them. When the breath is expired to such an extent that no more coughing is possible, there is a rapid intake of air, and the coughing continues. Each inspiration during the paroxysm is accompanied by a peculiar crowing sound or "whoop." The course of the disease is from six weeks to several months.

There is no natural immunity to whooping cough, and 70 percent of the deaths from this disease occur before the age of 1 year. Consequently, the infant is desperately in need of vaccine protection as soon as possible. In unprotected children, whooping cough can have serious consequence: coughing can rupture lungs, permanently enlarge the bronchial tube, or even burst small blood vessels in the brain.

Immunization of infants against whooping cough is usually given in combination with diphtheria and tetanus toxoids (DPT). Three injections are given at 4- to 8-week intervals starting at 3 or 4 months of age. Single reinforcing injections should be given 1 year later and again before the child enters school.

MEASLES

Measles is a highly communicable disease induced by a rubeola virus. The disease has symptoms of a cold, bronchitis, fever and *Koplik spots*—bluish-white, pinpointed, surrounded by a red circular area on the mucous membranes of the mouth—which are important in the early diagnosis of measles before the rash appears on the skin. Following the spots a rash consisting of small dark-red papules, which increase in size and grow together, produce the appearance characteristic of measles.

During the active stage of the disease, the measles virus is present in the nose, the mouth, the throat, and the eyes. It is spread through contamination of the discharges of these areas from an infected person. It is communicable from the beginning of the respiratory symptoms, before the appearance of the rash, and slowly diminishes in communicability as the respiratory symptoms disappear.

Measles occurs chiefly in the late winter and the early spring. Infants under 6 months of age usually do not become infected with measles because of acquired congenital immunity from the mother. After about 6 months, the child's susceptibility at any age is very great, but the disease is most often contracted between 2 and 8 years of age. One attack usually protects permanently against a second attack.

Until 1963 there was no way to avoid measles. Indeed, it was considered by most to be one of the hazards of growing up. Overlooked was the fact that measles may produce many side effects. Before the introduction of the measles vaccines, which have proven to be some of the most effective vaccines ever developed, an average of 4 million children per year suffered from measles. Of infected children, 1 in every 15 will suffer serious side effects from middle-ear infections, which may cause lifelong deafness; pneumonia; and encephalitis, a brain inflammation which will send many children to mental institutions for the rest of their lives. One in each thousand infected children, according to the American Medical Association, dies of complications from this "hazard of growing up."

Measles vaccine should be given to infants at or soon after 9 months of age. Congenital immunity will protect them for a few months after birth; in fact, early injections of vaccine may be inactivated by congenital immunity.

There are two vaccines presently available—live attenuated virus vaccine and inactivated virus vaccine. The live attenuated measles vaccine is recommended by the majority of physicians. With this vaccine a single dose induces active immunity by producing a mild measles infection.

The inactivated measles vaccine is preferred in some situations where live attenuated vaccine would be too hazardous. It is given in three injections at monthly intervals and a fourth booster dose is given one year later. This fourth injection prevents antibodies from declining to an ineffective level. Insufficient information is presently available to suggest a definite measles booster schedule.

GERMAN MEASLES (RUBELLA)

German measles (3-day measles) is a contagious virus disease characterized chiefly by a skin eruption and mild associated symptoms. The disease itself is relatively unimportant because of the slight incapacity produced. It does not commonly occur in the first 6 months, but usually is found in the age group 2 to 15. The immunity produced by the disease is permanent; recurrences are rare.

The only complications of importance are congenital malformations of a fetus when the mother develops German measles. If a pregnant woman develops German measles during the first three months (first trimester) of pregnancy, the fetus may develop congenital cataract, deafness, or malformations of the heart, mouth, spinal cord, or extremities. Later in pregnancy German measles has no effect upon the fetus. As explained in Chapter 9, many physicians feel that a mother's having German measles in the first trimester of pregnancy may be grounds for a therapeutic abortion.

ROSEOLA (BABY MEASLES)

Roseola is a communicable disease of infancy and early childhood. The causative agent has not been identified, but probably is a virus. Roseola is also known as *roseola infantum* or *exanthema subitum*.

The disease occurs predominantly in infants, nearly always in those under 3 years of age, although a few cases in older children have been reported. The onset is abrupt, with a fever which rises to between 102 and 105°F. in a few hours and continues for approximately four days, with some morning remissions. When the fever ends, the characteristic eruption appears; then the child seems to be as well as ever. No isolation is required, because the communicability of the disease seems to disappear by the time the rash appears and the diagnosis is made. There are no known complications, but the disease is often confused with measles or scarlet fever.

CHICKENPOX

Chickenpox is a highly communicable disease produced by the varicella virus. The chief feature is a generalized breaking-out of a characteristic mature lesion, which is a small blister filled with clear fluid and surrounded by a red area. This vesicle dries gradually, becoming depressed at the center; later a flat crust forms. The crust falls off in from one to three weeks. The period of communicability is from about one day prior to the breaking out until the vesicles dry up. Since infectivity precedes the onset of symptoms, little is gained by isolation of patients, but they should be kept out of school for about one week after the appearance of the rash.

The disease is usually induced at the first exposure after 6 months of age. It is most frequent between 2 and 8 years of age. The principal serious complications, which are rare, are encephalitis and pneumonia.

The chief public health importance of chickenpox lies in its possible confusion with smallpox. Also, the virus seems identical to the virus which causes *herpes zoster,* also known as *shingles,* an inflammation of certain nerve ganglia which produces small vesicles on the skin in the areas supplied by the infected nerves. The differences in response to the same virus seem to depend in some way upon localization of the virus and its persistence in the tissues.

MUMPS

Mumps is an acute virus disease affecting chiefly the salivary glands, especially the parotid salivary glands. The swelling of these glands appears abruptly and slowly subsides over a 1- or 2-week period. The disease produces moderate symptoms of fever, headache, and vomiting, which precede the swelling by one or two days. The swelling causes pain in the back and the neck when the victim opens his mouth.

The infectious process of mumps may affect not only the salivary glands but also the pancreas, testes, and ovaries, as well as the central nervous system and other organs. Symptoms of extension to other glands and structures usually develop from four to seven days after the onset of the swelling of the salivary glands, when this swelling is beginning to subside. Such extensions most often occur in males 15 to 25 years old. An affected testis may shrink to some extent and lose its ability to produce sperm, but complete sterility seldom is produced since both testes are rarely involved. The analogous infection of the ovaries in mature females is much less frequent, but does occur.

The largest number of children are attacked by mumps in the early school years, owing to their greater opportunity for exposure at this time. The age distribution of mumps is somewhat older than that for the other childhood diseases, and it is not unusual for individuals to escape infection until young adult life. Contracting of mumps in adult life is dangerous because of the greater risk of infectious extension at this time. Immunity is generally lifelong, but a second attack is reported frequently.

Vaccination has been shown to have protective value. But the degree and duration of protection conferred has not been well determined. Consequently, it is not yet desirable to vaccinate children, since having the disease in childhood is preferable to escaping it then and possibly acquiring it in adult life when the protection by a vaccine has been lost.

HEMOLYTIC STREPTOCOCCI

The streptococci are a large group of bacteria which have in common the properties of roundness and ability to form chains during the process of reproduction (see Chapter 15). These organisms are of great importance in human disease, particularly in childhood diseases.

The streptococci that are of major importance in disease produce *hemolysis,* the separation of hemoglobin from red blood cells, with the destruction of the red cell. The hemolytic streptococci have been subdivided into about a dozen groups (Groups A, B, C, etc.). Only the ones in Group A are important in human disease.

There are approximately 46 types of Group A hemolytic streptococcal bacteria; they cause a wide variety of diseases, which are usually differentiated according to (1) portal of entry, (2) the tissue in which the infectious agent is localized, and (3) the presence of a scarletinal rash. The more important conditions are *scarlet fever* and *streptococcal sore throat* (streptococcal tonsillitis, streptococcal pharyngitis). Rheumatic fever is also caused by this group of bacteria.

Scarlet fever (scarlatina) and streptococcal sore throat.   Scarlet fever is a streptococcal sore throat in which the infectious organism is capable of producing a toxin which in turn produces the characteristic scarlet fever rash. If the patient is immune to the toxin, there will be no rash or scarlet fever, but a streptococcal sore throat will result.

Scarlet fever rarely occurs in the first year of a child's life. Most commonly it occurs in children between 5 and 8 years, after which age it decreases in incidence. It occurs chiefly in the fall and winter months, rarely in summer.

The onset of scarlet fever is sudden, with sore throat, vomiting, and fever. The child's temperature remains elevated continuously for several days, then gradually declines, reaching normal in from 10 to 14 days after the onset. Great variations in the severity of scarlet fever have been observed. In one instance, the disease may be so mild that it is difficult to recognize; in another, so severe that the child dies in a few days, sometimes before a rash appears. There are also many complications from the high fever, the toxins, and the streptococcal bacteria. In general, scarlet fever is less severe today than it was in former years; few deaths now result directly from its effects.

The isolation period should be based on the persistence of streptococci in the throat. In uncomplicated cases, transmission is possible mainly during the incubation and fever stage of the disease, which is approximately 10 days. Also, adequate treatment with penicillin will eliminate, within 24 hours, the ability to transmit the disease, although the streptococci may still be present much longer. With the occurrence of complications, the child remains a source of infection for months or even years.

The toxin which produces the rash in scarlet fever is *erythrogenic* (rash-producing or Dick toxin). Consequently, a small amount of this toxin may be injected under the skin. If a small local rash occurs, the result is positive, and the person is susceptible to scarlet fever. This test just gives information as to the susceptibility to the rash and associated scarlet fever; it does not indicate the person's susceptibility to streptococcal infections in general.

Rheumatic fever. Rheumatic fever is a systemic disease that causes characteristic involvement of many organs and tissues. The most important effects of rheumatic fever are upon the heart (see Chapter 13). Other common characteristics are joint pains, various skin eruptions, and chorea (St. Vitus' dance), a convulsive nervous condition.

The primary underlying factor in rheumatic fever is infection in the throat with a Group A hemolytic streptococcus. Continued infection, or repeated reinfection by these organisms, causes the body to become sensitized. After sensitization, repeated infection leads to allergic response, the response varying in nature and degree according to the degree of sensitization. Before sensitization, the throat infection had no systemic effects. All or any one of these streptococcal infections may be unapparent or unrecognized before the onset of rheumatic fever.

Because of the process needed to produce this disease, it is rare in the first years of life, not because infections are uncommon, but because the development of the allergy requires time. The incidence increases from about 5 years of age to between 7 and 10, and then declines. The disease is most prevalent in the temperate zones of the world and in those seasons of the year during which respiratory infections are most frequent. Rheumatic fever has a high family incidence, occurs more in lower socioeconomic groups, and is affected by environment, living conditions, and nutrition.

Unlike many other communicable diseases, rheumatic fever carries with it the threat of future additional heart damage or other complications. Consequently, an individual who has it must maintain a high degree of vigilance for the greater part of his life. Prophylactic dosages of antibiotics should be used before any type of medical or dental work is performed upon him; otherwise he may become contaminated with streptococcal organisms. Colds, influenza, and sore throats are also constant threats of reinfection.

Appendix A includes a list of the more common childhood diseases. The appendix explains these diseases, their symptoms, when they may be passed on, chances of reoccurrence, available immunizations, and other specific information valuable to a parent. Since this check list is a very valuable aid to a family, it should be retained as a ready reference.[1]

IMMUNIZATIONS

Disease prevention through immunization may be achieved in two ways: (1) *Active immunity* is produced through the injection of weakened or killed antigens, which stimulate the body to produce antibodies against a specific disease (see Chapter 15). This method is used before the person is exposed to the disease in question in order to impart long-lasting protection against that disease. (2) *Passive immunity* is achieved through the injection of antibodies which have already been produced by some other animal or person. This is strictly an emergency procedure useful when a person has already been exposed to a disease. The immunity thus obtained is of relatively short duration, as no natural production of antibodies occurs, but it is very useful in certain situations.

SCHEDULES OF IMMUNIZATIONS

Immunization should be started at the proper age. Since some infants will have limited immunity response, the recommended booster doses are intended to insure or maintain immunity. The current practice is to begin active immunization during the second month of life with a triple vaccine (DPT injection), and either a concurrent feeding of oral poliovaccine (OPV or Sabin vaccine), or a concurrent injection of inactivated poliovaccine (IPV or Salk vaccine). These four immunizations should be given in a series, as shown in Appendix C. A routine for recall or booster injections throughout life is outlined also.

Unfortunately, deaths from whooping cough are very common among infants from birth up to 2 months of age, which is about the earliest date DPT injections can be safely started. Consequently the best protection

[1] Further information about any specific disease can be found in reference books such as *Control of Communicable Diseases in Man* (paperback), published by the American Public Health Association, 1790 Broadway, New York, N.Y.; *The Merck Manual,* published by Merck and Company, Rahway, N.J.; *Physicians' Desk Reference,* published by the Medical Economics Corporates, Oradell, N.J.; or *Diseases of Children* (also in paperback), published by Davis Publications, Inc., 44 Portland St., Worcester, Mass.

for the very young infant is to be sure all older children are properly immunized.

RECALL OR BOOSTER INJECTIONS

Recall or booster injections will give a very rapid re-increase in antibody level, as contrasted with the slow increase during and after the initial series. The first recall injection, after the initial series, is of such great importance that it may be considered part of the basic immunizations.

When children up to 6 years of age who have received DPT as infants are exposed to whooping cough, booster injections of whooping cough vaccine should be given. Administration of booster doses of diphtheria toxoid, poliomyelitis, or smallpox vaccine is to be given according to the standard schedule at any age.

IMMUNIZATION HISTORY

Because of the constant movement of families, each family should take it upon itself to originate and maintain an immunization record for each child. This will serve as a reference in an emergency situation and also as a means of keeping all immunizations up to date. Physicians' records of individual immunizations are not forwarded when a family changes doctors or moves to another locality. Consequently, the establishment of a personal health record, such as that in Appendix C, will prove to be a valuable tool.

PRECAUTIONS IN IMMUNIZATIONS

Under some conditions immunizations should be delayed. Injections should be postponed if the person has an acute respiratory infection. Children with eczema or other acute dermatitis ordinarily should not be vaccinated against smallpox because of the risk of generalized vaccinia (cowpox infection).

The initial vaccination against smallpox and poliomyelitis should preferably be done in cool weather during the latter half of the year. An interval of a month or more is desirable between doses of live virus antigens such as smallpox, measles, and poliomyelitis.

ISOLATION AND QUARANTINE

A child who is suspected of having a contagious disease should be separated from others until a diagnosis can be made. One who has the disease should be isolated until the danger of transmitting it to others no longer exists.

There is a distinction between isolation and quarantine. Quarantine consists of compulsory stoppage of travel or movement from, or into, the place of confinement. A ship coming into port is held in quarantine until the port health officer is satisfied, through inspection, that communicable disease is not present. Passengers and crew are confined to the ship and no visitors are permitted. Such a strict quarantine is employed in homes for very few diseases. Home quarantine is of less value than port quarantine since it is seldom strictly enforced. It is customary to quarantine against smallpox until all contacts have been vaccinated or are shown to be immune. In the case of diphtheria, the members of the household commonly are quarantined until they are shown not to be carriers. For certain other diseases such as whooping cough, measles, chickenpox, mumps, and scarlet fever, exposed children are merely excluded from school.

An appropriate period of isolation depends on the duration of communicability (Appendix A) of the disease. For some diseases, this period is determined by the presence or absence of the causative agents. Statistical studies have shown that after a certain time has elapsed, the child no longer transmits the disease to susceptible persons. By means of such observations, suitable isolation periods have been established for each disease.

DISEASES OF ANY AGE GROUP

THE COMMON COLD

The common cold stands today as the most common infectious disease in the United States and probably in the entire world. No other infectious disease causes as much absenteeism from work and school, personal inconvenience, and discomfort. Yet the cold remains the least preventable and treatable infectious disease.

It is believed that 50 or more different viruses can cause the symptoms known as "the common cold"—sore throat; stuffy, runny nose; sneezing; coughing; and watery eyes. The first symptoms usually include a scratchy feeling in the throat, a chilly feeling at a normally comfortable temperature, and a fatigued feeling. A high fever is *not* a normal symptom of a cold; when it accompanies cold symptoms, a physician should be consulted, as it may indicate a dangerous secondary infection.

Colds are "caught" by transfer of the virus from the nose and mouth discharges of an infected person. This transfer may be through direct contact; through droplets released in sneezing, coughing, or talking; or indirectly through contact with eating utensils or other articles contaminated by an infected person. Colds often seem to arise quickly after chilling or rapid cooling off after overheating. Such environmental factors may act by causing changes in the mucous membranes, which allow invasion by viruses already present. Colds are most contagious during their early stages, especially the first day. No transmission occurs beyond five days after the onset of symptoms. In fact, any cold symptoms remaining after five days are usually not the result of the original cold virus, but of secondary bacterial infection of the virus-damaged mucous membranes.

PREVENTION

Unfortunately, no suggestions can be given which will guarantee the prevention of the common cold. Even if all reasonable precautions were taken, the average person could expect at least one cold a year and possibly two or three. It is only common sense, however, to take certain precautions such as avoiding unnecessary contact with people having colds, maintaining general good health through adequate rest and nutrition, and dressing for the weather—neither too much clothing nor too little. No effective immunization against colds has been developed so far, probably because of the many viruses which can cause colds, the high incidence of mutations among these viruses, and the slight degree of active immunity (if any) which results from actually having a cold.

TREATMENT

Despite the introduction each year of "miraculous" nonprescription cold remedies, there is still no specific cure for the common cold. The apparent effectiveness of the cold remedies stems from their psychological effect and from the fact that many colds terminate spontaneously while still in the early stages. Most of the folk remedies (they are too numerous to list) prove worthless upon scientific investigation.

Although we commonly speak of "fighting a cold," the best advice to the person with an early cold is "don't fight it." The best treatment for a cold is still to stay in bed during the early stages. Aspirin often helps relieve some of the discomfort at this time. The result of "fighting" a cold is often severe secondary bacterial infection, especially of the ear or sinuses. The symptoms of these secondary infections may linger for weeks. Though antibiotics are useless against the virus stage of a cold, they may be necessary to clear up the secondary bacterial infections.

INFLUENZA

The word "influenza" or "flu" is commonly applied to many conditions as well as to the actual disease. Virus infections of many types and even bacterial intestinal infections are sometimes incorrectly called "flu." The true influenza is a virus infection of the respiratory tract characterized by very rapid onset of fever, chills, headache, muscular aches, and severe coughing. Marked prostration is typical, and after several days the symptoms may resemble those of a cold. Recovery usually occurs in two to seven days. Influenza often occurs in massive epidemics, sometimes sweeping over the entire world. The importance of influenza lies in the great numbers of people disabled at the same time—so many that the functioning of the community is disrupted. Uncomplicated influenza rarely leads to the death of an otherwise healthy person, but the death rate always rises during epidemics. A recent epidemic in the United States resulted in 57,000 deaths in excess of the normal death rate, mostly of elderly persons or those already suffering from some chronic disease. In such persons, influenza often leads to bacterial pneumonia, which is the actual cause of death.

Many types and strains of viruses have been associated with influenza. The types are called A, B, and C. Types A and B are the most common; several strains of each type have been isolated. The Asian influenza virus is one of the Type A viruses. Influenza is transmitted through virus contained in the discharges from the nose and mouth of infected persons.

The best prevention for influenza is vaccination followed by annual booster vaccinations. Vaccination is especially important for older persons, pregnant women, persons with chronic diseases, persons who have much public contact, and persons engaged in essential community services.

TETANUS

Tetanus (lockjaw) is a disease resulting from an exotoxin, produced by the bacterium *Clostridium tetani*. This bacillus is commonly found in the soil and fecal discharges of man and animals.

The organism is harmless when growing in the digestive tract, but when introduced into the body by way of a wound, it is able to grow and induce the disease tetanus. Its growth in a wound produces no local tissue damage and no characteristic lesion, but it does produce the exotoxin. This exotoxin has a special affinity for nervous tissue, finds its way into the central nervous system, and induces the characteristic signs and symptoms of tetanus. The effects of the toxin are shown by an early difficulty in opening the mouth (lockjaw), convulsions, spasms in the back muscles, and later a rigid neck. One-half to two-thirds of the victims die.

Tetanus is not contagious nor transmissible directly from one person to another. Contamination of a wound is the only means of inducing the disease. There is no natural immunity against tetanus, but the artificial immunizing process is one of the most effective procedures known. Consequently, immunization of all children and adults, with the goal of providing protection against tetanus for the entire population, should be encouraged.

The duration of immunity is temporary and varies from person to person. However, it is recommended that routine booster injections of tetanus toxoid be administered with diphtheria (adult TD booster) on a 5-year basis, but it is felt that even 10-year intervals would be adequate for most persons, and 15-year for some.

The spores of the tetanus bacillus are highly resistant; they may survive in nature for years. Tetanus bacilli are found in the intestinal tract of many animals, even occasionally in man, accounting for their abundance in the soil, especially if it has been manured. Because of their great abundance and small size, spores are blown in the air and may settle in household dust, street grime, or on a sharp object, a refuse heap, or a great variety of other objects. Burns, compound fractures, or *any wound* in which there may be soil or dust contamination is likely to produce tetanus. Many tetanus deaths occur among auto accident victims who are not immunized. Cases of tetanus in women are on an increase because of the increased activity of women in outdoor sports.

Nonimmunized individuals may be prevented from developing tetanus by an injection of an antitoxin as soon as possible after an injury. A decision as to which wounds require antitoxin is sometimes difficult to make; in cases of doubt the antitoxin should always be given. The antitoxin is prepared in horses; the fluid portion is the serum of the blood of the horse. Unfortunately, horse serum often causes violent and, at times, deadly allergy reactions. Consequently, an individual should always be tested for his sensitivity to horse serum before the antitoxin is given. A *human donor blood* antitoxin is now available that reduces the effect of reactions; unfortunately, this human serum is rare and very expensive. In the long run, an initial series of tetanus injections and *routine boosters* provide the easiest and cheapest means of tetanus protection.

INFECTIOUS HEPATITIS

Infectious hepatitis is a virus infection of the liver, leading to symptoms that include fever, loss of appetite, nausea, and general ill feeling; it may be followed later by jaundice (yellowing of the skin). Infectious hepatitis is more severe in adults than in children, but is rarely fatal. Many cases in children are probably not diagnosed, owing to their mild symptoms. Severe cases in adults are often followed by a long convalescent period. This disease is of worldwide occurrence.

The sources of infection are the feces, urine, blood, and probably the nose and throat discharges of infected persons. Transmission is through close personal contact, blood transfusions, or contaminated needles used for injections. Epidemics have been traced to sewage contamination of water, milk, or food, especially raw oysters and clams.

A similar disease, serum hepatitis, is characterized by the same symptoms, but is transmissible only through blood or blood products (including contaminated injection needles). The incubation period of serum hepatitis is usually 80 to 100 days; that of infectious hepatitis is about 25 days. Apparently two different viruses are involved.

The preventive measures for infectious hepatitis will also provide protection against serum hepatitis. Good personal hygiene and sanitary sewage disposal are important in the prevention of infectious hepatitis. Careful selection of blood donors and thorough sterilization of syringes, needles, and finger puncture stylets is important in the prevention of either type. Skin tattooing instruments are often responsible for hepatitis transmission, as are the injection needles and instruments of drug addicts. Exposed persons can be temporarily protected from infection through the use of gamma globulin.

INFECTIOUS MONONUCLEOSIS

Infectious mononucleosis is a viral infection, centering in the lymph glands and characterized by sore throat, fever, and swelling of the lymph glands. The white blood cell count rises markedly, especially the count of the large monocytes. The disease is rarely fatal, but often results in a general weakness lasting from a few weeks to several months. In children the disease is generally mild and difficult to recognize. The most severe cases usually occur in young adults. Infectious mononucleosis is worldwide in distribution, occurring most commonly in college students and military personnel.

Infectious mononucleosis is believed to be transmitted through contact with the respiratory discharges of infected persons. Since kissing is one good method of transmission, and since the disease is rather common on college campuses, it is sometimes called the "kissing disease." No preventive methods are known.

BACTERIAL MENINGITIS

Bacterial meningitis is an infection of the meninges (membranes covering the brain and spinal cord) by the meningococcus, *Neisseria meningitidis*. The symptoms of such infection include sudden onset of fever, intense headache, nausea, and often a rash. Delirium and coma often follow. The previous fatality rate of 40 to 50 percent has been reduced to about 5 percent through antibiotic therapy.

Meningitis is of worldwide occurrence. Sporadic cases are reported throughout the year, with epidemic waves starting every 7 to 11 years and lasting 2 to 3 years. Meningitis reaches its highest incidence among military personnel and other persons living under crowded conditions, such as in barracks and institutions.

A high degree of natural resistance exists among the general population, resulting in many exposed persons' becoming *symptomless carriers*. During nonepidemic periods it is estimated that from 10 to 25 percent of the population may be healthy carriers; during epidemics more than half of the members of a military command may become carriers. Symptomless carriers are important as sources of infection, as their nose and throat discharges carry the bacteria. Transmission of the disease requires direct or fairly close contact, since the meningococcus (like the closely related gonococcus) is rapidly killed through chilling or drying.

Preventive measures include avoiding direct contact and droplet infection and prevention of overcrowding in living quarters, working places, and public transportation. During epidemics, mass treatment with protective drugs is sometimes used to reduce the incidence, but drug-resistant strains of meningococcus are reducing the effectiveness of such treatment.

STAPHYLOCOCCAL INFECTIONS

The many strains of *Staphylococcus aureus* are among the most widespread and common bacteria infecting man. The staphylococci produce a great variety of infections ranging from tiny skin pustules to massive blood-borne infections of the entire body, leading to death. Staphylococcal ("staph") infections are usually characterized by the formation of pus and abscesses (pus-filled cavities). The infective ability of each strain of staph depends upon the type and quantity of enzymes and toxins it produces. The known strains range from nonpathogenic to highly virulent.

Some commonly occurring staphylococcal infections of the skin include boils, abscesses, carbuncles, impetigo, and infected cuts and abrasions. In more severe cases the bacteria may infect the lungs or be carried by the blood to infect the bones, joints, inner lining of the heart, or even the brain.

Staphylococcal infections are a major problem in hospitals, especially in nurseries and surgical sections. If a pathogenic strain is introduced into the hospital nursery, it may spread rapidly through the highly susceptible population. Most infants suffer only skin infections, but more serious infections sometimes occur. Staphylococcal infection following surgery has increased in importance as surgical procedures have become more complex and the patients more elderly. The patient who has a chronic illness is often highly susceptible to staph infection.

Hospital-acquired staph infections are often introduced into the

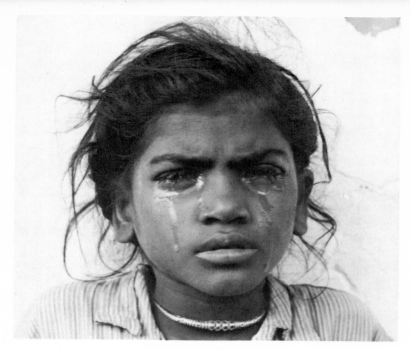

Fig. 17.1 Untreated trachoma. The eyes show serious inflammation which, if untreated, may lead to permanent blindness. (From *World Health,* the Magazine of the World Health Organization.)

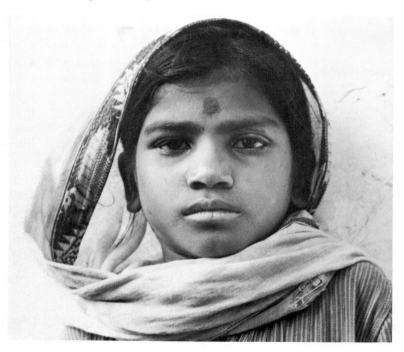

Fig. 17.2 Treated trachoma. The eyesight of this child has been saved by prompt treatment with antibiotics. (From *World Health,* the Magazine of the World Health Organization.)

home, where infections may alternate between members of the family for many months. Newborn infants are more likely to bring home such infections than are adults. A major obstacle in treating hospital-acquired staph infections is their high degree of resistance to drugs. Over 90 percent of such infections involve strains of bacteria that are resistant to penicillin or other commonly used antibiotics.

The most important source of infectious staphylococci is the pus and other discharges from staph infections. Transmission may be direct or through contact with contaminated articles. Potentially dangerous staph organisms can be found almost everywhere, since 30 to 40 percent of all healthy persons carry pathogenic staphylococci in their nasal cavities. Such persons may infect themselves or others.

Preventive measures applicable in the home include strict personal cleanliness (soap and water), avoidance of shared use of towels or other toilet articles, prompt treatment of any infections which appear, and careful disposal of dressings or other objects contaminated with discharges from infections. Hospitals should strictly enforce rules designed to reduce the danger of infection (too numerous to elaborate here), and patients and visitors should respect and follow these rules. Certain highly potent antibiotics should be reserved for use only for resistant staphylococcal infections, as their widespread use would hasten the development of staph strains resistant to even these drugs.

DISEASES OF WORLDWIDE IMPORTANCE

TRACHOMA

Trachoma is a chronic viral infection of the eyes, which, because of its serious threat to vision, is the world's most important eye infection (Fig. 17.1). Trachoma is worldwide in occurrence. High prevalence is usually associated with poverty, poor sanitation, and crowded living conditions, especially in dry, dusty areas. In the United States today, the disease remains a problem only among North American Indians and Mexican immigrants in the Southwest.

The virus of trachoma is spread through the eye discharges of infected persons. The disease produces extreme inflammation of the eye, with deformity of the eyelids and damage to the cornea, leading to visual disability and blindness. In some parts of the world, 5 percent of the population are blind or near-blind as the result of trachoma.

The prevention of blindness includes the finding and prompt treatment of all infected persons (Fig. 17.2). In addition, improved basic sanitation is required, including the use of soap, water, and clean personal towels and other toilet articles. Children should be taught to always wash their hands before touching their faces.

MALARIA

Although great strides have been made in the control of malaria in many countries, including the United States, it is still a major problem in many tropical and subtropical areas, such as parts of Africa, Asia, Central and South America, and the Southwest Pacific. Malaria is the result of infection by protozoa (several species of *Plasmodium*), which are transmitted from man to man only by certain species of *Anopheles* mosquitoes (Fig. 17.3). Such mosquitoes are common almost everywhere in the world. No direct man-to-man transmission is possible, except through blood transfusions or contaminated hypodermic needles.

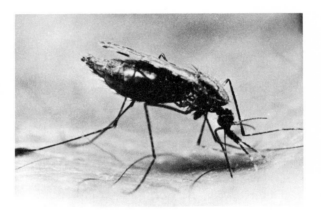

Fig. 17.3 Anopheles mosquito. This mosquito, shown puncturing the skin of a person, is of a malaria-transmitting species. (From *World Health,* the Magazine of the World Health Organization.)

An untreated case of malaria may last for years and is characterized by repeated cyclic attacks. Each attack is usually accompanied by weakness, chills, fever, headache, nausea, and profuse sweating. Long-term results include anemia and general weakness, with up to a 10 percent fatality rate. However, fatalities are rare in treated cases. Many effective drugs are available for treatment, but the development by some strains of *Plasmodium* of resistance to the newer antimalarial drugs has forced a return to the older drug quinine in treating some cases of malaria.

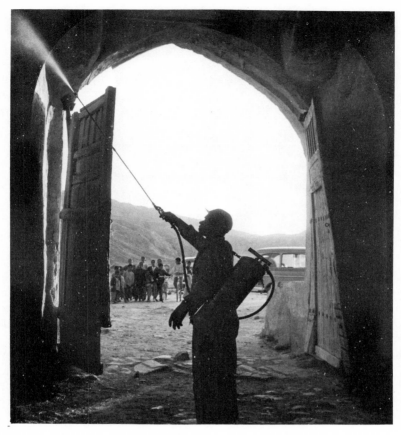

Fig. 17.4 Malaria control. A mosquito-spraying operation in Persia for the control of malaria-transmitting mosquitoes. (From *World Health,* the Magazine of the World Health Organization.)

The prevention of malaria is primarily through mosquito suppression, including elimination of breeding places, chemical control of larvae and adult mosquitoes, screening of houses, and use of repellents (Fig. 17.4). In certain situations, antimalarial drugs are used as a preventive measure.

YAWS

Yaws is a tropical disease, particularly common in equatorial Africa, the Philippines, Southeast Asia, Indonesia, and throughout the South Pacific Islands. Yaws, also known as *frambesia,* is usually contracted during childhood; an untreated case lasts for many years. The infective agent of yaws is a spirochete very similar to that of syphilis. Although a nonvenereal disease, yaws is in some ways similar to syphilis. Infection occurs through direct contact with the skin of an infected person. About a month after contact, a lump called a "mother yaw" appears at the point of infection. Within a few weeks or months, mild generalized lesions develop over the skin and bones. Successive crops of such lesions occur for several months or years. After 5 or 10 years, the late stage occurs, with permanently destructive lesions of the skin and bones, resulting in crippling and disfiguration. Unlike syphilis, the central nervous system and other vital organs are not involved and there is no congenital transmission. Yaws is not usually fatal.

The most successful approach to the control of yaws has been through mass treatment of all persons in heavily infected communities and selective mass treatment of infected persons and their contacts in less heavily infected localities. A single injection of long-acting penicillin can cure yaws. Also important in prevention of yaws are improved sanitation and social and economic conditions.

TUBERCULOSIS

Historically, tuberculosis has been a major cause of death in most of the countries of the world. For many years, tuberculosis (then called *consumption*) was the number one cause of death in the United States. Today, the death rate from tuberculosis has been reduced to a low level in the United States and many other economically fortunate countries because of improvements in housing, nutrition, working conditions, and the general standard of living of the masses. But tuberculosis remains a major cause of death in countries and regions with a low standard of living and among the underprivileged classes of many other countries.

Tuberculosis is a chronic infection by a rod-shaped bacterium, *Mycobacterium tuberculosis*. The usual site of infection is in the lungs, but *any* part of the body may be infected. The principal source of infection is bacteria carried by the respiratory discharges (through coughing, sneezing, or talking) of infected persons. These bacteria are more resistant to drying and chemical agents than are most pathogens, but can be destroyed by exposure to direct sunlight, high temperature (not lukewarm dishwater), and certain disinfectants. They can remain alive for long periods of time in dried sputum in a dark place. Dried respiratory droplets containing the bacteria may be suspended in the air as dust. Infection most commonly occurs when the bacteria are inhaled into the lungs. Drinking unpasteurized milk from tuberculous cows may cause infection of the digestive system.

Following lung infection, the disease may take one of several courses. Rarely does the infection spread rapidly through the lungs, leading to the swift death of the person. More commonly the infection spreads slowly through the lungs and, if left untreated, leads to death after a period of years. Many people have the ability to confine a tuberculosis infection to a small area of the lung where the bacteria may remain alive but inactive for several years. Such resistive ability is thought to depend upon many factors, including nutritional state, fatigue, and race. Inactive cases sometimes become active at a later time when the physical condition of the infected person is weakened.

Despite the reduced incidence of tuberculosis in the United States, it remains an important personal responsibility to prevent or detect tuberculosis infection. Personal prevention today consists mainly of avoiding contact with known or suspected active cases and avoiding places frequented by such individuals. Skid-row alcoholics have a very high incidence of tuberculosis; any place frequented by these derelicts is likely to be contaminated with tuberculosis bacteria. Maintenance of a high level of general health and nutrition is important for resisting infection when exposure does occur.

Several tuberculosis vaccines have been produced and have had widespread use in several countries, but they have never been extensively used in the United States, owing to their limited effectiveness, possible hazards, and interference with skin tests for tuberculosis (see below). The use of BCG (bacille Calmette-Guerin) vaccine is, however, recommended for high-risk individuals, such as nurses and children in contact with active tuberculosis cases.

DIAGNOSIS

There are two methods of tuberculosis screening in common use today, each having its advantages and limitations. These are chest X rays and tuberculin (skin) tests. Chest X rays are important in detecting tuberculosis and other lung disorders, although they may not reliably distinguish tuberculosis from the other disorders nor active from inactive tuberculosis. Nor will chest X rays detect tuberculosis in other areas of the body.

In tuberculin testing, a purified extract of killed tuberculosis bacteria (called *tuberculin*) is injected into the skin. If the person has, *or has ever had,* tuberculosis, a local inflammation will occur at the point of the injection. The tuberculin reaction becomes positive about four to six weeks after the first tuberculosis infection and remains positive; thus tuberculin testing cannot distinguish between active and inactive cases. The tuberculin test described above is the Mantoux test, the most widely used of the tuberculin tests. In other variations of tuberculin testing, the material is scratched or punched into the skin. When both the X-ray and tuberculin tests indicate possible tuberculosis, the confirming test for active tuberculosis is the bacteriologic examination of the sputum or other secretions for the presence of tuberculosis bacteria.

TREATMENT

Despite the vast improvement that has been made in the treatment of tuberculosis, its complete cure remains a very slow process. Active cases should be isolated and preferably hospitalized to prevent infection of family and other contacts. The sputum usually becomes free of bacteria within six months after treatment begins; the person is then no longer infective. A complete cure takes much longer, however.

YELLOW FEVER

Yellow fever is an often-fatal virus disease transmitted only by certain mosquitoes. Fortunately, yellow fever has been entirely eliminated from many countries where it was once common or epidemic. Many years have passed since the last epidemic occurred in the United States. Yellow fever occurs today primarily as sporadic cases in the jungle areas of Mexico, Central and South America, and Africa, with occasional outbreaks in cities bordering upon jungles.

Yellow fever is an acute disease, lasting just a few days, but having a 5 to 40 percent fatality rate. The higher death rate is characteristic for persons born in areas where yellow fever does not occur and who travel into a yellow fever area. Apparently over the years a selection for yellow fever tolerance has taken place among native populations of disease areas.

The yellow fever virus attacks the liver, causing severe jaundice; there is bleeding from many areas of the body, possibly through destruction of the platelets necessary for the clotting of blood. There is typically bleeding from the nose and mouth and vomiting of blood. Those persons surviving yellow fever are left with a lifelong immunity to the disease.

The reduction in the incidence of yellow fever has been partly the result of intensive control measures directed against its mosquito vectors, especially *Aedes aegypti*. This mosquito, which breeds primarily in artificial containers around human dwellings (Fig. 17.5), has been completely eliminated from some areas; an ambitious program is now underway for its eradication from the world. Also of prime importance in the reduction of yellow fever has been the widespread use of effective vaccines, which provide an immunity lasting at least 17 years. Vaccination is important for all persons living in or traveling through yellow fever areas and is required by law by many countries for travelers coming from or through yellow fever zones.

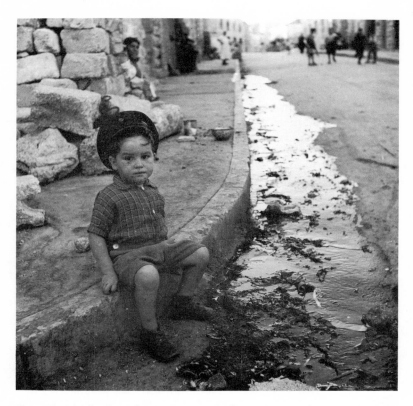

Fig. 17.5 Aedes breeding situation. *Aedes aegypti* is the most domesti-
cated of all mosquitoes. This mosquito multiplies abundantly
in small quantities of water resulting from human activities.
Notice the bites on this small boy. (From *World Health,* the
Magazine of the World Health Organization.)

DENGUE (DENGUE FEVER)

Dengue is a virus disease transmitted by mosquitoes of the genus
Aedes. Explosive epidemics of this disease occur in the Pacific islands,
Southeast Asia, Indonesia, India, and northern Australia. The last outbreak in the United States was in the Rio Grande Valley of Texas in
1942.

The fatality rate of dengue is very low, but the disease is very dis-
abling, the suffering intense, and the recuperation period long. Symptoms of dengue include fever, rash, and pain in the muscles and joints.

Dengue is currently best prevented by control of *Aedes* mosquitoes.
Research is being done on vaccines, but none is yet commercially available.

SMALLPOX

It is hard to visualize the terror in which people must have lived when smallpox raged unchecked. Smallpox was once as common throughout the world as chickenpox is today, but with a death rate of 30 to 40 percent of all cases (Fig. 17.6). After its introduction into the Western Hemisphere by the Spaniards, smallpox wiped out 50 percent of all American Indians. Periodic epidemics throughout the world killed millions (an estimated 60 million Europeans died of smallpox during the seventeenth century).

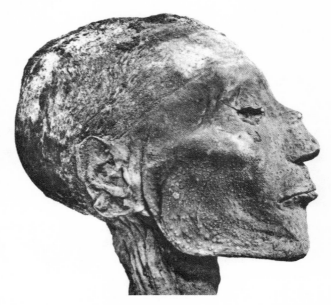

Fig. 17.6 Smallpox. Smallpox struck not only the common people, but also the great. The mummified face of the Egyptian Pharaoh Ramses V shows clear traces of smallpox. (From *World Health,* the Magazine of the World Health Organization.)

Although Edward Jenner, the imaginative English physician, developed smallpox vaccination from cowpox (vaccinia) virus in the 1790s, much of the world's population is still threatened by this dread disease. During a recent year there were 100,000 cases of smallpox, leading to 25,000 deaths. The problem lies in the need for revaccination every three to five years in order to maintain maximum protection against smallpox. Even in the medically enlightened United States, *very few adults* are up to date with their smallpox vaccinations. All that might be required for an epidemic would be one infected person entering and traveling through the United States. On several occasions infected persons have entered the country, but intensive efforts by public health authorities have *so far* prevented mass epidemics.

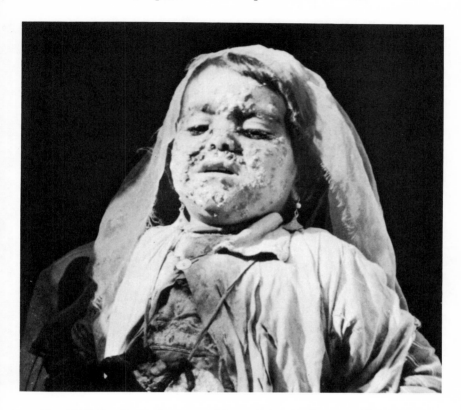

Fig. 17.7 Smallpox. A young girl struck by smallpox in Afghanistan. Her parents have dressed her in her finest clothes as if to protect her from evil. (From *World Health,* the Magazine of the World Health Organization.)

Smallpox is a highly communicable disease caused by the variola virus, which is present, during the course of the disease, in lesions of the skin (Fig. 17.7) and mucous membranes of the nose and throat and in the digestive tract, the blood, the feces, and the urine.

This disease is contagious from the beginning of the earliest symptoms until all the lesions have healed. It is transmitted by direct contact with the skin lesions; by droplets from the nose and throat lesions being projected from the respiratory tract of an infected individual through breathing, coughing, or spitting; and also by dried infectious material from healing lesions being suspended in airborne dust particles. Indirect transmission takes place through contamination of bed clothes, drinking glasses, eating utensils, or other personal articles.

Smallpox may occur in any exposed person, regardless of age, who is not immune because of a previous attack or by vaccination. If it were not for vaccination, smallpox would be chiefly a disease of childhood.

Three major types of the variola-vaccinia virus group have been recognized: (1) variola major, or smallpox; (2) variola minor, or alastrim; and (3) vaccinia, or cowpox. These viruses are closely related and have essentially the same physical characteristics and properties; they may be distinguished by the reactions they produce in man and experimental animals. Exposure to any one of the three produces immunity for the complete group. Consequently, the vaccination for smallpox consists of introducing vaccinia virus into the skin for the purpose of inducing cowpox in order to prevent smallpox. Cowpox, a disease normally affecting cattle, but communicable to man, is less virulent and less serious for both cattle and man than is smallpox for man.

CHOLERA

Cholera is a very serious acute disease resulting from the infection of the digestive tract by a bacterium, *Vibrio cholerae*, also called *Vibrio comma*. In past centuries, cholera has swept over most of the world. Today it is still a great scourge in parts of India, Iraq, and southern China, and in recent years epidemics have occurred in parts of Egypt, Thailand, Indonesia, the Philippines, Hong Kong, Macao, Korea, Taiwan and Malaysia. No cases have been reported in the United States for many years.

The incubation period for cholera is only a few hours or days. The disease is marked by a very profuse diarrhea, persistent vomiting, cramps, and profound sweating. The stools consist of little more than water with flakes of mucus and occasionally streaks of blood. In many outbreaks, most of the patients die, although proper care reduces the fatality rate. Death is the result of dehydration.

The source of infection of cholera is the feces and vomitus of infected persons, transmitted through contaminated water, contaminated food, flies, and direct contact.

Prevention of cholera involves sanitary sewage disposal, protection and purification of water supplies, pasteurization of milk, sanitary preparation of foods, and fly control. Cholera vaccine is available for use in epidemics, for persons traveling into cholera areas, and for those subject to unusual risk. The immunity produced, however, is of short duration—not more than six months.

TYPHOID FEVER

Typhoid fever has a worldwide distribution and is a major public health problem in many countries. In the United States its incidence has dropped considerably to about 600–700 cases per year. Typhoid fever is caused by the bacterium *Salmonella typhosa*. This bacterium invades the entire body, producing fever, general ill feeling, loss of appetite, and headache. The pulse is slow and rose-colored spots appear on the body. A fatality rate of about 10 percent can be reduced to 2 or 3 percent with antibiotic therapy.

The source of infection is the feces and urine of infected persons. Symptomless carriers are a problem with this disease. The bacteria may live in the gall bladder for many years, being passed with the feces. Transmission of the bacteria is through direct or indirect contact with patients or carriers, contaminated food or water, and flies.

Prevention of typhoid fever involves sanitary sewage disposal, safe water supplies, fly control, and vaccination.

LEPROSY (HANSEN'S DISEASE)

The fear of leprosy is almost without parallel, owing to the body mutilations produced by the advanced disease, exaggeration of its infectiousness, and ignorance of the benefits of modern treatment. Leprosy is a chronic, moderately communicable, bacterial infection of the skin, with infiltration of nerves, muscles, and bones (Fig. 17.8). Atrophy and deformity of the extremities occurs in advanced cases (Fig. 17.9). The progress of the disease is very slow, and death seldom results from it.

The number of cases of leprosy (also called Hansen's disease) is estimated at 5 to 12 million. Most of these cases occur in the tropics and subtropics, especially in Africa and Asia. A small number of cases occur in the United States, primarily in Hawaii and southeastern Texas.

The infectious agent of leprosy is the bacterium *Mycobacterium leprae*, related to the one which produces tuberculosis. Leprosy is transmitted through contact with the bacteria-laden discharges from the lesions of infected persons. Among persons living in the same household with a leprosy victim, about 30 percent of the males and 15 percent of the females will contract the disease. Leprosy is unique in its long incubation period—usually three to five years or longer.

In controlling leprosy, the old policy of isolating infected persons in hospitals or colonies is being replaced with out-patient treatment. Drugs are available which render a person noninfective in a short period of time and which over a longer period often lead to a complete cure

Fig. 17.8 Early leprosy. Like many other diseases, leprosy is more easily cured if detected in its early stages. (From *World Health,* the Magazine of the World Health Organization.)

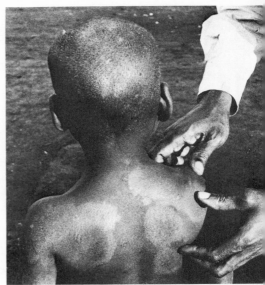

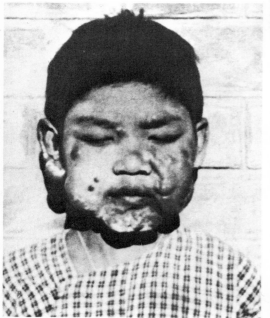

Fig. 17.9 Advanced leprosy. This 8-year-old girl in Burma already has an advanced, seemingly hopeless case of leprosy. (From *World Health,* the Magazine of the World Health Organization.)

Fig. 17.10 Treated leprosy. This is the same girl seen in Fig. 17.9, now 13 years old and entirely free of symptoms after several years of drug treatments. (From *World Health,* the Magazine of the World Health Organization.)

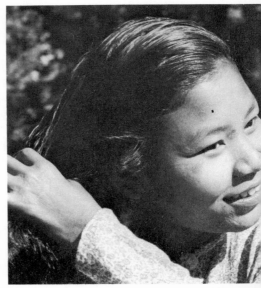

(Fig. 17.10). The compulsory segregation of infected persons formerly acted as an obstacle to leprosy control, since leprosy was often concealed to avoid forced separation of the sufferer from home and friends.

PARASITIC WORMS

The majority of all persons living on earth today are infected by one or more types of parasitic worms. Such parasites are partially responsible for the slow rate of development of many of the nations of the world. Parasitic worms seldom cause the total disability or sudden death of a person, but instead sap him of the strength necessary for progress, individual or national. The infected person needs all his available strength just for the day-to-day processes of living. His life span is decreased considerably, as is his ability to enjoy life while it lasts.

Fortunately, most of the parasitic worms we shall discuss are now relatively scarce, localized, or totally absent in the United States. But with international travel so commonplace and rapid, there is always the possibility that some kinds of parasitic worms will turn up in any town in the United States. The factors which help to minimize the worm problem in the United States include a temperate climate (many worms are favored by tropical climates), good nutrition (important in resisting worm infection), education (knowing what is dangerous and why), sanitary water supplies, sewage and garbage disposal, decent housing, wearing of shoes, and elimination of insect vectors or carriers of the worms. If parasitic worms are to be reduced in importance in other countries, these are the problems which must be solved. People will have to change their eating and living habits. Practices such as eating raw fish and meat or using the same river for bathing, excreting, and drinking will have to be stopped. Certain religious practices and beliefs may have to be revised.

A few of the parasitic worms of great world importance will be discussed below. These discussions are arranged by the method of transmission to man—from person to person, from insect vectors, and from animals to man.

WORMS TRANSMITTED FROM PERSON TO PERSON

HOOKWORMS

Hookworms are small roundworms, less than $\frac{1}{2}$ inch long and quite slender, which attach themselves by oral hooks into the inner lining of the small intestine. There they remain for 5 to 10 years, constantly sucking blood and laying eggs. The effect on man of hook-worm infection is chronic anemia and weakness. These symptoms are usually serious only when the infected person is poorly nourished. A good diet not only prevents anemia from developing, but also enables a person to develop a degree of immunity which results in resistance to infection and loss of worms already harbored.

The eggs of hookworms pass from the intestine with the feces, hatch in the ground, and develop into an infective larval (immature) form. These larvae wait on the soil or vegetation until a barefooted person comes by. The larvae burrow through the skin of the foot into a blood or lymph vessel. They are carried by the blood to the right side of the heart, then into the capillaries of the lungs, where they burrow out into the air sacs. The larvae are then carried by the cilia of the bronchial tubes or coughed up into the throat, where they are swallowed. When they reach the intestine, they attach themselves, develop into adults, and the cycle repeats itself.

The prevention of hookworm infection thus involves three phases: (1) good diet, (2) sanitary disposal of feces, and (3) wearing of shoes. Hookworms remain a problem today only in the economically depressed areas of the southeastern United States, where diet is apt to be poor, sewage disposal inadequate, and shoes worn only occasionally.

ASCARIASIS

Ascariasis is the infection of man by large worms of the genus *Ascaris*. This roundworm often exceeds a foot in length. About two-thirds of the world's population is infected by ascaris worms, probably the most widespread worm infection. The adult ascaris normally lives in the small intestine, where it feeds on partly digested foods and probably sucks some blood. The infected person suffers from loss of appetite and weight; when the worms are abundant (thousands have been removed from a single person), the intestine may be completely blocked, leading to death if the worms are not surgically removed. Toxic products of the worms cause such conditions as nervousness, swelling, convulsions, delirium, and coma. Other complications occur when the worms "wander" into ducts and cavities. They often invade the bile and pancreatic ducts and may travel to the gall bladder or liver.

Ascaris worms lay tremendous numbers of eggs (200,000 per female per day), which pass from the intestine with the feces. In moist soil, the eggs remain alive for up to six years. Infection of man usually occurs when the eggs are swallowed with raw vegetables or from contaminated hands. The eggs hatch in the small intestine, but the larvae take a little tour of the body before settling down. They burrow into the blood vessels of the small intestine; are carried with the blood to the liver, the heart, and the lungs; burrow out into the air sacs; travel up to the throat; and are swallowed in a manner similar to hookworms. When the small intestine is reached the second time, the worms mature into adults, living for nine months to a year.

Like hookworm infection, ascariasis is most common in moist tropical countries. In the United States the disease is most prevalent in the South. The prevention depends upon the use of sanitary toilet facilities, the training of children to wash hands after defecation and before eating and not to eat food dropped on the floor. Washing of raw vegetables is of some importance. Similar worms infect many dogs and almost all pigs, but their infection of man is believed to be uncommon.

PINWORMS

Pinworms, or seatworms, are the most common parasitic worms infecting children in the United States. The Caucasian race is the most susceptible to pinworm infection. Few members of this race manage to get through life without being at some time infected with pinworms. Pinworms are very slender, white roundworms about $\frac{1}{8}$ to $\frac{1}{2}$ inch in length. The worms live in the large intestine and rectum. Mature females emerge from the anus at night, lay eggs around the anus, and retreat back into the rectum, although some worms remain on the skin around the anus.

Pinworm infections are acquired through ingestion of the eggs. An infected child usually scatters the eggs throughout his environment. His hands, clothing, and bed linen are all likely to be contaminated. Carpets, draperies, and furniture are also frequently contaminated. The microscopic eggs are even airborne as dust particles. The air in classrooms containing infected children has been found to carry *hundreds* of pinworm eggs. It is not unusual for an entire family or class to become infected.

The results of a pinworm infection are usually more irritating than serious. The migration of the worms in the anal region causes intense itching, leading to loss of sleep, restlessness, nervousness, and even hysteria. In girls, the worms may cause vaginal inflammation. Contrary to popular belief, pinworms are not a common cause of appendicitis.

Suspected cases of pinworms are sometimes diagnosed by pressing Scotch tape around the anal region early in the morning. If worms are present, the physician can detect the eggs stuck to the tape and will prescribe an effective treatment. All members of the family should be tested.

Pinworm prevention must include use of sanitary toilet facilities, teaching children to wash hands after defecation and always before eating. Children should be discouraged from nail biting or otherwise putting fingers in the mouth or nose. When there is a known infection in a family, all clothing and bed sheets should be laundered daily in *hot* water (washing with warm water can spread the infection). Floors should receive frequent washing or vacuuming. Some authorities feel, however, that extreme efforts to eliminate pinworms completely may lead to a "pinworm neurosis" that is worse than a mild pinworm infection.

PARASITIC WORMS TRANSMITTED BY INSECT VECTORS

FILARIASIS

Filariasis leads to the condition which most people call *elephantiasis*. This disease is common in many tropical countries, but is not present in the United States. Filariasis is caused by microscopic, hairlike roundworms called filaria, which are transmitted from man to man only by mosquitoes of several species. These minute worms live in the lymph ducts and lymph glands of man, causing an allergic reaction producing chills, fever, aches, and pains. In old infections the flow of lymph through the lymph ducts is blocked, causing fluid to build up in the tissues. The result is elephantiasis—a tremendous and grotesque swelling of the arms, legs, breasts, and particularly the scrotum. If left untreated for several years, this swelling becomes permanent.

Filaria worms cannot complete their life cycle without mosquitoes. The female worms give birth to living young, which are carried in the bloodstream of the infected person, but these young worms cannot mature into adults without being taken up by a mosquito. Thus to become heavily infected, a person must be bitten by many infected mosquitoes. Since filariasis is transmitted only by mosquitoes, its control is through elimination of mosquitoes, breeding places, control of adult mosquitoes, screening of houses, and use of insect repellents. Prompt treatment of infected persons also helps to break the chain of infection.

PARASITIC WORMS TRANSMITTED FROM ANIMALS TO MAN

TAPEWORMS

Few human parasites are the subject of as much folklore and misinformation as the tapeworms. Tapeworms are almost paper-thin flatworms, each of which possesses a head bearing hooks and suckers plus a long chain of segments. Some species attain a length of over 30 feet. The adult forms of most species of tapeworms infecting man live in the small intestine, causing digestive disturbances, loss of weight, insomnia, nervousness, and abdominal pain. Each of the several species of tapeworms which commonly infect man will be discussed individually below.

Pork tapeworm. The pork tapeworm (*Taenia solium*) infects man in any part of the world where pork is eaten without being cooked thoroughly. The adult pork tapeworm lives in the small intestine of man. The larval (immature) worms form cysts (knotlike structures) in the flesh of pigs. The cysts are oval, whitish bodies from one-quarter to one-half inch long. When such cysts are eaten by man in poorly cooked pork, the larva attaches itself to the wall of the small intestine and in two or three months grows into a mature tapeworm. A man infected with a pork tapeworm passes several hundred mature segments per month with the feces, each segment containing thousands of eggs. If the eggs are consumed by a pig, then the cycle is completed, and the flesh of that pig will become infected with cysts. The pork tapeworm is particularly dangerous because if the eggs are consumed by man, as on contaminated vegetables, cysts are formed in the muscles, brain, eye, heart, or other vital organs of man. This condition commonly occurs in Mexico and other countries where sanitation is poor. In heavy infections, the fatality rate is high. Thorough cooking of all pork will prevent infection in man.

Beef tapeworm. The beef tapeworm (*Taenia saginata*) has a life cycle similar to the pork tapeworm's, except that cattle rather than pigs serve as the larval host, and only the adult worms, not the larvae, will infect man. The distribution of this tapeworm is worldwide. Thorough cooking will kill the larvae in beef, as will thorough salt curing.

Dwarf tapeworm. The dwarf tapeworm (*Hymenolepis nana*) is the smallest adult tapeworm found in man, seldom exceeding four inches in length, but is the most common tapeworm infecting man. Its distribution is worldwide. This worm differs from almost all other tapeworms in its ability to complete its entire life cycle in the same host. In addition to man, rats and mice are commonly infected. Most human infections are believed to result from contamination of food with rat, mouse, or human feces. The worm eggs consumed with these feces will hatch in the small intestine, pass through several larval stages, and mature into adults. The eggs of this worm sometimes hatch while still in the intestine of an infected man and this may result in massive secondary infection. The dwarf tapeworm does form minute cysts in fleas or grain beetles which have eaten worm eggs from rat or mouse feces. Consumption of these insects by man in contaminated food can lead to an intestinal infection of adult worms. Prevention of infection by the dwarf tapeworm is mainly through control of rats and mice, especially where their feces might contaminate food.

Dog tapeworm. The dog tapeworm, *Dipylidium caninum,* is an extremely common parasite of dogs and cats all over the world. Its cysts are formed in fleas and mature into adults when the fleas are eaten by a dog or cat. Most human infections are in children who have accidentally eaten fleas while playing with a dog or cat. Children are sometimes infected by having their faces licked by a dog just after the dog has nipped a flea. Therefore, it is important that pets be kept free of fleas.

Fish tapeworm. The largest tapeworm infecting man is the fish tapeworm, *Diphyllobothrium,* which often exceeds 30 feet in length. The number of worms infecting a single person may be over 100. The infection is acquired by eating raw or poorly cooked fish infected with the larvae of this worm. Infected fish are found primarily in the cold fresh waters of the northern hemisphere, including the Great Lakes region of the United States. In some parts of Alaska, nearly 100 percent of the population is infected. Fortunately, the symptoms of infection are usually mild or absent, although some persons develop severe anemia or toxic symptoms. Fish species commonly infected include pike, salmon, trout, perch, pickerel, burbot, and eel. The life cycle of the fish tapeworm is complex. The adult worm lives in the small intestine of man or other fish-eating mammals. Eggs passed with the feces hatch in fresh water, releasing a larva that must be swallowed by a small crustacean to continue its development. The crustacean must in turn be eaten by a fish, in the flesh of which the worm larva forms a cyst. If the fish is eaten by a man or other mammal, the cycle is complete. The obvious prevention for a fish tapeworm infection is to cook all fish before eating it. As an alternative, freezing of fish for several days at 0°F will kill the encysted larvae. Inspection of fish for cysts is impractical.

TRICHINOSIS

Trichinosis is the invasion of human flesh by the larvae of a parasitic roundworm, *Trichinella spiralis.* Man is infected by eating the poorly cooked flesh of animals containing the encysted larvae of the worm. The usual source of infection is pork, although bear or any meat-eating mammal may carry these larvae. After a man (or any flesh-eating mammal) has eaten diseased flesh, the larvae are freed from their cysts by the digestive juices, pass into the small intestine, become sexually mature, and give birth to living larvae, which penetrate the walls of the intestine. The larvae are then carried by the blood to all parts of the body. Almost every organ and tissue is invaded, but further development of the larvae takes place only in the muscles, where cysts are produced, completing the cycle.

The severity of the symptoms of trichinosis in man depends upon how many larvae are consumed. The disease may range from mild to fatal. The first symptoms occur as early as 24 hours following ingestion of infected meat; they include nausea, diarrhea, and abdominal pain—all resulting from the intestinal activity of the worms. Beginning about seven to nine days later, and continuing for several weeks, the larvae penetrate the muscles and other organs. It is during this period that the serious or fatal symptoms may appear. These symptoms commonly include fever, weakness, muscle soreness and pain, swelling of eyelids, chills, sweating, and difficulty in breathing. When death results, it is usually the result of invasion of the heart muscle. Muscular pains and weakness may continue for several months.

Trichinosis is worldwide in occurrence and is particularly common in the United States. About one in six Americans are infected at some time during their lives. The most effective and cheapest preventive measure is the thorough cooking of all pork or pork products. Butchers should carefully clean pork from meat grinders before grinding beef. Uncooked garbage fed to pigs may be infected by infected pork scraps contained in the garbage; most states outlaw this practice, but enforcement on small farms is virtually impossible. Meat inspection for trichinosis is impractical, costly, and not reliable. Freezing of pork at very low temperature effectively kills the larvae, but home freezers cannot be depended upon to reach these temperatures (20 days at 5°F, 10 days at −10°F, or 6 days at −20°F).

SCHISTOSOMIASIS

About 150 million persons are currently infected with schistosomes or *blood flukes*. These are small, slender flatworms, about ¼ to ½ inch long. Blood flukes are common in Africa, South America, and the Orient, but do not occur in North America. There are several species of blood flukes, each of which prefers to live in specific veins, usually those leading from the large intestine, rectum, and bladder. The symptoms of infection depend upon the veins infected and may be slight or severe. Among the more typical symptoms are fever and dysentery.

The life cycle of each species of schistosome requires a snail (Fig. 17.11) for its completion. The worm eggs leave the body of an infected person with the urine or feces. The egg hatches in water and the larva must then burrow into a suitable species of fresh-water snail. After several weeks, the larva begins to produce thousands of larvae of another form (cercariae), which leave the snail and swim freely through the water. A man entering the water will be infected by the cercariae which penetrate directly through the skin. The larvae enter the blood stream, grow to maturity in the blood vessels of the liver, then migrate as adults into the abdominal veins. Through destruction of tissues, the eggs escape into the urinary bladder or large intestine to leave the body with the urine or feces. Infection of man is also possible through drinking of water containing the cercariae larvae.

Preventive measures include sanitary disposal of feces and urine; drainage of swamps; chemical control of snails; and providing pure water for drinking and bathing, protective clothing for persons who

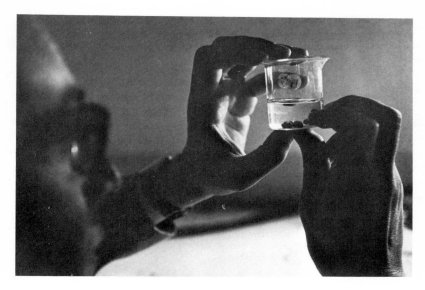

Fig. 17.11 Schistosomiasis. A scientist examines one of the species of water snails serving as hosts for the larvae of blood flukes. New irrigation projects in some parts of the world are increasing the problem of schistosomiasis. (From *World Health,* the Magazine of the World Health Organization.)

must enter contaminated water, and education for persons living in areas of contaminated water.

LIVER FLUKES

A serious health problem in many areas of the Far East (especially Japan, Korea, and China) is *clonorchiasis,* Oriental liver fluke disease. Liver flukes are slender, oval flatworms from one-half inch to one inch long that live in the bile ducts of the liver. In light infections the symptoms may be mild or absent. Severe infections may cause digestive disturbances or liver damage, but seldom lead to death. Infection sometimes lasts for 20 years or more. Man is infected with liver flukes through eating incompletely cooked fish (fresh, dried, salted, or pickled). The life cycle (Fig. 17.12), like that of blood flukes, involves snails. Worm eggs laid in the bile ducts leave the body of man with the feces. The eggs hatch after being eaten by fresh-water snails, which are in turn eaten by fish. The worm larvae form cysts in the flesh of the fish, and man is infected by the infected fish. The best preventive measure, obviously, is to thoroughly cook all fresh-water fish before eating them.

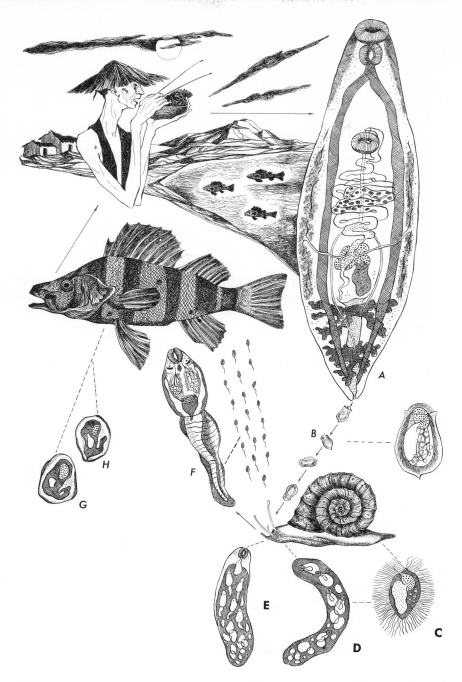

Fig. 17.12 Life cycle of the liver fluke. The adult fluke (A) lays eggs in the human liver and these eggs pass through the bile duct to the intestine and thence to the outside; (B) when the eggs are eaten by a certain species of freshwater snail, they hatch and go through larval stages (C–E) in the snail's body. The tadpole-like cercariae (F) leave the snail and form cysts (G) and (H) in the muscles of a fish. These cysts infect human beings who eat the infected fish. (From W. G. Whaley *et al., Principles of Biology,* New York, Harper & Row, 1964, p. 583.)

OCCUPATIONAL DISEASES

THE PAST

Occupational diseases are diseases which arise as a result of occupational exposure to some harmful element. In the strictest sense, this term includes only those diseases which are specific to a given occupation and are not found among the general public. In a broader sense, many diseases which do occur in the general population may be considered occupational diseases if their incidence is greatly increased within a given occupation.

In years past, it was accepted that many occupations had particular hazards and persons working within those occupations accepted the probability that eventually they would suffer from that occupational disease. Naturally, they did not like the idea, but such hazards were considered to be an unavoidable aspect of the struggle to make a living. Miners, for example, accepted lung diseases as an inevitable part of their way of life. Corporations, large and small, either showed no concern for the health of their employees or lacked the technical ability to overcome occupational hazards.

THE PRESENT

The incidence of occupational diseases has dropped considerably during the past forty to fifty years. This fortunate decrease may be attributed to several important developments. First, technical advances have been made which have either eliminated certain hazardous occupations completely or have increased the safety of the employee. Second, industrial safety laws have been passed to force the improvement of working conditions, and labor unions have often been successful in correcting occupational hazards for their members. Perhaps the most important development has been the realization by most corporation administrators that the health of their employees has a great influence upon the corporation's profit. An experienced, vigorous employee is worth much more to an employer than the same man weakened by an occupational disease or his inexperienced replacement in the event he became completely disabled.

Despite the improvements which have been made, many occupational disease hazards do remain in the United States today. Such hazards may be classified in the following manner.

CHEMICAL HAZARDS

Many occupational diseases result from exposure to chemical substances such as solvents, dusts, and gases. Almost every occupation involves some exposure to potentially dangerous chemicals. Even the office secretary is exposed to such solvents as type cleaners and duplicating fluids. The main portals of entry into the body for occupational chemicals are the lungs for the dusts, gases, and vapors, and the skin for many of the solvents. Although the employer is responsible for providing ventilation and other basic protections against chemicals, it is the duty of the employee to *learn* and *follow* the safety precautions for every chemical with which he has contact. Absence of poisoning symptoms is not proof of adequate protection, since many chemicals will cause *permanent damage to vital organs* long before any noticeable symptoms of poisoning develop.

PHYSICAL HAZARDS

Certain occupational diseases result from physical factors of the environment, such as temperature, noise, and radiation. The effects of temperature extremes depend upon how high or low the temperature is, the humidity, the length of exposure, and the degree of exertion. Exposure to extreme noise, such as that which occurs in factories of many types, may cause a temporary hearing impairment, recovery from which may take days or months, or may result in permanent hearing loss, which reaches a maximum after 5 to 10 years of exposure. The degree of hearing loss depends upon the pitch (frequency) of the sound and its intensity (measured in decibels). Damage begins to occur at 85 to 120 decibels, depending upon the pitch. Some typical noise intensities are:

Jet engine	up to 140 decibels
Drop hammer	up to 130 decibels
Boiler shop	up to 105 decibels
Punch press	up to 105 decibels

Among those types of radiation from which protection must be provided for the employee are gamma ray, X ray, ultraviolet ray, intense visible light, infrared ray, laser, microwave, and the atomic or particulate radiations. As the industrial use of many of these forms of radiation has become widespread, it has become important for the individual employee to learn and observe carefully all safety precautions relating to their use. Some of the harmful effects of overexposure to the forms of radiation are:

Gamma rays, X rays, atomic particles: Same effect. All are ionizing radiations causing permanent damage or death of cells. Chromosome damage leads to abnormal cell division. Effects of repeated small doses are cumulative. Mutations and cancer are produced. Any tissue of the body may be damaged. Large doses are always fatal.

Ultraviolet: Little penetrating ability. Affects only skin and eyes. Burns skin, produces tanning, thickens skin. Causes skin cancer. Inflammation of conjunctiva of eye. Clouding and ulcers of the cornea (usually temporary). Possible clouding of lens (cataract) not proven.

Intense visible light: Inflammation of conjunctiva and cornea. Temporary or permanent loss of vision through damage to retina.

Infrared: Burning of skin. Temporary or permanent damage to retina of eye. Possible cataracts of lens of eye.

Laser beams: Skin burns. Heat injury to any part of eye, especially the retina.

Microwaves (e.g., radar):   Main effect is the production of heat in tissue where absorbed. Cataracts produced.

The precautionary measures which apply to these types of radiation are too numerous and specific for discussion at this point. For further information the reader is directed to Chapter 18. Any person working with or near any radiation should *learn and observe* the precautions applying to that type of radiation.

MECHANICAL FACTORS

Among the mechanical factors which may lead to occupational disease are exposure to high or low atmospheric pressure, physical strain, and unusual movements. In exposure to high or low pressures, the considerations must include not only the effect of the unusual pressure, but also the effect of a sudden *change* in pressure. The effect of a sudden decrease in pressure may be the development of nitrogen bubbles in the blood, causing severe pains, called "the bends," and leading to possible rapid death or permanent physical damage. The nitrogen cannot be held in solution at the lower pressure, so the bubbles appear just as bubbles appear in a bottle of soda after it is opened.

Certain vibrating tools such as drills, grinders, riveters, and sanders may cause spasms of the blood vessels or inflammation of the joints. The most damaging vibrations are those from 2000 to 3000 cycles per minute. Improper lifting and carrying of loads is the most common cause of back trouble. The back should never be bent when lifting, but should be held straight while the knees are bent. Other problems can result from prolonged work in one position, especially prolonged standing still or bending.

INFECTIOUS AGENTS

Some jobs, especially in agriculture, expose a person to infectious disease agents. Several diseases can be contracted from animals or animal products. Certain lung-invading fungi are commonly contracted by agricultural or construction workers through airborne spores of the fungi. Most of these infectious diseases are discussed at other points in this book.

PSYCHOLOGICAL FACTORS

Often underrated as occupational diseases are the psychological factors inherent to certain types of employment. Few generalizations can be made here because a job might be ideally suited to the psychological makeup of one person yet be totally unacceptable to another. The person who is very shy or withdrawn might suffer greatly from a job which required considerable public contact or persuasion. Conversely, the very outgoing person would suffer from a job which involved constant isolation. Fortunately, there are both types of people and both types of work; but it is important that they are suitably matched. Much of the illness for which people miss days of work is believed to be the psychosomatic (psychogenic) result of jobs which are either consciously or subconsciously disliked. As an escape mechanism the person develops a physical illness, which rescues him from his misery for a few days. Industrial accidents are another common result of psychological problems. The accident-prone person may subconsciously want to be hurt. Many large corporations now hire psychologists or psychiatrists to deal with the emotional problems of their employees.

THE FUTURE

New technical advances will bring solutions for many of the occupational hazards of today, but will at the same time produce new hazards. Increased use of various types of radiation and of new and more exotic chemicals will require the observance of safety precautions more rigid than those in the past. More than ever before, the hazards will be obscure or invisible to many employees, who will have to blindly follow regulations which often seem needless to them. Precautions will require an almost military sense of discipline.

WORLD HEALTH ORGANIZATION (WHO)

The World Health Organization, an agency of the United Nations, was organized in 1946 and formally established in 1948, in recognition of the fact that diseases do not respect national boundaries. With today's large numbers of international travelers and the speed of such travel, a disease outbreak may jump from continent to continent in a few hours' time. In addition to fighting infectious diseases, the World Health Organization seeks the improvement of the general level of health of the world's population. Since the infectious diseases have been reduced in importance, the WHO, to achieve its goal, has put greater emphasis upon the problems brought about by the rapid increase in population.

The constitution of the World Health Organization lists its purpose as being

1. To assist governments upon request in strengthening health services.
2. To promote improved standards of teaching and training in the health professions.
3. To provide information, counsel, and assistance in the field of health.
4. To promote improvement in nutrition, housing, sanitation, working conditions, and other aspects of environmental hygiene.
5. To promote among scientific and professional groups cooperation related to health.
6. To promote maternal and child health and welfare.
7. To promote activities in the field of mental health, especially those affecting the harmony of human relations.
8. To promote and conduct research in the field of health.
9. To study social techniques affecting public health.

As world health problems have changed through the years, the World Health Organization has correspondingly shifted the emphasis of its programs and has played an important role in improving the health of the world's population.

SUMMARY

   I. Childhood Diseases and Hazards
     A. Prevention pointers
       1. Periodic physical examination.
       2. Proper nutrition.
       3. Physical fitness.
       4. Immunization program.
       5. Accident prevention.
       6. Parent guidance.
     B. Accidents—rank first as the cause of death in children after the age of infancy.
     C. Diseases
       1. Poliomyelitis
         a. Caused by one of three types of viruses.
         b. Prevented through immunization.
       2. Diphtheria
         a. Caused by the bacillus *Corynebacterium diphtheriae*.
         b. Prevention is by immunization in DPT vaccine.
       3. Whooping cough (pertussis)
         a. Caused by the bacillus *Hemophilus pertussis*.
         b. Prevention through DPT vaccine.
       4. Measles (rubeola)
         a. Caused by the rubeola virus.
         b. Protection by one of the highly effective vaccines available.
       5. German measles (rubella)
         a. Caused by the rubella virus.

       b. May cause congenital malformations if contracted by a woman in the first three months of pregnancy.

    6. Roseola (baby measles)—probably caused by a virus.

    7. Chickenpox

       a. Caused by the varicella virus.

       b. Same virus is the cause of shingles.

    8. Mumps

       a. Causative agent is a virus.

       b. Vaccines are still in developmental stage.

    9. Hemolytic streptococci

       a. Streptococci bacteria which destroy red blood cells are *hemolytic*.

       b. Important results of these bacteria include:

          (1) scarlet fever

          (2) "strep" throat

          (3) tonsilitis

          (4) rheumatic fever

  D. Immunizations

    1. Active immunity—produced through the injection of antigens which stimulate the body to produce its own antibodies.

    2. Passive immunity—achieved through the injection of antibodies which were produced by some other animal or person.

    3. Schedules of immunizations:

       a. Should be started at the proper age.

       b. Recall or booster injections should be given according to the schedule in Appendix C.

       c. Every family should maintain an Immunization Record for each member of the family (a form for this purpose provided in Appendix C).

II. Diseases of Any Age Group

  A. Common cold—remains as the most common and least preventable communicable disease.

  B. Influenza—a virus infection of the respiratory tract characterized by fever, chill, headache, muscular aches, and coughing.

  C. Tetanus (lockjaw)

    1. Result of an exotoxin produced by the bacterium *Clostridium tetani*.

    2. Immunization with tetanus toxoid provides highly effective protection.

    3. Booster injections at 5-year intervals are necessary to maintain immunity.

    4. Nonimmunized individuals may be given temporary protection after an injury with injection of tetanus antitoxin.

  D. Infectious hepatitis—virus infection of the liver.

  E. Infectious mononucleosis—virus infection of the lymph glands showing a marked rise in white blood cell count.

  F. Bacterial meningitis—infection of the meninges by the meningococcus, *Neisseria meningitidis*.

  G. Staphylococcal infections—common "staph" infections include:

    1. Boils.

    2. Abscesses.

    3. Carbuncles.

    4. Impetigo.

    5. Infected cuts and wounds.

III. Diseases of Worldwide Importance
    A. Trachoma—chronic viral infection of the eye.
    B. Malaria
        1. Result of infection by protozoa of the genus *Plasmodium*.
        2. Transmitted only by mosquitoes of the genus *Anopheles*.
    C. Yaws—a nonvenereal tropical disease caused by a spirochete similar to that of syphilis.
    D. Tuberculosis
        1. Caused by the bacillus *Mycobacterium tuberculosis*.
        2. Remains a major cause of death in countries and regions with low standard of living.
    E. Yellow fever—an often-fatal virus disease transmitted only by *Aedes aegypti* mosquitoes.
    F. Dengue
        1. A virus disease.
        2. Transmitted by *Aedes* mosquitoes.
        3. Epidemics are explosive, but fatality is low.
    G. Smallpox
        1. Caused by the variola virus.
        2. Effective vaccine has been available since about 1800.
        3. Revaccination is necessary every three to five years.
    H. Cholera—results from the infection of the digestive tract by the bacterium *Vibrio cholerae (Vibrio comma)*.
    I. Typhoid fever
        1. Cause is the bacterium *Salmonella typhosa*.
        2. Symptomless carriers are problem with this disease.
    J. Leprosy (Hansen's disease)—results from an infection by a bacterium related to the tuberculosis organism.

IV. Parasitic Worms
    A. Worms transmitted from person to person:
        1. Hookworms—roundworms, less than one-half inch long, living in the small intestine.
        2. Ascariasis—infestation of the intestine of man by the ascaris worm.
        3. Pinworms:
            a. Commonly infect children in the United States.
            b. Live in the large intestine and deposit eggs at the anus.
    B. Parasitic worms transmitted by insect vectors—filariasis (elephantiasis):
        1. Microscopic roundworms transmitted by mosquitoes.
        2. Worms live in the lymph ducts, causing grotesque swelling of the arms, legs, breasts, and scrotum.
    C. Parasitic worms transmitted from animals to man:
        1. Tapeworms
            a. Pork tapeworm—man infected by eating larval cysts in poorly cooked pork.
            b. Beef tapeworm—man infected by eating larval cysts in poorly cooked beef.
            c. Dwarf tapeworm—infection of man usually through food contaminated with rat, mouse, or human feces.
            d. Dog tapeworm—most human infections are in children who have accidentally eaten fleas from a dog or cat.
            e. Fish tapeworm—infection of man is through eating poorly cooked fish containing the larvae of this worm.

2. Trichinosis
a. The invasion of human flesh by the roundworm *Trichinella spiralis.*
b. Man is infected by eating animal flesh containing the encysted larvae of the worm.
3. Schistosomiasis (blood flukes)—man infected when he enters infected water, drinks such water, or eats contaminated water plants.
4. Liver flukes—man infected through eating incompletely cooked fish.

V. Occupational Diseases—diseases which arise as a result of occupational exposure to some harmful element.
A. Occupational diseases once accepted as an unavoidable aspect of the struggle to make a living.
B. Despite improvements that have been made, occupational disease hazards do remain in the United States today.
C. New technical advances will bring solutions for many of the occupational hazards of today, but will also produce new hazards.

VI. World Health Organization (WHO)
A. An agency of the United Nations, organized in 1946 and formally established in 1948.
B. Goal is improvement of the general level of health of the world's population.

Glossary

If you cannot find the word you wish in this glossary, check the index for text and glossary references.

abscess (ab′ses) (L. *ab,* away; *cedere,* to go). A localized collection of pus in a cavity formed by the disintegration of tissues.

Aedes (ā ē′dēz) (G. *aedes,* unpleasant). A genus of mosquitoes that includes many important vectors of yellow fever, dengue, and encephalitis.

Anopheles (ə nof′ə lēz) (G. *anopheles,* hurtful). A genus of mosquitoes that includes many vectors of malaria.

anoxia (an ok′ sē a) (G. *a-,* absence; oxygen). Absence or lack of oxygen.

Ascaris (as′kə ris) (L. *ascaris*). A genus of roundworms living as intestinal parasites in man and other animals.

booster dose. An injection of vaccine or toxoid administered at some time after primary immunization in order to maintain immunity.

Bordetella (bor də tel′ə) (Jules Jean Bordet, Belgian bacteriologist, 1870–1961). A genus of bacteria to which belongs the organism causing whooping cough.

carrier (kar′ē ər). An individual who harbors somewhere in his body the pathogens of a specific disease without suffering symptoms of that disease.

cercaria (sər kair′ē ə) (pl. *cercariae*) (G. *kerkos,* tail). The final free-swimming larval stage of certain parasitic flukes.

cholera (kol′ə rə) (G. *chole,* bile). A condition marked by severe diarrhea and vomiting.

clonorchiasis (klō nor kī′ə sis) (G. *klon,* branch; *orchis,* testis). The state of being infected with liver flukes of the genus *Clonorchis.*

Clostridium (klo strid′ē əm) (G. *kloster,* spindle). A genus of rod-shaped, spore-forming, generally anaerobic bacteria that includes species responsible for tetanus, botulism, and other diseases.

Corynebacterium (kor'ə nē bak tēr'ē əm) (G. *koryne,* club; *bakterion,* little rod). A genus of bacteria that includes the organism producing diphtheria.

cyst (sist) (G. *kystis,* sac). A sac.

Diphyllobothrium (dī fil ō both'rē əm) (G. *di,* two; *phyllon,* leaf; *bothrion,* pit). A genus of tapeworms that includes the fish tapeworm.

Dipylidium (dĭ'pi lid'ē əm) (G. *dipylos,* having two entrances). A genus of tapeworms that includes the common dog tapeworm.

eczema (ek'zə mə) (G. *ekzein,* to boil out). A skin inflammation disease, characterized by lesions with watery discharge and the development of scales and crusts.

elephantiasis (el ə fən tī'ə sis) ("elephant disease"). A common name given to the enlargement of body parts resulting from filariasis of the lymphatic ducts.

encephalitis (en sef'ə lī'tis) (G. *enkephalos,* brain; *-itis,* inflammation). Inflammation of the brain.

erythrogenic (e rith'rō jen'ik) (G. *erythros,* red; *gennan,* to produce). 1. Producing erythrocytes. 2. Producing a rash.

exanthema (ek san thē'mə) (G. *exanthema*). Any disease characterized by eruption or breaking out of the skin.

filariasis (fil ə rī'ə sis) (L. *filum,* thread). A diseased state due to the presence of filaria (thread-like parasitic roundworms) in the body.

hemolysis (hē mol'i sis) (G. *haima,* blood; *lysis,* dissolution). The separation of the hemoglobin from red blood cells.

hepatitis (hep ə tī'tis) (G. *hepar,* liver; *itis,* inflammation). Inflammation of the liver.

herpes (hur'pēz) (G. *herpes*). An inflammatory skin disease characterized by the formation of clusters of small vesicles.

Hymenolepis (hī mə nol'ə pis) (G. *hymen,* membrane; *lepis,* rind). A genus of tapeworms to which belongs the dwarf tapeworm.

jaundice (jawn'dis) (Fr. *jaune,* yellow). Deposit of bile pigment in the skin with resulting yellow appearance of the patient.

Koplik's spots (Kop'liks) (Henry Koplik, pediatrician, 1858–1927). Small, irregular, bright red spots on the tongue and mouth lining, each with a minute bluish white speck in the center, indicative of early measles.

larva (lahr'və) (L. *larva,* early stage). An immature stage in the life history of an animal in which it is unlike the parent.

Mantoux test (man too') (Charles Mantoux, French physician, 1877–1947). The injection of tuberculin into the skin as a diagnostic procedure for tuberculosis.

meninges (mə nin'jēz) (G. *meninx,* membrane). The three membranes that cover the brain and spinal cord.

meningitis (me nin jī'tis) (G. *meninx,* membrane; *itis,* inflammation). Inflammation of the meninges.

Mycobacterium (mī'kō bak tēr'ē əm) (G. *myces,* fungus; *bakterion,* little rod). A genus of rod-shaped bacteria, to which belong the organisms causing tuberculosis and leprosy.

papule (pap'yool) (L. *papula*). A small solid elevation of the skin.

paroxysm (par'ək sizm) (G. *paroxysmos,* attack). A sudden attack or recurrence of symptoms.

Plasmodium (plaz mō'dē əm) (G. *plasma,* anything formed; *eidos,* form). A genus of protozoa, parasitic in red blood cells; the malaria parasites.

pneumonia (nyoo mō'nē ə) (G. *pneumon,* lung; *-ia,* pertaining to). Inflammation of the lungs.

pseudomembrane (soo'dō mem'brān) (G. *pseudes,* false). A false membrane.

quarantine (kwor'ən tēn) (It. *quarantina,* 40 days). To detain or isolate in order to prevent transmission of a disease.

roseola (rō zē ō'lə) (L.). In its general sense, any rose colored rash; specifically roseola infantum (baby measles).

rubella (roo bel'ə) (L. *ruber,* red). German measles.

rubeola (roo bē ō'lə) (L. *ruber,* red). Measles.

Schistosoma (shis'tə sō'mə) (G. *schistos,* split; *soma,* body). The blood flukes. Formerly called bilharzia.

schistosomiasis (shis'tə sō mī'ə sis) (G. *schistos,* split; *soma,* body). The state of being infected with flukes of the genus Schistosoma. Formerly called bilharziasis.

Taenia (tē'nē ə) (L. *taenia,* tape). A genus of common tapeworms to which belong the pork and beef tapeworms.

tetanus (tet'ə nəs) (G. *tetanos,* stretched). 1. Continuous steady contraction of a muscle. 2. An acute infectious disease caused by the toxin of *Clostridium tetani,* resulting in spasm of various body muscles.

toxin (tok'sin) (G. *toxikon,* poison). A poison.

toxoid (tok'soid). A weakened bacterial toxin which has lost its toxic properties while retaining its ability to cause production of antitoxins; used in immunization.

trachoma (trə kō'mə) (G. *trachoma,* roughness). A viral disease of the conjunctiva and cornea of the eye, leading to visual disability and blindness.

Trichinella (trik i nel'ə) (G. *trichinos,* of hair). A genus of parasitic roundworms to which belongs the worm causing trichinosis.

trichinosis (trik i nō'sis). A disease condition due to the infection of the body by *Trichinella spiralis* worms.

tuberculin (tyoo bur'kyə lin) (L. *tuberculun,* a small nodule). A liquid extracted from the tuberculosis bacillus for use in tuberculosis skin testing.

vaccine (vak sēn') (L. *vaccinus,* of cows). A preparation of killed or attenuated microorganisms for use in immunization.

vaccinia (vak sin'ē ə). A virus disease (cowpox) of cattle communicated to man in order to confer immunity against smallpox.

variola (və rī'ə lə) (L.). Smallpox.

Vibrio (vib'rē ō) (L. *vibrare,* to shake). A genus of short, curved, rod-shaped bacteria, species of which cause cholera and similar diseases.

yaws (yawz). Infection of man by *Treponema pertenue,* resulting in destructive lesions of the skin and bones.

CHAPTER 18   RADIATION

ENVIRONMENTAL   CONSERVATION

HEALTH   SUMMARY

Chapter 17 discussed occupational diseases, the conditions which have been recognized as causing such diseases, and the biological damage to individuals who work in direct contact with such substances. Until a few years ago, knowledge of occupational conditions was largely limited to man's concern with his immediate working environment. However, research into these occupational conditions led to the realization that such conditions can also affect the total environment. The chemical substances that plagued man during working hours were also spilling out into the air, soil, and water that surrounded him 24 hours a day. Some products produced and used by man were found to pollute and make useless great amounts of soil, water, and air that he depended upon. Slowly, man has been able to identify these pollutants and measure their amounts, and effort now is being expended toward eliminating them.

Pollution has been the by-product of the tremendous industrial advancement that has taken place in the past years. Many of these substances are here to stay. Some we are able to replace with other pollutants that are not as dangerous to man; others we must learn how to live with or how to dispose of in a sophisticated and effective manner.

At the same time man has found ways to use other chemicals to his advantage to kill unwanted pests, to enhance and improve his foods, and to improve his standard of living. Man's overriding concern in this dynamic age should be how he can maintain and improve his health so that he can best contribute to effective and productive living.

RADIATION

To explain radiation and the effects of radiation, the authors would need to use technical terms which would require explanation. But it is beyond the scope of this book to discuss the physical nature of radiation in great detail. Such discussions can be found in a large number of books written on sophisticated physical and mathematical levels. Books devoted to radiation and its effects are available in college libraries for students who seek more detailed information.

NUCLEAR CONCEPTS AND TERMINOLOGY

As late as the latter part of the nineteenth century, physicists, chemists, and other scientists believed that the atom was the smallest unit of matter, that it was indivisible. Such a concept was proven erroneous with the discovery, by Pierre and Marie Curie, of an extraordinary element which was named radium. This element was found to give off radiations of energy, continuously and without the aid of any outside energy source. It was found that because of this discharge of energy, the element radium was slowly in the process of changing into a completely different element, lead. During this change the atoms of radium emitted the radiating energy particles, and in doing so changed into lead atoms. Atoms thus proved to have a complex subatomic structure of their own.

The atom is now known to be made up of many transitory particles that change during atomic reactions and three basic particles—*electrons, protons,* and *neutrons.* The configuration, or physical placement of these three particles is now known to resemble the general configuration and structure of a miniature solar system. In the center there is the atomic nucleus, compounded of protons and neutrons, which may be likened to the sun in the solar system. In the space around the nucleus are a number of electrons, spinning in orbits much like those of the planets spinning about the sun. The number of electrons in orbit around the nucleus is a characteristic of each atom. Also, the protons of the nucleus carry a *positive* electromagnetic charge, and the electrons, in orbit, carry a *negative* electromagnetic charge; these balance one another in charge and number. The neutrons do not carry a charge but are neutral.

The protons and neutrons are extremely heavy in comparison to the electrons. In fact, the electron is so light that it has only about 1/1840 the mass of one proton or neutron. Consequently, the weight of an atom is concentrated in the nucleus. The lightest atom, and the simplest, is ordinary hydrogen. It has one proton in the nucleus and one electron rotating in orbit. With one proton, the hydrogen atom is said to have an atomic weight of approximately 1.008. The weight of the electrons is considered to be negligible. All of the naturally occurring elements range in complexity and weight from hydrogen (atomic number 1) to uranium (atomic number 92), which is the heaviest (atomic weight 238) element found in nature. It contains 146 neutrons, 92 protons, and a balance of 92 electrons. The elements which have been discovered during atomic reactions are all heavier and more complex than uranium. None of these occur in nature.

These three particles of an atom are not completely fixed; they may be displaced and thrown about. When an electron is displaced from its orbit around the nucleus of an atom, it leaves a positively charged atom, which is termed a *positive ion*. When such an electron is displaced from its orbit, it will fly at an enormous speed into the surrounding space, where it hits other atoms. Such an electron, traveling at near the speed of light, is termed a *beta particle*. This free electron will collide with and rapidly attach itself to a neutral atom, and in turn will produce a negatively charged atom, a *negative ion*. This process, producing positive and negative ion pairs, is termed *ionization;* any radiation which is able to perform this task is termed *ionizing radiation*. Many forms of radiation are found in nature; few are ionizing radiations. Radiation is a continuum of wave lengths. X rays are a part of the radiation spectrum, visible light is another part, and radio waves are still another. The properties of radiation depend upon the length of its waves. As the wave lengths shorten, the amount of energy rises. Thus, visible light has relatively little energy, ultraviolet light is a little more powerful, and X rays and gamma rays are very powerful. X rays and gamma rays are known as *high-energy radiations*.

In certain instances the fast-moving electron (*beta particle*), when it collides with a stable atom, will displace many electrons and also disintegrate the nucleus into units containing two protons and two neutrons which in turn radiate into space, crashing into other atoms, causing more ionization. Such units of two protons and two neutrons are similar to the nucleus of the element helium; they are termed *alpha particles.*

In summation, there are five particles or waves which are produced during ionization (alpha particles, beta particles, gamma rays, X rays, and neutrons) and these are the particles which in turn also produce ionization. Now to explain the unique qualities of each of these five particles and waves.

ALPHA PARTICLES

Alpha particles, as mentioned earlier, consist of 2 protons, carrying 2 positive charges of electricity, and 2 neutrons. Alpha particles are emitted as a single unit in the disintegration of certain radioactive elements called *alpha emitters*. There are 30 such elements naturally occurring in nature. These particles are extremely large by nuclear standards; they travel at about one tenth the speed of light and they are not deeply penetrating.

The first layer of skin on an exposed body will stop alpha particles. But alpha particles contain tremendous amounts of energy when traveling very short distances and will produce large amounts of ionization. This abundance of ionization makes them especially hazardous, because they can do much damage to local organs and tissues. Consequently, great care should be exerted to prevent inhalation or ingestion of alpha emitters, because, after entering the body, they may travel only a short distance in the body, but will produce tremendous biological havoc in the process. But the damage from external alpha radiation is negligible because of its short range and failure to even penetrate skin.

BETA PARTICLES

Beta particles are actually high-speed electrons carrying a negative electrical charge. The penetrating power of beta particles is about 100 times that of alpha particles, but still only a small fraction of that of gamma rays. A thin sheet of paper will stop alpha particles, an inch of wood or 1.25 inches of aluminum will stop a beta particle, but it takes several inches of lead to stop gamma rays.

At least 90 percent of all radioactive isotopes (atoms) are beta emitters. In the list of radioactive isotopes in frequent use for medical and biological research, diagnosis, and treatment, at least 17 are well-known beta emitters. Internal emitters of beta particles can cause damage at low levels, but such damage is considered only a potential side reaction when such isotopes are used medically.

Externally emitted particles will penetrate deeply enough into the skin to cause radiation damage in the form of beta burns. These burns are similar to X-ray and gamma ray burns, but because the beta particles, only penetrate a few centimeters, such burns are superficial. They are less painful and heal much more rapidly than X-ray and gamma ray burns. But injury from commercial use of beta radiation is becoming more common in industry.

GAMMA RAYS

Gamma and X rays, although of different origin, have precisely the same characteristics. They occupy different wavelengths and energy levels but are close enough to perform the same functions. They penetrate and pass through matter in the same way, and therefore can be used in diagnosis, therapy, and industrial radiography.

Because of their great power of penetration and production of ionization, gamma rays are a potential biological hazard. Gamma and X rays cause radiation damage to cells and tissues; produce radiation illness; and, if the exposure is great enough, lead to the death of the individual.

X RAYS

X rays are also called *roentgen rays*. They were first discovered by a German physicist, Wilhelm Conrad Roentgen, in 1895. The properties of such radiations were mysterious enough at that time for them to be called X rays—"X" designating the unknown nature of the rays.

X rays, like gamma rays, produce ionizations. But because they are without electrical charge, they are much less likely to interact when they pass in the vicinity of an electron. They penetrate very deeply, at times completely through the body. The biological damage as a result of exposure to X rays may take a number of forms depending on the cumulative or total dose. Local skin reactions—ulcers, and carcinoma of the skin—are specific examples of this damage. Acute radiation illness, sterility, early aging, shortening of life, leukemia, cancer, and death may also be due to the direct effects of a single dose or accumulative body of radiation over long periods of time. Such irradiation may also cause mutations, leading to genetic death or abnormal offspring.

Use of X-ray machines and the fluoroscope in medical and dental practice accounts for the greatest amount of radiation exposure to most people. The main risk involved is to the gonadal (ovaries and testes) areas of the body. Here irradiation may affect the reproductive cells in such a manner as to produce sterility or to alter the genetic constitution of individuals not yet conceived. This *genetic dose* is cumulative; it begins at the time of that individual's conception and ceases with the end of his reproductive period. Such a risk varies with the type of examination; for example, a diagnostic X ray of the head would give a very small *gonadal dose* whereas an X ray of the oviduct or uterus of a woman would give a very large gonadal dose. But in spite of the slight risk, the continued use of X ray for diagnosis and treatment is essential in modern medicine and dentistry. Such use of X rays, however, should be held to a minimum, being used only when necessary.

NEUTRONS

Neutrons have effects of their own. When atomic nuclei disintegrate, neutrons are quite frequently ejected. These may travel at a fast or slow speed. They have no electric charge and can rush or drift right through the electronic orbits of other atoms. Eventually they are "captured" by the nuclei of other atoms. For unknown reasons, certain numerical combinations of protons and neutrons are unstable; they undergo spontaneous nuclear disintegration. Such disintegration is termed *fission*. It results in the ejection of additional neutrons, which are captured, creating more fission; more capture, more fission; and so on—in a *chain reaction*. A chain reaction may be slow and controlled (as in atomic piles) or almost instantaneous and of great violence (as in atomic or fission bombs).

RADIOLOGICAL UNITS OF MEASUREMENT

The effects of radiation upon a living cell or a living body depend upon the amounts of energy the living substance absorbs from this radiation. Consequently, it is important to be able to measure the quantities of radiation produced by a source and then relate this information to the biological effects produced.

ROENTGEN

The most useful unit of measurement of exposure to X rays or gamma rays is the roentgen, which is usually abbreviated as "r." This measurement is made quite easily with the aid of a dosimeter. The roentgen can only be used to measure X ray and gamma radiation.

RAD

The measurement of types of radiation other than that from X rays and gamma rays is more involved. It is therefore becoming general practice to specify the "absorbed dose" of an ionizing radiation. One unit of absorbed dose is termed a *rad*.

REM (ROENTGEN-EQUIVALENT FOR MAN)

In practice, the biological effects of radiations are measured by equating them with effects produced by a given dose of X rays as measured in roentgen. This unit is termed a *rem*.

RELATIVE BIOLOGICAL EFFECTIVENESS (RBE)

Equal absorbed doses of different types of radiation do not necessarily cause the same biological effects. What is known as the Relative Biological Effectiveness of a radiation is defined as the biological effect of one rad of the radiation in question. For X rays, gamma rays, and electrons, the RBE is approximately 1, but for alpha particles, protons, and neutrons, it can be as high as 20.

HALF-LIFE

The time taken for half the radioactive atoms of a particular radioactive element to disintegrate is called the half-life. Its value may lie between seconds (or less) up to millions of years. The activity of any radioactive material falls to half of its initial value at the end of one half-life period; it falls to one-quarter at the end of two half-lives, and so on. The recognition of half-life is of great importance in the therapeutic use of radioactive isotopes, since, if its life is too long, the material may be carcinogenic if injected; if it is too short, it cannot be effectively administered. For medicine the usefulness of a radioactive isotope has been set at 10 days as an upper limit and 12 hours as the lower limit of half-life.

CURIE

When a radioactive atom disintegrates, it emits energy in the form of gamma rays and/or alpha or beta particles. The rate at which tissues receive radiation from deposited radioactive substance is slowing as the quantity of deposited substance is disintegrating. A unit, named after Madame Curie, has been devised for such a condition. A *curie* is defined as that quantity of a given radioactive material in which 3.7×10^{10} disintegrations occur per second. This number was chosen because it is the rate at which 1 gram of radium disintegrates, and therefore 1 curie of radium is 1 gram of radium. The rate of disintegration cannot be changed by any means. But the weight of different substances varies with the rate of disintegration, which in turn depends upon the half-life. For example, 1 curie of polonium, which has a half-life of 130 days, is only 0.2 milligrams.

COMPARATIVE RADIOSENSITIVITY

Within a few years after the discovery of X rays, it became apparent that ionizing radiations had deleterious effects on the body. With the advent of radioactive isotopes and the extensive use of ionizing radiations in medicine, industry, research, and the military, the effects assumed increasing importance. But many of these effects are not immediately apparent in the body. The principal sources of radiation are as follows.

NATURAL BACKGROUND RADIATION

All forms of life have been subjected to low levels of radiation from natural sources throughout their evolution. In assessing the hazards of radiation, we have found it useful to compare these levels with those of man-made radiations.

EXTERNAL SOURCES

Radiations from naturally occurring radioactive substances in the ground, air, building materials, and water are constantly bombarding man. Also, cosmic radiation from space may play an important part in background radiation.

INTERNAL SOURCES

Potassium 40, carbon 14, and other naturally occurring radioactive elements such as radium and thorium are constituents of substances which enter the body through food, drinking water, or air. These are accumulated in the body throughout life.

MAN-MADE RADIATION

The degree of hazard in man-made radiation varies from high doses of radiation delivered in a short time—that coming as directly after the explosion of a nuclear weapon, as a result of an accident, or from radiotherapy—to low doses comparable with the natural background, but delivered over a long period of time. These radiations may come from an external source or internally from radioactive isotopes which have gained entry into the body. Some of the major man-made radiation sources are outlined below.

Radiotherapy. This is the use of radiation (usually X and gamma radiation) as means of diagnosis and treatment in medicine and dentistry. This is the major source of man-made radiation in the world today.

Radioactive isotopes. These are atoms of radioactive elements used in research, in medical diagnosis and treatment, and in industry.

Industrial X rays. These are X rays used in industry for radiography of welds, castings, and products where flaws could impair the quality of the product.

Radioactive fallout. This is the result of the explosion of nuclear devices, as in the testing or use of nuclear weapons.

Radioactive wastes. These are produced from the use and processing of radioactive materials, fission products, and the possible accidental release of radioactive substances. Some of these affect only individuals who are subjected to radiation because of their occupation. Others constitute a hazard to the whole population by pollution of the environment.

EFFECTS OF RADIATION ON THE BODY TISSUES

Large doses of all types of radiation will kill cells. With smaller doses of radiation, recovery of the cells can take place and they can continue to function. However, recovery may not be complete and there may be malignant changes later. In general, certain cells are more readily affected by radiation than are others, and tissues which are actively regenerating, with constant cell division and multiplication—such as embryonic tissue, intestinal mucosa, blood-forming tissue, gonadal germ cells, and skin—are the more vulnerable. These various types of tissue damage may be simplified into two main classes.

SOMATIC TISSUE EFFECTS

Somatic tissue is the general tissue of the body. Early damage produces effects resulting in the death of tissue cells. The extent of cell death will produce either abnormalities of structure, burn lesions, or death to the individual. Later in life radiation may accumulate but not appear until its effects involve altering cell functions, possibly producing cancer or leukemia. The early effects of radiation on tissue will show damage directly upon irradiation, but later effects may appear in tissues which did not show any changes at first (Table 18.1).

GENETIC EFFECTS

Genetic effects are effects upon the germ or reproductive cells carried on to affect the descendants of the irradiated person. No damage will appear in the individual receiving the radiation, but the effects of the radiation upon the person will appear in his offspring as abnormalities of form and function. Such genetic effects may be caused by small doses of radiation; therefore, *all* radiation must be considered as deleterious to a greater or lesser degree.

RADIOACTIVE FALLOUT

Fallout is the return to earth of radioactive material which had been carried up into the atmosphere by the detonation of a nuclear device. It also refers to any resulting contamination of food, drink, soil, air,

TABLE 18.1   EFFECTS ON THE WHOLE BODY OF PENETRATING RADIATION

The Acute Radiation Syndrome

The mean lethal dose, for a single whole body exposure lasting for minutes or a few hours, in all mammals, lies between 200 r and 900 r. With very high doses of the order of 2000 r, gross tissue destruction occurs and the patient passes into a shocklike state and dies within a matter of hours.

With doses of 500 r to 1000 r the patient usually survives long enough to show the features of the acute radiation syndrome:

Phase 1: A short latent period when no effects are absorbed.

Phase 2: Nausea and vomiting coming on a few hours after irradiation but passing off within 24 hours. Followed by general non-specific symptoms persisting for a few days.

Phase 3: A period of comparative well-being. Low-grade fever.

Phase 4: The hair starts to drop out abruptly at about the 17th to 21st day.
At about 21 days an increased feeling of discomfort and rising temperature occur.
The patient complains of pain in the throat and gums.
Signs of agranulocytic angina are found.
The general condition slowly deteriorates, with chronic diarrhea and emaciation, resulting in death.

SOURCE: Adapted from K. Williams, C. L. Smith, and H. D. Chalke, *Radiation and Health,* Boston, Little, Brown and Company, 1962.

or building materials resulting from such fallout. Environmental contamination produced by the worldwide dispersion of radioactivity from nuclear weapon tests has been a source of both internal and external radiation.

Distribution of a fallout pattern is determined by yield, height, and location of the detonation, and by meteorological conditions. The dose rate and the accumulated dose from fallout depend not only upon the amount of radioactive fallout but also upon the ionization effects of the radiation products.

In the process of detonation of a nuclear device, for every megaton of fission, yield will be about 110 pounds of intensely radioactive substances. Fortunately, many of the substances formed have extremely short radioactive half-lives and thus have little significance other than in local fallout. The isotopes remaining one hour after detonation decay, approximately, by a factor of ten for every sevenfold increase in time after detonation time plus one hour. As shown in Table 18.2, seven hours after a nuclear explosion, the radioactivity has decreased to one-tenth of what it was at one hour. In 49 hours the radioactivity is only one one-hundredth of what it was at one hour. In two weeks the radioactivity is only one-thousandth, and in three months, only one-ten-thousandth of its initial one-hour level.

Radioactive products from bomb tests—which contaminate food, drink, and the atmosphere—are introduced into the body, and some are retained. The most important of these radioisotopes (*radionuclides*) are *strontium 90, yttrium 90, strontium 89, caesium 137, iodine 131,* and *carbon 14*. Gamma-emitting fission products deposited in soil and elsewhere also provide an external source of radiation.

TABLE 18.2   FADING RADIATION HAZARD

Contamination in Curies of Radioactive Material	Time after Formation of Fission Products	Radiation Intensity from Fission Products (Roentgens per Hour)
1000	1 hour	10,000
100	7 hours	1,000
10	49 hours (2 days)	100
1	14 days (2 weeks)	10
0.1	14 weeks (3 months)	1

SOURCE: Adapted from C. W. Shilling, *Atomic Energy Encyclopedia,* Philadelphia, W. B. Saunders Company, 1964.

It has been shown that the total dose to bone marrow from artificial sources of radiation in technically advanced countries is approximately equal to the typical natural background dose. In children under five, fallout probably accounts for some 5 to 10 percent of the artificial dose to bone marrow. With the advent of a test ban treaty, this dosage will decrease in younger children. The genetically significant dose from artificial sources annually is probably about 3 percent of the natural background. Fallout, during atmospheric testing, was responsible for about one-fifth of the total artificial dose. The major effects of the more important radionuclides found in fallout are explained in the following sections.

STRONTIUM

Strontium and calcium have similar effects on biological behavior and metabolism. Strontium usually concentrates in food normally high in calcium, such as in milk; and deposits within the body in areas high in calcium, such as bones.

STRONTIUM 89

This radionuclide is an important antibiological hazard from fallout in the period of from one week to one year after detonation of an atomic device. It emits beta particles of low energy and has a very short half-life of about 53 days.

STRONTIUM 90

Strontium 90 is considered, biologically, the most important of all fission products in fallout, because of the amount of strontium 90 in fallout and its long half-life of 28 years. Particularly, it is important because it is metabolized by the body and deposited in large concentrations in bone tissue and the same way as calcium. This element and the daughter element, yttrium 90, which it decomposes into, are both weak beta emitters and do damage by the constant internal emission of beta particles.

CAESIUM AND POTASSIUM

These elements are absorbed by the body and distributed in approximately the same manner. They are widely distributed constituents of tissue; the average individual will have about 245 grams per 70 kilograms adult body weight of potassium and caesium according to their availability. The radioactive isotopes of these two elements are not considered major sources of internal radiation because of their feeble beta-emitting powers. However, because of their wide distribution within the body tissue, they still may be genetically significant for their effects on the gonadal area.

CARBON 14

Carbon 14, although not a fission product, is generated in nuclear explosions by the interaction between escaping neutrons and the nitrogen nuclei in the atmosphere. The carbon 14 level in the atmosphere, during the period of atmospheric nuclear testing, increased about 10 percent as the result of such testing. Due to the long effective half-life of carbon 14 (radioactive half-life is 5760 years; effective half-life, 40 days), it is considered one of the most important radioisotopes. The total number of mutations produced over many generations of mankind as a result could be large; this large total, however, will still be a very small fraction of the number of mutations produced by natural radiation over the same period.

Natural carbon 14 is formed as the result of cosmic ray bombardment of the nitrogen in the atmosphere and is present in atmospheric carbon dioxide. By this action carbon 14 is produced in nature in amounts estimated from seven to ten kilograms per year.

IODINE 131

Iodine 131 has been detected in human thyroid glands after bomb tests, but owing to its short physical half-life (eight days), the affinity of iodine for the thyroid glands of the neck, and the intermittence of major bomb tests, concentrations in the air are widely variable. Iodine 131 enters the body mainly by inhalation in air directly after a nuclear explosion. The main hazard could be that continued exposure to iodine 131 will injure and kill the cells of the thyroid glands; therefore its presence on a continuing basis would be undesirable.

DISPOSAL OF RADIOACTIVE WASTE

Radioactive wastes from industry vary so much that there is no single solution to their management or disposal. The solution depends upon such factors as the specific nature (radioactive half-life or type of radiation), *concentration* (quantity of radioactive material involved), and the *specific environment* in which disposal is being considered. The problem of disposal of radioactive wastes is that there is no way to destroy the radioactivity immediately; time alone with its radioactive decay serves to render the waste stable and harmless or of very low radioactivity and, therefore, nontoxic.

The magnitude of the waste disposal problem far outweighs the problems of fallout, or operation of a reactor. Waste disposal is potentially the greatest hazard to public safety. And the time of this danger is *now!* Many reactors are not currently in use, or are being run at reduced capacity, because of the many tons of high-level radioactive waste *already* stored. Yet no satisfactory method for disposal has been developed. As the nuclear power program builds up, the disposal of fission products in a manner that will not be injurious to health will need to have particular attention.

Spent fuel elements are now removed from reactors and shipped to one of the major United States Atomic Energy Commission processing sites. Here they are "cooled" for 90 days to allow decay of radioactive isotopes with short half-lives. They are classified as to energy level (high, medium, or low energy level) and disposed of in the following manners.

High-level radioactive wastes must be handled by containment in tank storage to allow time for radioactive decay. Suggestions for final disposal of high-level wastes include conversion of liquid wastes to solids and permanent storage in geological strata, with major sites being salt beds. Or liquids could be put directly into geological strata, either in deep wells or salt beds. Or both solids and liquids could be disposed of in the sea.

Medium-level radioactive wastes are usually held in trenches, in artificial ponds, or in tanks to allow for radioactive decay to a level at which they may be discharged into the environment. Some wastes with radioisotopes of reasonably short half-lives (weeks to months) are discharged directly into the ground. Some medium-activity wastes have been incorporated into concrete in steel drums, which have been buried in trenches or dumped at sea.

Low-level radioactive wastes, defined as having a radioactivity concentration in the range of one microcurie per gallon, are usually disposed of by dilution with water and released directly into the environment—in air, land, or sea. These wastes include things such as the reactor cooling water used in nuclear-powered ships and submarines.

Various other forms of waste processing, including chemical processing, are being used or experimented with, in an attempt to find a more economical and satisfactory method of waste disposal.

CONSERVATION

For years, conservation in this country was concerned with just maintaining the delicate balance between the needs of our people and the natural resources of our land. In recent decades, however, conservationists have been increasingly interested in a newer, more positive, more difficult approach—actually improving on the natural heritage that has been handed to us from the past.

The early pioneer coming to this country found a new land abounding in resources of every kind. Yet every one of these treasures was available to him only insofar as he made efforts to obtain them. Gradually the waters and land gave up their secrets as men learned how to master them. The federal government's concern for conservation in this country was expressed in three important periods.

1. The first great concern over conservation came during the time of Theodore Roosevelt. This first approach was primarily to preserve natural resources and to prevent their exploitation by the giant monopolies of that day. This was the first example of public management and regulation of use of natural resources. The primary concern was largely over the wholesale destruction of wildlife in the West and of the forests in the East.

2. The second period came during the days of Franklin Roosevelt. Conservation during this time was used as a depression-years' aid to economic and manpower recovery. Its practices and programs such as the W.P.A. (Works Projects Administration) and the C.C.C. (Civilian

Conservation Corps) contributed to the giant defense build-ups of World War II.

3. The third major thrust has come during the decade of the 1960s. Under the direction of John F. Kennedy, new impetus was given to existing programs and new programs were instituted to replace conservation of single resources with the preservation and development of the "American environment."

This new turn of events in conservation is technically called "applied ecology," which means the relationship of living things to their total environment. It means not just setting aside priceless and irreplaceable natural resources or using them in the wisest manner, but understanding the relationships between all living things on earth. It is becoming increasingly clear that man's position is safe only insofar as the broad base of lower life supporting him is also taken care of.

It has been estimated by conservationists that the needs of the present U.S. population for the basic resources of water, copper, and iron to sustain them during their remaining years of life are greater than the total amounts of these materials used by *all* men who have ever lived at any place on the earth. The future needs of this country's population are most difficult to project. In 1947 it was projected that the U.S. population would be 153 million in 1960. In actuality the 1960 population turned out to be almost 180 million. It is estimated at the present time that the population in A.D. 2010 will be near or in excess of 400 million. It becomes hard, if not impossible, to determine the demand, by that time, that will be placed on our natural resources.

Already water supplies in many parts of our country are a source of concern. In some places the underground resources have already been overdrawn. The day is swiftly coming when clouds will not carry sufficient water to meet our needs. Then, even after all of the industrial, domestic, irrigation, hydroelectric, and recreational usefulness has been extracted from the water, there still will be a shortage. More and more water will need to be reused and more will have to be gotten through desalination of salt waters. Thus, its purity and adequacy of supply will require the best efforts we can make.

What is said for water must be repeated for all other resources—fuels, minerals, and building materials. Conservation accordingly means more than an isolated wildlife preserve; it has become a universal necessity. Just as devastation of these resources will be universal, so can the quality of our use and conservation of them have universal advantage.

The total picture of conservation also relates to the urban environment and the ghetto. Polluted air, like polluted water, affects masses of people. Pure air must be achieved for the urban masses now living under the threatening cover of polluted air. Conservation of pure air is an important step toward achieving good health for our people.

Unfortunately, much remains to be done before we will be able to see *creative* conservation of all of our natural resources. Man still continues to pollute his environment in many ways. The most pressing contamination problems revolve around pollution of air, water, and food.

POLLUTION OF THE AIR

A man can live without food for five weeks, and without water for five days, but he cannot live without air for five minutes. Accordingly, air is the most vital of the resources.

For many years people have been treating the atmosphere as if it were a sewer, exhausting different kinds of waste products into it—gases, dusts, fumes, vapors, and smoke. Since the atmosphere is so vast, and since until recent years the amount of contamination had been small in terms of the amount of atmosphere, little real trouble was created. In recent years, however, this contamination is proving harmful to man, animals, and plants. In a study in France from 1950 to 1955, according to the World Health Organization, the incidence of deaths from bronchitis decreased in the rural areas by 18.7 percent, while it increased by 38 percent in Paris, where air pollution was increasing. The problem is well defined by Julien Custers, Minister of Public Health in Belgium, who, in speaking to a World Health Organization conference, stated "Since man has improved his means of transportation, concentrated his industries, and considerably developed the sources of energy available to him, atmospheric pollution has become one of the major worries of health authorities."

Air pollution involves different air contaminants in different areas. By general definition, pollution could be defined as the introduction of materials into the air as the result of man's activity. This definition would exclude from our discussion air pollutants from natural sources such as volcanoes, hot springs, and dust storms. There are other pollutants, such as smoke from forest fires, which may have started from either natural or human causes. Pollution, as discussed here, will imply the *possibility of control*.

Based upon their physical state, air pollutants can be considered in two categories—the aerosols and the gases.

GASEOUS POLLUTANTS

Gaseous pollutants exist as simple molecular entities and behave like the air itself. They do not settle out. Principally the product of industrial and domestic combustion, they arise from two general sources, combustion of fuels and the handling and processing of chemicals.

1. *Sulfur oxides.* These are widely prevalent and in some concentrations are of physiological significance. Low concentrations of sulfur dioxide (SO_2), for instance, cause irritation of the nose and throat.

Sulfur dioxide has been the suspected cause in several air pollution disasters, among them those of Donora, Pennsylvania, and London, England. Most fuels contain small amounts of sulfur, which is converted into sulfur dioxide during combustion. The sulfur oxides also result from smelting and other metallurgical operations.

2. *Nitrogen oxides.* Of the nitrogen oxides, nitrogen dioxide and nitric oxide appear to be the only ones of probable health importance as air pollutants. Health effects are usually noticeable only when comparatively high concentrations are found in enclosed areas. In addition, these oxides contribute to the nuisance effects of photochemical smog (smog conditions resulting from the action of sunlight on certain chemicals in the air) under certain weather conditions. The most important sources of nitrogen oxides in the atmosphere are combustion of fuels and certain chemical manufacturing operations. When anything is burned, some of the nitrogen in the air combines with some of the oxygen to form nitric oxide (NO), which will combine with more oxygen to form nitrogen dioxide (NO_2). The action of nitrogen dioxide and olefinic hydrocarbons produce eye-irritating products; vegetation damage; and, under intense sunlight, ozone.

3. *Ozone.* Ozone is formed from the photochemical reaction of nitrogen dioxide and olefinic hydrocarbons in the air. It shows the usual eye-irritating ability and is also thought to produce pulmonary fibrosis after long exposure.

4. *Carbon monoxide.* Carbon monoxide (CO) is a highly poisonous gas produced by the incomplete combustion of carbon and its compounds. Often considered an asphyxiant because of its strong combining powers with hemoglobin in the blood, it has caused many deaths in homes and garages where it has been released in closed spaces. Generally, its chief atmospheric source is the combustion of automobile fuels. Automobile exhaust is by far the most important source.

5. *Other gases.* Other gaseous air pollutants could be cited. Hydrocarbons such as methane and ethylene, in themselves nontoxic, help to lower the oxygen content of the air when they are in large quantities. Other pollutants include organic compounds, such as alcohols and esters, halogens, sulfur oxides, and aldehydes. Some of these may be strong eye irritants and rather toxic.

AEROSOLS

Aerosols are finely divided solid or liquid droplets, the larger of which will settle out of a gas. The finer particles can be buoyed up by the slightest air movement and may never settle out. Aerosols may consist of many things, but commonly include dusts (silica, iron, coal, uranium), fumes, mists, and smoke.

Dusts are solid particles of natural or industrial origin. *Fumes* are solid particles generated by the condensation of vapors in various ways. *Mists* are liquid particles which may arise from vapor condensation or chemical reactions.

An aerosol is the particle of matter during the time it is suspended in the air. Although the particle is an air pollutant only during the time it is in the air, it will be a nuisance both as an aerosol and as settled or deposited matter. Aerosols are most common over cities and least common over the ocean. The amount of problem depends on the concentration of the particles, their size, their chemical composition, and their rate of settling or dustfall.

The sources of aerosols are many. Fuel burning, incineration, agricultural operations, crushing and grinding operations, construction, mining, spraying, and sandblasting represent some common sources.

A new and very serious type of pollution to the atmosphere is radioactive aerosols. These materials are a source of concern because they cannot be detected by taste, smell, or the other human senses, and also because there is no way of neutralizing their radioactivity. It is important that they be kept out of the air. Possible sources include uranium mining operations, atomic laboratories, nuclear reactors, and radioactive waste disposal. Most concern has been shown over radioactive dusts and gases from atomic bomb tests, particularly strontium 90, which has a half-life of 28 years.

Aerosols can affect people in various ways. Some cause patches of irritation on the membranes lining the nasopharyngeal passage; such irritation may lead to lung damage, other bronchial diseases, cancer, or asthma.

Gases may contribute to bronchitis, asthma, allergy, eye irritation, pulmonary edema, pulmonary emphysema, other respiratory ailments, and cardiac diseases, as well as aggravating conditions that already exist from other causes, particularly among the old, the infirm, and infants.

THE EFFECTS OF AIR POLLUTION

The effects of air pollution may be considered in several rather broad categories, including (1) property damage, (2) vegetation damage, (3) soiling of surfaces, (4) sky-darkening, (5) limiting visibility, (6) annoyance to human senses, and (7) damage to health. The effects on plants, though economically important, is not often dramatic. Air pollution can cause leaf lesions and reduced productivity. Air pollution is of major concern to animal owners. Arsenic from smelting operations, for instance, may settle on vegetation and poison grazing cattle. Excessive absorption of fluorides may cause fluorosis in animals.

Of primary concern to us is the effect of air pollutants on man. This effect is not completely clear, but some things are known. The unburnt substances found in smoke are of particular importance. Benzpyrene, one of them, may play a role in cancer. The aerosols are so fine they may easily penetrate the lungs. And, in addition to being harmful themselves, they may also act as carriers of microbes and viruses. Mass attacks by air contaminants on people may be triggered by accidental escapes of large quantities of gases or dust. Although such acute episodes may be disastrous, as was the London attack in 1952 in which 4000 people died as the result of air pollution, these tragic situations represent unique meteorological conditions.

More common, however, are the subacute, noxious gases more or less always present in the air. *Smog* is such a condition. A word coined in England, combining the words "smoke" and "fog," smog is basically a smoke problem of various particles or gases which is made worse by fog. It is a phenomenon common to many metropolitan areas in this country, particularly those along seacoasts. In some places the smog conditions have become unique, owing to weather conditions that restrict diffusion of certain innocuous gases and at the same time slow their exposure to sunlight (photochemical smog), as in the Los Angeles area; others are of the smoke-fog variety in which the pollutants themselves, unaffected by light, are innocuous. Although the effects of either type of smog are not specific, some persons suffering from lung and heart ailments, as well as some infants or aged persons, have been affected. Whether or not atmospheric pollution is responsible for the development of certain forms of cancer has not been established. On the other hand, air pollution levels do seem to be correlated with chronic bronchitis, emphysema, lung cancer, and other respiratory diseases. Generally, it appears that persons in good health are not adversely affected, except for experiencing some degree of eye irritation.

CONTROL OF AIR POLLUTION

The control or prevention of air contamination is a complex problem and often expensive. Some authorities believe it is now possible to achieve almost complete elimination of such pollution, but each locality must decide how clean its air must be and how much its people are willing to pay for smog control. At the present time, the toleration levels for only a few contaminants are known and can be specified. Ideally, however, pollution should be eliminated at the source.

In some places the answer lies in reducing the source of pollution by substituting certain heating procedures with nonpolluting methods. In other cases, as with motor vehicles, the problem is to insure proper combustion through regulating the operating conditions of vehicles. In all places the problem involves whether control measures are feasible both economically and practically.

Also involved are the legal and regulatory aspects. A person must be free to use his property, yet at the same time he must be prevented from doing harm to others. The atmosphere will continue to receive various gases and aerosols, yet some must be eliminated in such a way as not to interfere with the health and function of society. Conflicts of interest must be overcome. To date, the greatest success in control has come in small areas—cities, villages, or counties—where the problem could be easily attacked. The first step is the control of air pollution; the second, more difficult one is its eradication, where feasible. Everyone needs the air to dispose of some wastes. Therefore, the problem of air pollution control affects everyone and is one for which everyone must take some degree of responsibility.

POLLUTION OF WATER

Water in its natural state is never 100 percent pure. As soon as it condenses as rain it begins gathering impurities which it carries until it is purified or until it evaporates. Much of this impurity is not sufficient to spoil the usefulness of water; some materials and substances, however, do limit its usefulness.

By definition, "water pollution" means the presence in water of any substance that impairs any of its legitimate uses—for public water supplies, recreation, agriculture, industry, the preservation of fish and wildlife, and esthetic purposes.

The principal forms of pollution are domestic wastes, industrial wastes, and silt. Domestic wastes include everything going down the drains of a city into its sewer system—used water from toilets, bathtubs, and sinks; and washings from restaurants, laundries, hospitals, hotels, and mortuaries. Industrial wastes include the acids, chemicals, oils, greases, and animal and vegetable matter discharged by factories; these wastes are discharged either through some sewer system or through separate outlets directly into waterways. Silt includes the soil that is washed into streams which muddies waters and fills up reservoirs and waterways. In addition to these principal forms of pollution there can be other pollutants, such as heat, radioactive substances, pesticides, and detergents.

The extent of pollution in a given body of water can be measured to some degree by the amount of organic wastes in it. The amount of organic waste in U.S. waters has increased sixfold in the first six decades of this century. Organic wastes can generally be destroyed by biochemical action, either naturally in a free-flowing stream or artificially in a waste treatment plant.

Not all pollutants can be so removed, for example, minerals and acids from industrial operations or from mining. Some, such as radioactive substances, silt, pesticides, detergents, and various oil products, are highly resistant to breakdown. If any breakdown of these occurs, it must be by other than ordinary methods.

Most uses to which water is put can be affected by pollution. Surely, to begin with, we want water for drinking and other domestic needs to be pure. Beyond this, though, water is the most used of all raw materials in industry. It is needed for making steel, synthetic yarns, woolens, and even aviation gasoline. The availability of pure water determines the location of many industries. Since its lack discourages many industries from locating in that area, pure water becomes an economic asset for most communities.

There are other economic considerations. Crops irrigated with polluted water may well transmit disease. Certain forms of industrial pollution in irrigation waters can damage crops. Fish often cannot survive in excessively polluted waters. Because of polluted water, beaches are closed to swimmers, boating is made undesirable, and outdoor water recreation is limited—all of which restrict certain forms of income in those localities, altering their economy.

The future demands on our country's water may well outstrip the supply. It is felt that only by the reuse of water will future needs be supplied. This reuse cannot occur, however, if polluted water cannot be reclaimed. Thus it becomes of utmost importance that answers be found to cope with the present pollution problem.

PURIFICATION PROCESSES

There are two primary methods of purifying water, either by natural processes or by the specific treatment of domestic and industrial sewage.

1. *Natural processes.* Water can purify itself by natural means up to the point where a stream cannot handle the pollution load. Such self-purification can be brought about by chemical, physical, and biological factors. The rate of self-purification will depend upon the water body's local features.

The time required will depend upon both the degree of pollution and the character of the water. Organic wastes are broken down by the action of bacteria present in the water. Their action in turn depends upon the amount of dissolved oxygen in the water. This is available either from direct absorption from the air over the surface of the water or from the oxygen given off by respiring water plants. But the more oxygen used up in this purification process, the less available for fish and other aquatic life. In addition to the presence of aquatic plants as an oxygen source, the nature of the water body will largely determine the amount of oxygen present. Oxygen replenishment will take place rapidly in a fast-flowing active stream, where the splashing action of the water allows for more air contact. The more motionless and sluggish a stream, or the greater its depth, the more time required to replenish its oxygen supply.

Because sunlight is restricted in polluted water, few water plants will grow in it; thus its oxygen supply is reduced. This reduction in turn leads to fewer bacteria in the water and an increased pollution problem, resulting in foul-smelling, unattractive water that cannot support fish or other aquatic life. The solution here is reduction of incoming wastes to a point where the stream can handle them through self-purification. This level will differ from stream to stream depending upon the stream's characteristics.

2. *Sewage treatment.* Sewage treatment is designed to reduce the pollutional effect of wastes before they are discharged into public waterways. Such treatment may be carried out by industries or by municipalities. Industrial treatment may be an in-the-plant process in which the water is treated for reuse.

In municipal treatment of sewage, the process may involve either a primary treatment or a primary-secondary type of treatment. In the so-called primary process, about 35 percent of the pollution is removed. The organic material is settled out from the water, which is then chlorinated to kill bacteria and discharge into a stream. The settled sludge is removed or dried, made harmless, and then burned or used for fertilizer, soil conditioners, or landfill.

Greater reduction of pollution is required when the water is to be reused. In this event, a further settling-filtering process is involved. The amount of pollution reduction required will determine the intensification of this secondary treatment. Pollution reduction up to almost 100 percent is possible to attain.

The more intense the treatment, the more cost is involved. The kind of treatment of local wastes will be determined, therefore, not only by the downstream water use, but also by the economy of the community involved. Of course, the amount of pollution at a source, as well as the degree of pollution reduction through natural stream processes, will determine the final nature of the sewage treatment decided upon.

Unfortunately, at the present time, the number of sewage treatment facilities in the nation are far behind the number of pollution sources. Many cities provided with sewer systems still dump their wastes directly into rivers and lakes rather than through sewage treatment facilities. Although various cities and many industries have made substantial expenditures in constructing waste-treatment plants, the growing U.S. population, along with the mounting industrialization, give evidence, in many areas, of worsening pollution conditions. Construction of new treatment plants will have to be stepped up in order to catch up with the needs.

FEDERAL CONTROLS

Federal responsibilities are primarily of a supporting nature designed to strengthen state programs. They include research, technical assistance, promotion of interstate action, and some enforcement of interstate pollution control. Federal action has come in the wake of inadequate state action. Since many waterways border on two or more states, action has been needed to unify the controls.

Starting in 1924 with the Oil Pollution Control Act to regulate the discharge of oil from ships in coastal waters, further action was taken by Congress in 1948 through the Water Pollution Control Act. Administered by the Public Health Service, it provides for enforcement authority, technical assistance, long-range planning, and loans to cities for construction of treatment plants. In 1961 the Congress strengthened this Act by giving it greater powers.

A great backlog of municipal sewage treatment needs still exists. Metropolitan areas will need to construct major sewer lines from urban areas to central treatment plants. Along with this phase of the problem are those relating to recreational needs (i.e., swimming, marinas, fishing); drainage from undeveloped land, streets, and farm lands; and siltation problems. The only solution is comprehensive action covering not only pollution from a single city, but also the total pollution along the entire length of a stream or lake. Unless water pollution is controlled, the country's health and economy will suffer.

POLLUTANTS IN FOOD

One of the favorite topics of discussion today among people concerned with maintaining health is the matter of substances added to food. On one side are people who claim that all types of chemical substances are being added to food without due regard to the consequences. On the other, food industry spokesmen are quick to point out that purposely added substances (additives) are used with justification. Such additives retard spoilage, enhance flavor, improve color, improve consistency, retard drying, or help to retain crispness. Some are added as nutritional supplements, such as thiamine to bread, iodine to salt, fluoride to water, or vitamins A and D to milk.

Some substances gain entrance into foods accidentally and unintentionally, including insecticides, hormones, antibiotics, and disinfectants. Some of these are substances which get into the food from the wrappers or containers where packaging materials touch the food.

Great efforts are made on the part of certain federal agencies to protect the consumer against injurious substances. Before we point out these areas of concern, however, we should define several terms as they will be used here. A *food additive* is a substance, other than a basic food stuff, which is present in food as a result of any aspect of production, processing, storage, or packaging. This definition does not include chance contaminants. *Toxicity* is the capacity of a substance to produce injury. *Safety* is the practical certainty that injury will not result from use of a substance in a proposed quantity and manner. *Hazard* is the probability that injury will result from use of a substance in a proposed quantity and manner.

TOXICITY OF PESTICIDES AND RESIDUES IN FOOD

Most pesticides are poisons. They are poisons because their proper usage is to kill insects. No one likes to use pesticides and their application is expensive to the producer, costing many millions of dollars each year. But they are necessary because insects, if uncontrolled, interfere with crop production by destroying crops, increase loss by spoilage, and lower the usefulness and attractiveness of the food. If pesticides were not used, the wholesomeness of many foods would be impaired.

These same pesticides, however, can be poisonous to humans if used incorrectly. Excessively heavy and too frequent application, improper timing, or improper formulation may lead to trouble. As a safeguard, no new pesticide may be legally sold for use on crops or soil until a safe method for its use is carefully established. If any amount of the pesticide remains on any part of the plant as a *residue,* the legal amount allowed as a residue must be well within the *safety* limit established by the federal government.

All pesticides must be registered with the United States Department of Agriculture (U.S.D.A.) before interstate marketing is allowed. Registration is granted only after the safety of a proposed chemical usage is conclusively proven. The Federal Food and Drug Administration (F.D.A.) carefully watches the levels of pesticide residues in foods. Normally the F.D.A. insists upon a residue safety margin of a hundredfold; in other words, only 1/100 of the safety level of concentration is allowed in consumer foods.

Generally, very little food pollution occurs as the result of improper pesticide usage. Federal laws and regulations very carefully control both the use of pesticides and the sale of foods containing pesticide residues (Miller Pesticide Amendment of 1954). Pesticide toxicity results primarily from improper use, from accidental exposure, or from deliberate ingestion with suicidal intent. The American public can be assured that no harm will result from pesticides through foods available in their markets.

FOOD ADDITIVES

It is wise here to make some comment regarding food additives. Although they are no longer considered pollutants by food authorities and the federal agencies responsible for pure foods, there are still some laymen who mistakenly propagandize against them as pollutants. The present state of federal control regarding pure foods should thus be properly noted.

Several laws have helped us to reach our present level of food safety. Laws in 1906 and 1938 were written to protect the public against injurious food additives. These laws required the federal government to test suspected injurious additives. They allowed a manufacturer to use a food additive until the government could test it, but during the delay, of course, people ran the risk of being injured. The 1958 food additives amendment, however, required that all new additives be tested for safety and such reports submitted to the government for acceptance *before* the additive could be used. These prior tests are conducted on animals, with results submitted to the F.D.A., whose scientists in turn independently scrutinize the findings and run their own tests. If the additive is passed, the Department of Health, Education, and Welfare permits its use.

With the 1958 amendment, the country has the best safeguards it has been possible to develop against polluted foods. New advances in food technology are allowed for without risk to human health. Each person today can be assured that the additives going into food are there to improve the food and bring it to the housewife in better condition and in a more convenient form.

RADIOACTIVE POLLUTION OF FOODS

The problem of man-made contamination of foods with radioactivity is rather new. So far, the responsible governmental agencies have made studies when they have seemed necessary. Large-scale studies have not yet been conducted because so far the present and potential hazard, according to the National Research Council, has not warranted the expenditure of money and effort. Studies to date, however, have sufficed to show the order of the hazard.

The radionuclides of strontium, particularly strontium 90, have been of some concern. Its behavior in the body is regulated by the amount of calcium present. Calcium appears to reduce the amount of strontium 90 that may be deposited in the body. This relation is referred to as the strontium-to-calcium ratio. This calcium standard is handy because the calcium levels in many important tissues and secretions are reasonably constant, regardless of dietary intake. Strontium 90 is absorbed into the body from the food and then deposited in the bones. High concentrations of it can cause bone cancers and possibly leukemia. The amount found to date in human beings is small compared with what is considered to be a permissible limit.

In the strontium-to-calcium ratio it appears that the higher the body levels of calcium, the lower the level of strontium 90. From data presently on hand, it appears that high intakes and body reserves of calcium serve as a built-in body protection against absorbed radioactivity. Fortunately, the body absorbs strontium 90 less readily than it absorbs calcium, and it excretes the strontium more readily than it does the calcium. Also it appears that although the radioactive contamination of foods varies considerably from place to place in this country, analysis of the various radioactive contaminants indicates that contamination to date is still well below the levels considered to be hazardous.

OTHER FOOD CONTAMINANTS

Outbreaks of food-borne diseases continue to be reported. By prompt inquiry into the circumstances in each particular case, Public Health Service epidemiologists are often able to pin down the particular disease organisms causing the outbreak, the food involved, and the way in which the food became contaminated. Causes of food-borne infections include species of *Salmonella* and *Clostridium*. Ways to prevent this contamination include elimination of flies (*Salmonella*); high-temperature sterilization (*Clostridium*); and freezing, washing of food, and proper cooking of food before eating. All of these safeguards will reduce the bacterial count.

SUMMARY

I. Introduction—pollution is the by-product of industrial advancement. Some pollutants:
  A. May be replaced with less dangerous pollutants.
  B. Must be disposed of in an effective manner.
  C. We must learn to live with.

II. Radiation
  A. Nuclear concepts and terminology.
    1. Three basic particles of an atom:
      a. Electron—negative electromagnetic charge which balances the proton in number and charge.
      b. Proton—positive electromagnetic charge and balances the electron.
      c. Neutron—carries no charge, but is neutral.
    2. Atomic weight—weight of one atom of an element.
    3. Electron, proton, and neutron particles are not completely fixed and may be displaced and thrown about.
      a. Positive ion—positively charged atom, produced when an electron is displaced from its orbit.
      b. Negative ion—negatively charged particle produced by a free electron rapidly attaching itself to a neutral atom.
      c. Ionization—process of producing positive and negative ion pairs.
      d. Ionizing radiation—radiation that is able to produce ionization.
    4. Five particles or waves produced during ionization:
      a. Alpha particles—two protons and two neutrons, which are emitted as a single unit.
      b. Beta particles—high-speed electrons.
      c. Gamma rays—released by a nucleus when it disintegrates or when electrons are knocked from an atom.

      d. X rays (roentgen rays)—waves of short length containing no electric charge.

      e. Neutrons—particles of no electrical charge ejected when atomic nuclei disintegrate.

        (1) Such neutrons travel until captured by the nuclei of other atoms.

        (2) Certain numerical combinations of protons and neutrons are unstable and undergo spontaneous nuclear disintegration, called fission.

        (3) A process of fission, capture; fission, capture; etc., is a chain reaction.

B. Radiological units of measurement

  1. Roentgen (r)—the amount of leakage of electricity from a charged object.

  2. Rad—one unit of absorbed dose of ionizing radiation.

  3. Rem (roentgen-equivalent for man)—the biological effects of radiation equated with the effects produced by a given dose of X rays measured in roentgens.

  4. Relative biological effectiveness (RBE)—the biological effects of one rad of the radiation being used.

  5. Half-life—time taken for half the radioactive atoms of a particular radioactive element to disintegrate.

  6. Curie—that quantity of a given radioactive material in which 3.7×10^{10} disintegrations occur per second, the rate at which one gram of radium disintegrates; therefore one curie of radium is one gram of radium.

C. Comparative radiosensitivity

  1. Natural background radiation—low levels of radiation from natural sources.

    a. External sources—radiation from naturally occurring radioactive substances.

    b. Internal sources—radioactive elements which are constituents of substances entering the body.

D. Effects of radiation on body tissues.

  1. Somatic tissue effects—radiation produces death of general body tissues and cells.

  2. Genetic effects—the effects upon germ or reproductive cells.

E. Radioactive fallout—the return to earth of radioactive materials which had been carried up into the atmosphere by the detonation of a nuclear device.

F. Waste disposal

  1. Solution of waste disposal depends upon:

    a. Specific nature of material—radioactive half-life or type of radiation.

    b. Concentration of radioactive material.

    c. Quantity of radioactive material.

    d. Specific environment of disposal.

  2. Wastes classified as:

    a. High-level radioactive wastes—allowed to decay while buried in salt beds, in deep wells, or while sunk in the sea.

    b. Medium-level radioactive wastes—held in trenches, in artificial ponds, or in tanks to allow for radioactive decay to a level at which they may be discharged into the environment.

c. Low-level radioactive wastes—disposed of by dilution with water and released directly into the environment.

III. Conservation

A. No longer limited to forests and mountains, but also extends to the urban environment.

B. Pollution of the environment—involves contamination problems which resolve around pollution of:

1. Air—introduction of pollutants into the air as the result of man's activity.

2. Water—the presence of any substances that impair the legitimate uses of water.

3. Food—addition of food additives and of substances accidentally and unintentionally added to food.

Glossary

If you cannot find the word you wish in this glossary, check the index for text and glossary references.

aerosol (air′ə sol) (G. *aer,* air or gas; *(hydro)sol,* a suspension of a solid in a liquid).   A system consisting of solid particles dispersed in a gas; a smoke, or fog.

agranulocytic angina (ā gran′yə lō sit′ik an ji′nə) (G. *a,* without; L. *granulum,* a little grain; G. *kytos,* a hollow vessel; L. *angina,* something choked).   Condition marked by destructive ulcerative lesions of the throat and other mucous membranes, producing suffocative pains.

alpha particle (al′fə) (G. *alpha,* first letter of Greek alphabet).   A fast-moving, positively charged, stable group of two protons and two neutrons, emitted as a single unit in the disintegration of the nucleus of certain radioactive isotopes. It has the same composition as a helium nucleus, but differs in origin and motion.

amenorrhea (ā men′ə rē′ə) (G. *a,* without; *men,* month; *rhoia,* flow).   Absence or abnormal stoppage of the menses.

anencephaly (an′ən sef′ə lē) (G. *an,* without; *enkephalos,* brain).   Abnormal development of the brain characterized by absence of the cranial vault and cerebral hemispheres completely missing or reduced to small masses.

anode (an′ōd) (G. *ana,* up; *hodos,* way).   The positive pole of an electric source.

anticathode (an′ti kath′ōd) (G. *anti,* opposite; *cathod,* a going down, descent).   The part of a vacuum tube opposite the cathode; the target.

atom (at′əm) (G. *atomos,* indivisible).   Any one of the ultimate particles of a molecule or of any matter.

beta particle (bā′tə) (G. *beta,* second letter of Greek alphabet).   A high-speed electron ejected from a disintegrating nucleus.

dosimeter (dō sim′i tər).   A meter for measuring X-ray output.

electromagnetic (i lek′trō mag net′ik) (G. *elektron,* amber; *magnes,* a magnet).   Magnetic attraction or repulsion produced by an electric current.

electron (i lek′tron).   Unit of negative electricity.

element (el′ə mənt) (L. *elementum,* element).   Any one of the simple substances that make up all compounds.

emaciation (i mā'shē ā'shən) (L. *emaciare,* to make lean).   A wasted condition of the body.

erythema (er i thē'mə) (G. *erythema,* redness).   A redness of the skin due to congestion of the capillaries.

fibrosis (fī brō'sis) (G. *fibrous,* tissue; L. *osis,* a condition of).   A condition marked by an increase of fibrous tissue.

fission (fish'ən) (L. *fissio,* to split).   The splitting into two parts, as the splitting of the nucleus of an atom, releasing a great quantity of energy.

fluoroscope (floor'ə skōp) (From *fluorescence,* first observed in fluor spar; G. *skopein,* to examine).   A device used for examining deep structures of the body directly by use of X rays.

gamma rays (gam'ə) (G. *gamma,* third letter of Greek alphabet).   A type of radiation (similar to X ray but of a shorter wave length) emitted by certain radioactive substances.

genetic dose (jə net'ik).   The amount of irradiation needed to affect the gonads, germ cells, or embryos produced by an individual.

half-life.   The time in which the radioactivity originally associated with an isotope will be reduced by one half through radioactive decay.

ion (ī'on) (G. *iōn,* going).   An atom or group of atoms having a charge of positive (cation) or negative (anion) electricity.

ionization (ī'ə ni zā'shən) (G. *ion,* going).   The dissociation of a substance into ions.

isotope (ī'sə tōp) (G. *isos,* equal; *topos,* place).   An element of identical chemical character as another element occupying the same place in the periodic table, but differing from it in other characteristics, as in radioactivity or in the mass of its atoms.

megaton (meg'ə tun) (G. *megas,* large).   A million tons.

microcephaly (mī'krō sef'ə lē) (G. *mikros,* small; *kephale,* head).   Abnormal smallness of the head, with smallness of the cerebral hemispheres.

molecule (mol'ə kyool) (L. *molecula,* little mass).   A unit of matter; the smallest portion of an element or compound that retains chemical identity.

necrosis (ne krō'sis) (G. *nekrosis,* deadness).   Death of a cell or of a group of cells which is in contact with living tissue.

neutron (nyoo'tron) (L. *neuter,* neither).   An electrically neutral or uncharged particle of matter.

nucleus (nyoo'klē əs) (L. *nucleus,* a kernel).   In nuclear technology, that part of an atom in which the total positive electric charge resides. It contains the protons and neutrons.

organogenesis (or'gə nō jen'i sis) (G. *organon,* organ; *genesis,* generation).   The development or growth of organs.

photochemical (fō'tō kem'i kəl) (G. *photos,* light; chemistry).   Pertaining to the chemical properties of light.

pollution (pə loo'shən) (L. *pollutio,* to defile).   Act of defiling or making impure.

proton (prō'ton) (G. *protos,* first).   An elementary particle of positive charge equal to the negative charge of an electron. Has approximately the atomic weight of one.

radiation (rā dē ā'shən) (L. *radiatio,* to emit rays).   The emission and propagation of energy through space or through a material medium in the form of waves or particles. Examples: sound waves, elastic waves, or electromagnetic waves and atomic particles.

radionuclide (rā' dē ō nyoo'klīd). A condensation for *radioactive nuclide*. Radioactive isotopes which upon spontaneous decomposition of an atom emit alpha, beta, or gamma rays. There are 50 or 60 naturally occurring radionuclides; those produced artificially as fission products number well over 900.

radioresistant (rā'dē ō ri zis'tənt) (L. *radio,* ray; *resistere,* standing back). Resisting the effects of radiation.

radiotherapeutic (rā'dē ō ther'ə pyoo'tik) (L. *radio,* ray; *therapeia,* cure). The treatment of disease by X ray, radium rays, etc.

toxicity (tok sis'i tē) (G. *toxikon,* a poison). Quality, state, or degree of being toxic or poisonous.

X ray (Named by German physicist Wilhelm Conrad Roentgen in 1895 because he did not know the nature of the rays). Also called *roentgen rays.* Penetrating electromagnetic waves of radiation.

CHAPTER 19

POPULATION
DYNAMICS

WORLD RESOURCES

WORLD POPULATION
PROBLEMS

UNITED STATES
POPULATION PROBLEMS

SUMMARY

Discussion of the population problem often centers on two issues, *space* and *food*, as though resolution of this problem rests on finding enough standing room and enough food per person for survival. Such oversimplification misdirects the vastness of the problem because:

1. Most of the world's people live so poorly today that it is not sufficient for food production merely to keep pace with population growth.
2. World output of everything, not only food, must be stepped up sharply to meet any *reasonable* needs and demands of people to live adequately.
3. Frustration of the growing desire among all people for decent living conditions, education, and economic opportunity is creating tremendous political and social tensions.
4. The world is *not* one big, unified reservoir of space, skills, resources, knowledge, and capital from which nations can procure their respective needs.

5. There is a wide gap between what is technologically or theoretically possible and its universal application.[1]

WORLD RESOURCES

The world population problem is the total of widely differing problems in the major regions and countries of the world. The problem in an individual country depends largely upon its particular stage of development. Consequently, the base of the population problem is the vast one of resources and the *alarming differentials in consumption of these resources* between different regions and nations of the world. Furthermore, a society devoted to supporting maximum numbers at a bare subsistence level is incompatible with the values of modern civilization.

POPULATION AND HEALTH

Public health, in its many forms, has effectively waged a battle against long-established infectious agents. Through measures such as its anti-malarial program, it has been able (for example, in Ceylon) to open huge areas for habitation and cultivation that were formerly uninhabitable. Public concern over health problems has resulted in improved sanitation; purer and more adequate water supplies; and prevention and control of communicable diseases through immunization, insecticides, antibiotics, and increased attention to nutritional disorders. These improvements have contributed toward a lowered death rate and an increased life expectancy.

It is mistakenly assumed by some that the present world population problem is due to the great efficiency of health programs. It is true that as countries develop economically, better living conditions and improved nutrition usually result. These in turn lead to a drop in death rates. In addition, however, after a lag of several generations of better conditions, the birth rate also tends to decline. In the past, owing to infant mortality, parents have conceived more children than they expected to raise to maturity. For example, parents conceived six children in order to raise four to maturity. As available medical services improve, infant mortality drops. It takes time for parents to realize that they can be assured of survival of most, if not all, of their children. If this lag could be reduced from several generations to a single generation, the total population growth in economically developing countries would be lessened.

Health programs, therefore, provide the *best* rather than the worst

[1] D. L. Nortman, *The Population Problem*, New York, National Educational Television, 1965, pp. 7–8.

prospects for solving the population problem. Family planning might well be decided upon and practiced where parents feel secure in the health of their children. As a result of this logical relationship between health programs and population control, national family planning programs are commonly assigned to health services. These have been pioneered in Japan, India, Korea, Taiwan, Pakistan, Egypt, Turkey, Tunisia, Czechoslovakia, and Poland.

The success of these programs, however, lies in sufficiently motivating the entire population. Historically, when conditions have become bad enough, people have voluntarily controlled population with methods normally considered objectionable or immoral. During the potato famines in Ireland a century ago, the excessive population was solved by both emigration and inheritance legislation favoring eldest sons. Japan currently legalizes abortion as a principal method of population control, with abortions exceeding live births. In mainland China there is indication of a return to the old custom of female infanticide. These examples lead some authorities to believe that a "standing room only" prophecy for the people of the earth has little chance of ever becoming reality. In preference to such practices, however, people must be motivated to accept the techniques of using contraceptives in family planning.

Various factors influence motivation—religious scruples, traditions, family relationships, and a family's view of its socio-economic condition. Some families have to realize they are living below subsistence levels before they are willing to limit family size. Unfortunately, some families realize their economic limitations only after their number of children has exceeded their resources.

Ample instruction for obtaining and using contraceptive devices needs to be promoted. One of the best devices in recent years has been the oral contraceptives, "the pill." Women in some parts of the world, however, have trouble in remembering when to take the pills, cannot count, or are unable to afford them. A device of more promise is the intrauterine contraceptive device (IUD), which can be used continuously with almost 100 percent effectiveness. These devices may provide the kind of technical breakthrough needed to effectively counter overpopulation in countries with severe human congestion and limited food and other resources.

At the same time the study of world health has expanded far beyond its former concerns with bacterial agents, insect vectors, parasitism, food supply, water pollution, fertility, and contraception. Today it includes also the study of the influence of patterns of human behavior such as cigarette smoking, compulsive striving, and the influence of social processes such as cultural change or occupational mobility. The patterns of men's lives are greatly interwoven with their health and behavior.

POPULATION AND FOOD

The majority of people living on the earth today do not have enough food to eat. More than half of the people in the world today live on less than 2200 calories per person per day, although the Food and Agricultural Organization (FAO) of the United Nations recommends a daily minimum of 2650 calories. The amount of calories in food is only one consideration. Equally important is how well the diet is balanced with the various kinds of foods. Generally the low-calorie diets of the world consist primarily of plant foods, which cannot be considered balanced diets. The American enjoys not only a high-calorie diet, but also one including liberal amounts of both plant and animal products (Table 19.1).

TABLE 19.1 LEVELS OF DAILY PER CAPITA CONSUMPTION OF FOOD BY REGIONS AND GROUPS OF COUNTRIES[a]

Regions	Calories	Total Protein (grams)	Animal Protein (grams)
Far East	1910	54	6
Near East	2190	70	14
Africa	2100	61	15
Latin America	2380	67	29
Europe	2870	91	31
Northern America	3120	90	60
World	2260	66	18

[a] The postwar levels of consumption were used.

SOURCE: Stuart Mudd, ed., *The Population Crisis and the Use of World Resources*, Bloomington, Ind., Indiana University Press, 1964.

Most of the world's population increase is occurring in areas that are already short of food and are poorly developed—Asia, Africa, and Latin America. To *blindly* believe that God will "provide for His flock" regardless of how large it becomes is a form of utopianism. This argument is unsatisfactory because it overlooks the fact that more than a billion people already in the world today are not provided with even the minimum dietary standards; in other words they are starving.

The basis for all food production is land. It must be both available and of good quality. Eroded soil which lacks minerals and organic mulch is unable to produce food in either quality or quantity. The techniques used to keep the soil in good condition, as well as techniques used to increase yield per acre per year, are essential to meeting food needs for populations.

Mineral fertilizers applied to the soil increase crop productivity. The high agricultural production of countries such as Japan and Western Europe has been due to the liberal use of mineral fertilizers. Improved control of insect pests and plant diseases have reduced waste and loss of plants. Advances in plant breeding have helped increase both the quality and amount of food crops produced per acre. Although these advances have been very obvious in certain countries, in much of the world there has yet been little increase in the yields per acre of the major crops. In spite of an increase in number of acres devoted to grain production during the past 40 years, the increase in world population has more than offset any gains made in providing more food per person. Between 1910 and 1950, the world population increased more than 30 percent, whereas world food production increased only about 15 percent. We would have to double the world's present food production to provide an adequate diet for the expanding world population. This expansion might be provided by increasing the yield of food per acre or by putting new lands into productivity.

TABLE 19.2 **PRODUCTION OF ORGANIC MATTER PER YEAR BY THE VEGETATION OF THE EARTH**

Type of Vegetation	Area in Millions of Square Kilometers	Net Production Per Year	
		Grams of Carbon per Square Meter	Millions of Tons of Carbon
Cultivated	13.31	204	2,728
Forest	44.41	874	48,100
Grassland	36.90	103	3,286
Other (Desert, swamp, etc.)	53.90	178	2,706
Total			
Land	148.5	373 (mean)	56,820
Sea	371.0	90 (mean)	33,400

SOURCE: From "The Human Population" by Edward S. Deevey, Jr. Copyright © 1960 by *Scientific American, Inc.* All rights reserved.

How much food can be produced throughout the world? Table 19.2 shows the production of *organic matter per year* by the vegetation of the earth; thus it indicates the earth's ultimate food-producing capacity. Cultivated vegetation is shown to be less efficient than forests and yielding a smaller over-all output. Thus we can see how inefficient cultivated vegetation is; yet this is the type of vegetation which will supplement the others for the production of food. Also, land vegetation leads sea vegetation in efficiency and in net tonnage. This comparison implies that reaching into the sea is not the answer to ultimate food production.

Since the most easily cultivated land is already in use, cultivation of new lands involves higher costs for irrigation, drainage, fertilization, and clearing of virgin lands. Higher yields, as well as conservation of existing lands, offer the best route for increased food production. However, efforts made to feed the present hungry peoples of the world will mean little if the world's population continues to rise unabated. The best hope lies both in increased food production and in reducing birth rates to replacement levels.

POPULATION AND ENERGY—MINERAL RESOURCES

The earth's capacity to provide raw materials and land is limited. Many minerals and most of the sources of energy in current use are nonrenewable. In some places the scarcity of forest stands is limiting the use of wood and wood products. More and more cities are having to curtail their water service or find new and more remote sources of fresh water.

If the entire world is to develop industrially on a level comparable to that of the United States and Europe, our known reserves of coal, petroleum, and natural gas will not be able to provide sufficient energy. It has been forecast that the high point in petroleum production will be reached in the relatively near future—sometime before the year 2000. The fossil fuels—natural gas, petroleum, and coal—are expected to provide the world's energy needs for no more than several hundred years.

Our sources of energy are water (for about 10 percent of our electrical power), coal, gas, and oil. By fulfilling an ever-increasing demand for power by burning these fossil fuels we are depleting stores which are not being replaced. These are nonrenewable natural resources and, in time (an alarmingly short time if the demand grows as it has for the past quarter of a century), these fuels will be gone. However, there are two energy sources that may replace fossil fuels; one is radiation from the sun (solar energy) and the other is nuclear energy—that derived from the fission of heavy atoms and the fusion of light ones (see Chapter 18).

It would seem that capturing solar energy directly would be preferable to utilizing atomic energy, with all its inherent dangers. However, the practical utilization of solar energy at present is restricted to rather small solar batteries. It is possible that this source of energy will be developed, but at the moment atomic energy is far in the lead.

There now appear to be only two paths to utilization of the energy locked within the nucleus: (1) fission of heavy nuclei—the controlled "A-bomb" reaction and (2) fusion of light nuclei—the controlled "H-bomb" reaction. In its present state the nuclear theory gives no hint that there are more spectacular reactions than fission or fusion. Yet it must be pointed out that the nuclear theory is in an incomplete and unsatisfactory state.

FISSION POWER

Theoretically, the fission process releases less than 0.1 percent of the energy of the ounce of uranium used in a reaction. Also, uranium, in the form of a fuel element (compound of uranium and other materials ready to be used in a reactor) for a nuclear reaction gives up no more than approximately 10 percent of that 0.1 percent theoretically available before the fuel element must be either discarded or reprocessed.[2] The tremendous wastes that would be produced in widely used fission reactors could become the restricting factor in the use of fission reactions as a source of power (see Chapter 18).

If the world fission fuel reserve was computed simply on the basis of the amount of fissionable uranium known to be readily extractable from the earth's crust, the total energy available from this source would be only about 15 percent of that of the remaining fossil fuels. But atomic fuel may in the future be used in many different forms. Happily it appears that the technology of reactors is advancing to a point where nonfissionable thorium and uranium could be transformed into fissionable forms of uranium (breeder reaction). It will be necessary to expand technology before this energy is unlocked, but when it is available, the known sources of uranium and thorium would be enough to supply the world's electrical power needs for several centuries.

FUSION POWER

Any discussion of fusion power must be riddled with "What if . . . ?" The feasibility of this second avenue to nuclear power is being explored in many laboratories throughout the world. Research on the problems involved has made slow progress.

In contrast to the fission reaction, which can take place at room temperature, the fusion reaction requires temperatures of millions of degrees. The construction of vessels to contain and control such a reaction is extremely complicated and expensive. If fusion power be-

2 *Ibid.,* p. 491.

comes a reality, deuterium, the naturally occurring heavy isotope (Chapter 18) of hydrogen will be the chief fuel. Tritium, the heavier, manmade isotope of hydrogen may also be needed, but this rare substance would be regenerated by the fusion reaction itself.

Deuterium is present in nature as 0.015 percent of all hydrogen. Even at this low concentration the ocean waters are estimated to contain a million billion tons of deuterium. Known processes are capable of extracting deuterium from the ocean at extremely small costs. Consequently, the deuterium present in the oceans is essentially inexhaustible.

Theoretically, fusion power has further advantages over fission power. A "runaway accident" of fission reactors would not be possible in the fusion reactors. Nor would disposal of the waste products of fusion reactors be anywhere near as difficult a problem as it is with fission reactors, since comparatively little radioactivity would be produced in the fusion reactors.

It is clear that nuclear power offers no cure-all for the world's energy problems. The adoption of fission power will be slow and its rate will depend ultimately on the exhaustion of fossil fuel reserves. Fusion power, while potentially having many advantages over fission power, including an inexhaustible fuel supply of negligible cost, has not yet been established as feasible and its costs cannot be readily assessed.

Since in the past the most easily obtained minerals and sources of energy have been used, the continued mining of less accessible deposits will cost this country increasingly more than they have in the past. Yet, even this low-yield extraction has its limits. Each of the acts mentioned above represent an unnecessary *borrowing on the future*.

Borrowing on the future is being done with the resources in the United States, as well as with those elsewhere in the world. Although Americans have 6 percent of the world's population, they consume half of the world's production of major minerals; they consume twice as much commercial energy per person as the British and four times as much as the people of India. It is estimated that each year the average American utilizes an amount of natural resources equal to that used by 25 to 30 Indians. In these terms the increase in *this country's population* appears frightening. In light of the aspirations of many parts of the world for better living standards, it can be questioned whether it will be justifiable for the 6 percent of the world's population in the United States to continue consuming 40 to 50 percent of the world's resources.

Discovery of new reserves, more efficient methods of extraction and use, and thoughtful conservation should help prolong the world's reserves of energy and minerals. On the other hand, the continued increase in demands placed on these resources through unlimited population increases will present an increasingly critical situation. Our choice is whether vast numbers of people will be limited to living poorly at low standards or whether fewer people will live well—a choice between *quantity* and *quality*.

POPULATION PRESSURE

The poorer populations of the world, whose expectations are not fulfilled, form the core of an increasingly larger group. They feel today the hardships of their low level of living more keenly than ever before, even though they may actually be living at a better level than they did in the past.

Table 19.3 shows the disparities between populations and industrial output of the world. Thirty percent of the world's population enjoy 90 percent of the industrial output. The remaining 70 percent of the population produces only 10 percent of the world's industrial products. There is a per capita ratio of the developed to the developing areas of 21:1. From such differences it is clear that even in the absence of population growth, the emerging areas face enormous problems of economic development.

TABLE 19.3 POPULATION AND INDUSTRIAL PRODUCTION AS PERCENT OF WORLD TOTAL

	Industrialized Areas	Nonindustrialized Areas
Population	30	70
Industrial Production	90	10
Mining	75	25
Manufacturing	91	9
Light	87	13
Heavy	93	7
Electricity	91	9

SOURCE: D. L. Nortman, *The Population Problem,* New York, National Educational Television, 1965, p. 9.

From the standpoint of creating tensions between nations, it is not absolute poverty that provides people with the strongest motives to support political aggression; it is the feeling that they do not have enough land or other resources to use so that they can live as well as other people. People must have some standard of comparison before they are aware of their own poverty and before they begin to feel the pressure of population as a motive for supporting national action to relieve this pressure. It requires only a little imagination and some knowledge of the actual living conditions in most of the developing countries of the world to make one realize that the growing feelings of deprivation can be a weapon ready-made for aggressive ideologies.

WORLD POPULATION PROBLEMS

During the past centuries, man's increase in numbers has been governed by the three regulators—*disease, war,* and *starvation.* Man's increasing control of disease has greatly freed him from one of these controls. War and famine, however, still act as biological checks upon populations in those parts of the world where they occur.

At the same time, man is gradually learning how to separate sexual gratification from reproduction through employing effective forms of contraception, or voluntary fertility control. And for the first time in history, modern man has the means of directing the course of his own population. Need for birth-control information is clear. Most animal species, including man, are endowed with the capacity to produce offspring in numbers far in excess of available supplies of food, natural resources, and space. As man continues to gain control over the operation of the traditional biological checks—war, disease, and starvation—he must demonstrate his ability to control his reproductive potential.

Although the means are at hand, mankind is still having trouble facing the realities of an important biological law—*any species that multiplies without limit eventually faces stark shortages of food.* Man must choose one of the two biological checks upon increase in number—*higher mortality or a lowered fertility.*

THE PAST AND PRESENT

Only fragmentary data are available to indicate the past rate of growth of the population of the world. A regular census of population was not conducted prior to 1800, although registers had been maintained for small population groups prior to that time. The commonly accepted population figures of the world prior to 1800 are only informed guesses. Nevertheless, it is possible to piece together a consistent series of estimates of the world's population during the past two centuries. This information, supplemented by rough guesses of the number of persons alive at selected earlier periods, is the background for Fig. 19.1, which contains estimates of the population of the world from A.D. 1 to A.D. 2000. This graph reveals a spectacular spurt during recent decades in the increase of the world's population.

A rough approximation can be made of the length of time required for the population of the world to reach one-quarter of a billion persons, which is the beginning of the *Christian era.* During the second United Nations World Population Conference in 1965, John Durand

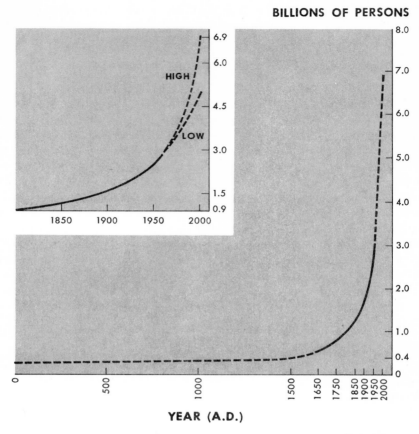

Fig. 19.1 Estimated population of the world, A.D. 1 to 2000. (Harold F. Dorn, "World Population Growth: An International Dilemma," *Science*, Vol. 135, pp. 283-290, 26 January 1962. Copyright 1962 by the American Association for the Advancement of Science.)

presented a paper analyzing the evolution of the world population between the years 1750 and 2000. This paper points out that the world reached its first billion inhabitants in 1810, the second in 1925, and the third in 1960. The fourth will doubtless be attained in 1980, and the fifth by 1995. The varying time spans required for each *increase of one billion people* are as follows:

1st billion	several hundred thousand years
2d billion	115 years
3d billion	35 years
4th billion	20 years
5th billion	15 years

According to two well-known authors on world demography (Carr-Saunders and Wilcox) the growth rates of Asia and Europe prior to 1900 were quite different. The population of Europe increased more than fourfold between 1650 and 1900, whereas Asia's population increased only about $2\frac{1}{2}$ times. Moreover, the population in the area of European settlement (including Europe and the Americas) increased about five times. As a result of these differential rates of growth in Asia and Europe, the proportion of the world's population living in Asia declined from around 60 percent in 1650 to about 55 percent in 1900. Since 1900 the proportion of the world's population living in Asia has been increasing and, according to the United Nations, in 1955 it amounted to 55.3 percent; the proportion living in Europe has been declining, and in 1955 constituted only 15.2 percent of the world's total.

During the past decade, 6 out of every 10 persons added to the world's population live in Asia; another 2 out of 10 live in Latin America and Africa. Undoubtedly, this increase will change the world's balance of power and influence world affairs in coming years. Everywhere there seems to be growing impatience with the conditions that limit improvement in the standards of living. This impatience can result only in political unrest and change. The results of human reproduction are no longer the concern only of the country where the people are citizens. Such a problem in one part of the world affects, in some manner, the health and welfare of those in even the wealthiest nations.

In the past each major upward step in population followed some major discovery or invention, such as agriculture, the initiation of urban life and trade, the harnessing of nonhuman power, or the technological revolution. As a more sophisticated and economically responsible society was achieved, the ability to maintain a higher population became a reality. But in the present century the decline in mortality is not only independent of economic development but is a positive obstacle to it. The most decisive factor in increasing population during this time is of a different sort—the application of scientific medicine, or what may be called "death control."

The discoveries of sulfa drugs and especially of the antibiotics, insecticides, and other means of combating disease-carrying organisms radically altered the situation of population dynamics. It became possible to lower mortality irrespective of economic development. This was man's first major victory over death. Within a few years, this victory was to be responsible for the rapid population explosion that jeopardizes the economic growth of all developing areas and the world itself.

In the Western world the reduction of the death rate came gradually and its effect on population growth was buffered by factors which tended at the same time to reduce the birth rate—namely, a rising standard of living and industrialization, which made children no longer an economic asset. The death rates in these advanced countries have been reduced from the traditional 35 or 40 per thousand to less than 10 per thousand. The average life span (life expectancy at birth) has almost doubled in the Western World since the mid-nineteenth century (Table 19.4). It now stands at over seventy years in Europe and North America, and, as shown in Table 19.5, this process of lengthening life has begun to get under way in the developing areas of the world.

TABLE 19.4   LIFE EXPECTANCY AT BIRTH[a]

Year	Life Expectancy at Birth in Years
1840	41.0
1850	41.5
1860	42.2
1870	43.5
1880	45.2
1890	47.1
1900	50.5
1910	54.3
1920	58.3
1930	61.7
1940	64.6
1955 to present	+71.0

[a] The average of six European countries and one state in the United States. The countries are Denmark, England and Wales, France, the Netherlands, Norway, and Sweden; the state in the United States is Massachusetts.

SOURCE: *Population Bulletin of the United Nations*, No. 6, United Nations Publication Sales No. 62. XVII.2, Table IV.1.

The reduction of the death rate has been a different matter in the developing countries of the world. Here death control was introduced with startling speed. Ancient diseases were brought under control or totally abolished in the space of a few decades or even a few years. Consequently, all are now in a stage of explosive expansion. As shown in Table 19.6, the developing countries at the present time are showing an annual population increase of 2 percent; some, such as Latin America, are increasing over 3 percent per year. If this increase continues as predicted through the year 2000, Europe will have a population of about 527 million and Asia will expand to better than 3 billion, 394 million inhabitants (Table 19.7).

Just as Thomas Malthus, at the end of the eighteenth century, could not foresee the tremendous changes that have taken place in Europe,

TABLE 19.5 LIFE EXPECTANCY AT BIRTH IN SIX DEVELOPING COUNTRIES

Country	Life Expectancy at Birth		
	1940	1950	1960
Mexico	40.2	50.3	57.2
Taiwan	44.8	58.0	65.4
Mauritius	38.4	50.8	58.4
Trinidad and Tobago	50.6	56.2	63.4
Singapore	43.1	56.0	66.8
Malaysia	–	51.0	59.6

SOURCE: Jean Bourgeois-Picbat, *Population Growth and Development,* New York, Carnegie Endowment for International Peace, 1966, p. 65.

TABLE 19.6 ANNUAL AVERAGE CHANGES (PERCENT/YEAR) IN THE POPULATIONS OF DEVELOPING REGIONS[a]

	1920 to 1930	1930 to 1940	1940 to 1950	1950 to 1960	1960 to 1970	1970 to 1980	1980 to 1990	1990 to 2000
All developing countries	1.1	1.3	1.3	2.1	2.3	2.3	2.1	2.0
East Asia	0.7[a]	0.7[b]	0.8[b]	1.6[b]	1.5	1.4	1.2	1.0
South Asia	1.3	1.5	1.4	2.3	2.7	2.7	2.3	2.1
Africa	1.5[b]	1.7[b]	1.6[b]	2.3[b]	2.7	3.0	3.1	3.1
Latin America	2.0	2.1	2.5	3.0	3.3	3.2	3.1	2.8

[a] Medium variant estimates.

[b] Estimates insecure.

SOURCE: United Nations, *Provisional Report on World Population Prospects, as Assessed in 1963,* New York, United Nations Doc. ST/SOA/SER.R/17.

we, today, cannot clearly foresee the final effects of an unprecedented rapid increase in population.

The rate of human reproduction in any part of the globe directly or indirectly affects the health and welfare of the rest of the human race. The increase in the world's population at the present time is occurring far more rapidly in some places than in others. The birth rates in Africa, Asia, and Latin America are presently around 40 births per thousand population, whereas their death rates are about 20 to 25 per thousand. The most rapid increase of population in the world today is reported to be in Costa Rica, where a birth rate of 50 per thousand

TABLE 19.7 **DECENNIAL CHANGES IN THE POPULATION OF**

Regions and Countries	1920	1930	1940	1950
Europe	327.0	355.0	380.0	392.0
Asia	1023.0	1120.0	1244.0	1381.0
Latin America	90.0	108.0	130.0	163.0
Africa	143.0	161.0	191.0	222.0

and a death rate of 8.5 per thousand is causing an increase of 4 percent per year. Similar rapid increases are taking place all over Latin America, where the population is expected to double within the next 26 years if the present rate of increase continues.[3]

This population increase intensifies the existing imbalance between the distribution of the world's population and the distribution of wealth, resources, and the use of nonhuman energy. It seems inevitable that the breaking up of world domination by northwest Europeans and their descendants will continue and that the centers of power and influence will shift toward the population centers of the world.

Probably for the first time in human history there is universal aspiration for rapid improvement in the standard of living and a growing impatience with conditions that appear to stand in the way of its attainment. Millions of persons in Asia, Africa, and Latin America now are aware of the standard of living enjoyed by Europeans and North Americans. They are demanding the opportunity to attain the same standard and resisting the idea that they must be permanently content with less. But continuation of the present high rate of human multiplication in these areas will act as a brake on the already painfully slow improvement in the level of living. This will increase political unrest and possibly bring about changes in governments.

The capital and technological skills that the nations of Africa, Asia, and Latin America require to produce enough food for a rapidly growing population and simultaneously to raise per capita income exceed their existing national resources and ability. An immediate supply of capital in the amounts required is available only from the wealthier nations which do not have the desire to extend such large amounts of capital to support the economic development of the less advanced nations. Even if such support should be accepted, it is not as yet clear how long the wealthier nations would be able to support the uncontrolled breeding of the populations receiving assistance. General acceptance of such a foreign aid program will only postpone for a few decades the

[3] Ronald Freedman, ed., *Population: The Vital Revolution*, Garden City, N.Y., Doubleday, 1964.

SELECTED AREAS OF THE WORLD IN MILLIONS

Populations 1960	1970	1980	1990	2000
425.0	454.0	479.0	504.0	507.0
1651.4	1999.5	2414.2	2872.6	3394.4
212.0	282.0	374.0	488.0	624.0
273.0	346.0	449.0	587.0	768.0

SOURCE: Derived from *Provisional Report on World Population Prospects, as Assessed in 1963*, New York, United Nations Doc. ST/SOA/SER.R/17, Chapters 8, 9, and 14. The same decennial increase has been assumed for 1990 to 2000 as for 1970 to 1980.

inevitable reckoning with the results of uncontrolled human multiplication.

THE FUTURE

When looking toward the future, we must wonder about the present. Is this present spurt in population growth a temporary phenomenon that will shortly cease, with the birth rate falling to near the level of the death rate, or will it continue until the former biological regulators—war, disease, and famine—once again take control?

The future populations of individual nations, or of regions, or even of the entire world cannot be predicted for more than a few decades with more than a moderate degree of certainty. Such projections prepared by the United Nations are presented in Table 19.7. The actual population growth since these projections were published (1963) indicate that even the highest projected values will be vast underestimates of the population in the year 2000. The estimated increase in the population of Asia will be approximately equal to the total population of the world in 1958. The increase in the population of Latin America during the last half of this century may equal the total increase in population of man during all of the time from his origin until 1650, when the first colonists were settling New England.[4] Numerical increase of this magnitude will create problems that may be beyond the ability of the nations concerned to solve.

A situation favorable equally to a rapid improvement in the level of living and a sharp increase in population does not appear likely to arise for the people now inhabiting Latin America, Africa, and Asia. Although there are many thinly populated areas in the world, their existence is testimony to the fact that, until now, they have been regarded as undesirable living places. The expansion of population

4 Philip M. Hauser, ed., *The Population Dilemma*, Englewood Cliffs, N.J., Prentice-Hall, 1963, p. 11.

to the remaining open areas would require large expenditures of capital for irrigation, drainage, transportation facilities, control of insects and parasites, and other purposes—capital that the rapidly increasing populations which will need these areas do not possess.

The future may witness a dramatic increase in man's ability to control his environment. Man has been able to modify or control many natural phenomena, but he has not yet discovered how to evade the consequences of biological laws. No species has ever been able to multiply without limit. There are two biological checks upon a rapid increase in number—high mortality and low fertility. Unlike other biological organisms, man can choose which of these checks shall be applied, but one of them *must* be. Whether or not we use scientific knowledge to guide the future more wisely than the blind forces of nature, only the future can reveal.

UNITED STATES POPULATION PROBLEMS

DOES OVERPOPULATION THREATEN THE UNITED STATES?

It is apparent that overpopulation is already a reality in many of the world's countries and a threat to many more. But does the United States, with its powerful economy and vast resources, need to concern itself with its own increasing population? In the opinion of the authors, the answer is a resounding *yes*.

Let us briefly consider some of the arguments given by those who maintain that the United States is *not* threatened by overpopulation. One such argument hinges upon food supply and reminds us that in the United States farmers are often paid for not growing certain crops. Our answer to this argument is that, although the margin between surplus and shortage of food is more narrow than many people realize, we do not feel that food supply alone should determine the optimum population level in a highly developed country. Other factors are likely to begin to interfere with human welfare before the food supply becomes critical.

Another argument heard is that a vigorous rate of population growth is essential in order to maintain a prosperous national economy. Theoretically, greater population should mean greater demand for the products and services of industries, and therefore greater profit and prosperity for all. Seldom considered by those who make this argument are the following factors: First, the highest birth rate occurs in the lowest-income families and additional births in these families result in little additional expenditure for goods and services. In fact, births in these families often result in larger welfare checks, putting a greater drain on the economy rather than having a stimulating effect. Children born into such circumstances are likely to receive inadequate education and to remain an economic burden, possibly for life. Another commonly overlooked factor is that as the population increases, there are more individuals present to share in any increased prosperity. Since many of our national resources are fixed in abundance, there would actually be *less* prosperity per individual.

In further discussion of possible United States overpopulation let us not concentrate on the threat of starvation, since it is likely that other population pressures would curtail the birth rate before the point of starvation was reached in this country. But it is quite possible that our fertility spree will continue until the *quality* of living is greatly reduced.

As the country becomes more crowded, life will gradually become less and less pleasant. Technical advances promise us more free time in the future, but population pressures threaten to eliminate much land from possible recreational use and to vastly overtax the recreational facilities that do remain. The miles of shoreline, lakefront, and rivers available for recreational use are fixed, but the need for these facilities is increasing. It will become increasingly difficult to "get away from the crowd" as the population increases.

Stress will play an ever-larger role in our lives. The more we are crowded, the more we feel stress. The result will be more emotional illness, accompanied by the many physical problems that stress causes or aggravates.

As discussed in the previous chapter, the problem of pollution of the environment is directly related to population. The greater the level of population, the less is the right of the individual to pollute his environment. For example, as the number of automobiles in the country continues to increase, the individual owner finds increasing restrictions of his "right" to pollute the air. In the future, we may find ourselves restricted from many of our current "rights."

The population of the United States still fits the country fairly comfortably, but the threat of overpopulation does exist. Let us now consider the nature of the population in the past, the present, and as it may be in the future.

THE PAST

During the early years of the United States the rate of population growth was a source of great pride. With seemingly limitless resources and room for westward expansion, the fertility rate reached levels seldom exceeded anywhere on earth. During the colonial period the average family included about eight children. Even with the high death rate, the

TABLE 19.8 **HISTORY OF POPULATION**

Year	Fertility Rate[a]	Birth Rate[b]	Death Rate[c]	Natural Increase[d]
1790				
1800	278	—	—	—
1810	274	—	—	—
1820	260	55.2	—	—
1830	240	—	—	—
1840	222	51.8	—	—
1850	194	—	—	—
1860	184	44.3	—	—
1870	167	—	—	—
1880	155	39.8	—	—
1890	137	—	—	—
1900	130	32.2	17.2	15.0
1910	126.8	30.1	14.7	15.4
1920	117.9	23.7	13.0	10.7
1930	89.2	18.9	11.3	7.6
1940	79.9	19.4	10.8	8.6
1950	106.2	24.1	9.6	14.5
1960	118.0	23.7	9.5	14.2

a Fertility rate is the number of births per 1000 women ages 15 through 44. Figures prior to 1900 for white population only; 1900 and subsequent for all races.

b Birth rate is the number of births per 1000 total population.

c Death rate is the number of deaths per 1000 total population. Few states registered deaths prior to 1900.

d Natural increase is the number of births less the number of deaths per 1000 population.

e Exclusive of Alaska and Hawaii. Major land acquisitions completed by 1850.

SOURCE: Various U.S. Census Bureau Reports.

population more than doubled in every generation. At this time a large family was considered a definite asset. The more children a family produced, the more land it could clear and cultivate.

In addition to this high fertility rate, the United States for many years practiced an open-door immigration policy. Prior to the 1921 Immigration Act about 35 million immigrants entered the country, accounting for about one third of the population growth to that time. Since 1921, immigration has accounted for less than 10 percent of the population growth.

But long before 1921 the women of the United States slowly began to limit the size of their families. Actually, neither the government nor the women had yet become concerned about the threat of overpopula-

GROWTH IN THE UNITED STATES

Millions of Immigrants in Preceding Decade	Total U.S. Population in Millions	Persons per Square Mile[e]	Percent Annual Population Growth
—	3.9	4.5	—
—	5.3	6.1	3.0
—	7.2	4.3	3.1
—	9.6	5.6	2.9
0.1	12.9	7.4	2.9
0.6	17.1	9.8	2.8
1.7	23.2	7.9	3.1
2.6	31.4	10.6	3.0
2.3	38.6	13.4	2.0
2.8	50.2	16.9	2.6
5.2	63.0	21.2	2.3
3.7	76.2	25.6	1.9
8.8	92.2	31.0	1.9
5.7	106.0	35.6	1.4
4.1	123.2	41.2	1.5
0.5	132.2	44.2	0.7
1.0	151.3	50.7	1.4
2.5	179.3	60.1	1.7

tion. The government restricted immigration because of the diminishing need for unskilled labor. The women restricted their family size because their interests were beginning to extend beyond the farm, kitchen, and nursery toward the city, school, and labor force. By the middle 1920s the average family size had dropped to 2½ children.

During the decade of the 1930s the birth rate dropped still further toward a low of just over two children per family. Although the low birth rate of the 1930s is commonly attributed to the economic depression that characterized those years, a study of Table 19.8 shows this rate to be the culmination of a trend which began in 1880. Actually, then (as now) poor economic conditions have been a slight deterrent to large family size, since traditionally the poorest families have the most children. At what point the birth rate might have leveled off without the Depression is purely a matter of speculation. In any event, even at this low birth rate the population of the country continued to grow significantly.

After World War II a temporary surge in the birth rate was expected in order to make up for births "postponed" during the war years. But the birth rate, rather than rising and then returning to "normal," continued to rise year after year until in 1957 it reached a peak which was resulting in an average family size of almost 3.8 children. Station wagons and four-bedroom houses suddenly became very popular. After 1957 the birth rate started dropping, at first slowly, then sharply during the 1960s. Possible future trends will be discussed later in this chapter.

THE PRESENT

In addition to the total rate of population growth, it is significant to compare the relative birth rates of various segments of the population. Some of the groups we should examine for possible differences are those of differing racial composition, financial level, and educational background.

BIRTH RATE AND RACE

Let us first consider birth rate in relation to race alone, neglecting possible differences in education or income between the groups compared. The only racial breakdown made here is white and nonwhite. In 1960, 88.5 percent of the population was white, 10.5 percent was Negro, and 1 percent was other nonwhite races, including primarily North American Indians and Orientals.

TABLE 19.9 **FERTILITY RATE IN THE UNITED STATES FOR YEAR 1963, BY RACE AND AGE GROUP (NUMBER GIVEN IS THE NUMBER OF CHILDREN BORN PER 1000 WOMEN IN EACH AGE GROUP DURING THAT YEAR)**

Race	Age Groups								
	10–14	15–19	20–24	25–29	30–34	35–39	40–44	45–49	15–44
White	0.4	68.2	224.9	181.2	102.3	48.8	13.4	0.8	103.7
Nonwhite	4.0	139.9	278.1	211.2	128.9	68.9	21.0	1.5	144.8

SOURCE: *Vital Statistics of the United States,* Vol. 1, *Natality,* Washington, D.C., U.S. Department of Health, Education, and Welfare, Public Health Service, 1963, Table 1–6.

Table 19.9 is a comparison of the fertility rates of white and nonwhite women of various age groups. The fertility rate is the number of children born per 1000 women within a given group. From the table it can be seen that in all age groups the nonwhite women produced more children than the white women. These figures, of course, do not indicate whether the greater fertility is due to greater inherent fertility, desire for a larger family, or less effective use of contraceptive measures.

TABLE 19.10 FAMILY SIZE AND INCOME (AVERAGE NUMBER OF CHILDREN EVER BORN PER MARRIED WOMAN OF TWO AGE GROUPS, BY FAMILY INCOME AND RACE, FROM 1960 CENSUS)

Family Income	Age 30–34 White	Nonwhite	Age 35–39 White	Nonwhite
Under $2,000	3.21	4.40	3.32	4.43
$2,000–$3,999	2.95	3.59	3.05	3.54
$4,000–$4,999	2.78	3.19	2.81	3.21
$5,000–$5,999	2.70	2.97	2.75	3.10
$6,000–$6,999	2.61	2.70	2.68	2.81
$7,000–$9,999	2.41	2.40	2.52	2.53
$10,000–$14,999	2.29	2.11	2.38	2.33
$15,000 and over	2.50	2.42	2.60	2.41
Average of all incomes	2.61	3.32	2.67	3.32

SOURCE: U.S. Census Bureau, 1960 Census of Population, Report P.C. (2) 3A.

BIRTH RATE AND INCOME

For many decades in the United States it has been a common observation that low income is often accompanied by large family size ("the rich get richer and the poor get children"). Table 19.10 indicates that in 1960, the last year for which such figures are available, this relationship still held true. Those families with the lowest income had the most children. As incomes increased, family size decreased until an income of over $15,000 was reached. At this level there was an upturn in family size. The apparent significance of these figures is that the middle-income families either desired smaller families or else made more effective use of contraceptive measures than did the lower income groups. Possible reasons may include greater motivation to control family size; better education, enabling more efficient use of contraceptives; household conditions more favorable to the application of contraceptives; and income sufficient to engage medical assistance in the selection and prescription of contraceptives. The increase in family size above $15,000 income probably relates to the ease with which these families could afford to have additional children and raise them in comfort and with convenience.

Another significant trend shown by Table 19.10 is that the higher-income nonwhite families actually have fewer children than white families of the same income level. It is possible that this difference is due to the unusually high motivation levels that are often associated with those members of minority races who attain the higher income levels.

BIRTH RATE AND EDUCATION

Table 19.11 relates the number of children born to the educational level of the woman. The relationship here is similar to that between income and number of children. The higher the level of education, the fewer children are produced. Unlike the income comparison, no upturn in number of offspring exists at the upper end of the scale. The racial breakdown is also similar to that found in the income comparison. The poorly educated nonwhite woman has more children than the similarly educated white woman. The well-educated nonwhite woman has fewer children than the similarly educated white woman. Among women who reach high school graduation the number of children produced by the two racial groups is about equal.

TABLE 19.11 FAMILY SIZE AND EDUCATION (AVERAGE NUMBER OF CHILDREN EVER BORN PER WOMAN OF TWO AGE GROUPS, BY EDUCATION AND RACE, FROM 1960 CENSUS)

Woman's Educational Level	Age 30–34 White	Age 30–34 Nonwhite	Age 35–39 White	Age 35–39 Nonwhite
Elementary—1 to 4 years	3.21	3.54	3.46	3.67
Elementary—5 to 8 years	2.77	3.41	2.88	3.36
High school—1 to 3 years	2.58	3.01	2.58	2.93
High school graduate	2.29	2.31	2.32	2.28
College—1 to 3 years	2.22	2.13	2.28	2.05
College—4 or more years	1.84	1.37	2.03	1.51
Average of all levels	2.40	2.85	2.47	2.90

CURRENT TRENDS IN POPULATION GROWTH

The rate of population growth for the United States has been dropping in recent years (Table 19.12). In 1960 the population increased by 1.75 percent; by 1966 the annual rate of increase had dropped to about 1.1 percent and was continuing to drop. But even this seemingly low rate of population growth is still too high to be maintained on an indefinite basis without severe restriction of the standard of living of the country.

In addition to growth in total numbers, several significant changes are taking place in the geographic distribution of the population. Most of these trends began many years ago, but they are now assuming greater importance in light of the increasing total population and the speed with which these changes are occurring. Professor Donald Bogue of the University of Chicago considers the following trends to be important:

TABLE 19.12 RECENT POPULATION GROWTH IN THE UNITED STATES

Year	Fertility Rate[a]	Birth Rate[b]	Death Rate[c]	Total U.S. Population on July 1 (millions)	Percent Annual Population Growth
1960	118.0	23.7	9.5	179.3	1.8
1961	117.2	23.3	9.3	183.1	1.7
1962	112.1	22.4	9.5	185.9	1.5
1963	108.0	21.6	9.6	188.7	1.4
1964	105.6	21.2	9.4	191.4	1.4
1965[d]	96.7	19.4	9.4	193.6	1.3
1966[d]	93.2	19.1	9.5	195.7	1.1

[a] Fertility rate is the number of births per 1000 women ages 15 through 44.
[b] Birth rate is the number of births per 1000 total population.
[c] Death rate is the number of deaths per 1000 total population.
[d] Figures for years 1965 and 1966 are provisional.
SOURCE: U.S. Public Health Service and Bureau of Census Reports.

1. *Rapid depopulation of rural areas.* Farming areas and small towns are losing population, while the total population grows. Between 1950 and 1960 almost half of the nation's counties *lost* population. Hundreds of small towns are dead or slowly dying.

2. *Heavy movement toward metropolitan areas.* It has been predicted[5] that by 1985 half of the nation's population will be concentrated into three "strip cities," one extending from San Francisco to San Diego, one from Chicago to Buffalo, and one from Boston through Washington, D.C.

3. *Extensive migration from low-income areas to regions of greater economic opportunity.* Among the results of this move is loss of the economically vital and dynamic younger portion of the population from these depressed areas, leaving only the older persons and those lacking the ambition to move to more prosperous regions. Another problem is the readjustment of those who do migrate.

4. *A flow of middle- and upper-income population from the North and East into the South.* Bogue sees this as a very beneficial trend, weakening the caste system and improving the political and economic conditions of the South.

5. *A great migration to the Pacific Coast of people from all strata and all regions.* Bogue suggests that the economy of California may be based upon a rather weak foundation of population growth and government contracts.

[5] "What's Ahead in the Population Boom," *U.S. News and World Report*, May 6, 1963, pp. 68–71.

6. *The dying central city and the suburban sprawl.* Almost all the population growth of the metropolitan areas has been concentrated at their suburban edges. The suburbs of one metropolitan area often meet back-to-back with the suburbs of an adjacent metropolitan area. Simultaneously, the middle-class population of the central city has moved out to the suburbs in search of space, privacy, newer housing, and neighbors of similar interests. In the central city, housing deteriorates into slums, major business follows the money to the suburbs, and crime rises.

7. *Concentration of the Negro population into the deteriorated central portions of the cities.* In less than 30 years, as the need for farm labor has decreased, the Negro population has shifted from being primarily rural to being primarily urban. Today, over three-quarters of the Negro population is concentrated in cities, and this move from rural areas still continues. For most of the migrating Negroes, the move is advantageous, leading to higher income, better housing, better health, and better schools. But for many it is merely a change from rural exploitation to even worse exploitation in the city. Pay is low, rent is high, and commodities and services are priced well above similar goods or services in the suburbs.

THE FUTURE

In predicting future population sizes, we would be in error to merely take the past or present rate of population growth and project this rate of growth out to a given year. For example, the average annual rate of population growth in the United States from 1790 to 1964 (174 years) was 2.2 percent per year. Simply projecting this rate of growth for another 174 years (until the year 2138) would give a population of 8.8 billion, several times the current population of the entire world. Obviously, long before this population level is reached, drastic measures would be taken to curtail reproduction. Actually, the point at which the population of the United States will level off may lie as low as 300 to 400 million people.

Our most immediate future population concern lies in the "boom babies" born between 1950 and 1960. In 1960 there were 11 million women in the 20–30 year age group. In 1980 there will be 20 million women in this prime reproductive age group. This statistic is not just a guess or a rough speculation—these females have already been born and are now growing up. The only question remaining is the rate at which they will reproduce. Will the current trend toward smaller families continue, or will a larger family again become fashionable? If the latter takes place, the baby boom of the 1950s will compare to the baby boom of the 1980s as a cap gun compares to a cannon.

Effective contraceptive methods will certainly not be lacking in 1980. The better contraceptive methods of today, such as oral hormones and intrauterine devices, are already adequate for the maintenance of population growth at an acceptable level. It is likely that even more effective methods will be available in 1980, perhaps based upon entirely new principles. It is also likely that by 1980 family planning information will be so widely available in the United States that any woman with the desire to control her fertility will find the means to do so readily attainable at a cost she can easily afford to pay.

Thus, in 1980 it would seem that the only factor determining the average family size will be the attitudes of the parents regarding the ideal number of children. As the suburbs become increasingly crowded and as the cost of raising and educating a child continues to rise, the trend toward smaller families may definitely continue. Indeed, as more women are better educated and are interested in careers outside the home, many more married couples may decide to remain childless. The feeling that children are needed to insure security in the parents' old age has largely disappeared through improved pension plans and government programs for the health and other needs of elderly persons.

Thus it is possible that a stable population may be reached through the voluntary decisions of married couples to limit their family sizes. It has been mathematically determined that if, with our present low death rate and high proportion of marriages, each family had on the average only a fraction over two children, our population could be maintained at its present number.

If individuals do not control the birth rate voluntarily, it may eventually become controlled through legal regulation. A first step might be the revision of tax laws to favor the small family rather than the large family, which currently receives tax relief. If the population reached a high enough level, measures such as compulsory sterilization, which seem repulsive today, might find widespread support. It is hoped that voluntary family limitation will preclude the need for more radical means of population control in future years.

SUMMARY

    I. World Resources
        A. World population problem extends beyond adequate food and space.
        B. Population and health—must be concerned with birth rate as well as death rate and include population control programs.
        C. Population and food
            1. Majority of people subsist on diets deficient in both calories and essential food elements.
            2. Cultivation of new lands involves high costs for clearing, drainage, irrigation, and fertilization.
        D. Population and energy-mineral resources
            1. Earth's capacity to provide raw materials and land is limited.
            2. Nuclear power offers no cure-all for the world's energy problems.

E. Population pressure
  1. Disparity in standards of living between countries of the world is increasing rather than decreasing.
  2. This disparity creates tensions which tend to create and support political aggression between nations.

II. World Population Problems
  A. Past regulators of population have been:
    1. Disease.
    2. War.
    3. Starvation.
  B. Man must now choose between two biological checks upon population
    1. High mortality through war and starvation.
    2. Lowered fertility through voluntary fertility control.
  C. Past and present
    1. Significant increases in world population have taken place only during the most recent few decades.
    2. Rate of population increase is not uniform over the world; it is most rapid in:
      a. Latin America.
      b. Asia.
      c. Africa.
    3. Population problems anywhere in the world affects the welfare of even the wealthiest nations.
  D. Future
    1. Population growth cannot be predicted with certainty.
    2. No species is able to multiply without limit.

III. United States Population Problems
  A. Although starvation is unlikely in the United States, overpopulation would greatly reduce the quality of living.
  B. Past situation
    1. Early rate of population growth was source of great pride.
    2. Prior to 1921 United States practiced open-door immigration policy.
    3. Long before overpopulation became a concern, women of the United States began limiting family size.
  C. Present situation
    1. Birth rate and race—fertility rate of nonwhite women is higher than that of the corresponding white women.
    2. Birth rate and income—families with the lowest income have the most children.
    3. Birth rate and education—higher the level of education, the fewer children produced.
    4. Current trends in population growth
      a. Rate of population growth for United States has been dropping in recent years, but remains too high.
      b. Other population changes are occurring; including:
        (1) rapid depopulation of rural areas.
        (2) heavy movement toward metropolitan areas.
        (3) migration to regions of greater economic opportunity.
        (4) flow of middle- and upper-income groups from North and East to the South.
        (5) great migration to Pacific Coast.
        (6) dying central city and birth of suburban sprawl.

(7) concentration of Negro into deteriorated central portions of cities.

D. Future
1. Possible that stable population may be reached through voluntary decisions to limit family sizes to an average of a fraction over two children.
2. If individuals do not control birth rate voluntarily, it may eventually become necessary to control it through legal regulation or economic pressures.

Glossary

If you cannot find the word you wish in this glossary, check the index for text and glossary references.

demographic (dē′mə graf′ik) (G. *demos,* people; *graphein,* to write). The science of vital and social statistics.

deuterium (dyoo tēr′ē əm) (G. *deuteros,* second). An isotope of hydrogen, having twice the mass of hydrogen; heavy hydrogen.

fission (fish′ən) (L. *fissio,* to cleave). The splitting of the nucleus of an atom, releasing a great quantity of energy.

fusion (fyoo′zhən) (L. *fusio,* from *fundere,* to pour). The union of material into one body or mass.

infanticide (in fan′ti sīd) (L. *infans,* infant; *caedere,* to kill). The murder or murderer of an infant.

intrauterine contraceptive device (in′trə yoo′tə rin kon trə sep′tiv) (IUD) (L. *intra,* within; *uterus,* womb). A mechanical device placed within the uterus which prevents conception or impregnation.

solar (sō′lər) (L. *sol,* sun). Pertaining to the sun.

thorium (thor′ē əm). A radioactive metallic element.

tritium (trit′ē əm). An isotope of hydrogen having an atomic weight of three.

uranium (yoo rā′nē əm) (G. *ouranos,* sky). A hard and heavy radioactive metallic element.

APPENDIXES

DISEASES IN BRIEF

This appendix provides condensed information on many infectious diseases for quick reference or review. For more complete information, refer to Chapters 15, 16, and 17 of this text, or the references listed with each of these chapters.

Chancroid

Caused by:	*Hemophilus ducreyi,* a bacillus.
Usual Age Infected:	15 to 30.
Mode of Transmission:	Predominantly through sexual intercourse.
Incubation Period:	Usually 3 to 5 days.
Early Signs:	An open, red sore, oozing pus, painful, on or near the genitalia; swelling of local lymph glands.
Length of Disease:	Usually self-limiting within 1 month; may be chronic.
Contagious Period:	Until healed.
Permanent Aftereffects:	None.
Immunity:	None.
Prevention:	Chancroid can be definitely prevented by the proper use of soap and water immediately after exposure.

Chickenpox

Caused by:	Varicella virus. Same virus causes herpes zoster (shingles) in adults.

Usual Age Infected:	2 to 8 years.
Mode of Transmission:	Direct or indirect contact with discharges from skin lesions or nose or throat of infected person or airborne.
Incubation Period:	10 to 21 days, usually 14 to 16.
Early Signs:	Slight fever, skin eruption.
Length of Disease:	9 to 14 days.
Contagious Period:	From 1 day before eruption until 6 days after.
Permanent Aftereffects:	Very rare—death due to encephalitis or pneumonia.
Immunity:	One attack confers long immunity.
Prevention:	None.

Common Cold

Caused by:	Over 50 types of viruses.
Usual Age Infected:	Any.
Mode of Transmission:	Direct or indirect contact with nose or throat discharges of infected persons.
Incubation Period:	12 to 72 hours, usually 24 hours.
Early Signs:	Sore throat, running nose, chilliness, aches.
Length of Disease:	3 to 5 days.
Contagious Period:	From 24 hours before onset until 3 to 5 days after.
Permanent Aftereffects:	None.
Immunity:	Little or none.
Prevention:	Avoid infected persons.

Diphtheria

Caused by:	*Corynebacterium diphtheriae,* the diphtheria bacillus.
Usual Age Infected:	Under 15 years.
Mode of Transmission:	Contact with nose or throat discharges of a patient or carrier.
Incubation Period:	1 to 6 days.
Early Signs:	Sore throat, mild fever, running nose.
Length of Disease:	Highly variable—possibly several weeks.
Contagious Period:	Variable—usually from 3 days before until 10 days after onset of symptoms.
Permanent Aftereffects:	5 to 10 percent of cases fatal. Toxin may permanently damage heart or nervous system.
Immunity:	Congenital immunity lasts for several months. The actual disease sometimes confers lasting immunity.
Prevention:	Immunization with DPT shots according to the schedule in Appendix C.

German Measles (Rubella)

Caused by:	Rubella virus.
Usual Age Infected:	2 to 15 years.

Mode of Transmission:	Direct or indirect contact with nose or throat discharges of infected person, or airborne.
Incubation Period:	10 to 28 days, usually 14 to 21.
Early Signs:	Slight fever, swelling of lymph glands, rash.
Length of Disease:	1 to 4 days.
Contagious Period:	From one week before until end of rash.
Permanent Aftereffects:	Rare, except for damage to fetus in early pregnancy.
Immunity:	One attack usually confers permanent immunity.
Prevention:	Vaccines are being developed. Deliberate exposure of female children recommended until release of effective vaccine.

Gonorrhea

Caused by:	*Neisseria gonorrheae,* the gonococcus.
Usual Age Infected:	15 to 30 years.
Mode of Transmission:	Sexual intercourse. Infection of eyes of newborn during childbirth.
Incubation Period:	3 to 5 days, sometimes 9 days or longer.
Early Signs:	Male—discharge of pus from urethra, burning urination.
	Female—slight discharge from vagina, slight burning in urination.
Length of Disease:	Indefinite—until properly treated.
Contagious Period:	Indefinite—as long as discharges persist.
Permanent Aftereffects:	Sterility in male or female; occasional damage to joints or heart lining.
Immunity:	None.
Prevention:	Avoidance of casual sexual contacts, case-finding programs, antibacterial drops in eyes of newborn infants. Personal prophylaxis before, during, and after exposure is of some value.

Granuloma Inguinale

Caused by:	The Donovan body (probably a bacterium).
Usual Age Infected:	20 to 40 years.
Mode of Transmission:	Sexual intercourse.
Incubation Period:	From 8 to 100 days.
Early Signs:	Deep, red, open sores, starting on the genitalia and spreading to surrounding areas.
Length of Disease:	Indefinite—until treated.
Contagious Period:	As long as skin lesions persist.
Permanent Aftereffects:	The untreated disease may lead to destruction of the genital organs. On rare occasions the disease may become generalized and lead to death.
Immunity:	None.
Prevention:	Avoidance of casual sexual contacts, personal cleanliness, case-finding programs.

Infectious Hepatitis

Caused by:	A virus.
Usual Age Infected:	Any.
Mode of Transmission:	Fecal contamination, contact with patient, contaminated food or water.
Incubation Period:	2 to 7 weeks, commonly 3 to 4 weeks.
Early Signs:	Fever, mild headache, chilliness, fatigue, jaundice.
Length of Disease:	Variable—often 2 to 4 weeks.
Contagious Period:	Unknown—believed to be from 1 week before onset until 1 week after.
Permanent Aftereffects:	Rarely death or permanent liver damage.
Immunity:	Second attacks are rare.
Prevention:	Good sanitation and sewage disposal, sterile injection syringes and needles, gamma globulin after exposure to disease.

Infectious Mononucleosis

Caused by:	A virus.
Usual Age Infected:	2 to 20 years.
Mode of Transmission:	Unknown—believed to be direct contact with nose or throat discharges of infected person.
Incubation Period:	2 to 6 weeks.
Early Signs:	Fever, sore throat, fatigue, enlarged lymph nodes.
Length of Disease:	Variable—1 week to several months.
Contagious Period:	Probably from several days before symptoms until end of sore throat.
Permanent Aftereffects:	None.
Immunity:	Infection with or without symptoms is believed to confer lasting immunity.
Prevention:	None.

Influenza

Caused by:	Several types of influenza viruses; new strains frequently develop.
Usual Age Infected:	Any.
Mode of Transmission:	Direct or indirect contact with nose or throat discharges of infected persons, possibly air-borne.
Incubation Period:	1 to 3 days.
Early Signs:	Sudden fever, chills, headache, muscular pain, marked prostration, dry cough.
Length of Disease:	3 to 10 days.
Contagious Period:	1 day before onset until 4 days after.
Permanent Aftereffects:	Rare, except predisposes elderly or weakened persons to pneumonia. The general death rate rises during epidemics.

Immunity:	Infection produces immunity of unknown duration to the infecting virus, but not necessarily to other influenza viruses.
Prevention:	Annual immunization with vaccine based upon prevailing strains of viruses.

Lymphogranuloma Venereum

Caused by:	A virus.
Usual Age Infected:	15 to 30.
Mode of Transmission:	Primarily through sexual intercourse, also indirectly through contaminated articles and clothing.
Incubation Period:	Usually 7 to 12 days, may be several months.
Early Signs:	Small lesion on genitalia, swelling of lymph nodes and genitalia.
Length of Disease:	Indefinite.
Contagious Period:	Variable—from weeks to years.
Permanent Aftereffects:	Rarely fatal, but may cause great disability.
Immunity:	Recovered persons may be immune.
Prevention:	Avoidance of casual sexual contacts, cleanliness.

Measles

Caused by:	Rubeola virus.
Usual Age Infected:	2 to 8 years.
Mode of Transmission:	Direct or indirect contact with nose or throat discharge of infected person; also airborne.
Incubation Period:	7 to 14 days, usually 10 to 12.
Early Signs:	Gradually increasing fever, cold symptoms, severe cough, conjunctivitis, running nose. Rash appears on third or fourth day.
Length of Disease:	6 to 12 days.
Contagious Period:	From 4 days before until 5 days after rash appears.
Permanent Aftereffects:	Occasional death and brain damage due to encephalitis.
Immunity:	Congenital immunity lasts a few months. The disease usually confers permanent immunity.
Prevention:	Immunization with live measles vaccine.

Meningitis (Bacterial)

Caused by:	*Neisseria meningitidis,* the meningococcus, several types.
Usual Age Infected:	Any.
Mode of Transmission:	Direct contact with patient or carrier. Indirect contact not important.
Incubation Period:	2 to 10 days, commonly 3 to 4.
Early Signs:	Fever, headache, nausea, irritability, delirium, coma.

Length of Disease:	Usually 1 to 3 weeks.
Contagious Period:	Until 24 hours after treatment with proper drug.
Permanent Aftereffects:	Fatality rate about 5 percent with proper treatment, 40 to 50 percent without treatment. Brain damage is frequent.
Immunity:	Over half of the population exhibits natural immunity, becoming healthy carriers upon exposure. Degree and duration of immunity after attack unknown.
Prevention:	Personal hygiene, prevention of overcrowding, mass treatment in epidemics.

Mumps

Caused by:	Mumps virus.
Usual Age Infected:	2 to 14 years.
Mode of Transmission:	Direct or indirect contact with nose or throat discharges of infected person.
Incubation Period:	12 to 28 days, usually 16 to 20.
Early Signs:	Fever; swelling and tenderness of salivary glands.
Length of Disease:	4 to 10 days.
Contagious Period:	7 days before swelling until end of swelling.
Permanent Aftereffects:	Very rarely brain damage; atrophy of one testis (rarely both) in about 25 percent of males over age 15. Ovarian infection in females much less frequent.
Immunity:	The disease usually confers lifelong immunity.
Prevention:	Vaccines currently available have limited value and are rarely recommended for children as their use may delay infection until after puberty.

Poliomyelitis (Polio)

Caused by:	Three types of polio viruses.
Usual Age Infected:	Any, but most common among children.
Mode of Transmission:	Direct contact or close association with infected persons, indirectly through fecal contamination or nose or throat discharges of infected person.
Incubation Period:	3 to 28 days, usually 7 to 12.
Early Signs:	Fever, headache, sore throat, nausea, muscle pain, and weakness.
Length of Disease:	Highly variable—up to several months.
Contagious Period:	Maximum period from one week before to three months after onset of symptoms; usually from 3 days before to 10 days after onset.
Permanent Aftereffects:	2 to 10 percent fatality rate in paralytic cases; paralysis may be permanent.
Immunity:	Most cases are nonparalytic and result in immunity to the specific type of virus responsible, but not to the other two types.

Prevention: Oral polio vaccine administered according to the
                                schedule in Appendix C.

Rabies

Caused by: Rabies virus.
Usual Age Infected: Any.
Mode of Transmission: Bite or scratch of infected animal (all mammals
                                are susceptible). Airborne spread from bats to
                                man in bat caves has been reported.
Incubation Period: Usually 4 to 6 weeks. May be shorter or longer.
Early Signs: Headache, anxiety, fever, muscular pain.
Length of Disease: About one week.
Contagious Period: Not contagious from man to man, except possibly
                                through saliva.
Permanent Aftereffects: Almost always fatal.
Immunity: No natural immunity. Few survivors.
Prevention: 1. Vaccination of bitten person for 14 to 21 con-
                                   secutive days, beginning soon after bite. Passive
                                   immunization with serum is often also used.
                                2. Vaccination of all dogs.
                                3. Avoidance of contact with sick bats or other
                                   mammals.

Scarlet Fever

Caused by: Over 40 types of Group A hemolytic streptococcal
                                bacteria.
Usual Age Infected: 1 to 9 years.
Mode of Transmission: Direct or indirect contact with patient or carrier.
Incubation Period: 1 to 5 days.
Early Signs: Fever, sore throat, nausea, rash.
Length of Disease: 4 to 10 days.
Contagious Period: Highly variable—from one week to several months.
Permanent Aftereffects: Kidney disease or rheumatic heart disease.
Immunity: Second attacks of scarlet fever are rare, but re-
                                peated attacks of streptococcal infection are com-
                                mon.
Prevention: Prompt treatment of streptococcal infections;
                                pasteurization of milk, strict sanitary precautions
                                in doctors' offices and hospitals.

Smallpox

Caused by: Smallpox or variola virus.
Usual Age Infected: Any.
Mode of Transmission: Direct or indirect contact with throat or skin dis-
                                charges of infected person. Airborne transmission
                                over short distances.

Incubation Period:	7 to 16 days.
Early Signs:	High fever, headache, prostration, skin eruption.
Length of Disease:	1 to 7 weeks.
Contagious Period:	From 4 to 5 days before rash until rash disappears.
Permanent Aftereffects:	From 1 to 40 percent of cases die; blindness, brain damage, scars.
Immunity:	Second attacks are rare.
Prevention:	Vaccination according to the schedule in Appendix C.

Syphilis

Caused by:	*Treponema pallidum,* a spirochete.
Usual Age Infected:	15 to 30 years.
Mode of Transmission:	Sexual intercourse, other close direct contact; congenital transmission across placenta.
Incubation Period:	10 days to 10 weeks, usually about 3 weeks.
Early Signs:	The chancre.
Length of Disease:	Usually persists until proper treatment.
Contagious Period:	During primary and secondary stages (see Chapter 16).
Permanent Aftereffects:	Death; damage to brain, heart, other vital organs.
Immunity:	Develops only after long-term infection.
Prevention:	Avoidance of casual sexual contacts, premarital and prenatal blood testing, intensive case-finding programs. Personal prophylaxis before, during, and after exposure is of limited value.

Tetanus

Caused by:	*Clostridium tetani,* the tetanus bacillus.
Usual Age Infected:	Any.
Mode of Transmission:	Tetanus spores infect the body through a wound.
Incubation Period:	Commonly 4 days to 3 weeks.
Early Signs:	Painful contractions of muscles.
Length of Disease:	Variable—several weeks.
Contagious Period:	Not contagious directly from man to man.
Permanent Aftereffects:	Fatality rate averages about 35 percent. Usually no permanent damage in patients who recover.
Immunity:	Second attacks are known to occur.
Prevention:	Immunization according to the schedule in Appendix C.

Tuberculosis

Caused by:	*Mycobacterium tuberculosis,* the tubercle bacillus.
Usual Age Infected:	Any.
Mode of Transmission:	Contact with patients, airborne, indirect contact through contaminated articles, unpasteurized milk.

Incubation Period:	4 to 6 weeks.
Early Signs:	None.
Length of Disease:	Indefinite.
Contagious Period:	As long as disease is active.
Permanent Aftereffects:	Death; destruction of lungs, bones, kidneys, skin.
Immunity:	Immunity conferred by healed infection is very limited.
Prevention:	Avoidance of crowding, proper nutrition, intensive case-finding programs, testing of cattle, pasteurization of milk, BCG vaccine for high-risk individuals.

Whooping Cough (Pertussis)

Caused by:	*Bordatella* (*Hemophilus*) *pertussis,* the pertussis bacillus.
Usual Age Infected:	Birth to 10 years.
Mode of Transmission:	Direct or indirect contact with nose or throat discharges of an infected person.
Incubation Period:	5 to 16 days, usually 7 to 10 days.
Early Signs:	Gradually increasing dry cough, especially at night.
Length of Disease:	2 to 10 weeks, usually 4 to 6 weeks.
Contagious Period:	Variable—usually first two weeks.
Permanent Aftereffects:	In infants, death or brain damage.
Immunity:	No congenital immunity. Second attacks of the disease occasionally occur.
Prevention:	Immunization with DPT shots according to the schedule in Appendix C.

RECOMMENDED DAILY DIETARY ALLOWANCES[a]

Designed for the maintenance of good nutrition of practically all healthy persons in the U.S.A.

[*Allowances are intended for persons normally active in a temperate climate*]

Persons	Age in Years[d] (From)	(Up to)	Weight in Pounds	Height in Inches	Food Energy[b] (Calories)	Protein (Grams)
Men	18	35	154	69	2,900	70
	35	55	154	69	2,600	70
	55	75	154	69	2,200	70
Women	18	35	128	64	2,100	58
	35	55	128	64	1,900	58
	55	75	128	64	1,600	58
Pregnant (second and third trimester)					+200	+20
Lactating					+1,000	+40
Infants[e]	0	1	18		lb. $\times 52 \pm 7$	lb. $\times 1.1 \pm 0.2$
Children	1	3	29	34	1,300	32
	3	6	40	42	1,600	40
	6	9	53	49	2,100	52
Boys	9	12	72	55	2,400	60
	12	15	98	61	3,000	75
	15	18	134	68	3,400	85
Girls	9	12	72	55	2,200	55
	12	15	103	62	2,500	62
	15	18	117	64	2,300	58

[a] The allowance levels are intended to cover individual variations among most normal persons as they live in the United States under usual environmental stresses.

[b] Tables 1 and 2 and Figures 1 and 2 in Publication 1146 (see Source) show calorie adjustments for weight and age.

[c] Niacin equivalents include dietary sources of the preformed vitamin and the precursor, tryptophan. 60 milligrams tryptophan represents 1 milligram niacin.

[d] Entries on lines for age range 18 to 35 years represent the 25-year age. All other entries represent allowances for the midpoint of the specified age periods, i.e., line for children 1 to 3 is for age 2 years (24 months); 3 to 6 is for age 4½ years (54 months), etc.

[e] The caloric and protein allowances per pound for infants are considered to decrease progressively from birth. Allowances for calcium, thiamine, riboflavin, and niacin increase proportionately with calories to the maximum values shown.

NOTE: The Recommended Daily Dietary Allowances should not be confused with Minimum Daily Requirements. The Recommended Dietary Allowances are amounts of

Calcium (Grams)	Iron (Milligrams)	Vitamin A (International units)	Thiamine (Milligrams)	Riboflavin (Milligrams)	Niacin Equivalent[a] (Milligrams)	Ascorbic Acid (Milligrams)	Vitamin D (International units)
0.8	10	5,000	1.2	1.7	19	70	
0.8	10	5,000	1.0	1.6	17	70	
0.8	10	5,000	0.9	1.3	15	70	
0.8	15	5,000	0.8	1.3	14	70	
0.8	15	5,000	0.8	1.2	13	70	
0.8	10	5,000	0.8	1.2	13	70	
+0.5	+5	+1,000	+0.2	+0.3	+3	+30	400
+0.5	+5	+3,000	+0.4	+0.6	+7	+30	400
0.7	lb. ×0.45	1,500	0.4	0.6	6	30	400
0.8	8	2,000	0.5	0.8	9	40	400
0.8	10	2,500	0.6	1.0	11	50	400
0.8	12	3,500	0.8	1.3	14	60	400
1.1	15	4,500	1.0	1.4	16	70	400
1.4	15	5,000	1.2	1.8	20	80	400
1.4	15	5,000	1.4	2.0	22	80	400
1.1	15	4,500	0.9	1.3	15	80	400
1.3	15	5,000	1.0	1.5	17	80	400
1.3	15	5,000	0.9	1.3	15	70	400

nutrients recommended by the Food and Nutrition Board of National Research Council, and are considered adequate for maintenance of good nutrition in healthy persons in the United States. The allowances are revised from time to time in accordance with newer knowledge of nutritional needs.

The Minimum Daily Requirements are the amounts of various nutrients that have been established by the Food and Drug Administration as standards for labeling purposes of foods and pharmaceutical preparations for special dietary uses. These are the amounts regarded as necessary in the diet for the prevention of deficiency diseases and generally are less than the Recommended Dietary Allowances. The Minimum Daily Requirements are set forth in the *Federal Register,* vol. 6, No. 227 (Nov. 22, 1941), beginning on p. 5921, and amended as stated in the *Federal Register* (June 1, 1957), vol. 22, No. 106, p. 3841.

SOURCE: Adapted from Recommended Dietary Allowances, Publication 1146, 59 pp., revised 1964. Published by National Academy of Sciences—National Research Council, Washington, D.C., 20418. Price $1.00. Also available in libraries.

PREVENTIVE MEDICINE SCHEDULE

The modern trend in medicine is toward the prevention of diseases. The following tables are combined into a schedule which, if followed, would further this trend of preventive medicine.

TABLE 1 TYPICAL IMMUNIZATION SCHEDULE

Age	Preparation
2 months	DPT (diphtheria, whooping cough, tetanus) Trivalent OPV (oral polio vaccine combining types I, II, and III)
3 months	DPT Trivalent OPV
4 months	DPT Trivalent OPV
9 months	Smallpox vaccine
12 months	Live measles vaccine
15 months	DPT Trivalent OPV
4 years	DPT
6 years	Smallpox vaccine Trivalent OPV
8 years	DT (adult type diphtheria and tetanus booster)
12 years	DT Smallpox vaccine
16 years	DT
Over 16 years	Smallpox and tetanus boosters every 5 years for life

NOTE: This schedule is recommended as a flexible guide which may be modified within limits to meet the needs of the individual patient or physician.

TABLE 2 TYPICAL EXAMINATION AND TESTING SCHEDULE

Age	Recommendation
14 days or under	Exam, urinalysis (for infection or diabetes), PKU test
1 month	Exam
2 months	Exam
3 months	Exam, second PKU test
4 months	Exam
5 months	Exam
6 months	Exam
9 months	Exam
12 months	Exam, hemoglobin test, urinalysis, tuberculin test
18 months	Exam
2 years	Exam, urinalysis, tuberculin test Regular dental care to begin
3 years	Exam, hemoglobin test, urinalysis, tuberculin test
4 through 18 years	Yearly—exam, urinalysis, tuberculin test
19 through 40 years	Yearly—chest X ray or tuberculin test Every five years—exam, blood count, urinalysis
40 years and up	Yearly—exam, blood count, urinalysis, check for rectal cancer, check eyes for glaucoma, chest X ray Every five years—electrocardiogram
20 through 50 years	Females—yearly pelvic exam and pap smear for cancer of the cervix
50 years and up	Females—pelvic exam and pap smear every six months

NOTE: This schedule is recommended as a flexible guide which may be modified within limits to meet the needs of the individual patient or physician.

TABLE 3 **IMMUNIZATION RECORD**

		Father	Mother	Children's Names
Names				
Birth Dates				
Polio	First			
	Second			
	Third			
	Fourth			
	Boosters			
Diphtheria + Tetanus + Whooping Cough: (DPT)	First			
	Second			
	Third			
	Boosters			
Smallpox	First			
	Second			
	Boosters			
Measles	First			
	Boosters			
Influenza	First			
	Boosters			

Other immunizations

_____

_____

_____

_____

_____

_____

The Human Body

A Harper & Row Dissectograph

PLATE 3

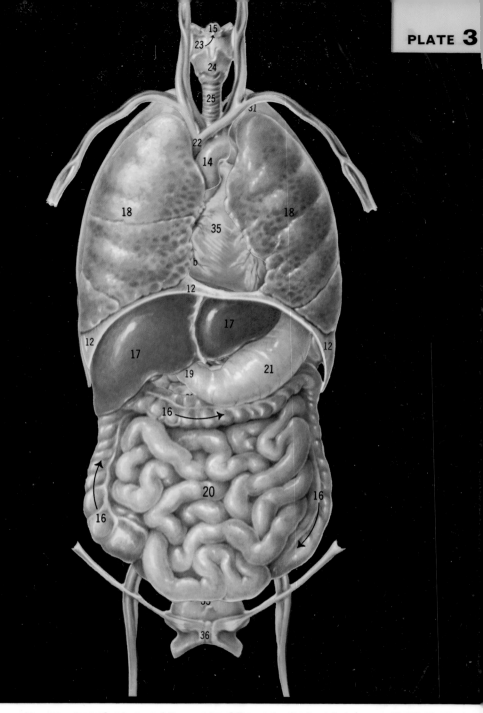

Here you see a front view of the organs of the neck, chest, and abdomen. **12. Diaphragm.**
14. Aorta. The arched part shown is the beginning of this main blood vessel (artery).
15. Epiglottis. 16. Large Intestine (Colon). It ascends on the right side, crosses over,
and descends on the left side. **17. Liver. 18. Lungs. 19. Pylorus. 20. Small Intestine.**
21. Stomach. 22. Superior Vena Cava. This is the great collecting blood vessel (vein) for
the upper parts of the body, except for the lungs. **23. Tongue Bone (Hyoid Bone).** It supports the root of the tongue. **24. Voice Box (Larynx). 25. Windpipe (Trachea).** Its cavity
is kept open permanently by incomplete rings of cartilage.

PLATE **6**

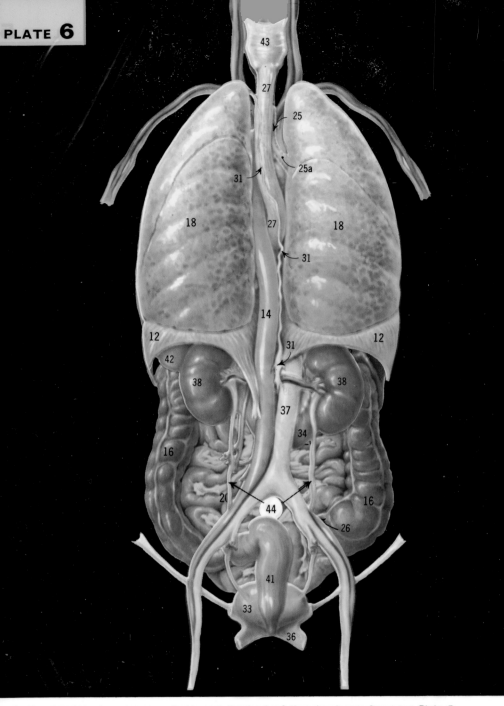

In the drawing above, you are looking at the back of the structures shown on Plate 5.
12. Diaphragm. 14. Aorta. 18. Lungs. 25. Windpipe (Trachea). The branch to the right lung
(bronchus) is shown, 25a. **27. Esophagus.** It lies between the windpipe and the muscles of
the backbone. **31. Lymphatic Vessel (Thoracic Duct).** Note its beginning below the diaphragm. **33. Bladder. 34. Duodenum. 36. Hipbone. 37. Inferior Vena Cava (Postcava).**
38. Kidneys. Note the blood vessels to the kidney. **41. Rectum.** The end of the large intestine
is attached to it. **42. Spleen. 43. Throat (Pharynx).** Only part of the back wall is shown.
44. Ureters. These connect the kidneys with the bladder.

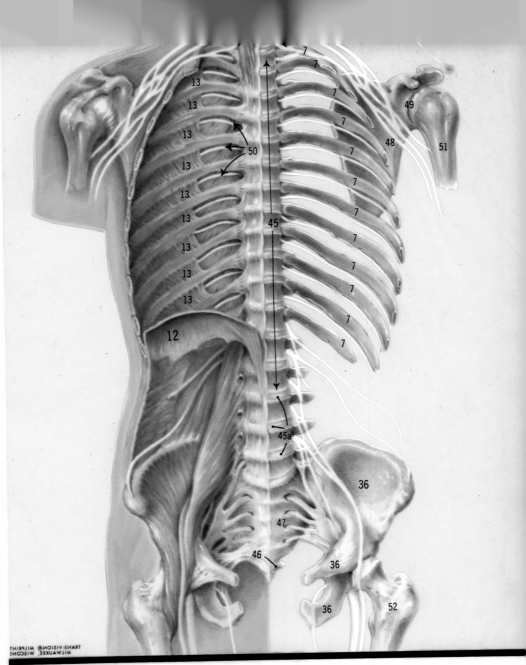

This plate shows the spinal nerves, the front view of muscles, and parts of the skeleton near the back. The last two ribs are too far back to be included in the section of the chest wall on the right side. **7. Ribs.** All twelve ribs are shown on the left side. **12. Diaphragm. 13. Rib Muscles. 36. Hipbone. 45. Backbone (Vertebral Column).** It consists of many small bones *(vertebrae)* which are separated by pads of cartilage, 45a, except near the hip. **46. Coccyx. 47. Sacrum. 48. Shoulder Blade (Scapula). 49. Shoulder Joint.** The ligaments are shown on the right shoulder joint. **50. Spinal Nerves. 51. Upper Arm Bone (Humerus). 52. Upper Leg Bone (Femur).**

The paintings and anatomical drawings in the Harper & Row **Dissectograph**
are by Arnold Ryan Chalfant, science illustrator.

*The paintings and anatomical drawings in the Harper & Row **Dissectograph**
are by Arnold Ryan Chalfant, science illustrator.*

HEALTH CAREER FIELDS

Today there are opportunities of many kinds in the health fields. Owing to the expanding and aging population in this country, rising awareness of health in the population, the explosion of health insurance plans, and the health care provisions under federal and state medical programs, the urgent need for many more health workers will continue. These professions cover all types of work and interests related to hospitals, clinics, laboratories, phar-

Vocation	Nature of the Work	Education
Cytological Technician	He does microscopic analysis of exfoliated body cells to determine presence or absence of cancer, evaluates estrogen, and stains slides.	At least 2 years of college work with emphasis on biology courses, followed by a 6-month clinical training in an approved hospital.
Dental Assistant	She greets patients and prepares them for examination or treatment, prepares dental materials, takes and	Often training is given on the job. Some colleges are now giving a 1–2 year training program

macies, private offices, industrial plants, and nursing homes. They may require training from a few months to many years and may be either routine or highly creative.

The following chart lists information regarding the various health careers. It has been designed to help a person decide if he belongs in one of these health fields.

Where Employed	Employment Opportunities	Where to Find Additional Information
Hospitals, clinics or public health laboratories.	Increasing demand as cancer-diagnosing techniques improve. Some become laboratory supervisors.	American Society of Cytology, 1012 Walnut St., Philadelphia, Pa., 19107. National Committee for Careers and Medical Tech., 1785 Massachusetts Ave. N.W. Washington, D.C., 20036.
Dental offices and dental clinics.	Opportunities are easy to find. Advancements are limited.	American Dental Assn., Council on Dental Education, 222 E. Superior St., Chicago, Ill., 60611.

Vocation	Nature of the Work	Education
	processes X rays, handles records, and serves as a receptionist.	following high school graduation.
Dental Hygienist	She cleans and polishes teeth, massages gums, charts conditions of decay and disease for diagnosis by a dentist, provides dental health education.	Usually a 2-year training program following high school leading to a dental hygiene certificate. A state board examination is required in most states, which, if passed, entitles one to become a Registered Dental Hygienist (R.D.H.).
Dental Laboratory Technician	He makes artificial dentures of all kinds upon prescription from a dentist. (Some do only selected kinds of work.) He may work for one or several dentists and have no patient contact.	Commonly trained on the job—usually in a laboratory or dental school for 3–4 years. A few schools offer a 1–2-year training program.
Dentist	He fills cavities in the teeth, straightens teeth, X rays the mouth, extracts teeth, substitutes artificial dentures, and treats gum diseases. Most dentists are in general practice. A few do research or teach,	Two to 3 years of college work followed by 4 years of dental training leading to the degree of Doctor of Dental Surgery (D.D.S.) or Doctor of Dental Medicine (D.M.D.). State board examinations re-

Where Employed	Employment Opportunities	Where to Find Additional Information
A profession consisting entirely of women, who work in private dental offices, public health agencies, industrial plants, or public school systems.	Future is increasingly good as dental care becomes more important. With a college degree, openings are good in public health.	American Dental Hygienists Association, 100 E. Ohio St., Chicago, Ill., 60611.
Commercial laboratories with 1–10 men handling orders from many dentists. Some employed by private dentists, in hospitals, or by governmental agencies.	Job futures very good as dental care expands. Opportunities are good to set up one's own laboratory.	American Dental Assn., Council on Dental Education, 222 E. Superior St. Chicago, Ill., 60611. National Association of Dental Laboratories, Inc. 500 Walker Bldg., Washington, D.C., 20005.
Mostly in private practice, others in armed services, dental schools, hospitals, and public health.	Demand for dentists is growing faster than the supply for private practice, public health, research, and dental college faculties.	American Dental Association, Council on Dental Education, 222 E. Superior St., Chicago, Ill., 60611. American Association of Dental Schools, 840 N. Lake Shore Drive, Chicago, Ill., 60611.

Vocation	Nature of the Work	Education
	either part-time or full-time.	quired in most states. Advanced training required for dental specialties.
Dietician	They plan and supervise food preparations and meal planning, usually in hospitals, schools, or industry. Some are administrators, others are therapeutic dieticians, teachers, or research workers.	A bachelor's degree with a major in foods and nutrition or food management. Often an internship program is required, as with medical therapeutic dietary work.
Food Technologist	He is concerned with all phases of food production, processing, packaging, distribution and utilization of foods. He checks food spoilage and quality control. He may teach or give consultation.	Generally a bachelor's degree in food technology. Some schools offer graduate programs.
Hospital Administrator	In charge of the hospital management, its smooth running and the carrying out of policies of the board.	New men in the field have master's or Ph.D. degrees in hospital administration, law, or business

Where Employed	Employment Opportunities	Where to Find Additional Information
Work in hospitals, school systems, colleges, industrial plants, public health departments, and private food service companies.	Need will continue to be good for a number of years as public health programs rapidly increase. Number of men in field is small, but slowly increasing.	The American Dietetic Association, 620 N. Michigan Ave., Chicago, Ill., 60611.
Canning factories and research departments of food industries and manufacturers.	Field rather new and a number of routes of work are open. The better the training the better the job opportunities.	American Home Economics Association, 1600 20th St., N.W., Washington, D.C., 20009.
Hospitals of all kinds and related institutions, both private and governmental.	Jobs increasing as number of new hospitals increase. First jobs are often as assistants or in small	American College of Hospital Administrators, 840 N. Lake Shore Dr., Chicago, Ill., 60611.

Vocation	Nature of the Work	Education
	In charge of all departments, staff members, and facilities. Responsible for hiring, training, budgets, planning, purchasing, and accounting.	administration. Some must be physicians or registered nurses. Internships required in some states.
Industrial Hygienist	Watches factory environment for anything of possible harm to employees and recommends necessary changes.	Bachelor's degree with major in physical sciences. Some go on for master's degree in public health.
Inhalation Therapist	Aids physicians in administering medical gases and in resuscitative procedures. Checks hospital's supply of oxygen and the safety rules in its use.	Following high school graduation, a 9-month in-service training program to a 2-year college program.
Medical Assistant	Helps prepare patients for examinations, sterilizes instruments, records information, and runs routine tests. Works under a nurse or physician. If in a laboratory, she probably works under a technologist or a pathologist.	Often expected to have some college training in biological sciences. Some junior colleges offer 2-year programs with special work in medical records, terminology, and laboratory procedures.
Medical Record Librarian	She keeps complete and accurate records of all patients while in the hospital, their X-ray reports, laboratory reports, progress	Preferred training is 2–4 years of college work plus a 1-year course in medical record library service. Some hospitals offer

Where Employed	Employment Opportunities	Where to Find Additional Information
	hospital, and then eventually to full administrators in a large hospital if work is acceptable.	
Governmental health agencies, industry, insurance companies, consultant companies, and universities.	Profession is uncrowded. Work is demanding and calls for a responsible person.	American Public Health Association, 1790 Broadway, New York, N.Y., 10019.
Hospitals, clinics, research laboratories, and offices.	Opportunity will depend on the size of the hospital and the kind of work called for.	American Association of Inhalation Therapists, 332 S. Michigan Ave., Chicago, Ill., 60604.
Hospitals, clinics, and physicians' offices.	Always openings in private physicians' offices. Better chance for advancement in hospitals or laboratories as supervisors.	American Medical Assn. Council on Medical Education and Hospitals, 535 N. Dearborn St., Chicago, Ill., 60610.
Hospitals, clinics, public health agencies, medical departments of insurance agencies, and industrial firms.	Many hospitals lack trained record librarians. Field is quite short of enough trained librarians. Mostly women, but a	The American Association of Medical Record Librarians, 840 N. Lake Shore Dr., Chicago, Ill., 60611.

Vocation	Nature of the Work	Education
	notes, etc. She checks, organizes, and files them; compiles statistics; and summarizes the medical records.	in-service training programs. Librarians who are graduates of approved schools may take a national registration examination, and, if passing, are Registered Record Librarians (R.R.L.).
Medical Social Worker	She helps patients and families with personal problems resulting from illness or disability. She helps with new job placement,, convalescence, and any other needs.	Need bachelor's degree plus 2 years of graduate study in medical social work (often leading to a master's degree).
Medical Technologist	Does laboratory procedures of all kinds under the guidance of a physician or a pathologist as a part of the diagnosis of diseases. Some work in laboratories; others do new drug research or administer laboratories.	New students should take 3 years of college work in the sciences, plus 1 year of specialized laboratory training. Graduates of AMA-approved schools may take an examination to qualify for certification by the Registry of Medical Technologists of the American Society of Clinical Pathologists (ASCP). Some states license medical technologists.
Nurse's Aide	Shares in the actual care of patients, such	No formal preparation required.

Where Employed	Employment Opportunities	Where to Find Additional Information
	small number of men in the field.	
Hospitals, clinics, public and private health centers and departments. Some in teaching.	Many more openings than available workers.	National Commission for Social Work Careers, 345 E. 46th St., New York, N.Y., 10017.
Hospitals, private physicians' offices, clinics, public health laboratories, private laboratories, and drug manufacturers.	Demand is great. Good chance for advancement as supervisor or researcher. Fits in well as a part-time job. Mostly women in the field.	American Society of Medical Technologists, Suite 25, Herman Professional Bldg., Houston, Texas, 77025. Registry of Medical Technologists of the American Society of Clinical Pathologists, P.O. Box 44, Muncie, Indiana, 47344.
Hospitals, nursing homes, and clinics.	Duties and responsibilities depend on	American Nursing Association, 10

Vocation	Nature of the Work	Education
	as answering calls, feeding and bathing, and adjusting beds. Male aides are called orderlies.	Hospitals provide on-the-job training. No licensing required.
Nurse, Licensed Practical (L.P.N)	Also known as a Licensed Vocational Nurse (L.V.N.), they assist in care of the physically and mentally ill under direction of physicians and registered nurses, such as taking temperatures, bathing, taking blood pressure readings, etc.	A 1-year training program and passing a state examination for licensing. Practical nurses having no formal training are not eligible for licensing. Thus only formally trained practical nurses may become L.P.N.'s.
Nurse, Registered (R.N.)	She provides nursing services for patients, either by direct care or through supervising allied nursing personnel. She administers drugs prescribed by a physician, observes and records patient information, assists in patient education and rehabilitation, instructs other personnel and students, or does administrative work.	Several programs may be followed: (1) a 2-year program with A.A. degree, (2) a 3-year program with diploma or A.A. degree; (3) a 4-year program integrated with academic work for bachelor's degree; (4) a 3-year program following the A.A. degree and leading to the bachelor's degree, or (5) a master's degree program in nursing following a liberal arts college major. A nurse may be registered by passing a state board examination (R.N.).

Where Employed	Employment Opportunities	Where to Find Additional Information
	size of hospital. Demand is constant wherever there are hospitals. Often a good job for young women seeking part-time work.	Columbus Circle, New York, N.Y., 10019.
Hospitals, public health agencies, private homes, physicians' offices, nursing homes, and similar institutions.	Great shortage. Future employment quite secure. Little chance for advancement except in specialized areas. A few men in field help provide care for men patients.	American Nurses Association, 10 Columbus Circle, New York, N.Y., 10019. National Federation of Licensed Practical Nurses, Inc., 250 W. 57th St., New York, N.Y., 10019.
Public and private hospitals, public health nursing, industrial nursing, nursing education, private duty, clinics, private physicians' offices.	Continuing excellent demand in all parts of the country. Work often begins as general duty nurse. Chances good for advancement to supervisory or administrative position.	American Nurses Association, 10 Columbus Circle, New York, N.Y., 10019. National League for Nursing, Committee on Careers, 10 Columbus Circle, New York, N.Y., 10019.

Vocation	Nature of the Work	Education
Nutritionist	Teaches people about food needs and helps special groups with adequate diets. She determines how food is utilized and its contents. She sees that scientific knowledge on foods is translated into simple, specific information people can understand and use.	College work with a home economics major, with special emphasis on foods, nutrition, and related sciences and with some work in the social sciences. Many have a year or more of graduate training.
Occupational Therapist	Works under a physician and uses creative, educational, and recreational activities to help people get well both physically and mentally and to acquire job skills. They recommend activities to patients in terms of their likes, dislikes, and abilities.	Four years of college training leading to B.S. degree in occupational therapy, or 18 months of training after a bachelor's degree in some other field. Training includes both academic and clinical phases. Passing of national registration examination entitles him to registration and use of initials O.T.R.
Optician	Interprets prescription of optometrist or ophthalmologist for the grinding and polishing of lenses. Advises on selection of frames and shapes of lenses in terms of the facial features. Fits and adjusts the finished glasses.	Most get informal on-the-job training. With an apprenticeship program of 4–5 years, he may become an optical dispenser. Several schools offer courses. Several states license the technician or the dispenser of eyeglasses.

Where Employed	Employment Opportunities	Where to Find Additional Information
In hospitals as dieticians, in teaching, or in extension work. Many of them work in local public nutrition programs as teachers or consultants. Also in research or in college or university teaching.	County extension departments, local health departments, food industries, or universities. Advancement depends on amount of training and experience.	American Home Economics Association, 1600 20th St., N.W., Washington, D.C., 20009.
Primarily a field for women, although men are entering it. Works in hospitals, rehabilitation centers, nursing homes, outpatient clinics, and research centers.	Need for many more registered therapists is extensive. Opportunities to move into research, administration, and teaching.	American Occupational Therapy Association, 250 W. 57th St., New York, N.Y., 10019.
Wholesale or large retail establishments or as dispenser owning one's own business. Some in optical laboratories.	Need will continue to increase as population expands. Advancement opportunities for supervisors or shop foremen in large establishments.	Guild of Prescription Opticians of America, 1250 Connecticut Ave., N.W., Washington, D.C., 20036.

Vocation	Nature of the Work	Education
Optometrist	Examines eyes and performs other services to safeguard and improve vision. Uses special instruments to find eye defects and measure them. Does not use drugs or do surgery.	Usually 2 years of college work followed by 3–4 years of optometry training leading to degree Doctor of Optometry (O.D.). Passing a state board examination is required in all states.
Orthotist and Prosthetist	The *orthotist* makes and fits braces and other supports; the *prosthetist* makes artificial arms and legs and adjusts them to fit amputees.	Apprentice training in a certified establishment where appliances are fitted and made. Can apply for certification after 4 years of work.
Osteopathic Physician	Treats illness and diseases, giving special attention to impairments of the musculoskeletal system. Makes major use of manipulative therapy along with drugs and surgery; uses other methods of prevention, diagnosis, and treatment, depending upon the individual patient.	Three to 4 years of preosteopathic training, followed by 4 years of professional training leading to degree Doctor of Osteopathy (D.O.) followed by 12 months' internship in a hospital; 2–3 years additional training required for specialties. Passing of state board examination required for practice.
Pharmacist	Specializes in science of drugs. Understands composition and effects of drugs, tests for purity and strength, and compounds them. Makes drugs and	Usually 1–2 years of college followed by 3–4 years of professional training leading to degree Bachelor of Science in Pharmacy, fol-

Where Employed	Employment Opportunities	Where to Find Additional Information
Usually self-employed. May start as an associate with established practitioner, be salaried in an industrial plant, or work in governmental agency.	Employment opportunities are good, particularly in private practice.	American Optometric Association, 7000 Chippewa St., St. Louis, Missouri, 63119.
Retail establishments, hospitals' shops, rehabilitation centers, or in small shops working alone or supervising other employees.	Employment is steady. Skilled fitters are needed more now than before. Opportunity to set up own shop and supervise other employees.	American Orthotic and Prosthetic Association, 919 18th St., N.W., Washington, D.C., 20006
Usually in private practice or in partnership in clinics.	Excellent, particularly in parts of the country where osteopathy is an accepted form of treatment. Advancement in terms of location and size of practice and degree of training.	American Osteopathic Association, 212 E. Ohio St., Chicago, Ill., 60611.
Many in retail pharmacies, either as owner or as salaried employee. Others in pharmaceutical manufacturing or wholesaling, in hos-	Great need for well trained pharmacists. Opportunities to acquire own business and supervise other employees as one gains experience.	American Pharmaceutical Association, 2215 Constitution Ave., N.W., Washington, D.C., 20037. American Council on

Vocation	Nature of the Work	Education
	medicines available and gives information on their use, as well as other kinds of medical supplies.	lowed by 1 year of practical experience under the supervision of a registered pharmacist. Some take advanced work. State board examination required in all states for a license to practice.
Physical Therapist	Helps persons with muscle, nerve, joint, and bone diseases or injuries. Under a physician's direction he helps patients overcome their disabilities through exercise, manipulation, or use of mechanical apparatuses. Teaches patients and families to perform exercises. Helps patients learn to live with limitations.	A 2–4 year training program, with some leading to a bachelor's degree or the master's degree. Many are required to have 1 year of supervised experience. License to practice required in most states after having passed a state board examination.
Physician	Diagnoses diseases and treats people who are ill or in poor health. Concerned with prevention of disease and rehabilitation of people who are injured or ill.	Three to 4 years of college work followed by 4 years of professional training leading to degree Doctor of Medicine (M.D.), followed by a 1-year hospital internship. Passing a state or national board examination required for a license to practice; 2–4 years more required for specialties.

Where Employed	Employment Opportunities	Where to Find Additional Information
pitals, research, or teaching.		Pharmaceutical Education, 77 W. Washington St., Chicago, Ill., 60602.
Hospitals, children's hospitals, nursing homes, rehabilitation centers, industrial clinics, schools for crippled children, armed forces, and public health services.	Rapidly growing field. Not nearly enough workers. Many advance to teaching, research, or supervision. Many therapists are women.	American Physical Therapy Association, 1790 Broadway, New York, N.Y., 10019.
Usually engaged in private practice. Others in armed services, veterans' hospitals, public health, industry, medical schools, state and local health departments, research, or professional organizations.	Opportunities are innumerable. Heavy demand for physicians. Good chance for advancement in many areas. A small percentage are women.	Council on Medical Education and Hospitals, American Medical Association, 535 N. Dearborn St., Chicago, Ill., 61610. Association of American Medical Colleges, 2530 Ridge Ave., Evanston, Ill., 60201.

Vocation	Nature of the Work	Education
Podiatrist	Sometimes also called chiropodist; he diagnoses and treats diseases and deformities of the feet. Performs foot surgery, uses drugs and therapy, prescribes proper shoes, fits corrective devices, and provides general foot care.	Two years of college followed by 4 years of professional training after which the degree Doctor of Podiatry (Pod.D.), Doctor of Podiatric Medicine (D.P.M.), or Doctor of Surgical Chiropody (D.S.C.) is awarded. A few states require a 1-year internship. License to practice granted upon passing of state board examination.
Psychiatric Social Worker	Attends patients in mental hospitals or clinics, often works in clinical teams with other kinds of professional personnel. Guides patients and families in understanding an illness and making social adjustments in homes and communities.	Bachelor's degree with a major in social sciences and a master's degree from a school of social work, which includes both academic and clinical study.
Psychologist	Studies the behavior of persons and groups, helps them to understand themselves and achieve a satisfactory personal adjustment.	Generally a master's degree in psychology and often a Ph.D. degree, plus 1 year of clinical internship.
Psychometrist	Specializes in administering tests under guidance of a psy-	Ordinarily a master's degree in psychology, including 1 year of

Where Employed	Employment Opportunities	Where to Find Additional Information
Usually in private practice. May be in hospitals, teaching, veterans' hospitals, the armed services, or industry.	Field is not over-crowded. Demand is growing. Advancement depends on size of practice. A few are women.	American Podiatry Association, 3301 16th St., N.W., Washington, D.C., 20010.
Mental hospitals and mental health clinics, child guidance centers, general hospitals, courts, and rehabilitation centers.	Openings are numerous and increasing. A few top administrative positions are open for one with sufficient experience.	National Commission for Social Work Careers, 345 E. 46th St., New York, N.Y., 10017.
Teaching, research, hospitals, public schools, counseling clinics, government agencies, and personnel work.	Good for well-trained persons. A few administrative positions with experience.	American Psychological Association, 1200 17th St., N.W., Washington, D.C., 20036.
Usually works in association with or under supervision of a psy-	Increasing need as more public schools administer placement	American Psychological Association, 1200 17th St., N.W.,

Vocation	Nature of the Work	Education
	chologist and in interpreting the score.	supervised experience.
Public Health Administrator	Directs professional health services. Work will vary considerably with nature of the service, but may consist of medical services in health agency, public service department, medical laboratory, or nursing service. Often works under a director to carry out general assignments.	Often bachelor's degree or master's degree in public administration, public health, or social sciences. May hold degree in specialized health fields such as medicine, nursing, or medical technology.
Public Health Educator	Specializes in getting health facts accepted and used. Works closely with community and professional groups to achieve projects and actions that maintain and improve health of the community.	Bachelor's degree in the sciences and the communication arts. Master's degree in public health if possible. Older health educators are often from other health fields.
Radioisotope Technician	Usually works in research center or medical laboratory. Prepares radioisotope materials, records their use, maintains safety precautions, and helps devise necessary apparatuses. In some places this	Usually 1–2 years of on-the-job training. A few schools offer a 1–2-year program of study.

Where Employed	Employment Opportunities	Where to Find Additional Information
chologist in schools, clinics, hospitals, and industry.	tests. Kind of advancement depends upon the nature of the particular job.	Washington, D.C., 20036.
Health agencies of all kinds.	All health agencies are looking for good managerial personnel. Advancement possibilities are excellent with training and successful experience.	American Public Health Association, 1790 Broadway, New York, N.Y., 10019.
Local, state, and federal health departments, international health programs, extension services, hospitals, clinics, and industry.	A relatively new field. Urgent need for more. Advancement chances are good for administration and consultantships.	American Public Health Association, 1790 Broadway, New York, N.Y., 10019.
Hospitals, clinics, research centers, and medical laboratories.	Growing need for this type of technician even though the field is relatively new. Often in the past it has been done by X-ray technicians or medical technologists.	The American Society of Radiologic Technologists, 537 S. Main Street, Fond du Lac, Wis., 54935.

Vocation	Nature of the Work	Education
	work may be handled by a specially trained X-ray technician.	
Sanitarian and Sanitation Technician	Determines standards and enforces regulations for food, milk, air, water, radiation, metropolitan planning, accident prevention, pesticide control, hospital sanitation, communicable disease control, insect and rodent control, housing, industrial hygiene, sewage and waste disposal.	Bachelor's degree in sciences, humanities, and communication arts. Master's degree in public health or related health field recommended.
X-ray Technician	Also called medical X-ray technologist; he operates X-ray equipment under general direction of physicians (radiologists). He prepares patients, positions them and films the desired body areas.	Usually a 2-year training program beyond high school or junior college in a hospital or medical school. Registration by the passing of an examination with the American Registry of Radiologic Technologists (ARRT) desirable.

Where Employed	Employment Opportunities	Where to Find Additional Information
Local, state, and federal health departments, industry, hospitals, schools and colleges, federal agencies (Public Health Service), and international agencies (Peace Corps, World Health Organization).	Relatively new field. Limitless opportunities with urgent need for more workers. Openings in public health, as educators, inspectors, and advisors.	National Association of Sanitarians, 1550 Lincoln Street, Denver, Colo. 80203.
Hospitals, medical laboratories, clinics, physicians' and dentists' offices, school systems, or governmental agencies.	The shortage of technicians is expected to continue as more hospitals and medical facilities are built.	The American Society of Radiologic Technologists, 537 S. Main St., Fond du Lac, Wis., 54935. The American Registry of Radiologic Technologists, 2600 Wayzata Blvd., Minneapolis, Min., 55404.

BIBLIOGRAPHY

A Lifetime of Health   CHAPTER 1

Kandle, Roscoe P., "Report of the Chairman of the Technical Development Board of the Governing Council 1959–1960," *American Journal of Public Health,* Vol. 52, No. 2, February 1961, pp. 287–294.

Common Emotional Problems   CHAPTER 2

Blain, Daniel, "Mental Health and Hospital Care in California," *California Medicine,* July 1963, pp. 70–74.

Closson, William G., and Robert A. Hall, "The Functioning of a Private Psychiatric Clinic," *California Medicine,* July 1964, pp. 30–41.

Dublin, Louis I., *Factbook of Man, From Birth to Death,* 2d ed., New York, The Macmillan Company, 1965.

Enelow, Allen J., "Drug Treatment of Psychotic Patients in General Medical Practice," *California Medicine,* January 1965, pp. 1–9.

English, O. Spurgeon, and Stuart M. Finch, *Introduction to Psychiatry,* 3d ed., New York, W. W. Norton & Company, Inc., 1964.

English, O. Spurgeon, and Gerald H. J. Pearson, *Emotional Problems of Living,* 3d ed., New York, W. W. Norton & Company, Inc., 1963.

Fullerton, Donald L., "Psychotherapy: Basic Principles," *American Family Physician,* February 1964, pp. 28–33.

Knox, Stuart C., "A Decade of Progress in Psychiatry," *Journal of the American Medical Association,* March 21, 1964, pp. 169–170.

Kramer, Morton, "Collection and Utilization of Statistical Data from Psychiatric Facilities in the United States of America," *Bulletin of the World Health Organization,* 1963, pp. 491–510.

Lewis, Frederick A., "Community Care of Psychiatric Patients Versus Prolonged Institutionalization," *Journal of the American Medical Association,* October 27, 1963, pp. 97–100.

Menninger, Karl A., Martin Mayman, and Paul Pruyser, *The Vital Balance: The Life Process in Mental Health and Illness,* New York, The Viking Press, 1963.

Mental Health Statistics, Current Reports, Washington, D.C., National Institute of Mental Health, Public Health Service, January 1966.

Rosen, Ephraim, and Ian Gregory, *Abnormal Psychology,* Philadelphia, W. B. Saunders Company, 1965.

Structure and Disorders of the Nervous System   CHAPTER 3

Asimov, Isaac, *The Human Brain: Its Capacities and Functions,* Boston, Houghton Mifflin Company, 1964.

Baker, A. B., *Clinical Neurology,* 2d ed., Vols. 1–4, New York, Hoeber-Harper, 1962.

Cardwell, Viola, *Cerebral Palsy: Advances in Understanding and Care,* New York, Association for Aid of Crippled Children, 1956.

Clinical Team Looks at Phenylketonuria, revised, Washington, D.C., Department of Health, Education, and Welfare, Children's Bureau, Welfare Administration, 1964.

De Gutierrez-Mahoney, C. G., and Estra Carini, *Neurological and Neurosurgical Nursing,* St. Louis, The C. V. Mosby Co., 1965.

Feiling, Anthony, *Modern Trends in Neurology,* New York, Hoeber-Harper, 1951.

Gardner, Ernest, *Fundamentals of Neurology,* 3d ed., Philadelphia, W. B. Saunders Company, 1958.

Grollman, Sigmund, *The Human Body: Its Structure and Physiology,* New York, The Macmillan Company, 1964.

Guthrie, Robert, and Stewart Whitney, *Phenylketonuria, Detection in the Newborn Infant as a Routine Hospital Procedure,* Washington, D.C., U.S. Department of Health, Education, and Welfare, Children's Bureau Publication No. 419–1964, Welfare Administration, 1964.

Guyton, Arthur C., *Textbook of Medical Physiology,* 2d ed., Philadelphia, W. B. Saunders Company, 1961.

Herskowitz, Irwin J., *Genetics,* 2d ed., Boston, Little, Brown and Company, 1965.

Hsia, D. Y., *Inborn Errors of Metabolism,* Chicago, Yearbook Medical Publishers, Inc., 1959.

Hull, Edgar, and Cecilia M. Perrodin, *Medical Nursing,* 5th ed., Philadelphia, F. A. Davis Company, 1954.

Langley, L. L., E. Cheraskin, and Ruth Sleeper, *Dynamic Anatomy and Physiology,* 2d ed., New York, McGraw-Hill Book Company, Inc., 1963.

Lennox, William G., *Epilepsy and Related Disorders,* Vols. 1 and 2, Boston, Little, Brown and Company, 1960.

Memmler, Ruth Lundeen, *The Human Body in Health and Disease,* 2d ed., Philadelphia, J. B. Lippincott Company, 1962.

Smith, Bernard H., *Principles of Clinical Neurology,* Chicago, Yearbook Medical Publishers, Inc., 1965.

Stern, Curt, *Principles of Human Genetics,* 2d ed., San Francisco, W. H. Freeman and Company, 1960.

Thompson, George N., "The Psychiatric Witness, Epilepsy, Psychomotor Epilepsy, Acute Pathological Alcoholic Intoxication and Sociopathic Personality, Medicolegal Considerations" (paper presented to the Los Angeles County Association of Deputy District Attorneys, through the Office of William B. McKesson, District Attorney, County of Los Angeles).

Understanding the Brain and Nervous System: Research Advances in Neurological and Sensory Disorders, U.S. Department of Health, Education, and Welfare, Public Health Service Publication No. 962, 1962.

Drug Abuse   CHAPTER 4

Andres, Goth, *Medical Pharmacology,* St. Louis, The C. V. Mosby Company, 1961.

Anslinger, H. J., and W. F. Tompkins, *The Traffic in Narcotics,* New York, Funk & Wagnalls, 1953.

Ausubel, D. P., *Drug Addiction,* New York, Random House, 1965.

Brown, T. T., *The Enigma of Drug Addiction,* Springfield, Ill., Charles C Thomas, Publisher, 1961.

Cohen, Sidney, *The Beyond Within: The L.S.D. Story,* New York, Atheneum Publishers, 1965.

Committee on Public Health Relations of the New York Academy of Medicine, *Conference on Drug Addiction Among Adolescents,* New York, The Blakiston Company, 1953.

Davenport, Lowrey F., *The Abuse of Codeine,* Boston, Mass., U.S. Public Health Service, U.S. Marine Hospital at Boston, Mass., 1938.

Drug Arrests and Dispositions in California, 1964, State Department of Justice, Sacramento, California Bureau of Criminal Statistics, 1965.

Extract from Treasury–Post Office Departments and Executive Office Appropriations, Washington, D.C., U.S. Treasury Department, Bureau of Narcotics, 1963.

Goldstein, N. L., *Narcotics 1952,* Albany, Department of Law, 1953.

Isbell, H., *What to Know About Drug Addiction,* Washington, D.C., U.S. Department of Health, Education, and Welfare, Public Health Service Publication No. 94, 1951.

Livingston, R. B., *Narcotic Drug Addiction Problems,* Washington, D.C., U.S. Department of Health, Education, and Welfare, Public Health Service Publication No. 1050, 1958.

Narcotic Clinic in the United States (pamphlet), Washington, D.C., U.S. Government Printing Office, 1955.

Narcotics in California, Usage, Trends, and Recommendations for Controls, California, Board of Corrections, 1959.

Prevention and Control of Narcotic Addiction, Washington, D.C., U.S. Treasury Department, Bureau of Narcotics, 1964.

Proceedings of the School and College Health Education Short Term Training Course X407, Los Angeles, University of California, 1963.

Proceedings White House Conference on Narcotic and Drug Abuse, State Department Auditorium, Washington, D.C., 1962.

Report of Assembly Interim Committee on Criminal Procedure, Vol. 22, No. 3, Sacramento, Assembly of the State of California, 1963.

State of California Narcotic Act, Sacramento, Division of Criminal Law and Enforcement, Bureau of Narcotic Enforcement, 1964.

Traffic in Opium and Other Dangerous Drugs, Washington, D.C., U.S. Treasury Department, Bureau of Narcotics, 1964.

Udell, Gilman G., *Opium and Narcotic Laws,* Washington, D.C., U.S. Government Printing Office, 1964.

United Nations, *Bulletin on Narcotics,* Vol. XVII, No. 1, Jan.–March, 1965.

Williams, Jesse F., *Narcotics: The Study of a Modern Problem,* California State Department of Education, Sacramento, California, 1952.

Williams, John D., *Narcotics,* Dubuque, Iowa, Wm. C. Brown Co., 1963.

Wright, H. N., and M. Montag, *Pharmacology and Therapeutics,* 7th ed., Philadelphia, W. B. Saunders Company, 1959.

Alcohol Abuse   CHAPTER 5

Bjerver, K., and L. Goldberg, "Effect of Alcohol Ingestion on Driving Ability," *Quarterly Journal of Studies on Alcohol,* Vol. 11, pp. 1–30, 1950.

Chafetz, Morris E., and H. W. Demone, Jr., *Alcoholism and Society,* New York, Oxford University Press, 1962.

Diethelm, O., ed., *Etiology of Chronic Alcoholism,* Springfield, Ill., Charles C Thomas, Publisher, 1955.

Jackson, J. K., "The Adjustment of the Family to the Crisis of Alcoholism," *Quarterly Journal of Studies on Alcohol,* Vol. 15, pp. 562–586, 1954.

Jellinek, E. M., *The Disease Concept of Alcoholism,* Highland Park, N.J., Hillhouse Press, 1960.

Jellinek, E. M., "Phases of Alcohol Addiction," *Quarterly Journal of Studies on Alcohol,* Vol. 13, pp. 673–678, 1952.

Keller, M., and V. Efron, "The Prevalence of Alcoholism," *Quarterly Journal of Studies on Alcohol,* Vol. 16, pp. 619–644, 1955.

Keller, M., and V. Efron, "The Rate of Alcoholism in the U.S.A., 1954–1956," *Quarterly Journal of Studies on Alcohol,* Vol. 19, pp. 316–319, 1958.

Loomis, T. A., and T. C. West, "The Influence of Alcohol on Automobile Driving Ability," *Quarterly Journal of Studies on Alcohol,* Vol. 19, pp. 30–45, 1958.

McCarthy, Raymond G., ed., *Alcohol Education for Classroom and Community,* New York, McGraw-Hill Book Company, Inc., 1964.

Pittman, D. J., and C. R. Snyder, eds., *Society, Culture, and Drinking Patterns,* New York, John Wiley & Sons, Inc., 1962.

Foods and Digestive System   CHAPTER 6

Grollman, S., *The Human Body,* New York, The Macmillan Company, 1964.

Lyght, Charles E., ed., *The Merck Manual,* 11th ed., Rahway, N.J., Merck & Co., 1966.

Miller, J. J., and C. R. Wells, *Your Teeth: And How to Keep Them,* New York, Lantern Press, 1951.

Miller, J. J., "Nutritive Value of Foods," rev., U.S. Department of Agriculture, Home and Garden Bull. No. 72, Washington, D.C., Government Printing Office, 1964.

Tuttle, W. W., and B. A. Schottelius, *Textbook of Physiology,* 15th ed., St. Louis, The C. V. Mosby Company, 1965.

Wohl, Michael G., and Robert S. Goodhart, *Modern Nutrition in Health and Disease,* 2d ed., Philadelphia, Lea & Febiger, 1960.

Diet and Weight Control   CHAPTER 7

"Adipose Tissue and Obesity," *Nutrition Reviews,* March, 1964, pp. 84–86.

"Appetite Suppressants and Treatment of Obesity," *Nutrition Reviews,* February, 1962, pp. 38–40.

American Institute of Baking, *The Wonder of You,* Chicago, 1961.

Batjer, Margaret Q., *et al., Meals for the Modern Family,* New York, John Wiley & Sons, 1961.

Byrd, Oliver E., *Nutrition Sourcebook*, Stanford, Calif., Stanford University Press, 1955.

"Diet and Drug Response," *Nutrition Reviews*, June 1962, pp. 187–189.

"Drug-Management-of-Obesity Controversy," *Nutrition Reviews*, July 1961, pp. 202–206.

Duegeon, L. T., "Buying Food for Your Family," *Food Marketing Leaflet 13*, rev. ed., Ithaca, N.Y., New York State Colleges of Agriculture and Home Economics, Cornell University, September, 1960.

Food, The Yearbook of Agriculture, 1959, Washington, D.C., U.S. Department of Agriculture, 1959.

Grollman, S., *The Human Body*, New York, The Macmillan Company, 1964.

Hein, Fred V., and Dana L. Farnsworth, *Living*, 4th ed., Chicago, Scott, Foresman and Company, 1965.

"How to Keep Your Weight Down," *U.S. News and World Report*, June 7, 1965, pp. 66–70.

Nutrition Service, Iowa State Department of Health, *The Simplified Diet Manual*, Ames, Iowa, Iowa State University Press, 1961.

Nutritive Value of Foods, Washington, D.C., U.S. Department of Agriculture, 1964.

Proudfit, Fairfax T., and Corinne H. Robinson, *Nutrition and Diet Therapy*, New York, The Macmillan Company, 1954.

Recommended Dietary Allowances, 6th ed., Washington, D.C., The National Research Council, 1964.

Sherman, Henry C., *Chemistry of Food and Nutrition*, 6th ed., New York, The Macmillan Company, 1941.

Stare, Frederick J., *Eating for Good Health*, Garden City, N.Y., Doubleday and Company, Inc., 1964.

Waldo, Myra, *Cooking for the Freezer*, Garden City, N.Y., Doubleday and Company, Inc., 1960.

Wright, C. E., *Food Buying, Marketing Information for Consumers*, New York, The Macmillan Company, 1962.

Success in Marriage   CHAPTER 8

Bell, Howard M., *Youth Tell Their Story*, Washington, D.C., The American Youth Commission of the American Council on Education, 1938.

Blood, Robert O., Jr., *Marriage*, New York, The Free Press, 1962.

The Book of the States, 1964–65, Vol. XV, Chicago, The Council of State Governments, 1964.

Bowman, Henry A., *Marriage for Moderns*, 4th ed., New York, McGraw-Hill Book Company, 1960.

Christensen, Harold T., *Handbook of Marriage and the Family*, Chicago, Rand McNally & Company, 1964.

Duvall, Evelyn M., and Reuben Hill, *Being Married*, Boston, D. C. Heath and Company, 1960.

Fishbein, Morris, and Ruby Jo Reeves Kennedy, *Modern Marriage and Family Living*, New York, Oxford University Press, 1957.

Harper, Robert A., *Marriage*, New York, Appleton-Century-Crofts, Inc., 1949.

Jacobson, Paul H., *American Marriage and Divorce*, New York, Holt, Rinehart and Winston, 1959.

Kinsey, Alfred C., Wardell B. Pomeroy, Clyde E. Martin, and Paul H. Gebhard, *Sexual Behavior in the Human Female*, Philadelphia, W. B. Saunders Company, 1953.

Kling, Samuel G., *The Complete Guide to Divorce*, New York, Bernard Geis Associates, 1963.

Lantz, Herman R., and Eloise C. Snyder, *Marriage, An Examination of the Man-Woman Relationship*, New York, John Wiley & Sons, 1962.

Peterson, James A., *Education for Marriage*, New York, Charles Scribner's Sons, 1956.

Pike, James A., *If You Marry Outside Your Faith*, New York, Harper & Row, 1954.

Poffenberger, Shirley, Thomas Poffenberger, and Judson T. Landis, "Intent Toward Conception and the Pregnancy Experience," *American Sociological Review*, Vol. 17, October 1952, pp. 616–620.

Statistical Abstract of the United States, 1964, National Data Book and Guide to Sources, 85th ed., Washington, D.C., U.S. Department of Commerce, Bureau of the Census, 1964.

Statistical Abstract of the United States, 1965, National Data Book and Guide to Sources, 86th ed., Washington, D.C., U.S. Department of Commerce, Bureau of the Census, 1965.

Venereal Disease Information for Educators, Sacramento, California State Department of Public Health, 1965.

Reproduction   CHAPTER 9

Anderson, Kenneth N., "Is 'The Pill' the Answer?" *Today's Health*, Vol. 43, No. 6, June 1965, pp. 28–34, 70.

Apgar, Virginia, "Drugs in Pregnancy," *American Journal of Nursing*, Vol. 65, No. 3, March 1965, pp. 104–105.

Barish, Natalie, *The Gene Concept*, New York, Reinhold Publishing Corporation, 1965.

Bates, Jerome E., and Edward S. Zawadzki, *Criminal Abortion*, Springfield, Ill., Charles C Thomas, Publisher, 1964.

Davis, Maxine, *Sexual Responsibility in Marriage*, New York, The Dial Press, Inc., 1963.

De Lee, Sol T., *Safeguarding Motherhood*, 5th ed., Philadelphia, J. B. Lippincott Company, 1962.

Dobzhansky, Theodosius, *Evolution, Genetics, and Man*, New York, John Wiley & Sons, Inc., 1955.

Eastman, Nicholson J., *Expectant Motherhood*, 3d ed., Boston, Little, Brown and Company, 1957.

Fuchs, K., S. Grunstein, and A. Peretz, "An Intrauterine Silkworm Gut Ring For Contraception," *Current Medical Digest*, Vol. 32, No. 2, Feb. 1965, pp. 135–138.

Gardner, Eldon J., *Principles of Genetics*, 2d ed., New York, John Wiley & Sons, Inc., 1964.

Gebhard, P. H., W. R. Pomeroy, C. Martin, and C. V. Christenson, *Pregnancy, Birth, and Abortion*, New York, Hoeber-Harper, 1958.

Goldfarb, Alvin F., "Ovulation Control," *Medical Science*, Vol. 14, No. 5, Nov. 1963, pp. 42–47.

Grollman, Sigmund, *The Human Body*, New York, The Macmillan Company, 1964.

Guttmacher, Alan F., *Planning Your Family*, New York, The Macmillan Company, 1964.

Guttmacher, Alan F., and editors of Consumer Reports, *The Consumers Union Report on Family Planning*, 2d ed., Mount Vernon, N.Y., 1966.

Guyton, Arthur C., *Function of the Human Body*, Philadelphia, W. B. Saunders Company, 1964.

Guyton, Arthur C., *Textbook of Medical Physiology*, 2d ed., Philadelphia, W. B. Saunders Company, 1961.

Hall, Judith G., and Hecht, Frederick, "The Autosomal Trisomies," *American Journal of Nursing*, Vol. 64, No. 11, Nov. 1964, pp. 87–91.

Herskowitz, Irwin J., *Genetics*, 2d ed., Boston, Little, Brown and Company, 1965.

King, Robert C., *Genetics*, 2d ed., New York, Oxford University Press, 1965.

Levine, R. P., *Genetics*, New York, Holt, Rinehart and Winston, Inc., 1962.

Newman, Lucile, "Abortion as Folk Medicine," *California's Health*, Vol. 23, Oct.–Nov. 1965, pp. 75–79.

Pace, Donald M., and B. W. McCashland, *College Physiology*, 2d ed., New York, Thomas Y. Crowell Company, 1964.

Pace, Donald M., B. W. McCashland, and P. A. Landolt, *Physiology and Anatomy*, New York, Thomas Y. Crowell Company, 1965.

Sonneborn, T. M., *The Control of Human Heredity and Evolution*, New York, The Macmillan Company, 1965.

Stern, Curt, *Principles of Human Genetics*, 2d ed., San Francisco, W. H. Freeman and Company, 1960.

Strand, Fleur L., *Modern Physiology*, New York, The Macmillan Company, 1965.

Sutton, H. Eldon, *Genes, Enzymes and Inherited Diseases*, New York, Holt, Rinehart and Winston, Inc., 1961.

Turner, C. Donnell, *General Endocrinology*, Philadelphia, W. B. Saunders Company, 1960.

Tuttle, W. W., and B. A. Schottelius, *Textbook of Physiology*, St. Louis, The C. V. Mosby Company, 1965.

Woodward, H. L., B. Gardner, and A. Overland, *Obstetric Management and Nursing*, 5th ed., Philadelphia, F. A. Davis Company, 1955.

Ziegel, Emma, and Carolyn Van Blarcom, *Obstetric Nursing*, 5th ed., New York, The Macmillan Company, 1964.

Choosing Medical Services CHAPTER 10

A National Program to Conquer Heart Disease, Cancer and Stroke, Vol. II, Washington, D.C., The President's Commission on Heart Disease, Cancer and Stroke, 1965.

"As Medicare Nears—A Crisis in Hospital Care," *U.S. News and World Report*, March 15, 1965, pp. 73–76.

Editors of Consumer Reports, *The Medicine Show*, rev. ed., Mount Vernon, N.Y., Consumers Union, 1963.

"Health: Are We the People Getting Our Money's Worth?" *The New Republic*, November 9, 1963.

Health Careers Guidebook, New York, National Health Council and The Equitable Life Assurance Society of the United States, 1955.

"Health Insurance: Why Spending Is Soaring," *Business Week*, June 24, 1961, pp. 144–166.

"Hospital Statistics," Part 2, *Journal of the American Hospital Association*, August 1, 1965, pp. 427–491.

"Is Your Hospital Safe?" *Good Housekeeping*, September 1961, pp. 74–75.

Occupational Outlook Handbook, 1963–64 ed., Washington, D.C., U.S. Department of Labor, 1964.

"Patients for Profit," *The Saturday Evening Post,* September 29, 1962, pp. 19–23.
"Your Health, Your Doctor, and Your Pocketbook," *Changing Times,* June 1961, pp. 5–24.

Quackery CHAPTER 11

Cook, James, *Remedies and Rackets,* New York, W. W. Norton & Co., Inc., 1958.
Editors of Consumer Reports, *The Medicine Show,* Mount Vernon, N.Y., 1963.
Food, the Yearbook of Agriculture, 1959, Washington, D.C., U.S. Department of Agriculture, 1959.
Fraud and Quackery Affecting the Older Citizen, Washington, D.C., Special Committee on Aging, United States Senate, 88th Congress, 1st Session, January 15, 1963.
Health Frauds and Quackery, Washington, D.C., Special Committee on Aging, United States Senate, 88th Congress, 2d Session, January 13, 1964.
Holbrook, Stewart H., *The Golden Age of Quackery,* New York, The Macmillan Company, 1959.
"What the Health Hucksters Are Up To," *Changing Times,* Vol. 18, No. 9, September 1964, pp. 24–29.
Your Money and Your Life, Washington, D.C., Food and Drug Administration, Publication 19, 1964.

Financing Medical Services CHAPTER 12

Angell, Frank Joseph, *Health Insurance,* New York, The Ronald Press Company, 1963.
Blue Cross and Blue Shield Fact Book, 1965, Chicago, Blue Cross Association and National Association of Blue Shield Plans, 1965.
Blue Cross and Private Health Insurance Coverage of Older Americans, Washington, D.C., A Report by the Subcommittee on Health of the Elderly to the Special Committee on Aging, U.S. Senate, July 1964.
Deceptive or Misleading Methods in Health Insurance Sales, Washington, D.C., A Hearing Before the Subcommittee on Frauds and Misrepresentations Affecting the Elderly of the Special Committee on Aging, U.S. Senate, May 4, 1964.
"Health Insurance: Why Spending Is Soaring," *Business Week,* June 24, 1961, pp. 144–166.
Materials from the Los Angeles County Health Department, Los Angeles, Division of Public Health Education.
The Older American: President's Council on Aging, 1963, Washington, D.C., U.S. Government Printing Office, 1963.
School and College Health Education, Proceedings of the School and College Health Education Training Course, School of Public Health, University of California, Los Angeles, August 26–30, 1963.
Source Book of Health Insurance Data, 1965, New York, Health Insurance Institute, 1965.
Troan, John, *What You've Got Coming from Medicare and Social Security,* Cleveland, Newspaper Enterprise Association, Inc., 1965.
Voluntary Prepayment Medical Benefit Plans with Charts and Graphs, 1965, Committee on Insurance and Prepayment Plans of the Council on Medical Services, Chicago, American Medical Association, 1963.

The Heart and Circulation CHAPTER 13

A Handbook of Heart Terms, Washington, D.C., U.S. Department of Health, Education, and Welfare, Public Health Service Publication No. 1073, 1964.

American Heart Association, 44 E. 23rd St., New York, N.Y. 10010.

    Heart Attack
    Heart Disease Caused by Coronary Atherosclerosis
    The Framingham Heart Study
    Heart Disease in Children
    High Blood Pressure
    Latest Mortality Data for the U.S.—1964 Estimates
    Heart Disease and Pregnancy
    Varicose Veins

A National Program to Conquer Heart Disease, Cancer and Stroke, Vol. II, Washington, D.C., President's Commission on Heart Disease, Cancer and Stroke, 1965.

Arey, Leslie Brainerd, *Developmental Anatomy,* 5th ed., Philadelphia, W. B. Saunders Company, 1946.

"Atherosclerotic Coronary Heart Disease—The Major Challenge to Contemporary Public Health and Preventive Medicine," *Medical Times,* February 1965, pp. 120–146.

Cecil, Russel L., and Robert F. Loeb, *A Textbook of Medicine,* 10th ed., Philadelphia, W. B. Saunders Company, 1959.

Evans, William, *Diseases of the Heart and Arteries,* Baltimore, The Williams & Wilkins Company, 1964.

Gefter, William I., Bernard H. Pastor, and Ralph M. Myerson, *Synopsis of Cardiology,* St. Louis, The C. V. Mosby Company, 1965.

Grollman, Sigmund, *The Human Body,* New York, The Macmillan Company, 1964.

Guyton, Arthur C., *Textbook of Medical Physiology,* 2d ed., Philadelphia, W. B. Saunders Company, 1961.

"The Heart, A Symbol of Life," *World Health,* June–July 1965, Special Issue, pp. 1–43.

Hull, Edgar, and Cecilia M. Perrodin, *Medical Nursing,* 5th ed., Philadelphia, F. A. Davis Company, 1954.

Langley, L. L., E. Cheraskin, and Ruth Sleeper, *Dynamic Anatomy and Physiology,* 2d ed., New York, McGraw-Hill Book Company, Inc., 1963.

MacBryde, Cyril Mitchell, *Signs and Symptoms,* 4th ed., Philadelphia, J. B. Lippincott, 1964.

Memmler, Ruth Lundeen, *The Human Body in Health and Disease,* 2d ed., Philadelphia, J. B. Lippincott Company, 1962.

"The Patient with Myocardial Infarction," *American Journal of Nursing,* November 1964, pp. C–1 to C–32.

Wood, Paul, *Diseases of the Heart and Circulation,* 2d ed., rev., Philadelphia, J. B. Lippincott Company, 1961.

Cancer as a Health Problem CHAPTER 14

Brecher, E., and R. Brecher, "Smoking and Lung Cancer," *Consumer Reports,* Vol. 28, No. 6, June 1963, pp. 265–280.

Cameron, Charles S., *A Cancer Source Book for Nurses,* New York, American Cancer Society, 1962.

Chronic Bronchitis: The Facts, National Tuberculosis Association, 1963.

Chronic Respiratory Disease: A Growing Menace, Washington, D.C., U.S. Department of Health, Education, and Welfare, 1966.

Emphysema: The Facts, National Tuberculosis Association, 1963.

Hammond, Cuyler E., "The Effects of Smoking," *Scientific American,* Vol. 207, No. 1, July 1962 (reprint).

Horn, Daniel, and Selwyn Waingrow, "What Changes Are Occurring in Public Opinion Toward Cancer: National Public Opinion Survey," *American Journal of Public Health,* Vol. 54, No. 3, March 1964, pp. 431–440.

Knapp, Margaret, *Cancer Nursing,* Washington, D.C., U.S. Department of Health, Education, and Welfare, National Cancer Institute, Public Health Service, 1955.

Koss, L. G., *Diagnostic Cytology,* Philadelphia, J. B. Lippincott Co., 1961.

Lyght, C. E., ed., *The Merck Manual,* 11th ed., Rahway, N.J., Merck & Co., 1966.

Morrow, Albert S., *Cancer,* New York, New York City Cancer Committee and the American Cancer Society, 1953.

National Program to Conquer Heart Disease, Cancer and Stroke: Report to the President, Vol. 1, Washington, D.C., U.S. Government Printing Office, 1964.

National Program to Conquer Heart Disease, Cancer and Stroke: Report to the President, Vol. 2, Washington, D.C., U.S. Government Printing Office, 1965.

Robinson, F. N., "Pulmonary Emphysema," *American Journal of Nursing,* Vol. 63, No. 9, September 1963, pp. 92–96.

Rodman, M. J., "New Drugs in the Fight Against Cancer," *RN,* November 1964, pp. 79–89.

Sartwell, P. E., *Preventive Medicine and Public Health,* 9th ed., Des Moines, Meredith Publishing Company, 1965.

Smoking and Health: Report of the Advisory Committee to the Surgeon General, Washington, D.C., U.S. Department of Health, Education, and Welfare, 1964.

Williams, Henry M., Jr., "Pulmonary Emphysema," *American Journal of Nursing,* Vol. 63, No. 9, September 1963, pp. 88–91.

Disease   CHAPTER 15

Carpenter, Philip L., *Immunology and Serology,* 2d ed., Philadelphia, W. B. Saunders Company, 1965.

Chandler, Asa C., *Introduction to Parasitology,* 9th ed., New York, John Wiley & Sons, Inc., 1955.

Pelczar, Michael J., and Roger Reid, *Microbiology,* 2d ed., New York, McGraw-Hill Book Company, Inc., 1965.

Wedberg, Stanley E., *Paramedical Microbiology,* New York, Reinhold Publishing Corporation, 1963.

Young, Genevieve G., *Witton's Microbiology,* 3d ed., New York, McGraw-Hill Book Company, Inc., 1961.

Venereal Disease   CHAPTER 16

Clark, E. G., "Natural History of Syphilis and Levels of Prevention," *British Journal of Venereal Diseases,* Vol. 30, No. 191, 1954.

Gonococcus, Procedure for Isolation and Identification, Washington, D.C., U.S. Department of Health, Education, and Welfare, Public Health Service (Communicable Disease Center), 1960.

The Eradication of Syphilis: A Task Force Report to the Surgeon General, Public Health Service On Syphilis Control in the United States, Washington, D.C., U.S. Department of Health, Education, and Welfare, Public Health Service, 1963.

Guthe, T., and R. R. Wilcox, "Treponematoses, a World Problem," *Chronicles,* World Health Organization, 1954.

Sartwell, P. E., *Preventive Medicine and Public Health,* 9th ed., New York, Appleton-Century-Crofts, 1965.

Stokes, J. H., *Modern Clinical Syphilology, Diagnosis Treatment and Case Study,* 3d ed., Philadelphia, W. B. Saunders Company, 1944.

Syphilis, Modern Diagnosis and Management, Washington, D.C., U.S. Department of Health, Education, and Welfare, Public Health Service (Communicable Disease Center), 1960.

V.D. Fact Sheet, Washington, D.C., U.S. Department of Health, Education, and Welfare, Public Health Service (Communicable Disease Center), annual.

"Venereal Disease," *Consumer Reports,* Vol. 28, No. 10, October 1963, pp. 496–499.

Other Diseases of Man   CHAPTER 17

Carpenter, Philip L., *Immunology and Serology,* 2d ed., Philadelphia, W. B. Saunders Company, 1965.

Chandler, Asa C., *Introduction to Parasitology,* 9th ed., New York, John Wiley & Sons, Inc., 1955.

Gordon, John E., ed., *Control of Communicable Diseases in Man,* 10th ed., New York, The American Public Health Association, 1965.

Sartwell, Philip E., ed., *Preventive Medicine and Public Health,* 9th ed., New York, Appleton-Century-Crofts, 1965.

Wedberg, Stanley E., *Paramedical Microbiology,* New York, Reinhold Publishing Corporation, 1963.

Environmental Health   CHAPTER 18

Air Pollution Manual, Part I, Evaluation, Detroit, American Industrial Hygiene Association, 1960.

A Place to Live, The Yearbook of Agriculture, Washington, D.C., U.S. Department of Agriculture, 1963.

Faith, W. L., *Air Pollution Control,* New York, John Wiley & Sons, Inc., 1959.

"Food Additives," *Nutritional Reviews,* August 1961, pp. 227–228.

Odum, E. P., and H. T. Odum, *Fundamentals of Ecology,* Philadelphia, W. B. Saunders Company, 1959.

Principles and Procedures for Evaluating the Safety of Food Additives, Publication 750, Washington, D.C., The National Research Council, Food and Nutrition Board, 1959.

Quest for Quality, The Conservation Yearbook, Washington, D.C., U.S. Department of the Interior, 1965.

Radionuclides in Foods, Publication 988, Washington, D.C., The National Research Council, Food and Nutrition Board, 1962.

Shillings, C. W., ed., *Atomic Energy Encyclopedia in the Sciences,* Philadelphia, W. B. Saunders Company, 1964.

"The Sky as a Sewer," *World Health*, February 1963, pp. 12–13.

"Some Comments on Silent Spring," *Nutritional Reviews*, January 1963, pp. 1–4.

"The Toxicity of Pesticides and Their Residues in Food," *Nutritional Reviews*, August 1965, pp. 225–230.

Wallace, B., and T. H. Dobzhansky, *Radiation, Genes, and Man*, New York, Holt, Rinehart and Winston, Inc., 1965.

Water: The Yearbook of Agriculture, Washington, D.C., U.S. Department of Agriculture, 1955.

Williams, K., C. L. Smith, and H. D. Chalke, *Radiation and Health*, Boston, Little, Brown and Company, 1962.

Population Dynamics   CHAPTER 19

Berelson, Bernard, and Ronald Freeman, "A Study in Fertility Control," *Scientific American*, Vol. 210, No. 5, May, 1964, pp. 29–37.

Bogue, Donald J., *The Population of the United States*, New York, The Free Press.

Bogue, Donald J., "Population Growth in the United States," *The Population Dilemma*, Englewood Cliffs, N.J., Prentice-Hall, Inc., 1963.

Bourgeois-Pichat, Jean, "Population Growth and Development," *International Conciliation*, No. 556, January 1966, pp. 1–81.

Carr-Saunders, A. M., *World Population*, Oxford, Clarendon Press, 1936.

Dublin, Louis I., *Factbook on Man from Birth to Death*, New York, The Macmillan Company, 1965.

Durand, John, *World Population Estimates, 1750–2000*, United Nations Doc., WPC/WP/289, 1965.

Facts of Life and Death, U.S. Department of Health, Education, and Welfare, Public Health Service Publication No. 600, 1965.

Freedman, Ronald, ed., *Population: The Vital Revolution*, Garden City, N.Y., Doubleday & Company, Inc. (Anchor Books), 1964.

Hauser, Philip M., ed., *The Population Dilemma*, Englewood Cliffs, N.J., Prentice-Hall Inc., 1963.

Hauser, Philip M., "Demography and Ecology," *Annals of the American Academy of Political and Social Science*, No. 362, November 1965, pp. 129–138.

"How U.S. Is Changing—People on the Move," *U.S. News and World Report*, Vol. 59, No. 20, November 15, 1965, pp. 74–78.

Huxley, Julian, "World Population," *Scientific American*, Vol. 194, No. 3, March 1956, pp. 64–76.

Landis, Paul H., *Population Problems*, 2d ed., New York, American Book Company, 1954.

Lewis, W. B., "A Canadian Views the U.S. Civilian Power Reactor Program," *Nuclear News*, Vol. 5, No. 5, 1962, pp. 3–10.

Mudd, Stuart, ed., *The Population Crisis and the Use of World Resources*, Bloomington, Indiana University Press, 1964.

Nortman, Dorothy L., *The Population Problem*, New York, National Educational Television, 1965.

Osborn, Fairfield, ed., *Our Crowded Planet: Essays on the Pressures of Population*, Garden City, N.Y., Doubleday & Company, Inc., 1962.

Putnam, P., *Energy in the Future*, Princeton, N.J., D. Van Nostrand Co., Inc., 1958.

Roosevelt, James, *United States Presents Views on Population Growth and Economic Development*, Department of State Bulletin, Vol. 54, No. 1388, January 31, 1966, pp. 175–178.

Sax, Karl, *Standing Room Only, The World's Exploding Population,* 2d ed., Boston, Beacon Press, 1960.

Scammon, Richard M. (interview), "What's Ahead in the Population Boom," *U.S. News and World Report,* Vol. 54, No. 18, May 6, 1963, pp. 68–71.

Taylor, Carl E., "Health and Population," *Foreign Affairs,* Vol. 43, April 1965, No. 3, pp. 476–486.

Thompson, Warren S., *Population and Progress in the Far East,* Chicago, The University of Chicago Press, 1959.

Wallace, B., and T. Dobzhansky, *Radiation, Genes, and Man,* New York, Holt, Rinehart and Winston, Inc., 1959.

"What's Ahead in the Population Boom," *U.S. News and World Report,* May 6, 1963, pp. 68–71.

Wilcox, Walter F., ed., *International Migrations,* 2 vols., New York, National Bureau of Economic Research, 1929–1931.

INDEX